PRINCIPLES OF
Immunology

PRINCIPLES OF

Immunology

SECOND EDITION

Edited by

Noel R. Rose, M.D., Ph.D.

Professor and Chairman, Department of Immunology and Microbiology,
Wayne State University School of Medicine, Detroit

Felix Milgrom, M.D.

Professor and Chairman, Department of Microbiology, and Member,
The Center for Immunology, School of Medicine,
State University of New York at Buffalo

Carel J. van Oss, Ph.D.

Professor of Microbiology, and Member,
The Center for Immunology, School of Medicine,
State University of New York at Buffalo

MACMILLAN PUBLISHING CO., INC.
New York
COLLIER MACMILLAN CANADA, LTD.
Toronto
BAILLIÈRE TINDALL
London

Macmillan Publishing Co., Inc.
866 Third Avenue, New York, New York 10022

Collier Macmillan Canada, Ltd.
Baillière Tindall · London

Library of Congress Cataloging in Publication Data
Rose, Noel R.

  Principles of Immunology.
  Includes bibliographies and index.
  1. Immunology. 2. Immunopathology. I. Milgrom,
Felix. II. Van Oss, Carel J. III. Title.
[DNLM: 1. Immunology. QW505 P957]
QR181.R59 1978   616.07′9   77–15780
ISBN 0–02–403610–2

Printing: 1 2 3 4 5 6 7 8   Year: 9 0 1 2 3 4 5

Preface to the Second Edition

Since publication of the first edition of *Principles of Immunology*, the growth of immunology has continued and even accelerated. Two parallel paths are evident. The first is the rapid development of molecular immunology and immunogenetics, especially concerning regulation of the immune response and the action of cell-surface molecules that control cellular interactions. Immunology has turned much more to the study of cellular recognition. The elucidation of genes and gene products that control cellular interactions makes it possible to combine immunology with developmental and somatic cell genetics. The technology of cellular hybridization and recombinant DNA now permits the immunologist to discern the sources of antibody diversity. An understanding of the molecular basis of the differentiation of immunologically competent cells can be expected. It is likely that the lessons learned in studies of cellular differentiation and cellular interaction will be applicable far beyond immunology and provide the groundwork for an understanding of similar phenomena in cell biology, developmental biology, and the neural sciences. Thus, immunology has rapidly taken a place at the forefront of the natural sciences.

At the same time, there has been increasing application of immunologic principles and methodology to clinical problems. Immunologic dysfunction is recognized in a great variety of diseases that fall within the traditional purview of such clinical specialties as hematology, rheumatology, gastroenterology, neurology, oncology, and surgery. Clinical immunology has inaugurated major advances in the diagnosis and treatment of such diverse and poorly understood disorders as systemic lupus erythematosus, myasthenia gravis, and mucocutaneous candidiasis. Increasing knowledge of immunologic regulation raises the possibility that improved methods for benefiting patients with these and many other diseases will soon become available.

Because of the many developments in immunology, the editors felt that extensive revision of *Principles of Immunology* was required. As before, the book is written with the beginning student in mind. Most of the chapters have had to be greatly altered and some rewritten entirely. The first part of the book is again devoted to the fundamental principles of immunology. Newer

knowledge of cellular interactions and genetic regulation has been emphasized. The second portion of the book, consisting of 13 chapters on clinical
applications of immunology, has also been extensively rewritten because of
the new fund of information presently available. A short third unit has been
added to bring together some of the many practical applications of immunology in medical diagnosis and treatment.

We thank our many colleagues and associates who have pointed out ways
in which *Principles of Immunology* could be improved; we hope they will find
this second edition even more useful than the first. We will be particularly
pleased if those colleagues who spent some time in Buffalo will, on reading
this book, recall the enthusiasm, wisdom, and scientific integrity of the
creator of the Buffalo School of Immunology, Ernest Witebsky.

N. R. R.
F. M.
C. J. v. O.

Preface to the First Edition

Only a few years ago, a textbook of immunology for students of medicine and other health sciences, graduate students of biomedical sciences, and clinicians would have had little justification. It is not that immunology is a new science; on the contrary, the readers of Chapter 1 will find that it is among the oldest of the natural sciences basic to medicine. Immunology has had, rather, the status of a collaborator of microbiology, pathology, biochemistry, clinical medicine, and other disciplines. This integration with other sciences has been a strength and, at the same time, a weakness. It has meant that immunologic approaches have been brought to bear on a great many biologic and medical problems, giving an extraordinary richness and versatility. Accordingly, immunology has enjoyed the stimulation of intimate links with other rapidly growing areas of science.

Yet too often biologists and physicians, unfamiliar with the basic principles of immunology, have failed to understand their real potential benefits. Young investigators have sometimes been more aware of techniques than principles; health practitioners have applied the methods of immunology without understanding their broader implications.

At the urging of the late Ernest Witebsky, Distinguished Professor of Bacteriology and Immunology, a Center for Immunology was chartered by the Trustees of the State University of New York in 1967 to meet the special needs of a science that had not yet found its proper academic setting. With responsibility to foster research and training in all aspects of immunology, it brought together immunologists in many different departments of the State University of New York at Buffalo, its affiliated hospitals, and the related Roswell Park Memorial Institute. The creation of this book was long the dream of Ernest Witebsky, and it culminates several years of close collaboration of the Buffalo group of immunologists. Dr. Witebsky's untimely death on December 7, 1969, cut short his participation.

In organizing this book, the editors have attempted to attain certain goals. The text is graduated, so that the beginning student can systematically build concept upon concept, chapter by chapter. Yet each chapter is entire in itself, thus allowing the more experienced reader to review a particular subject in a meaningful way. The editors have tried to avoid duplication by extensive cross-references among chapters, but have not hesitated to treat the same subject from several different viewpoints in various chapters to attain a more balanced or comprehensive presentation. The character of this book precluded any extensive list of references, but all chapters end with a succinct bibliography, as a guide to further information on each subject.

After a first chapter designed to give the uninitiated reader an overall perspective of immunology, the book is divided into two roughly equal parts: the first 15 chapters treat the basis of immunology, and the last 13 chapters pertain to applications of the subject. The book aims at providing the fundamentals of immunology for medical, dental, and graduate students, as well as for physicians and other biomedical scientists who wish to be brought abreast of this important and rapidly evolving discipline.

The Center for Immunology   N. R. R.
State University of New York at Buffalo   F. M.

                                                      C. J. v. O.

Contributors

C. John Abeyounis, Ph.D.   Professor of Microbiology, School of Medicine, State University of New York at Buffalo. Member, The Center for Immunology.

Boris Albini, M.D.   Assistant Professor of Microbiology, School of Medicine, State University of New York at Buffalo. Associate Member, The Center for Immunology.

Giuseppe A. Andres, M.D.   Professor of Microbiology, Pathology, and Medicine, School of Medicine, State University of New York at Buffalo. Member, The Center for Immunology.

Carl E. Arbesman, M.D.   Clinical Professor of Medicine and Microbiology, State University of New York at Buffalo; Director, Allergy Research Laboratory, and Consultant-Attending, Buffalo General Hospital. Member, The Center for Immunology.

Almen L. Barron, Ph.D.   Professor and Chairman, Department of Microbiology and Immunology, College of Medicine, University of Arkansas for Medical Sciences, Little Rock. Formerly Member, The Center for Immunology.

Albert A. Benedict, Ph.D.   Professor of Microbiology, University of Hawaii, Honolulu.

Ernst H. Beutner, Ph.D.   Professor of Microbiology and Dermatology, State University of New York at Buffalo; Director of the Immunofluorescence Testing Service, Buffalo. Member, The Center for Immunology.

Pierluigi E. Bigazzi, M.D.   Associate Professor of Pathology, University of Connecticut School of Medicine, Farmington. Formerly Member, The Center for Immunology.

Stanley Cohen, M.D.   Professor and Associate Chairman, Department of Pathology, University of Connecticut School of Medicine, Farmington. Formerly Member, The Center for Immunology.

Herald R. Cox, Sc.D.   Research Professor Emeritus of Microbiology, School of Medicine, State University of New York at Buffalo. Formerly Member, The Center for Immunology.

Howard C. Goodman, M.D.   Director, Tropical Medicine Center, The Johns Hopkins University School of Hygiene and Public Health, Baltimore.

Allan L. Grossberg, Ph.D.   Associate Chief Cancer Research Scientist, Department of Immunology Research, Roswell Park Memorial Institute; Research Associate Professor of Chemistry, Roswell Park Division of the Graduate School; Research Professor of Microbiology, School of Medicine, State University of New York at Buffalo. Member, The Center for Immunology.

Kyoichi Kano, M.D.   Professor of Microbiology, School of Medicine, State University of New York at Buffalo. Member, The Center for Immunology.

Joseph H. Kite, Jr., Ph.D.   Professor of Microbiology, School of Medicine, State University of New York at Buffalo. Member, The Center for Immunology.

Paul-Henri Lambert, M.D.   Professeur Associé; Head, WHO Immunology Research and Training Center, University of Geneva, Switzerland.

Robert T. McCluskey, M.D.   Mallincrodt Professor of Pathology, Harvard Medical School; Director, Department of Pathology, Massachusetts General Hospital, Boston. Formerly Member, The Center for Immunology.

Jacques Mauel, Ph.D.   Assistant Professor of Biochemistry, University of Lausanne Faculty of Medicine, Switzerland.

Manfred M. Mayer, Ph.D.   Professor of Microbiology, The Johns Hopkins University School of Medicine, Baltimore.

Felix Milgrom, M.D.   Professor and Chairman, Department of Microbiology, School of Medicine, State University of New York at Buffalo. Member, The Center for Immunology.

James F. Mohn, M.D.   Professor and Associate Chairman, Department of Microbiology, and Director, Blood Group Research Unit, School of Medicine, State University of New York at Buffalo; Director, Blood Bank, The Buffalo General Hospital. Director, The Center for Immunology.

Wolfgang Müller-Ruchholtz, M.D., D.D.S.   Professor of Microbiology, Hygiene Institut, Universität Kiel, West Germany.

Erwin Neter, M.D.   Professor of Microbiology, Department of Microbiology, and Professor of Clinical Microbiology, Department of Pediatrics, School of Medicine, State University of New York at Buffalo; Director of Bacteriology, Children's Hospital, Buffalo. Member, The Center for Immunology.

Russell J. Nisengard, Ph.D., D.D.S.   Professor of Periodontics-Endodontics, School of Dentistry, and Associate Professor of Microbiology, School of Medicine, State University of New York at Buffalo.

David Pressman, Ph.D.   Associate Institute Director, Roswell Park Memorial Institute; Research Professor of Chemistry, Roswell Park Division of the Graduate School; Research Professor of Microbiology, School of Medicine, State University of New York at Buffalo. Member, The Center for Immunology.

Robert E. Reisman, M.D.   Clinical Associate Professor of Medicine and Pediatrics, School of Medicine, State University of New York at Buffalo.

Noel R. Rose, M.D., Ph.D.   Professor and Chairman, Department of Immunology and Microbiology, Wayne State University School of Medicine, Detroit. Visiting Member and Formerly Director, The Center for Immunology.

Robert H. Swanborg, Ph.D.   Professor of Immunology and Microbiology, Wayne State University School of Medicine, Detroit.

Carel J. van Oss, Ph.D.   Professor of Microbiology, School of Medicine, State University of New York at Buffalo. Member, The Center for Immunology.

Yasuo Yagi, D.Sc.   Director, Nippon Roche Research Center, Kamakura, Japan. Formerly Member, The Center for Immunology.

Marek B. Zaleski, M.D.   Associate Professor of Microbiology, School of Medicine, State University of New York at Buffalo. Member, The Center for Immunology.

Contents

xiii

UNIT III.   APPLIED IMMUNOLOGY

UNIT I

Basic Immunology

I

Scope and Background of Immunity

NOEL R. ROSE, FELIX MILGROM, AND
CAREL J. VAN OSS

Immunity

Human beings are destined to spend their lives surrounded by microorganisms. The vast majority of these microorganisms are harmless. Most of them are free living or are saprophytes, growing on dead, decaying matter. A few live with man in a mutually beneficial, symbiotic relationship, while many others are commensals, depending upon their human host for support and nourishment. Less than 100 of the tens of thousands of microbial species are regularly capable of causing disease in the human host. Those organisms that can cause disease in man in many cases are not able to reinfect a given individual for an extended period of time after recovery from a particular infectious disease. People are then said to be "immune" (from the Latin *immunis*, meaning "exempt from duty"). Such a state of immunity from a particular disease is specific and does not apply to any other disease.

Natural (Innate) Resistance

Traditionally, defense mechanisms are divided into innate or native resistance and acquired resistance (Figure 1–1). Innate immunity, as the name suggests, is normally present from birth and provides the first line of

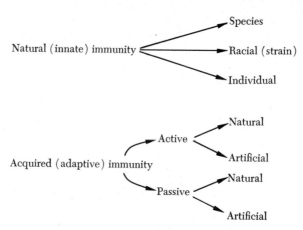

Figure 1-1. Defense mechanisms.

defense against microbial invasion. A lowered innate immunity is the most common event leading to infectious disease. The mechanisms providing natural immunity depend upon the species or even the strain within the species. For instance, body temperature itself determines to what diseases an animal may be susceptible. Almost a century ago, Pasteur showed that he could infect chickens with anthrax bacilli only by lowering their body temperature. Some microorganisms require special nutrients available in some tissues but absent from others. For example, *Brucella abortus* requires erythritol for growth; this carbohydrate is relatively abundant in the placenta of cattle but not in most other tissues. There are also genetic differences among members of the same species. By selective breeding, strains of mice have been derived that are much more susceptible to *Salmonella* infection than the average. Cross-breeds of susceptible and resistant mice are generally resistant, but analysis showed that resistance is due to several different genes.

The most important single organ providing innate resistance is the skin. It serves first as a mechanical barrier to invasion of microorganisms; second, fatty acids and other substances with potent antibacterial and antiviral activity have been discovered on the skin. Any event that interrupts the integrity of the skin, such as a wound or a burn, renders man considerably more susceptible to microbial invasion, even by microorganisms of low intrinsic virulence.

Those parts of the body not enveloped by skin are covered by mucous membranes. Although less of a mechanical barrier than skin, mucous membranes possess special mechanisms to control bacterial growth or penetration. Nasal hair, cilia, mucus, saliva, and tears are all important for control of infection. When ciliary action is interfered with by smoke or drugs, the individual becomes considerably more prone to respiratory tract infection. Chemical properties of the mucous membranes are also important in providing resistance. The low pH of gastric secretions is advantageous, since only a few species of bacteria can survive it. Secretions of the small intestine also prevent the growth of most microorganisms. In contrast, bacteria are abundant in the large intestine.

One interesting substance with antibacterial properties found in saliva and tears is lysozyme. Discovered by Fleming in 1922, it is an enzyme capable of dissolving the mucopeptide present in the cell wall of many bacteria. Lactoferrin is also found in saliva and other secretions and is lethal to several species of bacteria.

If microorganisms trespass the skin or mucous membranes, elements of the blood provide natural resistance. That serum has antibacterial properties was known as early as 1888 from investigations of Nuttall and of Buchner. A number of aspecific microbicidal and opsonizing factors have been identified in normal human and animal sera. Cells can be stimulated by infection or suitable chemicals to release interferon, which prevents proliferation of viruses and other organisms. Finally, the major phagocytic cells of the circulation, polymorphonuclear neutrophils, and of the tissues, macrophages, are important in innate resistance and also come into play in acquired immunity, as will be discussed later (Chapter 10).

Another important element in native resistance is competition among microorganisms. Under natural conditions, members of the normal microbial population of the gut hold each other in check. Agents that disturb the normal flora, such as broad-spectrum antibiotics or mixtures of antibiotics, predispose the patient to severe infection by antibiotic-resistant microorganisms. Drug-resistant staphylococci and candidae are notorious pathogens in such cases.

Acquired Immunity

Acquired immunity differs from innate resistance quantitatively in its greater potency and qualitatively in its specificity for the individual pathogenic microorganism. It develops after experience with the respective microorganism.

History records many early attempts to induce immunity by artificial means. Emanuel Timoni, a native of Italy who practiced medicine in Constantinople, first communicated to the Royal Society in 1713 the practice of inoculation for the smallpox, which had then already been in successful use in Turkey for 40 years. The inoculation of small volumes of fresh pus from pustules of young smallpox patients was made into several little wounds in the arms or legs of normal subjects, with the help of a needle. This procedure almost invariably gave rise to a very mild form of the disease, leaving no scars or pits on the face, and it conferred lasting immunity. Lady Mary Wortley Montagu, the wife of the British ambassador to Turkey, described the practice in 1717, and she subsequently was instrumental in making the method popular in England. However, between 5 and 30 of every 1000 inoculees contracted smallpox from the inoculation, and could then, in turn, infect others. Some inoculated individuals, without themselves showing clinical signs of the disease, also could infect other people with smallpox.

In 1798 the English physician Edward Jenner, having noted earlier in his medical practice in Gloucestershire that it was firmly believed locally that dairy workers who had contracted cowpox were thereby protected from a subsequent attack of smallpox, published the results of experiments he had conducted in 1796. He had procured material from a case of cowpox and injected it into several human volunteers. Cowpox (the Latin word is *vaccinia*, from *vacca*, "cow") usually produces only a few localized lesions in humans, but it conveys immunity against smallpox. Jenner verified this immunity by challenging his volunteers by inoculating them with smallpox pus. Jenner's important contribution was based on careful clinical observations. He had discovered the important principle of inducing immunity by inoculating humans with a naturally occurring virus of a low pathogenicity that establishes a state of immunity similar to that induced by the fully virulent infectious agent. Instead of biologic attenuation, Pasteur, 80 years later, used physical means to attenuate virulent organisms, by culturing anthrax bacilli at temperatures higher than body temperature.

It is convenient to distinguish two major groups of bacterial diseases with regard to mechanisms of host resistance. A few diseases are caused by specific toxins secreted by the microorganisms (Chapter 13). Usually these exotoxins are capable of producing well-defined lesions at sites distant from the infection. Examples of diseases that are mainly toxigenic are diphtheria and tetanus. In 1890, von Behring and Kitasato showed that guinea pigs receiving nonlethal doses of tetanus or diphtheria toxin acquired specific immunity to that respective toxin. Later, Ramon demonstrated that detoxified toxin (later called toxoid) could be prepared by aging or formalin treatment, and that toxoid induced active immunity as well as did the potent toxin.

Actively acquired antitoxic immunity usually requires more than one injection and takes weeks or months to develop. However, it lasts many years. Moreover, a second exposure to the same toxin or toxoid elicits a greater, more rapid response, referred to as the secondary (or anamnestic or memory) response. Active immunization with toxoid is still an effective method for preventing diphtheria and tetanus.

Von Behring and Kitasato discovered that the source of immunity in immunized animals is serum. By taking serum from immunized animals, they could protect untreated guinea pigs. They referred to this newly developed property of immune serum as antitoxin (Chapter 26). We now recognize antitoxin as one of the protective antibodies. Ehrlich demonstrated that antitoxin combines with and neutralizes toxin in the test tube. This procedure provided a means of standardizing antitoxin and permitted its use for the treatment of toxigenic diseases.

Most bacterial diseases are not due to a particular toxin but rather to invasion of tissues by the microorganisms. Soon after the investigations of von Behring, Pfeiffer and Issaeff immunized guinea pigs by injecting them with small numbers of cholera vibrios or some other bacilli. They later injected living organisms into the peritoneum of the immunized guinea pig and noticed that the bacteria swelled and dissolved. This lysis was specific for the particular organism. Protection could be transferred to normal guinea pigs by injections of the immune serum, indicating that protection is due to antibody in the bloodstream. A parallel effect was demonstrated in the test tube by Gruber and Durham by means of an agglutination reaction, in which the immune serum was mixed with the suspension of bacteria, or by Kraus using precipitation, in which the immune serum was mixed with a soluble extract of the microorganism (Chapter 6).

Immunoglobulins

Upon fractionation of an antiserum, antibody activity is found in the γ and β globulin fractions. The globulins carrying antibody activity are called immunoglobulins. There are at least five classes of immunoglobulins: IgG, IgM, IgA, IgD, and IgE. Antibodies of the IgG class are the most frequent. They have a sedimentation rate of 6 to 7 S. IgM antibodies are often the first antibodies to appear during immunization. They are approximately six times larger than IgG antibodies and their sedimentation rate is around 19 S. The IgA antibodies occur as monomers with a sedimentation rate of 7 S, as dimers with a sedimentation rate of 10 to 11 S, and even, in small amounts, as trimers and tetramers (13 S and 16 to 17 S). IgE has the unique ability to attach avidly to cells of the same species and to mediate hypersensitivity reactions. The immunoglobulins are discussed in Chapter 4.

Immunoglobulins of all classes have fundamentally the same structure, comprising (in their simplest, monomeric form) two heavy chains and two light chains. All classes share the same light chains (which themselves occur in only two types, κ and λ). The various immunoglobulin classes differ solely in the structure of their heavy chains.

Antibodies are the important mediators of acquired immunity. However, in most cases, antibodies cannot act alone. Sometimes, they cooperate with complement, a complex interactive series of plasma proteins that, when activated, exert enzymatic functions (Chapter 8). Complement can dissolve certain types of gram-negative microorganisms. In other instances, antibody cooperates with the phagocytic cells of the blood, polymorphonuclear neutrophils, to promote phagocytosis (Chapter 10). The ingested bacteria are usually destroyed by the phagocytes. The rapid mobilization of polymorphonuclear neutrophils is an early sign of infection in patients. This mechanism is important in defense against the pyogenic cocci, such as staphylococci and streptococci. In addition to the polymorphonuclear phagocytes of the blood, tissue macrophages are important phagocytes. They play a critical role in immunity to many chronic infections. Initially, macrophages have only limited capacity for phagocytosis; when activated they can exert considerably greater phagocytic power. The stimulation may be provided by factors released from the lymphocytes of immunized animals.

Cells of the Immunologic System

Although all cells have a certain capability for recognition, in vertebrates this function is the specialty of the immunologic system. Like other organ systems, the immunologic apparatus is structured to perform its function in a highly proficient fashion, utilizing interactions among several different types of cells. Unlike most other organs of the body, however, the immune system is not a localized structure but is diffused throughout the body, an arrangement that is particularly favorable for its job of searching out foreign molecules. Figure 1–2 illustrates our current understanding of the major cell types that comprise the immunologic system and describes their interactions in producing an immunologic response.

Lymphocytes

The most important cells specialized in immunologic functions are lymphocytes. The lymphocyte is endowed with a surface receptor or recognition site that allows it to pick out a particular three-dimensional molecular configuration known as an antigenic determinant. A single lymphocyte seems to be responsive to only one or at most two antigenic determinants. Initially the body has only a small number of lymphocytes programmed to react with any particular determinant at a given time. The encounter of a quiescent lymphocyte with its corresponding antigenic determinant perturbs the cell membrane. This event, in turn, triggers metabolic stimulation of the lymphocyte, which is soon followed by an increase in the level of DNA synthesis in the nucleus. The lymphocyte enlarges and eventually divides, giving rise to offspring with the same specific receptor as the parent cell. This process continues until a whole colony or "clone" of lymphocytes with the same recognition properties is produced.

B and T Lymphocytes. As Figure 1–2 shows, there are two major types of lymphocytes in the immunologic apparatus. The B lymphocyte derives directly from the bone marrow in adult mammals, but in birds its maturation depends on a unique lymphoid organ, the bursa of Fabricius. When it encounters an antigen for which it has a receptor, the B lymphocyte under-

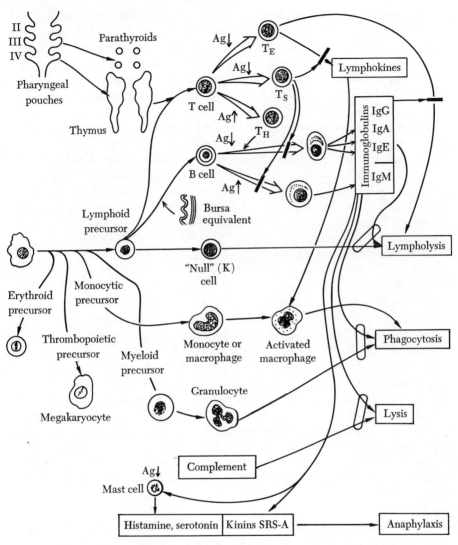

Figure 1-2. Schematic outline of the cellular interactions in the immune response. Abbreviations: Ag = antigen; T_E = effector T cell; T_S = suppressor T cell; T_H = helper T cell; K = "killer" cell.

goes proliferation and morphologic change, giving rise eventually to cells with characteristic marginal chromatin in the nucleus and a highly baso-philic cytoplasm, the plasma cell. Plasma cells secrete large amounts of the proteins detectable in the blood serum and other body fluids as immuno-globulins.

A few antigens, particularly large molecules with repeating subunits, are able to trigger proliferation of the B lymphocyte all by themselves. However, other antigens require cooperation of a T lymphocyte with a B lymphocyte for initiating antibody production (Chapter 3). After arising in the bone marrow, the T lymphocyte matures under the influence of the thymus, probably through the action of simple peptide hormones. Like the B lymphocytes, T lymphocytes are programmed to recognize a particular antigenic determinant. Proliferative differentiation of the T lymphocyte may proceed along several pathways. After encountering their counterpart antigenic determinant, some lymphocytes mature into helper T cells that cooperate with B lymphocytes in antibody synthesis. Other populations of T cells impede or suppress synthesis of immunoglobulin molecules by B cells. T cells are also involved in cell-mediated (in contrast to antibody-mediated) immunity (Chapter 11). These effector T cells produce the delayed hypersensitivity skin reaction. When they encounter their corresponding antigenic determinant on cell surfaces, the effector T lymphocytes are capable of destroying the target cell (Chapter 9).

Lymphokines.   After interacting with their specific antigen, the T lymphocytes secrete soluble factors that affect surrounding cells. These factors, which are released from stimulated activated lymphocytes, are called lymphokines. They can affect neighboring lymphocytes, causing them to proliferate. Another cell that is highly susceptible to lymphokine action is the macrophage. A macrophage-activating factor is secreted by immune lymphocytes when they come into contact with their specific antigen. This type of immunity, dependent upon immune lymphocytes and macrophages rather than upon antibody, is referred to as cell-mediated immunity (Chapter 11). Since antibody does not play a role in this form of immunity, determinations of antibody titer in the serum do not signal the immune status of the patient. Skin tests designed to measure delayed hypersensitivity (such as the tuberculin test) are the easiest means to demonstrate cell-mediated immunity in patients.

Macrophages.   Like the lymphocyte, the macrophage is produced mainly in the bone marrow. It is found in the bloodstream as a relatively quiescent monocyte and, in the tissues, as the histiocyte. The particular specialty of the macrophage is phagocytosis (Chapter 10). This function of the macrophage is relatively nonspecific in the sense that it is governed primarily by the physicochemical properties of the respective surfaces. After phagocytosis, the lysosomes in the cytoplasm of the macrophage increase. The activated macrophage is rich in the cytoplasmic hydrolytic enzymes that arise from its lysosomes. Most bacterial cells are readily digested by the lysosomal enzymes, while others are resistant to hydrolytic breakdown. A few microorganisms, such as tubercle bacilli, may survive and kill the macrophage.

Activated macrophages more vigorously engulf and destroy invading microorganisms than do circulating monocytes or quiescent histiocytes. Some of the lymphokines produced by the T lymphocyte have the ability to activate the macrophage even before they phagocytize invading microorganisms.

Certain classes of antibody, called cytophilic antibodies, are thought to attach strongly to the surface of the macrophage. These cytophilic antibodies may confer the ability to the macrophage to recognize particular antigens.

Other Lymphocytes. Many other types of cells play a role in the immunologic system. One cell in particular looks very much like a lymphocyte, but lacks the characteristic surface markers of either the T lymphocyte or the B lymphocyte; thus the name "null cell" (Chapter 3). Together with antibody, some of these cells seem to be able to kill certain cellular targets directly and are designated "killer" or K cells.

Polymorphonuclear Neutrophils

Another important member of the immunologic team is the polymorphonuclear neutrophil. As the most plentiful member of the circulating white cell population, it is capable of responding rapidly to tissue injury. The neutrophils leave the bloodstream and accumulate at the site of damage, where they go about their specialized duties of phagocytosis (Chapter 10). As with the macrophage, phagocytosis by the polymorphonuclear neutrophil is a physical phenomenon depending upon the relative surface properties of the phagocyte and the particle. Antibody acting on the surface of the particle, referred to as opsonizing antibody, increases phagocytosis. After the combination of some classes of antibody with their respective antigens, complement factors are activated that further favor phagocytosis.

Amplification Mechanisms

Complement is a group of circulating plasma proteins with complex stimulatory and inhibitory interactions, some of which have enzymatic functions (Chapter 8). After they are activated by splitting from their natural inhibitors, these enzymes are capable of weakening or dissolving (i.e., lysing) the walls of certain kinds of cells. Complement can be activated in a variety of ways, such as the alteration of certain immunoglobulins following combination with antigen. In lysis, the initial interaction of antigen with immunoglobulin provides specificity (Chapter 7). Once activated, complement is nonspecific in its action.

Complement exemplifies the several biologic systems that may serve to amplify and extend immunologic interactions. The kinin system of inactive proteolytic enzymes of the plasma and tissue may also be activated, as may be the clotting system. Antigen-antibody reactions (Chapter 5) on cell surfaces may stimulate the release of histamine, serotonin, and the slow-reactive substance of anaphylaxis (SRS-A), which exert local or systemic actions.

Integral Scope of the Immune System

In recent years, our concept of the significance of the immunologic response has broadened greatly. It not only provides protection against infection but is sometimes an important cause of disease. Immunologic diseases may be due to interactions of extrinsic antigens (for example, allergic and immune complex disease) (Chapters 18 and 19) or intrinsic antigens (autoimmune disease) (Chapter 25). Failure of the immunologic response or malignant change in lymphocytes may also be responsible for disease (Chapter 24). Protective immunity and disease production are both coincidental by-products of an even more fundamental function of the immune system, which is the physiologic recognition of molecules introduced into the body.

Bibliography

Alexander, J. W., and Good, R. A. (eds.): *Fundamentals of Clinical Immunology.* W. B. Saunders Company, Philadelphia, 1977.

Bellanti, J. A.: *Immunology* II. W. B. Saunders Co., Philadelphia, 1978.

Bolduan, C., and Ehrlich, P. (eds.): *Studies in Immunity.* John Wiley & Sons, New York, 1910.

Bordet, J.: *Traité de l'Immunité dans les Maladies Insectieuses.* Masson et Cie, Paris, 1939.

Coombs, R. R. A.; Gell, P. G. H.; and Lackmann, P. J. (eds.): *Clinical Aspects of Immunology,* 3rd ed. F. A. Davis Co., Philadelphia, 1975.

Freedman, S. O., and Gold, P. (eds.): *Clinical Immunology,* 2nd ed. Harper & Row Hagerstown, Md., 1976.

Fudenberg, H. H.; Stites, D. P.; Caldwell, J. L.; and Wells, J. V. (eds.): *Basic and Clinical Immunology,* 2nd ed. Lange Medical Publications, Los Altos, Calif., 1978.

Golub, E. S.: *The Cellular Basis of the Immune Response: An Approach to Immunology.* Sinauer Associates, Sunderland, Mass., 1977.

Holborow, E. J., and Reeves, W. G. (eds.): *Immunology in Medicine: A Comprehensive Guide to Clinical Immunology.* Academic Press, London, 1977.

Kabat, E. A.: *Structural Concepts in Immunology and Immunochemistry.* Holt, Rinehart & Winston, Inc., New York, 1976.

Landsteiner, K.: *The Specificity of Serological Reactions.* Dover Publications, Inc., New York, 1962.

Long, E. R.: *A History of Pathology.* Dover Publications, Inc., New York, 1965.

Metchnikoff, E.: *Lectures on the Comparative Pathology of Inflammation.* Dover Publications, Inc., New York, 1968.

Nossal, G. J. V.: *Antibodies and Immunity.* Basic Books, Inc., New York, 1969.

Roitt, I. M.: *Essential Immunology,* 3rd ed. Blackwell Scientific Publications, Ltd., Oxford; J. B. Lippincott Co., Philadelphia, 1977.

Samter, M. (ed.): *Immunological Diseases*, Vols. I and II, 2nd ed. Little, Brown & Co., Boston, 1971.

Sell, S.: *Immunology, Immunopathology and Immunity*, 2nd ed. Harper & Row, Hagerstown., Md., 1975.

Thaler, M. S.; Klausner, R. D.; and Cohen, H. J. (eds.): *Medical Immunology*. J. B. Lippincott Co., Philadelphia, 1977.

Wilson, G. S., and Miles, A. A. (eds.): *Topley and Wilson's Principles of Bacteriology and Immunity*, 6th ed. Williams & Wilkins, Baltimore, 1975.

2

Phylogeny of the Immune Response

ALBERT A. BENEDICT

Introduction

Although all vertebrate classes exhibit cell-mediated and humoral immune responses, and immunologic memory (anamnesis), the immune system shows an increasing degree of complexity in the phylogenetic progression from the more primitive vertebrate classes to the more advanced ones. In evaluating the evolution of the immune system it is important to keep in mind that, based on present-day animals and without a fossil record, only inferences can be made about the phylogenetic organization of the animal kingdom. The phylogenetic approach also is complicated by the adaptation of unrelated species confronted with similar ecologic pressures. In other words, certain aspects of immune responses might represent convergent evolution in unrelated groups of animals.

Despite the lack of precise relationships of structures and functions based on evolutionary data, the study of nonmammals provides simple immunologic model systems for unraveling the complex mammalian systems. For example, discrimination between self and nonself by specific cellular immune responses in invertebrates is not complicated by synthesis of humoral antibodies. Amphibians offer a good model for the study of tolerance to self-antigens because in metamorphosis new adult structures differentiate in contact with the already functional larval immune system. In birds there is a clear-cut delineation of T cells and B cells by virtue of the presence of a thymus and a recognized B-cell-generating lymphoid organ, the bursa of Fabricius.

Invertebrate Immunity

To date molecules structurally and functionally analogous to vertebrate immunoglobulins have not been recognized in invertebrates; nevertheless, many invertebrates to a certain extent recognize self and nonself. In addition to the survival value of producing a large number of progeny, survival among invertebrates may also depend on recognition systems for maintaining individual integrity, and for developing internal defense mechanisms, such as phagocytosis (Chapter 10). It is unlikely that the major histocompatibility complex (MHC) evolved in vertebrates just to confound the transplantation surgeon (Chapter 22). It is reasonable that a gene complex controlling histo-incompatibility exists in invertebrates. When tissues of two genetically different individuals come into contact, histoincompatibility reactions prevent fusion of their tissues. In the broadest sense histoincompatibility reactions occur in most multicellular organisms. Moving up the invertebrate phylo-genetic tree, histoincompatibility progresses in complexity until forms that resemble allograft reactions in vertebrates have evolved (Chapter 23). In vertebrates, the MHC has an all-pervading influence on both cell-mediated and humoral immune responses (Chapter 3).

In invertebrates, histoincompatibility reactions can occur in a variety of forms. Among the Porifera, dissociated cells of two different species of sponges will sort out and form specific separate aggregates when mixed. There is no sign of cell damage. Inhibition of aggregation between individuals of the same species does not occur; thus, allorecognition is not evident. This incompatibility and those found in protozoa probably depend on recognition of cell-surface molecules, probably glycoproteins, rather than on immuno-recognition mechanisms.

Among certain anemones and corals acute aggressive allo- and xenogeneic reactions* occur within minutes and hours after tissue contact. Hallmarks of immune mechanisms in vertebrates, specificity and memory, have not been demonstrated in these reactions. The mechanism of graft rejection in these animals is not known.

Transplantation immunity as manifested by graft rejection has not been observed in arthropods and mollusks. Nevertheless, encapsulation of foreign tissue or organisms occurs.

---

* Allogeneic reactions are directed to other members of the same species; xenogeneic re-actions are directed to members of other species (Chapter 22).

Specific allo- and xenograft rejections accompanied by cellular proliferative responses, and in some instances associated with at least short-term memory, appear in the advanced invertebrates, notably echinoderms, annelids, and the highest invertebrate form, the tunicates (protochordates). Earthworms, the most thoroughly studied invertebrates, produce accelerated second-set responses to tissue antigens after an initial priming of hosts, clearly demonstrating anamnesis.

There is a variety of cells, including lymphocyte-like cells, with which quasi-immunologic functions are associated. Coelomocytes or hemocytes are wandering phagocytes found in invertebrates with a coelom (annelids, mollusks, arthropods, echinoderms). In addition to their discrimination between self and foreign materials in their phagocytic function, these cells may utilize similar recognition mechanisms for handling allo- and xenografts. Coelomocytes found at the site of xenograft rejection in annelid worms have been shown to transfer immunity to xenografts in *nonimmune* animals. This is one of the best examples of a putative immune mechanism in invertebrates. The coelomocytes of earthworms also respond to mitogens by an increase of DNA synthesis. Indeed, the coelomocytes and hemocytes are good candidates for receptor cells analogous to vertebrate lymphocytes.

Tunicates, which are probably the evolutionary ancestors of vertebrates, have small undifferentiated blood cells, which bear striking morphologic and functional resemblance to vertebrate lymphocytes. These similarities are as follows: (1) sensitivity to x-irradiation, (2) blastogenic response *in vitro* to phytohemagglutinin, (3) stem-cell function for regeneration of new colonies, (4) infiltration in graft rejection sites, and (5) rosette formation with sheep red blood cells. Further study is needed to determine the structural and functional analogy of invertebrate blood leukocytes and vertebrate lymphocytes.

Poorly defined nonspecific humoral substances found in the hemolymph of coelomate invertebrates agglutinate foreign red blood cells, kill some bacteria, and inactivate ciliary movements. The physicochemical characterization of several hemagglutinins reveals protein molecules with similar structural properties and molecular weights of about 100,000 to 500,000. These hemagglutinins seem to have no functions analogous to vertebrate immunoglobulins. Opsonin-like humoral substances in crayfish hemolymph facilitate the uptake of particles by coelomocytes.

In summary, invertebrates do not have humoral substances structurally and functionally resembling vertebrate immunoglobulins. Immunorecognition seems to have evolved from primordial cell-mediated immune responses, primarily through histoincompatibility reactions involving recognition of self and nonself cell-surface components. These recognition reactions are characterized by phagocytosis and reactions that range from those without evidence of allorecognition or aggressive properties to those which resemble vertebrate allograft reactions. There is a good possibility that the histocompatibility genetic system evolved in invertebrates whose function in vertebrates causes lymphocyte proliferation, generation of effector cells, and production of serologically detectable antigenic determinants.

Vertebrate Immunity

Agnatha

The first true vertebrates that appear in the known fossil record belong to the fish class Agnatha (Figure 2–1). Members of this class, the hagfish and lamprey, have a limited repertoire of immune responsiveness associated with limited organization of lymphoid organs. The hagfish does not possess a thymus gland; however, phagocytic and antigen-reactive cells are associated with the pharyngeal muscles. These cells may represent the precursor of a thymus in higher vertebrates. Agnathans also lack a discrete spleen and bone marrow, but they have small hemopoietic foci in the lamina propria of the gut and in the anterior kidney that appear to carry out both myeloid and lymphoid cell development. In hagfish blood there are a variety of complex and specialized cells, including small lymphocytes similar to mammalian small lymphocytes. Plasma cells have not been found in either the hagfish or lamprey, thus implicating the small blood lymphocyte as an effector in humoral antibody production.

The agnathan immune responses are sluggish. First-set skin allografts are rejected at a much slower rate than in higher vertebrates. Repeat grafts also have prolonged survivals; however, somewhat accelerated rejection of repeat grafts indicates short-term memory. Indicative of B cell competence, antibodies are synthesized to cellular and soluble antigens, but the responses are not vigorous.

Only one immunoglobulin class exists in Agnatha, and in cartilaginous (sharks) and bony fishes as well. (Immunoglobulin classes are distinguished on the basis of antigenic and amino acid differences in the constant region of the heavy chains [Chapter 4].) Where a low molecular weight (LMW) immunoglobulin occurs in these animals, the heavy chain is antigenically indistinguishable from the high molecular weight (HMW) immunoglobulin heavy chain. More than one immunoglobulin class emerges at the level of amphibians.

The hagfish immunoglobulin has a molecular weight of about 1,000,000 and is of anodal electrophoretic mobility. This immunoglobulin appears to be a multimer composed predominantly of light chainlike polypeptides. In the lamprey, antibody activity has been associated with 7 S, 9 S, and 14 S molecules. The purified 7 S immunoglobulin has a molecular weight of 188,000, consists of heavy and light subunits with masses of 70,000 and 25,000 daltons, respectively, and lacks intersubunit disulfide bonds. The isolated 9 S molecule has a molecular weight of 320,000 with a unique structure consisting

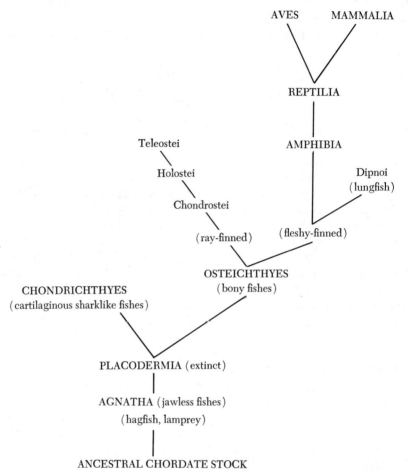

Figure 2-1. Vertebrate evolution. (Adapted from Romer, A. S.:
The Vertebrate Story. University of Chicago Press, Chicago, 1959.)

of four polypeptide chains of identical size and also lacks intersubunit disulfide bonds. A relationship between the 9 S immunoglobulin and invertebrate agglutinating glycoproteins has been postulated.

Fishes

Compared to the Agnatha, sharks (class Chondrichthyes—cartilaginous fishes) show slightly more vigorous rejection of skin allografts, which is evident in acute rejection of fourth-set grafts. Among bony fishes (class Osteichthyes) a transition from slow to rapid graft rejection is seen. The lower bony fishes (Chondrostei) show chronic allograft reactivity, whereas advanced bony fishes (Teleostei) elicit acute rejection of first-set scale grafts followed by accelerated rejection of second-set grafts.

All Elasmobranchean (sharks, skates, rays), Chondrostean (paddlefish, sturgeon), Holostean (gar, bowfin), and Teleostean (bass, trout, pike, carp, catfish, grouper) fishes possess only one class of immunoglobulin. This immunoglobulin is considered analogous to mammalian IgM. Whereas most of the representatives have two size classes (HMW and LMW), three species studied (gar, goldfish, and carp) possess only the HMW form. The HMW immunoglobulin exists as either a pentamer, tetramer, or dimer, whereas the LMW immunoglobulin is a monomer of the HMW structure and does not possess an antigenically unique heavy chain. Heavy chains of these immunoglobulins are characterized by a molecular weight of approximately 70,000 and a high carbohydrate content. In addition, the grouper and bowfish have a 5.7 S immunoglobulin with a molecular weight of approximately 120,000. The mass of the 5.7 S immunoglobulin heavy chain (40,000 daltons) is one immunoglobulin domain (10,000 to 12,000 daltons) less than the mammalian IgG heavy chain (50,000 daltons). With respect to the HMW immunoglobulin heavy chain, the 5.7 S immunoglobulin heavy chain does not have unique antigenic determinants and therefore does not represent a new immunoglobulin class. Molecules analogous to the mammalian J chain have been identified in association with the HMW shark immunoglobulins.

Amphibians

Amphibia represent a bridgepoint in the evolution of the lymphoid system. Less advanced forms, such as salamanders, have a simple lymphoid system equivalent to that of cartilaginous fishes. The more advanced amphibians (bullfrog and toad), in addition to possessing a thymus and spleen, also have multiple lymph node-like structures, lymphopoietic bone marrow, and gut-associated lymphoid tissues. A number of mammalian T cell and B cell functions are found in some amphibians. Lymphocyte heterogeneity (T and B cells?) is indicated by their different responses to several mitogens. Splenic lymphocytes and thymus cells undergo blastogenesis in response to allogeneic spleen cells. This latter response, known as the mixed leukocyte reaction (MLR), is under the control of a single genetic region. Recently the MLR in the toad (*Xenopus*) was shown to have a genetic relationship to graft rejection and to certain red blood cell antigens, thus giving evidence of the emergence of a major histocompatibility complex (MHC) analogous to the avian and mammalian MHC.

Collaboration between carrier-specific "helper" cells and hapten-specific antibody-secreting cells, a characteristic of many antibody responses in birds and mammals, has been reported in the newt. One would like to know more about the source of B cells, as the newt does not have lymphopoietic bone marrow or a known bursal equivalent. Related to this, early thymectomy in larval *Xenopus* depresses both cell-mediated and humoral responses. During early ontogeny most, if not all, of *Rana pipiens* peripheral lymphocytes are thymus derived.

Reflecting the evolutionary progression in amphibians, chronic allograft rejection is characteristic of lower groups whereas the more advanced amphibians show acute rejection.

Amphibians are particularly useful for studying the ontogeny of the immune response. Both larval and adult amphibians are immunocompetent. The larval stage is not confined to an *in utero* development, and it is readily available in the free-living stage.

Low environmental temperatures have a depressive effect on the immune responses in cold-blooded (ectothermic) classes of fish, amphibians, and reptiles. Studies on the effect of temperature on antibody production in carp and toads reveal that early events after primary stimulation with antigen are not temperature sensitive. The temperature-sensitive events may relate to cellular interactions and/or cellular differentiation.

Distinct classes of immunoglobulins emerge in amphibians. The HMW immunoglobulin is considered analogous to IgM, whereas the LMW 7 S immunoglobulin, with a molecular weight of 170,000, has an antigenically distinct heavy chain with a mass of 62,000 daltons. Immunoglobulins of this same molecular weight are also found in reptiles and birds. It should be noted again that the mammalian IgG and the γ chain have molecular weights of 150,000 and 50,000, respectively; therefore, the amphibian, reptilian, and avian 7 S immunoglobulin of intermediate molecular weight (170,000) probably is not an IgG molecule (Table 4-1, page 44).

Lungfish (Dipnoi) occupy a unique position in the scheme of vertebrate evolution. They possess many structural features resembling those of primitive amphibians but are not ancestral to higher vertebrates. Of particular interest, the African lungfish has the HMW, the intermediate molecular weight, and the 5.7 S immunoglobulins.

Reptiles

Although reptiles were among the first nonmammals to be used as experimental animals in immunology, they have not been studied as extensively as amphibians. The lymphoid complex of turtles and lizards show well-organized thymus, spleen, small lymph nodes, and intestinal and cloacal aggregates. Plaque-forming cells are found in the spleen and blood in some species. Plasma cells, as well as a variety of transitional cell types, have been demonstrated in turtles.

Representatives of reptiles elicit chronic rejection of first-set allografts not unlike those found in primitive fishes and lower amphibians. The evolutionary progression from chronic to accelerated graft rejection may actually represent weak transplantation antigens rather than a deficiency in the immune responses. Turtle spleen cells undergo graft-versus-host (GVH) reactions, the incidence of lethality and rapidity of which are greater at elevated temperatures (Chapter 23).

Unlike most lower vertebrates some reptilian species are capable of "maturation" of the immune response. That is, antibody affinity increases during the course of immunization. Reptiles have IgM-like immunoglobulins and a LMW immunoglobulin of intermediate molecular weight (170,000) similar to those of amphibians and birds. A 5.7 S immunoglobulin (120,000 daltons) synthesized in turtles does not seem to have unique antigenic determinants. Thus, as in amphibians, reptiles have two major immunoglobulin classes.

Birds

It has been proposed that mammals inherited their "warm-bloodedness" (endothermy) from therapsids (mammal-like reptiles evolved during the Permian) and that birds inherited their endothermy from dinosaurs. Thus, living birds may represent a continuing expression of basic dinosaur biology.

The chicken and duck immune systems are the best characterized among avian species. The most striking difference between the avian immune system and that of other animals is the presence of two well-organized primary (central) lymphoid organs, the thymus and the bursa of Fabricius. As in mammals, the thymus produces precursors of cells involved in cell-mediated immune responses. The bursa is responsible for B lymphopoiesis. Immunoglobulin synthesis by precursor cells begins early in ontogeny. B-stem cells first appear in the bursa about the twelfth day of embryonogenesis. Within 48 hours, these cells express surface HMW immunoglobulin. Later LMW and secretory-like (IgA) immunoglobulins arise in bursa follicles.

Chickens do not possess lymph nodes, whereas ducks do. In addition to the spleen, the most obvious secondary or peripheral lymphoid tissues in chickens are agglomerations of lymphoid cells along the gut, the largest being the coecal tonsil.

Birds have all of the cell-mediated responses exhibited by mammals. T and B lymphocytes are stimulated by the usual mitogens resulting in increased DNA synthesis. The chicken MHC is highly developed as it consists of a gene complex that controls a number of functions seen in mammals, namely, acute allograft rejection, MLR, GVH, response to certain immunogens (immune response genes), synthesis of lymphocyte and erythrocyte allo-antigens, and the level of blood complement. The chicken has MHC allo-antigens of approximately the same molecular weights as the mouse H-2D, H-2K, and Ia antigens (Chapter 22).

Functionally, the immune responses (both humoral and cellular) of birds —of at least some gallinaceous species—resemble mammalian responses. Unlike many lower vertebrates, but like mammals, birds manifest brisk antibody responses to a variety of antigens. In contrast to the sluggish responses seen in fishes, amphibians, and reptiles, antibodies are synthesized in birds in relatively high concentrations in short periods of time. Similarly, the affinity constants of chicken antihapten antibodies increase in time and approach the high values found in some mammals. In many lower

Table 2-1

EVOLUTION OF SOME IMMUNOLOGICALLY IMPORTANT CHARACTERISTICS

Immunologic Characteristics		Agnatha	Fishes		Dipnoi	Amphibians		Reptiles	Birds	Mammals
			SHARK-LIKE	BONY	LUNGFISH	PRIMITIVE	ADVANCED		CHICKEN	MAN
Graft rejection		C	C	A&C		C	A	C	A	A
Major histocompatibility complex (MHC)*			■	■	■	■	■		■	■
MHC—control of antibody responses (immune response genes)			■	■	■	■			■	■
Serologically detectable MHC antigens				▨			■			■
MHC—control of serum complement level							■			■
Complement		■	■	■	■	■	■	■	■	■
Lymphoid system	Lymphocytes	▨	■	■	■	■	■	■	■	■
	Plasma cells		■	■	■	■	■	■	■	■
	Macrophages	▨	■	■	■	■	■	■	■	■
	Thymus	▨	■	■	▨	■	■	■	■	■
	Spleen	▨	■	■	■	■	■	■	■	■
	Lymph nodes								■	■
	HMW (IgM-like)	■	■	■	■	■	■	■	■	■
	IMW	▨		▨	■	■	■			■
	LMW	▨		■	■	■	■	■	■	
Immunoglobulins	LMW (IgG-like)								■	■
	Secretory (IgA)								■	■
	IgE									■
	IgD									■
Number of classes		1	1	1	2	1	2	2 (3?)	3	5

22

C = Chronic.

A = Acute.

Empty boxes = absence of characteristic or knowledge.

Filled boxes = characteristic is typical in some representatives.

Stippled boxes = atypical or not fully developed.

HMW = high molecular weight.

IMW = Intermediate molecular weight (approximately 170,000 daltons).

LMW = low-molecular-weight monomer of the HMW immunoglobulin. The LMW and HMW heavy chains are antigenically indistinguishable. Another LMW immunoglobulin of approximately 120,000 daltons is found in the grouper and bowfish (bony fishes), lungfish, turtles, and ducks.

* = based on genetic association between allograft rejection and other functions, such as mixed leukocyte reaction and serologically detectable antigens.

vertebrates, antihapten antibodies have relatively lower binding constants, and "maturation" of affinity is a rather slow process.

Chickens have three major classes of immunoglobulins. The HMW immunoglobulin is the IgM-like molecule as found throughout the vertebrates. The LMW immunoglobulin is of intermediate molecular weight (170,000) and, as pointed out previously, is similar in size to the LMW immunoglobulins of some amphibians and reptiles. A secretory immunoglobulin, most likely the counterpart of the mammalian IgA, is found in low concentrations in serum and in high concentrations in biliary, intestinal, and respiratory secretions. Immunoglobulins similar to mammalian IgE and IgD have not been identified. However, hypersensitivity reactions occur in birds that are functionally similar to those caused by mammalian IgE. Ducks have three major immunoglobulins: the HMW, the intermediate-molecular-weight, and the 120,000-molecular-weight immunoglobulins. Whether or not birds have evolved multiple classes and subclasses of immunoglobulins as diverse as mammalian immunoglobulins should have important implications for our knowledge of the phylogeny of immunoglobulins.

The vast repertoire of immune responses in mammals mediated by T and B lymphocytes and the diversity of the mammalian immunoglobulins based on heavy- and light-chain variable and constant region differences are presented in Chapters 4 and 5.

The precise relationships of mammalian IgG, IgM, IgA, IgE, and IgD to the major immunoglobulins in lower vertebrates have not been determined. Also, immunoglobulin relationships between vertebrate classes are still puzzling. Three criteria have been used to evaluate these relationships. In order of importance these are (1) amino acid sequences and antigenic cross-reactivity; (2) relatively specific properties of an immunoglobulin, such as those associated with mammalian IgA and IgE; and (3) phenomena not necessarily unique to a single immunoglobulin, such as carbohydrate or amino acid composition, electrophoretic mobility, and molecular weight. Most of the data presented in this chapter are chiefly third-order criteria. Immunoglobulin homologies will be more firmly established when they can be based on amino acid sequences and precise antigenic analyses of the heavy chains.

Bibliography

Borysenko, M.: Phylogeny of immunity: an overview. *Immunogenetics*, **3**:305–26, 1976.

Cooper, E. L. (ed.): *Comparative Immunology*. Prentice-Hall, Englewood Cliffs, N.J., 1976.

Hildemann, W. H., and Benedict, A. A. (eds.): *Immunologic Phylogeny*. Plenum Press, New York, 1975.

Kubo, R. T.; Zimmerman, B.; and Grey, H. M.: Phylogeny of immunoglobulins. In Sela, M. (ed.): *The Antigens*, Vol. 1. Academic Press, New York, 1973, pp. 417–77.

Marchalonis, J. J. (ed.): *Comparative Immunology*. Blackwell Scientific Publications, Ltd., Oxford; J. B. Lippincott Co., Philadelphia, 1976.

Marchalonis, J. J.: *Immunity in Evolution*. Harvard University Press, Cambridge, Mass., 1977.

3

Origin of the Immune Response

PIERLUIGI E. BIGAZZI, STANLEY COHEN, AND
CAREL J. VAN OSS

Introduction

The central feature of the immune system is that it provides the organism
with a means for the specific recognition of foreign substances. These
substances, or antigens, when they contact the immune system result in the
activation and proliferation of sensitized cells, that is, lymphocytes with
antibody-like receptors on their surfaces. These cells serve three functions.
First, they may directly participate in certain reactions of cell-mediated
immunity (Chapter 11). Second, they may differentiate and become
antibody-producing plasma cells. Third, some of these cells may persist as
a reservoir of information-bearing machinery so that subsequent contact
with the same antigen leads to a greatly augmented response. This latter
phenomenon is known as immunologic memory.

A major question in immunology concerns the nature of the recognition
mechanism. There are two types of theories that attempt to explain
immunologic recognition. One type postulates that the antigen in some
manner penetrates into the antibody-producing machinery of the cell and
instructs it as to what sort of antibody to make. A second type of theory
proposes that this knowledge exists even before the first antigenic contact is
made and that the antigen *selects* the appropriate cells that have the capacity

to make antibody complementary to it. The latter view, which, as we shall see, is now the majority opinion, implies that a given antigen can interact with only a limited number of lymphocytes.

In any case, it has recently been shown that there is a necessity for cooperation among multiple cell types for an immune response to occur. This requirement must be taken into account in any discussion attempting to synthesize the current information relating to antibody formation.

Origin and Kinds of Lymphocytes

In mammals, the principal source of lymphocytes is the hematopoietic tissue in the bone marrow. *In utero* and in the early neonatal period, hematopoiesis can occur in various solid organs such as the liver, and lymphocyte production presumably can also occur in these locations.

The lymphocytes may be subdivided into two broad populations (Chapter 1). One group of lymphocytes migrates from the marrow to the thymus and there differentiates and proliferates. These cells are involved in cell-mediated immunity—i.e., delayed hypersensitivity, graft rejection, and graft-vs.-host reactions—and have been defined as "thymus dependent," "thymus derived" (an obvious misnomer), "thymus processed," or more simply T cells. Neonatal thymectomy in mice causes the virtual disappearance of lymphocytes from the periarteriolar regions of the spleen and the perifollicular and paracortical areas of the lymph nodes, of many lymphocytes from the thoracic duct, and of about half of the lymphocytes from the peripheral blood. Cell-mediated immunity does not develop in neonatally thymectomized or congenitally athymic mice, which is a similar situation to some congenital immune deficiency diseases of man, such as DiGeorge's syndrome and Nézelof's syndrome, characterized by depletion of lymphocytes and thymic aplasia or dysplasia (Chapter 17).

The second population of lymphocytes also arises in the bone marrow, but presumably does not require passage through the thymus to reach a differentiated form (Chapter 1). In birds, the controlling organ for these cells is the bursa of Fabricius, an organ closely associated with the intestinal tract. The bursa is responsible for the development of a population of bone marrow–derived cells that in the "peripheral" lymphoid organs become plasma cell precursors and are capable of antibody production. Manipulations of the bursa, such as the suppression of its development by testosterone administration, bursectomy at an early embryonic age, or neonatal bursectomy followed by irradiation, suppress antibody formation. A similar situation is observed in a congenital immune deficiency disease of man, sex-linked Bruton-type agammaglobulinemia (Chapter 17). In mammals, which lack the bursa of Fabricius, gut-associated lymphoid tissues (Peyer's patches, appendix) might be "bursa-equivalent" tissues. The cells that are programmed by the bursa or equivalent tissues are defined as "bursa dependent," "bursa equivalent derived," "bone marrow derived," "thymus independent," or more simply, B cells. B cells are localized mostly in the subcapsular, medullary areas and in the germinal centers of the lymph nodes and in the peripheral white pulp and the red pulp of the spleen.

Identification of T and B Cells

T and B cells cannot be distinguished by conventional light microscopy or by electron microscopy. Early investigations by scanning electron microscopy seemed to indicate that human B lymphocytes could be identified because of the presence of numerous small stubs and microvilli on their surfaces, whereas T cells had a rather smooth appearance. However, there is considerable overlap between the two populations, and recent evidence shows that the presence of microvilli is not characteristic of a special class of lymphocytes. The surface of lymphocytes, independently of their T and B nature, can be altered by various factors, among which are stage of cell cycle, temperature, and in general the method of preparation of the cells for scanning electron microscopy. T cells tend to have a higher electrophoretic mobility than B cells, but that property has hitherto been rarely used for their identification.

On the other hand, T and B cells can be identified because they express different surface markers and have different biologic behavior. Mouse T cells possess surface antigens that are lacking on B cells. One of the best investigated of these antigens is theta (θ) or Thy-1 which is expressed on approximately 95 to 98% of thymic lymphocytes and 70% of peripheral blood lymphocytes. Another surface component, the thymus leukemia or TL antigen, is expressed only on thymocytes and not on peripheral T cells. A more recently discovered set of surface markers is composed of the Ly antigens that are present on both thymocytes and T cells and absent on B cells. Their expression varies according to the various subpopulations of T lymphocytes (see below). Human T cells have been less easy to characterize than mouse T cells, because of the lack of the appropriate antisera. However, they spontaneously form rosettes when incubated with nonsensitized sheep red blood cells (E rosettes). By this procedure, it has been calculated that approximately 70% of peripheral blood lymphocytes in man are T cells.

B cells are usually identified because they possess surface immunoglobulins easily demonstrable by a variety of procedures. In contrast, T cells may possess only small amounts of immunoglobulin, which are less easy to detect. Approximately 15 to 30% of peripheral lymphocytes have been identified as B cells on the basis of the presence of surface immunoglobulins. There has been considerable variation in the literature regarding the class of surface immunoglobulins on B lymphocytes, but it now seems that IgM and IgD are the major classes present on the membrane of human B cells. Fc receptors, another type of surface marker initially thought to be present on B lymphocytes, macrophages, and neutrophils, may also be present on T lymphocytes. These receptors are components of the cell membrane that can combine with the Fc portion of immunoglobulin molecules and are associated with a variety of biologic functions such as antibody-dependent cytotoxicity and phagocytosis. In addition, B cells have complement receptors, which react with certain complement components in antigen-antibody-complement complexes. These are commonly detected using erythrocytes, anti-erythrocyte antibody, and complement (EAC). This leads to the formation of rosettes of red cells around the lymphocytes, which are defined as EAC rosettes.

T and B cells can also be distinguished on the basis of their different biologic behavior. Substances that induce proliferation, called mitogens, have been found to stimulate selectively different classes of lymphocytes. Even though this action is not as selective as initially thought, in general it can be said that concanavalin A (Con A) and phytohemagglutinin (PHA) are mitogenic for T cells, while pokeweed mitogen (PWM) and bacterial lipopolysaccharide (LPS) are mitogenic for B cells. Finally, different functions can be attributed to T and B cells: the former have helper, suppressor, or cytotoxic activity and produce soluble products capable of affecting other cells and called lymphokines, whereas the main function of B cells appears to be the production of antibodies. These functional distinctions are becoming less clear-cut. Thus, under certain experimental conditions, B cells can produce lymphokines *in vitro*. The appearance of serum lymphokine activity in certain neoplastic diseases of B cells suggests that this can also happen *in vivo*. Similarly, certain cytotoxic mechanisms may involve B cells rather than T cells. Finally, characterization of T and B cells on the basis of different properties does not always lead to the same subpopulations. In addition, there are certain lymphocytes that have marker properties of both T and B cells and, conversely, those that lack both (null cells).

Subpopulations of T and B Cells

There is some evidence in favor of the existence of subclasses of the two broad populations of lymphocytes. In the mouse, the θ alloantigen is present in different amounts on the surface of T cells: thymocytes have the most, and decreasing amounts are detected on mature thymus cells (T_1) and peripheral T cells (T_2). The opposite occurs with the H-2 antigen, which is more abundant on T_1 and T_2 cells than on thymocytes. As previously mentioned, immature cortical thymocytes express the TL antigen and, in addition, possess Ly123 antigens. On the other hand, peripheral T lymphocytes can be distinguished in two populations, one expressing Ly23 surface antigens and thus defined as Ly1− Ly23+, and the other expressing Ly1 surface antigen and defined as Lyl+ Ly23−. The first subpopulation has killer and suppressor functions, the second is programmed for helper function (see below). It has been shown that Lyl− Ly23+ and Lyl+ Ly23− subsets are derived from two separate lines of differentiation and are not sequential stages of a single differentiative pathway.

B cells also probably are a heterogeneous population, and indeed some investigators have presented evidence in favor of the existence of B_1 (precursor) and B_2 (secretory) cells.

Antigen Binding by Lymphocytes

Specific receptors capable of binding antigens are present on the surface of immunocompetent cells, from both normal and immunized individuals. This is important support for selective theories of antibody formation, and indeed had already been proposed many years ago by Paul Ehrlich.

Cells bearing antigen-binding receptors can interact with and be triggered by antigen and are, therefore, defined as antigen-reactive cells (ARC) or antigen-binding cells (ABC). These cells have been detected and quantitated by several techniques: immunocytoadherence, autoradiography using radio-labeled (iodinated) antigens, and the so-called "antigen suicide," i.e., elimination of antigen-binding cells by "hot" radiolabeled antigen. For one particular hapten-homologous protein conjugate such as 2,4-dinitrophenyl guinea pig albumin (DNP-GPA), approximately 40 ARC per 10^5 cells have been demonstrated in nonimmunized guinea pigs, whereas after immunization with DNP-GPA, their number is increased to approximately 4000 per 10^5 cells. This increase precedes the increase in antibody-secreting cells that is observed after immunization and that in its turn precedes the increase in circulating antibodies. It is now established that antigen-binding receptors are present on the surface of both B and T cells. The receptors on T cells are less easily demonstrated, possibly because their density on the surface is low or because they are "buried" in the surface. As far as the nature of the receptors is concerned, since both antigen-binding sites and immunoglobulins are on the surface of B lymphocytes and since antigen binding is inhibited by anti-immunoglobulin sera, it seems reasonable to deduce that antigen-binding receptors of B cells are immunoglobulin molecules. Circumstantial evidence suggests that the combining site of the receptor molecules present on ARC is similar to the combining site of the antibody produced in response to the antigen specific for the receptor. The number of antigen-binding receptors has been estimated to approximate 60,000 per cell.

On the other hand, the nature of the receptors on T cells is still rather obscure. They have been tentatively defined by some investigators as "IgX," an as yet unknown class of antibody, or "IgT." Alternatively, it has been postulated that T cells possess different and more primitive recognition structures, possibly related to the histocompatibility antigens or the Ir gene products.

Induction of the Immune Response

The first step in antibody formation is the introduction of an antigen into an animal. The antigen can be introduced by several routes, e.g., through mucosal surfaces, the skin, or the bloodstream. In nature, antibody formation is most commonly caused by microorganisms, but foods, pollens, and various other antigens can also initiate it. Experimentally, antibody formation is best obtained by parenteral injection, but other routes may also be used. Insoluble antigens generally elicit a stronger antibody response than soluble antigens.

The dose and physicochemical characteristics of an antigen, its distribution in the organism, and its catabolism are important factors in antibody production, as well as in the persistence of antibodies, their class, and their binding affinity. Persistent antigenic stimulation is equally necessary for continued antibody formation as well as for the phenomenon known as tolerance (Chapter 12).

Primary Response

The primary response is observed when an animal meets a previously uncontacted antigen and makes antibodies to it. The time required before antibodies are produced and before peak levels are obtained, the duration of the peak, etc., vary with the antigen, its dose, the route of administration, and the method used for antibody detection. Taking all these variables into account, one can say that in general antibodies are first detected within one or two weeks from the first immunization. The class of antibodies detected first is generally IgM, followed after a short interval by IgG. The production of IgM antibodies usually lasts for approximately 15 days, whereas IgG antibodies are produced for a much longer period.

Secondary Response

The secondary or anamnestic (memory) response is observed when an animal is exposed to the same antigen after the primary response. That exposure causes an enhanced reaction characterized by a reduction of the interval between contact with the antigen and antibody production and by the appearance of larger amounts of antibody for a longer period of time. The antibodies produced in the secondary response are mostly IgG. The first contact with antigen somehow conditions the animal for this enhanced secondary response. This state of augmented reactivity is intimately connected with immunologic memory.

Multiple mechanisms operate to generate memory. The simplest of these involves the consequences of antigen contact previously mentioned. This contact triggers a wave of proliferation of certain immunocompetent lymphocytes, not all of which are destined to become end-stage cells such as antibody-producing plasma cells or cells that mediate delayed hypersensitivity. Some of the proliferating cells remain available for future contact with antigen. Thus, the second, challenging dose of antigen finds a greatly augmented population of cells that can specifically respond to that antigen.

Adjuvants

Antibody formation can be increased by injecting the antigen together with certain substances known as adjuvants that aspecifically stimulate the immune system. The mechanisms of adjuvant action are not yet very clear. The stimulation of the immune system may occur via the activation of macrophages or other cells. Adjuvant also may provide for a slow, sustained release of antigen from the sites of administration. The adjuvants most commonly used in experimental immunization are the water-in-oil emulsions introduced by Freund (incomplete Freund's adjuvant). The antigen suspended in water is mixed with mineral oil and an emulsifier and then injected subcutaneously or intramuscularly. A much stronger and more persistent response is obtained when the adjuvant, besides mineral oil and emulsifier, contains killed mycobacteria (complete Freund's adjuvant). This mixture gives rise to granuloma formation and slower release of the antigen, for a period that in some cases may be several months. Other microorganisms such as *Bordetella pertussis, Corynebacterium parvum*, staphylococci, and streptococci have also been used as adjuvants. Alum (potassium aluminum sulfate) and aluminum hydroxide have been employed as adjuvants for human immunization with diphtheria or tetanus toxoids.

Passive Antibody Administration

In addition to factors such as memory or adjuvancy that enhance the immune response, there are feedback mechanisms for suppression of that response. This regulation is important to prevent the organism from completely depleting its immune system by massive responses to a single antigen. One of the best-known agents of such suppression is antibody itself. It has been shown that antibody administered passively to an immunized animal inhibits synthesis of that antibody. This observation suggests that endogenous antibody can control its own production.

Anatomy of the Immune Response

Following injection into a tissue, antigenic material penetrates through the afferent lymphatics into the draining lymph nodes, where it is phagocytized by macrophages in the sinusoids and in the germinal centers. When injected intravenously, the antigen enters into the spleen and is picked up by the macrophages of the germinal centers. Most of the antigen disappears in a few days, but small amounts persist for a longer period of time.

The germinal centers of the lymph nodes contain B cells beside the macrophages. B cells are also present in the subcapsular and medullary areas of the lymph nodes. A compact cuff of T cells surrounds the germinal centers, and other T cells are contained in the paracortical areas, located between the germinal centers and extending into the medulla. A similar situation exists in the spleen, where T lymphocytes are localized in the periarteriolar regions and around the germinal centers, whereas B cells are found within the germinal centers.

The close topographic relationship between antigen, macrophages, T cells, and B cells provides ample opportunity for interactions. Unfortunately, the mechanisms of these interactions are not yet clear. Macrophages may be nonspecific handlers of antigen or they may process the antigen and present it to the lymphocytes. On the other hand, lymphocytes stimulated by an antigen liberate mediators (e.g., MIF, Chapter 11) that interact with the macrophages. It seems rather well established that a collaboration between T and B cells is necessary for an antibody response to many antigens. T cells interact with B cells, facilitating antibody production. This could be accomplished as a result of antigen presentation to B cells by T cells, or through the elaboration by T cells of a substance capable of influencing antibody production by B cells. Once these interactions have taken place, plasma cells appear and migrate into the medullary cords of the lymph nodes or into the red pulp of the spleen and secrete immunoglobulins. Both T and B cells (including B cell-derived antibody-producing cells) can leave the lymph nodes through the efferent lymphatic ducts or the spleen through the splenic vein.

Genetic Control of the Immune Response

In the last few years considerable evidence has become available indicating that immune responses to a wide variety of antigens are under genetic control. Several autosomal dominant genes, each of which controls the response to a specific antigen, have been identified in guinea pigs and mice. Most of these genes, defined as "immune response genes" or Ir genes, are linked to a major (or in some cases a minor) histocompatibility locus (Chapter 22). An animal endowed with an Ir gene is capable of a strong immune response to the corresponding antigen and is, therefore, described as a "responder." An animal lacking the same gene does not respond or responds poorly to the antigen and is defined as a "nonresponder."

At present, several Ir genes have been well characterized in guinea pigs. The PLL gene controls responsiveness to poly-L-lysine, the GA gene controls the immune response to a copolymer containing L-glutamic acid and L-alanine, and the GT gene controls the reactions to another copolymer composed of L-glutamic acid and L-tyrosine. The response to bovine serum albumin in guinea pigs of the inbred strain 2 is controlled by the BSA-1 gene. The Ir genes identified in strain 2 guinea pigs (PLL, GA, BSA-1) are linked to the major locus controlling the histocompatibility specificities of strain 2. The GT gene found in strain 13 guinea pigs is similarly linked to a major histocompatibility locus of this strain.

In the mouse, the animal best investigated from a genetic point of view, Ir genes have been localized in a special part of the major histocompatibility complex that has been defined as the I region. This region codes for several cell-surface antigens (Ia antigens). They are glycoproteins with a molecular weight of approximately 30,000 daltons and their tissue distribution is more restricted than that of H-2 antigens: they are expressed on macrophages, B lymphocytes, and some T lymphocytes. Ia antigens are usually not detected on other cells, even though there have been a few reports about their presence on epithelial cells and spermatozoa. They may have a role in cooperation between various cells (macrophages, T and B lymphocytes) in the initiation of the immune response, but their importance and their relationship with Ir are not yet completely clear.

A correlation between response to thyroid antigens, both as autoantibody production and autoimmune thyroiditis, and H-2 type has recently been observed in some inbred strains of mice (Chapter 25). Correlations between the histocompatibility HLA type and some human diseases (e.g., systemic lupus erythematosus) have also been described. Specific Ir genes might, therefore, be capable not only of controlling immune responses to various antigens, but also of affecting the susceptibility of animals and man to a variety of autoimmune and possibly also neoplastic diseases.

Cell Cooperation in Antibody Formation

The large majority of antigens are thymus dependent; that is, T-B cell interaction is a prerequisite for antibody production. Some antigens, usually large polymers consisting of repeating units, may interact directly with B cells and induce antibody response. They are thus defined as thymus independent and include *Escherichia coli* lipopolysaccharide, polymerized flagellin from *Salmonella adelaide*, pneumococcal polysaccharide S-III, polyvinylpyrrolidone, dextrans, and levans. Many, if not all, of these substances are B cell mitogens, and their ability to induce proliferative responses directly in B cells may explain the lack of a requirement for T cell participation in the immune responses they trigger. Immune responses to thymus-dependent antigens are regulated in both a positive and negative sense by the operation of regulatory T lymphocytes. As previously mentioned, separate classes of T cells mediate the positive (helper) and negative (suppressor) functions. The regulatory action exerted by T cells is not just a simple negative or positive control of antibody responses in general, but seems to be much more complex and is reflected in a number of phenomena, such as differences in stimulation of IgG antibody versus IgM, the progressive selection of clones of cells secreting high-affinity antibody, and so forth. A subclass of T lymphocytes helps B lymphocytes in antibody formation and has thus been defined as "helper cells." T helper cells react with the carrier determinants on an antigenic molecule and B effector cells react with the hapten determinants. Antibodies to the hapten determinants will be produced only if T helper cells have reacted with the carrier determinants. There are several hypotheses on the nature of T cell help; i.e., T cells may focus antigen on B cells, have membrane interactions with B cells, or produce helper factors, antigen specific or nonspecific. Recent evidence seems to favor the latter hypothesis. Nonspecific factors of T cell origin behave as polyclonal B cell activators and stimulate syngeneic and allogeneic B cells to synthesize antibodies against a variety of antigens. Antigen-specific factors from T cells cooperate only with syngeneic B cells or B cells that share Ia determinants. Specific T cell factors do not contain parts of the constant region of heavy or light chains of immunoglobulins, but bear antigenic determinants coded in the I region of the major histocompatibility complex (Chapter 22). Some have antigen-binding activity and bear Ia determinants.

The relationship between the soluble nonantibody lymphocyte-derived factors and the lymphokines is unclear. However, at least the nonspecific helper factors might be related to either mitogenic factors, lymphocyte chemotactic factor, or both.

There is also abundant evidence that macrophages can participate in immune responses. They appear to have a helper function in antibody production, and antigen- and mitogen-induced lymphocyte proliferative responses, and lymphokine production. Their effects are thought to be mediated either by direct cell-to-cell contact, or by macrophage-derived soluble factors (so-called monokines).

Theories of Antibody Formation

As already outlined, there are two types of theories, selective and instructive. Paul Ehrlich proposed the first theory on the formation of antibodies in 1900. It was a selective theory, involving many different antibody-like receptors on the periphery of cells. Upon combination between these receptors and the antigens that fit them best, the cells are in some manner induced to produce and to secrete large quantities of these antibody-like receptors. However, the growing awareness of the impressive number of

Table 3–1

FACTS THAT IDEAL ANTIBODY-FORMING

	Diversity of Antigens to Which Antibodies Can Be Made	Possibility of Antibody Formation to Synthetic Chemical Antigenic Determinants That Do Not Occur in Nature	Amount of Informational DNA Needed per Antibody-Forming Cell	Accordance with Molecular Biology Laws of Synthesis of All Proteins
Instructive Theories				
Refolding template theory	Cells must make "uncommitted" globulins that after folding on the antigen rigidify and become specific antibodies		No excessive amount of informational DNA needed	Up to the postulated refolding step, the classical protein synthesis process is followed
		Antibodies presumably can be made to any conceivable antigen		
De novo synthesis template theory	Previously uncommitted antibody-forming cells must upon interaction with an antigen somehow start making antibodies specific to it		An extreme flexibility of informational DNA required such as has not hitherto been encountered in any system	In contradiction with all known protein synthesis processes
Selective Theories				
Clonal selection theory	Existence of a great multitude of cells, each producing antibodies of different antibody specificity, must be postulated. These many different cells may be presumed to originate from multiple somatic mutations		No excessive amount of informational DNA needed	Classical protein synthesis process followed
		Apparently difficult to accommodate. However, there are only a finite number of possible antigens (synthetic as well as natural)		
Germ line theory	Potential of every antibody-forming cell to make any of the different possible antibody specificities must be postulated		Very large amount of informational DNA needed; as high as, or higher than, 15% of total DNA	Variants of protein synthesis processes have been proposed for this theory, which are, however, within the realm of possibility

Tolerance to Self-Antigens (Self-Recognition)	Amino Acid Sequence (in the Variable Part) of Antibodies Differs for Each Antibody Specificity	Only One (or at Most Two) Specificities of Antibody Found per Single Antibody-Forming Cell	Genetic Control of Antibody Formation	Anamnestic Response
	Impossible to account for			
Difficult to account for		Difficult to account for	Difficult to account for	Difficult to account for
	Easy to account for			
		Required	Easy to account for	Easy to account for
Easy to account for by elimination of all cells making antibodies to self-antigens	Easy to account for			
		Possible to account for if special mechanism for repression of the synthesis of all other antibody specificities is postulated	Possible to account for	Possible to account for if special mechanism for the permanent repression of the synthesis of all other antibody specificities of committed cell line is postulated

possible antibodies with different specificities (even toward entirely synthetic antigens) compelled many investigators to abandon such selective theories and to devise various instructive theories. More recently the advances in biochemical knowledge of protein chemistry and the emergence around 1950 of molecular biology rendered the hitherto proposed instructive theories untenable. More sophisticated selective theories then evolved, of which the clonal selection theory and the germ line theory are the most important. Various aspects of selective and instructive theories are grouped in Table 3–1.

Instructive Theories

Refolding Template Theory.   According to this theory, uncommitted and aspecific globulins can become refolded upon the antigen, which serves as a template for it. The cell thereupon releases the complementary antibodies, which from then on with the help of appropriate disulfide bonds rigidly retain their shape. This theory had to be abandoned when it became clear that the specificity of antibodies in all cases is due to the particular arrangement of their primary amino acid sequence (see Table 3–1).

De Novo **Synthesis Template Theory.**   Template theories that recognize that antibodies must be synthesized amino acid by amino acid, in the proper and predetermined order, still have to contend with the well-nigh-insurmountable objection that, according to the molecular biology dogmas of protein synthesis, proteins cannot serve as informational models for the synthesis of other proteins (Table 3–1). It should be pointed out that the germ line theory, although discussed below under selective theories, still has many aspects that are closely akin to instructive theories.

Selective Theories

Clonal Selection Theory.   The most widely regarded selective theory is Burnet's clonal selection hypothesis, which postulates the presence of numerous antibody-forming cells, each capable of synthesizing its own predetermined antibody. One of these cells, after having been selected by the best-fitting antigen, multiplies and forms a clone of cells that continue to synthesize the same antibody. Provided that one accepts the existence of very many different cells, each capable of synthesizing an antibody of a different specificity, all known facts of antibody formation are easily accounted for (except possibly, in the opinion of some workers, the formation of antibodies to synthetic antigens, see Table 3–1). An important element of the clonal selection theory as proposed by Burnet is the hypothesis that the many cells with different antibody specificities arise through random somatic mutations, during a period of hypermutability, early in the animal's life. Also early in life, the "forbidden" clones of antibody-forming cells (i.e., the cells that make antibody to the animal's own antigens) are all wiped out after encounters with these autoantigens. This process then accounts for the fact that animals are tolerant toward their own antigens.

Jerne recently proposed an extension of the clonal selection theory, explaining the somatic generation of the large number of genes that the population of lymphocytes can express by the postulate that they initially are directed against a complete set of the species' histocompatibility antigens. The animal's own histocompatibility antigens, in the process of reacting with the cells that can form antibodies against them, cause these cells to mutate randomly early in life, thus giving rise to many clones of antibody-forming cells with new and different specificities. This theory not only proposes a mechanism for the required somatic mutations but also offers an explanation for the fact that the antibody production to certain antigens is linked to particular histocompatibility loci (see below).

If one admits that some such mechanism operates, it must nevertheless be pointed out that the animal still has other antigens beside the histocompatibility ones, to which the corresponding antibody-making cells must be eliminated. That elimination process may then, according to the same reasoning, also cause random mutations among antibody-forming cells, thus giving rise to further different clones of new antibody-forming cells.

Germ Line Theory. Germ line theories have been brought forward to obviate the necessity of endowing animals with multitudinous antibody-forming cells, each with a different specificity. Instead it is proposed that each antibody-forming cell be endowed with the potential of synthesizing all conceivable antibodies. A specific antibody is now selected by the antigen, and the antigen-antibody reaction then somehow suppresses the production of all other unrelated antibodies. In its simplest form the germ line theory fulfills about the same requirements as the clonal selection theory. However, it requires each cell to bear the very heavy burden of containing all the informational DNA to code for all possible antibody specificities (see Table 3–1).

Summary

The induction of an immune response represents a microevolutionary process in which appropriate cells are selected and allowed to multiply preferentially and accumulate. This process involves the participation of multiple cell types, and the macroscopic effect is induced differentiation which leads to new functional properties for the organism. Thus, antigenic challenge leads to the appearance of cells with specificity for the antigen, molecules with similar specificity (antibodies), and a wide array of regulatory factors that control the overall response. Although a complete theoretic framework for all these effects is not yet at hand, a great deal is known about the genetic, biochemical, and physiologic mechanisms involved. The subject is of great practical importance, not only because of the central role of immunologic functions in host defense, but because similar mechanisms are probably involved in biologic processes of growth and differentiation in general.

Bibliography

Ada, G. L.: Antigen binding cells in tolerance and immunity. *Transplant. Rev.*, **5**:105–29, 1970.

Benacerraf, B.; Green, I.; and Paul, W. E.: The immune response of guinea pigs to hapten-poly-L-lysine conjugates as an example of the genetic control of the recognition of antigenicity. *Cold Spring Harbor Symp. Quant. Biol.*, **32**:569–75, 1967.

Burnet, F. M.: *Self and Not-Self.* Cambridge University Press, Cambridge, 1969.

Coutinho, A., and Moller, G.: Thymus-independent B-cell induction and paralysis. *Adv. Immunol.*, **21**:113–236, 1975.

Dickler, H. B.: Lymphocyte receptors for immunoglobulin. *Adv. Immunol.*, **24**:167–214, 1976.

Golub, E. S.: *The Cellular Basis of the Immune Response.* Sinauer Associates, Inc., Sunderland, Mass., 1977.

Hood, L., and Talmage, D. W.: Mechanism of antibody diversity: germ line basis for variability. *Science*, **168**:325–31, 1970.

Jerne, N. K.: The somatic generation of immune recognition. *Eur. J. Immunol.*, **1**:1–9, 1971.

Shreffler, D. C., and David, C. S.: The H-2 major histocompatibility complex and the I immune response region: genetic variation, function, and organization. *Adv. Immunol.*, **20**:125–95, 1975.

Talmage, D. W.: Theories of antibody formation. In Abramoff, P., and La Via, M. (eds.): *Biology of the Immune Response.* McGraw-Hill Book Co., New York, 1970, pp. 304–31.

Warner, N. L.: Membrane immunoglobulins and antigen receptors on B and T lymphocytes. *Adv. Immunol.*, **19**:67–216, 1974.

4

The Immunoglobulins

CAREL J. VAN OSS

General Considerations

Introduction

All antibodies are immunoglobulins. These serum globulins are of relatively slow (β and γ) electrophoretic mobility. Although it has been known for more than a century that antibodies are soluble serum constituents, the certitude that they were proteins was only gained when Tiselius and Kabat demonstrated in 1937 that antibody activity was associated with the electrophoretic γ globulin fraction of human serum.

Due to the fact that the immunoglobulins of any one individual consist of molecules of many thousands of different antibody specificities, these immunoglobulins display a wide range of physical properties, exemplified by a particularly broad spectrum of electrophoretic mobilities. For that reason even purified immunoglobulins are impossible to crystallize. Because of this heterogeneity, it was long believed impossible to unravel the exact physicochemical makeup of the immunoglobulins. However, owing to the occurrence of homogenous immunoglobulins in some neoplastic immunoglobulin disorders (Chapter 17), it has become possible to obtain an exact picture of the primary as well as of the tertiary configuration of these proteins.

Fundamentally, all immunoglobulins consist of only two kinds of chains: heavy (H) chains of a molecular weight of 53,000 to 71,000, and light (L) chains of a molecular weight of about 23,000. In man, there are five major classes of immunoglobulins. Each of these five immunoglobulins has a different type of heavy chain, but all classes of immunoglobulins have only one type of light chain, which can fall into either one or the other of two subgroups. The immunoglobulins consist of two heavy and two light chains, or, in some cases, multiples thereof. The heavy chains are attached to one another by means of one or more disulfide bonds, and on each side a light chain is attached to a heavy chain by a disulfide bond (Figure 4–1). The antibody-specific sites of the immunoglobulins are situated near the amino-terminal end of each of the four chains, and it is in the aminoterminal region of the four chains that the greatest variability in amino acid sequence occurs from immunoglobulin to immunoglobulin. Much more constant amino acid sequences are found in the carboxyterminal regions of the immunoglobulin chains.

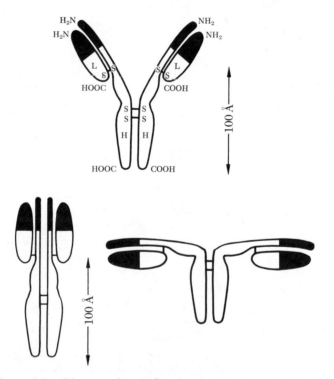

Figure 4-1.   Diagram of the IgG molecule, with the major disulfide bonds connecting the four chains and the carboxy- and amino-terminal ends indicated. The blackened parts at the aminoterminal ends of both H and L chains indicate the parts of variable amino acid composition. The diagram at the bottom shows how the unreacted, closed IgG molecule (left) can bend at the hinge region and open to a full 180°.

Both heavy and light chains, when separated and isolated, tend to form dimers, held together by weak, noncovalent forces. After separation from an intact immunoglobulin, the heavy and light chains from the *same* immunoglobulin will recombine, even when the formation of interchain disulfide bonds is prevented. The antibody specificity of both separated H and L chains persists, although with much weaker affinity for the antigen. Upon spontaneous recombination of the separated H and L chains the strong initial affinity for the antigen reappears. When separated H and L chains of two different immunoglobulins, 1 and 2, are mixed together, the H and L chains of immunoglobulin 1 will preferentially combine with one another, to reconstitute immunoglobulin 1, and so will the H and L chains of immunoglobulin 2, with little or no tendency for the formation of hybrids.

Classes of Human Immunoglobulins

Of the five known classes of human immunoglobulins, IgG is the major immunoglobulin. It occurs in the greatest quantities and is mainly a γ globulin; it is the one immunoglobulin that can pass the placenta. IgM, a macroglobulin, of much higher molecular weight than all the others, is the immunoglobulin type of antibody that is most often, although not exclusively, elicited during the primary antibody response. IgA is a serum immunoglobulin that can also occur as a dimer. In that form it is often encountered as a secretory immunoglobulin; i.e., it is secreted by many tissues into body

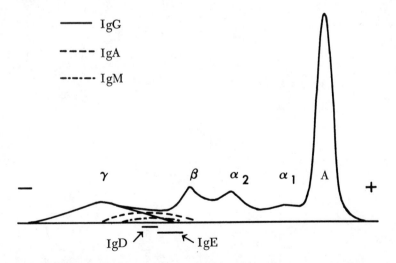

Figure 4-2. Electropherogram of normal human serum, showing the location and approximate quantities of the human immunoglobulins. IgG occupies practically the entire γ region. IgA and IgM are of an intermediary mobility, between γ and β, as are IgD and IgE. For the last two only the location is shown, as their quantities are too small to show on this scale.

Table 4-1
Properties of the Human Immunoglobulins*

	IgG	IgA	IgM	IgD	IgE
Normal adult serum concentration (in gm/100 ml)	1.0–1.4	0.2–0.3	0.04–0.15	0.003	10^{-3}–10^{-5} (average $\approx 10^{-4}$)
Distribution	Intravascular and extracellular fluid	Intravascular and internal secretions	Mainly intravascular	Mainly intravascular	Intravascular and skin, respiratory and GI tracts
Intravascular (%)	45	42	80	75	51
Electrophoretic mobility	γ	Slow β	Between β and γ	Between β and γ	Slow β
Sedimentation coefficient (in Svedbergs)	7 S	7 S (11.5 S for stgA)	19 S	7 S	8 S
Molecular weight	150,000	155,000 (395,000 for S-IgA)	900,000	185,000	187,000
Molecular weight of the H chains (MW of the L chains $\approx$ 23,000)	53,000	55,000	65,000	70,000	71,000
H chains	γ	α	μ	δ	ε
Molecular formula	$\gamma_2\kappa_2, \gamma_2\lambda_2$	$\alpha_2\kappa_2, \alpha_2\lambda_2$ 2 (monomer)	$\mu_{10}\kappa_{10}J, \mu_{10}\lambda_{10}J$	$\delta_2\kappa_2, \delta_2\lambda_2$	$\varepsilon_2\kappa_2, \varepsilon_2\lambda_2$
Valency	2	2	10	2	2
Normal H/L chain ratio	2/1	5/4	3/1	1/6	?
H chain subclasses	IgG1, IgG2, IgG3, IgG4	IgA1, IgA2	IgM1, IgM2	Ja, La	—

Approximate occurrence of the H chain subclasses (%)	75, 15, 7, 3	93, 7	—	85, 15	—
Number of domains per H chain	4	4	5	5	5
Allotypes (all the immunoglobulins with κ L chains have In V allotypes)	Gm	Am	Mm	—	—
Carbohydrate (%)	2.9	5–10	12	13	12
Synthetic rate (gm/day/70 kg)	2.3	1.7	0.1	0.03	2×10^{-4}
Half-life (days)	23	6	5	3	3
Complement binding (via the classic pathway)	+	—	+	—	—
Rheumatoid factor binding	+	—	—	—	—
Placental transport	+	—	—	—	—
Skin sensitization					
Heterologous	+	—	—	—	—
Homologous	—	—	—	—	+
Involvement in opsonization	+	—	+†	—	—
Other important biologic properties	Major Ig in antimicrobial defense; Ig with strongest precipitating capacity	Major Ig (in secretions) in antiviral defense	Major Ig produced in the primary response; Ig with strongest agglutinating capacity	Present on the surface of B lymphocytes of the newborn	Involved in atopic allergy; increased in parasitic infections

*Waldmann, T. A.; Strober, W.; Polmar, S. H.; and Terry, W. D.: IgE levels and metabolism in immune deficiency diseases. In Ishizaka, K., and Dayton, D. H. (eds.): *The Biological Role of the Immunoglobulins E System.* National Institutes of Health, Bethesda, Md., 1972, pp. 247–58.

van Oss, C. J.; Edberg, S. C.; and Bronson, P. M.: The valency of IgM. In Pressman, D.; Tomasi, T. B.; Grossberg, A. L.; and Rose, N. R. (eds.): *Third International Convocation on Immunology.* Karger, Basel, 1973, pp. 60–68.

Nisonoff, A.; Hooper, J. E.; and Spring, S. B.: *The Antibody Molecule.* Academic Press, New York, 1975.

van Oss, C. J.: General physical, chemical and biological properties of the human immunoglobulins. In Greenwalt, T. J., and Steane, E. A. (eds.): *Blood Banking,* Vol. II, *CRC Handbook Series in Clinical Laboratory Science.* CRC Press, Cleveland, 1977.

† In the presence of complement.

fluids other than serum. IgD is an immunoglobulin that occurs in very low quantities. IgE occurs in even smaller quantities, but it nevertheless plays an important role in atopic allergy. Figure 4–2 shows the location and the approximate quantity of the five immunoglobulins in a normal human serum electropherogram. As mentioned above, all five of the immunoglobulins differ in their heavy chains. The heavy chains are designated by the Greek letter corresponding to the Roman letter by which the entire immunoglobulin is characterized: thus, IgG has γ; IgM, μ; IgA, α; IgD, δ; and IgE, ε heavy chains. Any of these immunoglobulins has light chains of only one of two possible types, named κ and λ. Thus, any immunoglobulin, of whatever class its heavy chain may be, will have *either* κ or λ light chains. The nomenclature and principal properties of the five known human immunoglobulins are listed in Table 4–1. As will be seen, most of the major types of immunoglobulins are known to have heavy-chain subgroups.

Immunoglobulins of Other Species

Most mammalian species have immunoglobulins that roughly correspond to human IgG, IgA, and IgM but are not necessarily closely related to these human Ig classes. The species that have been most closely studied have generally been found to have one or two more major groups of immunoglobulins analogous to the above-mentioned three. Horse immunoglobulins contain what is known as a T component, a β globulin that nevertheless appears to be of the IgG type. Guinea pig and mouse immunoglobulins contain an IgG-like group of slow β mobility, which can passively sensitize the skin of an animal of the same species; these homocytotropic antibodies are responsible for anaphylaxis. Immunoglobulins of chickens contain a class that will best precipitate under conditions of much higher salt concentration than is optimal for the immune precipitation reactions with antibodies of other species.

Immunoglobulin G

General and Physicochemical Properties (Table 4-1)

IgG normally occurs in adult human serum in a concentration of 1.0 to 1.4 gm per 100 ml, and thus represents 12 to 18% of the total serum proteins. IgG is also distributed extravascularly (for about 55%). Its rate of synthesis is about 2.3 gm per day (for a weight of 70 kg), and its half-life is approximately 23 days. Its electrophoretic distribution ranges over the entire γ globulin area (Figure 4–2). The fact that this major immunoglobulin is a γ globulin has given rise to the tenacious but erroneous custom of alluding to all immunoglobulins as "γ globulins." The carbohydrate content of IgG is fairly low: 2.9%. The molecular weight of IgG is approximately 150,000, and its sedimentation coefficient is close to 7 S.

Structure

As seen in Figure 4–1 IgG has a symmetric structure: two heavy (H) chains (molecular weight about 53,000 each) are attached to one another by means of two or more disulfide bonds near the middle. Somewhat above the middle of each H chain (toward the aminoterminal ends), a light (L) chain is attached at a point close to its carboxyterminal end, by means of a disulfide bond. The L chains have a molecular weight of about 23,000. The pronounced spread in physicochemical properties and the large variety of different antibody specificities of IgG (and of all the other immunoglobulins) are due to the great variability in amino acid composition among different Ig molecules in the aminoterminal parts of all their chains; this applies to about half of the L chain amino acid sequence and to the first quarter of that of the H chain. The carboxyterminal sections of different Ig molecules are much more constant in their amino acid composition.

Amino acid sequencing studies of immunoglobulins have shown that the polypeptide chains consist of a number of globular "domains," or "homology units," comprising 110 to 120 amino acids. The domains are closed in a loop by a single disulfide bond. When detached from the intact immunoglobulin molecule, different domains do not tend to bind to each other except for pairs of homologous domains (e.g., C_κ and $C_\gamma 1$), which interact strongly with one another. The complement-binding site is associated with $C_\gamma 2$, as is the carbohydrate fraction of the IgG molecule. The sites that specifically bind to antigens are solely found in the V domains. The part of the IgG molecule that attaches to phagocytic cells is situated in the $C_\gamma 3$ domain (Figure 4-3).

At the variable, aminoterminal ends, the antibody specificity is situated. In any one immunoglobulin molecule the amino acid sequences of the two H chains are identical to one another, as are those of the two L chains. Thus IgG is divalent. As indicated above, an IgG molecule consists of two γ-type H chains and *either* two κ-type *or* two λ-type L chains. (λ-type L chains have the subgroup Oz+ and Oz−.) Thus, the two forms under which human IgG can occur are $\gamma_2\kappa_2$ and $\gamma_2\lambda_2$. In any one immunoglobulin molecule even the variable (V) sections of both the H and L chains have many amino acids in the same positions in common, which in all probability serves to enhance their collaborative affinity for the antigen.

Normally IgG is present in the closed conformation (bottom of Figure 4–1, left), but electron microscopic observations have shown that upon reacting with its antigen, both antibody-specific halves can fold out at the hinges as far as 180°. The hinge region is slightly above (in the direction of the aminoterminal ends) the major disulfide bonds that hold the two halves together at the H chains. Upon folding out, the H chain moieties below the hinge remain fairly close together but nevertheless undergo some configurational changes, which cause them to expose regions that hitherto remained hidden and that contain the reactive sites that are capable of fixing

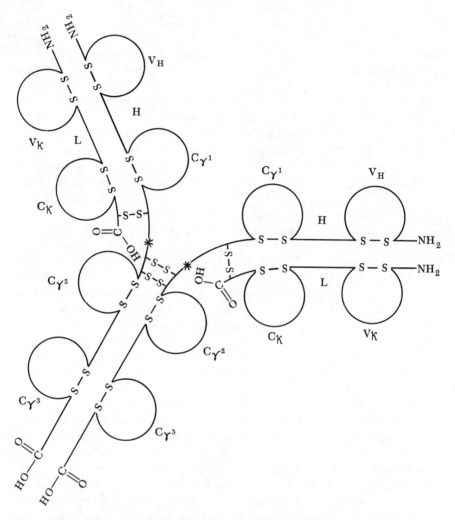

Figure 4-3. The domain structure of human IgGl(κ). The loops formed by the intrachain disulfide bonds are globular units designated as *domains* called V domains in the *variable* and C domains in the *constant* regions. IgG H chains have *three* C domains ($C_\gamma 1$, $C_\gamma 2$, and $C_\gamma 3$); IgA H chains also have *three* C domains, but IgM, IgD, and IgE H chains have *four* C domains. The L chains have one V and one C domain (V_κ and C_κ, and V_λ and C_λ). The hinge regions on the H chains are indicated by asterisks. (From van Oss, C. J.: Diagrammatic representation of the tetrapolypeptide IgCl molecule with light chains of the κ-type. In Greenwalt, T. J., and Steane, E. A. [eds.]: *Blood Banking*, Vol. II [CRC Handbook Series in Clinical Laboratory Science]. © CRC Press, Inc., Cleveland, 1977. Used by permission of CRC Press, Inc.)

complement (Chapter 8) and rheumatoid factor (Chapter 25). These two sites are close together; it has not yet been determined whether or not they are identical.

The ratio of κ to λ L chains in normal IgG is approximately 2/1.

Biologic and Immunologic Properties

IgG is the only human immunoglobulin that passes the placental barrier. After having reacted with its corresponding antigen it will fix complement. IgG and IgM are the only two immunoglobulins that will do so. Only IgG will bind rheumatoid factor. IgG and IgM are opsonizing immunoglobulins (Chapter 10). IgG antibodies are most efficient in the immune precipitation reaction; they are somewhat less efficient as agglutinating and particularly as hemagglutinating antibodies, although it is misleading to give them the label of "incomplete antibodies" (Chapter 6). IgG antibodies are most often, but not exclusively, formed as the secondary or anamnestic response to an antigenic stimulus. Owing to its unique placenta-passing properties, IgG is the most important immunoglobulin that lends protection to the newborn in the first months of life (Figure 4–4). It plays an important role in virtually all the immune defense reactions and is of crucial importance in the defense against microbial invasions. Heterocytotropic antibodies (e.g., human antibodies that can passively sensitize, or bind to, skin cells of animals of other species, such as rabbit and guinea pig) are of the IgG class, as are "blocking antibodies" i.e., antibodies that preferentially tend to combine with allergens and thus prevent their reaction with the homocytotropic IgE-type antibodies (see page 61 and Chapter 18).

IgG Fragments

Although techniques have been devised to decompose IgG molecules into their constituent chains (page 42) techniques of enzymatic digestion, resulting in various fragments that comprise pieces of both H and L chains, are so simple and have become of such general use that they must be briefly discussed.

In the top portion of Figure 4–5 the effect of papain on IgG is shown; it attacks the molecule at the hinge region, just above (toward the amino-terminal ends) the main disulfide bonds holding the two H chains together. This results in three fractions: two monovalent fractions with antibody activity, called Fab; and one fraction that is devoid of antibody activity, called Fc, consisting of two carboxyterminal halves of H chains still joined together by disulfide bonds. The Fab pieces contain all the variable (V) domains of both H and L chains. The Fab pieces can specifically react with the antigen, but, being monovalent, they can no longer cross-link antigen molecules or particles, so that they can neither precipitate nor agglutinate.

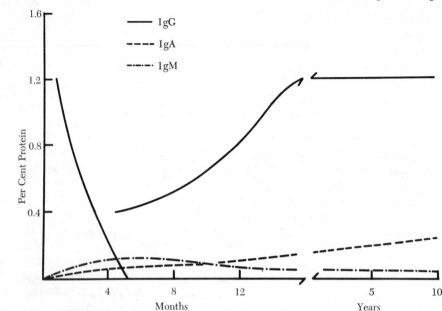

Figure 4-4.   Ontogeny of the three major human immunoglobulins. This diagram shows how the newborn individual is endowed with a normal adult concentration of IgG at birth, which, in the absence of significant new production, quickly decreases (its half-life is about 23 days), to rise again after the age of about four months, when the baby has started the production of significant amounts of IgG-type antibody in response to various antigenic stimuli. Adult IgM levels are reached and surpassed within a few months and decrease to normal adult levels at the age of about a year. IgA increases more gradually; adult levels are reached by the age of five to ten years. (Adapted from Fahey, J. L.: Antibodies and immunoglobulins. II. Normal development and changes in disease. *J.A.M.A.*, **194**: 255–58, 1965.)

The Fc piece, although without antibody specificity, still contains the sites for the fixation of complement and of rheumatoid factor. The Fc piece also contains the opsonizing part of IgG (Chapter 10). The Fc piece consists of the greater part of the constant (C) domain of the H chains.

In the bottom portion of Figure 4–5 the effect of pepsin on IgG is shown: it attacks the molecule *below* (in the direction of the carboxyterminal ends) the main disulfide bonds holding the two H chains together. This results in only one fraction; a bivalent piece with antibody activity, called F(ab′)$_2$, is still joined together by interchain disulfide bonds. The action of pepsin produces virtually complete digestion of the carboxyterminal halves of the H chains. Thus, the F(ab′)$_2$ piece, although it will specifically bind the antigen and can precipitate and agglutinate, has lost its sites for fixing

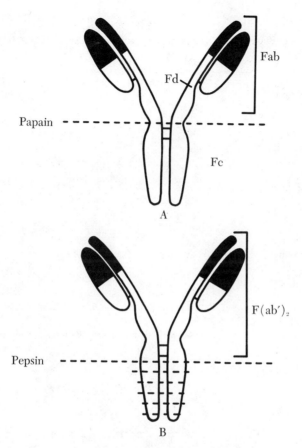

Figure 4-5. Diagrams of the fragments produced by enzymatic splitting of IgG. The top diagram shows the action of papain, leaving monovalent Fab pieces (with antibody activity) and the Fc piece (devoid of antibody activity). By chemical reduction, the Fab piece can be further dissociated into a free L chain and an Fd piece. The bottom diagram shows the action of pepsin, which irretrievably fractionates the Fc pieces but leaves a divalent $F(ab')_2$ piece with antibody activity, which is still capable of immune precipitation and agglutination.

complement and binding rheumatoid factor, as well as its opsonizing capacity.

The separation of H and L chains can only be achieved chemically, by reduction with mercaptoethanol (to break the disulfide bonds), followed by alkylation with iodoacetamide (to block the exposed sulfhydryl groups). By gel filtration in the presence of an organic acid (to keep H and L chains from recombining through van der Waals–London interactions), free H and L chains can then be collected separately.

Table 4-2
PROPERTIES OF THE HUMAN IgG SUBCLASSES*

	IgG1	IgG2	IgG3	IgG4
H chains	γ_1	γ_2	γ_3	γ_4
Approximate occurrence in serum (%)	70	20	7	≈ 3 (rather variable)
Half-life (days)	20	24	7	23
Electrophoretic mobility	Slow γ	Fast γ	γ	Fast γ
Complement binding	+ +	+	+ + + +	−
Rheumatoid-factor binding	+	+	±	+
Reaction with staphylococcal protein A	+	+	−	+
Involvement in opsonization	+	−†	+	−
Placental transport	+	±	+	+
Cytophilic properties				
Heterologous skin sensitization	+	−	+	+
Binding to macrophages and monocytes	+	−	+	−
Gm groups	1, 2, 4, 17, 22	23	5, 6, 13, 14, 15, 16, 21	−
Papain digestibility	Most readily	Only after reduction with mercapto-ethanol	Readily	After reduction with cysteine
Aggregation	+ (Fab only)	+ (Fab only)	+ + + (Both Fab and Fc)	+ (Both Fab and Fc)
Location of the interchain disulfide bonds				
Other chemical properties			γ_3 chains have an extended hinge region and a MW $> 60,000$; the complete IgG3 molecule has a MW $\approx 200,000$	
Other important biologic properties		Appears early in immunization; antiteichoic, antidextran, and anti-levan antibodies tend to be of this class		

Aggregation of IgG

By physicochemical means, part, but not all, of human IgG can be polymerized or "aggregated" to higher-molecular-weight complexes. These complexes can vary in molecular weight from 320,000 (sedimentation coefficient = 10 S) for dimers, to one to several million (sedimentation coefficients 20 to 40 S). Mild treatment of IgG, such as the alcohol precipitation process used in isolating it from human serum, results in the formation of 10 S IgG dimers of about 10 to 15% of the total IgG molecules. Heating IgG solutions at 63° C for ten minutes or more results in the formation of 20 to 40 S complexes. IgG thus aggregated has some of the same properties as untreated IgG when the latter is specifically combined with antigen; aggregated IgG fixes complement and combines with rheumatoid factor without the necessity for being bound to antigen. Thus, upon aggregation, the same configurational changes apparently occur, as with native IgG when it binds with antigen: the same hitherto secluded regions in the Fc part become exposed and contain the reactive sites for complement fixation and rhematoid-factor binding.

Only about 20% of all human IgG molecules are prone to aggregation. Once all the heat-aggregatable IgG has been removed from a given preparation, further heating (at 63° C) will not aggregate more IgG. All four subclasses of IgG contain aggregatable molecules; molecules of the IgG3 subclass aggregate quite strongly. Molecules of the IgG1 and IgG2 subclass aggregate solely through inter-Fab links, and IgG3 and IgG4 also seem to be able to attach through their Fc sections (Table 4–2).

IgG Subclasses

There are four subgroups of IgG: IgG1, IgG2, IgG3, and IgG4. Respectively they represent about 70, 20, 7, and 3% of normal human IgG. The proportion of IgG4 is fairly variable from person to person. IgG2 does not occur as a heterocytotropic antibody (see page 49). IgG3 has a shorter half-life than the other three subclasses; it has the strongest tendency to aggregate and possibly for that reason is the one that fixes complement most strongly. IgG3 also has a much bigger γ chain than the other subclasses, due to its extended hinge region (Table 4–2). When present in pathologically large amounts, IgG3 tends to give rise to clinically important hyperviscosity of the

* Kunkel, H. G., and Yount, W. J.: Heavy-chain subgroups of γG and γA globulins. In Merler, E. (ed.): *Immunoglobulins*. National Academy of Science, Washington, D.C., 1970, p. 137.
Stanworth, D. R., and Turner, M. W.: Immunochemical analysis of immunoglobulins and their subunits. In Weir, D. M. (ed.): *Handbook of Experimental Immunology*, Vol. 1. Blackwell, Oxford, 1973, 10.1.
Michaelsen, T. E., and Natvig, J. N.: Unusual molecular properties of human IgG, proteins due to an extended hinge region. *J. Biol. Chem.*, **249**; 2778, 1974.
van Oss, C. J.: General physical, chemical and biological properties of the four subclasses of human immunoglobulin G. In Greenwalt, T. J., and Steane, E. A. (eds.): *Blood Banking*, Vol. 11. CRC Handbook Series in Clinical Laboratory Science, CRC Press, Cleveland, 1977.
† IgG2 can be involved in opsonization by the prior fixation of complement.

serum. The differences between the four IgG subgroups are, of course, situated on the γ chains. Different sets of the various allotypic γ chain Gm groups (see below) are associated with each of the first three IgG subclasses.

The molecules of the four IgG subgroups differ in the number and/or in the location of their major disulfide bonds, and they thus also differ somewhat in their physicochemical properties, which makes possible their separation from one another, e.g., by gel electrophoresis. The optimal conditions for papain digestion of the four IgGs also vary according to each subgroup. The mode of aggregation also differs. Antibodies to certain antigens sometimes tend to be of a particular IgG subgroup. For instance, antiteichoic acid and antidextran antibodies of the IgG type tend to be IgG2.

IgG Allotypes

"Allotypes," a term initially used only for rabbit immunoglobulins, is now generally applied to genetically determined protein polymorphisms in other species.

L Chain Allotypes.   The light-chain allotypes are common to all immunoglobulins: they will be discussed here, but it must be clear that everything here stated on this subject also applies to light chains of all other Ig classes. The Km groups, formerly called In V groups, are solely associated with the κ-type L chains. The κ chains in Km(3) individuals have the amino acid valine in position 191, whereas the κ chains of Km(1,2) individuals have leucine in that position. Both Oz + and Oz − λ chains have serine in position 190. Although the Oz groups were initially thought to be allotypes, it is now established that λ chains of both types occur together in any one individual.

Gm Groups.   These are allotypic configurations associated with the γ chains of the first three IgG subgroups (Table 4–2).

The Gm groups are associated with the IgG subgroups in the following way: IgG1 can contain Gm (1), (2), (3), (4), (22), and (17); IgG2 can contain Gm (23); IgG3 can contain Gm (5), (6), (11), (13), (14), (15), (16), and (21); IgG4 has no Gm group activity. The Gm groups are of some anthropologic importance; e.g., Gm (3), Gm (21), and Gm (22) are rarely found among negroid populations. These allotypes are determined immunologically, with the help of typing antisera of human origin, generally rheumatoid-factor-containing sera.

Immunoglobulin A

General and Physicochemical Properties

IgA normally occurs in adult human serum in a concentration of 0.2 to 0.3 gm per 100 ml and thus represents 2.4 to 3.9% of the total serum proteins.

Its rate of synthesis is about 1.7 gm per day (for a body weight of 70 kg), and its half-life is about six days. IgA occurs for about 58% extravascularly. Electrophoretically it is a slow β globulin (Figure 4–2). Its carbohydrate content is 5 to 10%. Most of the serum IgA molecules occur as monomers, but a small proportion of them exist as dimers, trimers, and tetramers (in amounts that decrease with increasing molecular weight). The molecular weight of monomeric IgA is approximately 155,000, and its sedimentation coefficient is 7 S. The molecular weight of its H (α) chains is about 55,000. The approximate sedimentation coefficients of dimers, trimers, and tetramers are, respectively, 10.5 S, 13 S, and 16 to 17 S. These polymers can be dissociated into monomers by reduction with mercaptoethanol. It has not yet been established with certainty whether J chains (see also the section on secretory IgA, below) are involved in the linkage of these polymers (Tables 4–1 and 4–3).

Table 4-3
PROPERTIES OF HUMAN IMMUNOGLOBULIN A AND SECRETORY IMMUNOGLOBULIN A*

	IgA1	IgA2	sIgA
Nomenclature of the H chains	α_1	α_2	Both IgA1 and IgA2 can form SIgA
Approximate occurrence in serum (%)	85	14	1
Major Am groups	...	A2m(1) A2m(2)	...
Frequency among Caucasians (%)		98 2	
Location of the interchain disulfide bonds	*(diagram)*	*(diagram)*	*(diagram)* SIgA occurs as dimers of both α_1 and α_2 monomers, linked with a J chain and provided with a secretory component molecule
Molecular weight	154,000†	158,000†	> 395,000; MW of J chain > 15,000; MW of secretory component > 74,000‡
Molecular weight of H chains	54,000	56,000	
Electrophoretic mobility	β_2	β_1	
Other important biologic properties	...	...	Main secretory Ig; important in antiviral defense in the upper respiratory tract

* Mestecky, J., and Lawton, A. R. (eds.): *The Immunoglobulin A System.* Plenum Press, New York, 1973.
van Oss, C. J.: General physical, chemical and biological properties of the subclasses of human immunoglobulin A and of secretory immunoglobulin A. In Greenwalt, T. J., and Steane, E. A. (eds.): *Blood Banking,* Vol. II. *CRC Handbook Series in Clinical Laboratory Science.* CRC Press, Cleveland, 1977.
† May also occur in small amounts in serum as dimers or higher polymers.
‡ Secretory component also appears to be associated with IgM, in its secretory form.

Apart from its presence as circulating serum immunoglobulin, IgA occurs as the principal secretory, or exocrine, immunoglobulin (see below). Secretory IgA, however, occurs as a dimer that cannot be dissociated into the monomers by simple reduction.

The structure of monomeric IgA is similar to that of IgG (Figure 4–1); monomeric IgA is also bivalent. It can occur in the form of $\alpha_2\kappa_2$ and $\alpha_2\lambda_2$. As with IgG, the action of papain on IgA produces Fab pieces, but (unlike IgG) no intact Fc piece. IgA H chains have three C domains. The J chain is attached to $C_\alpha 3$ and the interchain disulfide bonds of IgA monomers connect between $C_\alpha 2$ domains. The ratio of κ to λ chains in normal human IgA is approximately 5/4. Two main subclasses of human IgA; IgA1 and IgA2; are present in a ratio of about 85/14. Analogous to the Gm allotypes of IgG, there are Am allotypes of IgA. In the A2m(1) variety of IgA2 the L-H disulfide bonds are lacking.

Biologic and Immunologic Properties

IgA does not pass the placenta, nor does it fix complement or rheumatoid factor. IgA seems to play no role in opsonization, but it does function in immune precipitation and agglutination. IgA is especially important in the organism's defense against viral infections. Its mechanism may be mainly based on the power of specific antibodies of the IgA type to coat viruses and thus to prevent them from penetrating the target cells. The nonopsonizing and noncomplement-binding properties of IgA may be of advantage in this function of preventing cell penetration by viruses. The presence of IgA seems to play no role in allergic reactions. The role of secretory IgA is discussed below.

Secretory IgA

Secretory or exocrine IgA (sIgA) is the principal immunoglobulin found in colostrum, saliva, tears, and bronchial, gastrointestinal, and nasal secretions. In this form IgA is dimeric and the two constituents monomers, which are bound together by disulfide bonds through the intermediate of a special "J" chain, are, in addition, combined with a secretory "piece," or "T" component, which has a molecular weight of 74,000. The J chain has a molecular weight of about 15,000. The total molecular weight of sIgA is thus around 305,000, and its sedimentation coefficient is about 11.5 S (Figure 4–6). The T component may be involved in facilitating the transport of IgA. It lends to IgA a pronounced resistance to enzymatic degradation, which is of undoubted advantage to an immunoglobulin that has to retain its activity in external secretions that are rich in proteolytic enzymes. sIgA is synthesized locally in oral, nasal, and gastrointestinal tract tissues in response to local antigenic stimuli. sIgA plays an important role in the defense against viral infections, such as by influenza virus, poliovirus, adenovirus, and rhinovirus (Chapter 15).

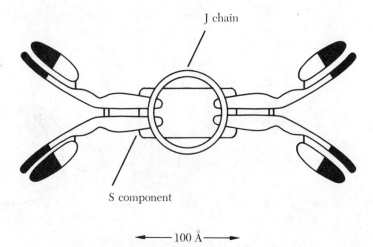

J chain

S component

←—— 100 Å ——→

Figure 4-6. Diagram of secretory IgA. The two parts of the dimeric molecule are held together by the J chain (for schematic reasons drawn here as a circular band). (See also Figure 4-7.) The T (or transport) component (or secretory piece) is also schematically indicated.

Immunoglobulin M

General and Physicochemical Properties

IgM normally occurs in adult human serum in a concentration of 0.04 to 0.15 gm per 100 ml and thus represents 0.5 to 1.9% of the total serum proteins. Hardly any IgM is found extravascularly. Its rate of synthesis is about 0.1 gm per day (for a weight of 70 kg), and its half-life is about five days. Electrophoretically it migrates between γ and β globulin (Figure 4–2). Its carbohydrate content is 12%. IgM has a molecular weight of about 900,000 and a sedimentation coefficient of 19 S; a small proportion occurs as dimers and an even smaller proportion as trimers, with sedimentation coefficient of, respectively, 29 S and 38 S. A 7 S variety of IgM has been found in a number of pathologic cases; in very small amounts it also occurs in normal serum (Table 4–1).

An important proportion of human IgM belongs to the class of euglobulins, i.e., globulins that are insoluble at low salt concentrations, at pHs near their isoelectric point (in the case of IgM at pH 5.5 to 6.0).

Structure

As seen in Figure 4–7, IgM has the shape of a star with five identical branches; each is roughly the shape of one entire IgG molecule, although slightly thicker and somewhat shorter.

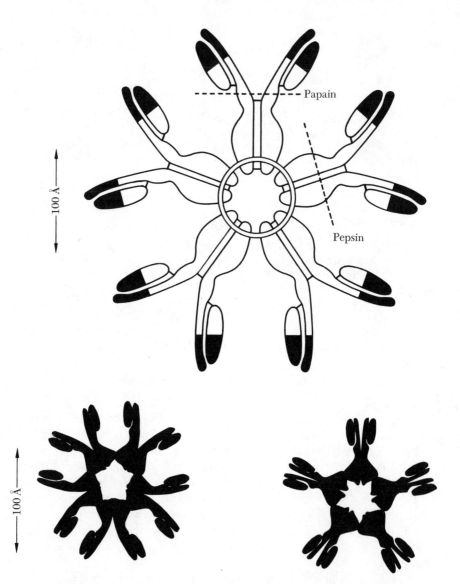

Figure 4-7. Diagram of the IgM molecule, with an indication of the loci of enzymatic attack by papain and pepsin. In the bottom diagrams IgM is shown in the closed position (left) and in the maximally open position (right). It is clear that, if IgM is largely planar, its branches cannot open nearly as wide as those of IgG (see Figure 4-1). The J chain, which aids in connecting the five subunits, is also (for schematic reasons) drawn as a circular band (see Figure 4-6).

The ratio of κ to λ chains in normal human IgM is approximately 3/1. There are two main subclasses of human IgM: IgM1 and IgM2. IgM is composed of 10 H chains of the μ variety, ten L chains, and one J chain; it thus occurs in the form of $\mu_{10}\kappa_{10}$ J and $\mu_{10}\lambda_{10}$ J (see below). Its starfish-like shape has become apparent from electron microscopic observations. When tested with antigens of fairly low molecular weight (M < 3000), the valency of antibodies of the IgM class can be shown to be 10. With antigens of larger molecular weight, however, the valency appears to be less than 10. This discrepancy is in all probability due to steric hindrance: there is reason to suppose that IgM has a planar configuration and that its ten branches thus cannot open to more than 36° in contrast to the 180° of which IgG is capable (compare Figures 4–1 and 4–7). Any large antigen bound to one antibody-active site of an IgM molecule will, therefore, tend to block at least one other neighboring antibody-active site, which produces the semblance of a lower valency (frequently 5). Antigen-binding studies with single fragments of IgM-type antibodies confirm the intrinsic decavalency of IgM. The heavy (μ) chains have a molecular weight of approximately 65,000. J chains have been found in IgM as well as in sIgA (see above) with the function in IgM of solidifying the C terminal ends of the 10 μ chains, to tighten them into a pentagonal structure. The J chain is attached to the $C_\mu 4$ domain of IgM. The interchain disulfide bonds of IgM monomers connect between $C_\mu 3$ domains. Secretory component (see above, under IgA) also appears to be associated with IgM in its secretory form; secretory component will spontaneously bind to pentameric IgM.

Biologic and Immunologic Properties

IgM does not pass the placenta. It does fix complement, but not rheumatoid factor—contrary to IgG, which fixes both (see above). IgM, like IgG, is an opsonizing immunoglobulin (Chapter 8). IgM-type antibodies are most efficient in agglutination; they are somewhat less efficient in the immune precipitation reaction. IgM-type antibodies are most often formed in the primary response to an antigenic stimulus. IgM-like antibodies are also the sole or the predominant antibodies among the more primitive vertebrates (Chapter 2).

Antibodies to polysaccharides tend to be predominantly of the IgM type, as is also the case with natural antibodies to blood group antigens. IgM-type antibodies play an important role in the defense against bacterial infections. Cold agglutinins tend to be of the IgM type; κ-type light chains are predominant in them.

Newborn babies possess only maternal IgG, acquired via the placenta. Inasmuch as their IgM level normally develops gradually, the demonstration of elevated IgM levels in infants is a strong indication of congenital or perinatal infection.

Rheumatoid Factor

Rheumatoid factor is a human immunoglobulin mainly, but not exclusively, of the IgM class. IgG- and IgA-type rheumatoid factors also occur in small amounts. Rheumatoid factor reacts with human IgG that either is aggregated or has been altered by reaction with an antigen. It occurs often among patients with rheumatoid arthritis and in certain other individuals (Chapter 25). Rheumatoid factor tends to form complexes of a sedimentation coefficient of 22 S when reacted with IgG. On occasion such 22 S complexes can be demonstrated to occur *in vivo* among rheumatoid arthritis patients. IgG easily absorbs onto polystyrene latex particles and becomes partly aggregated in the process; rheumatoid factor thus will agglutinate IgG-coated latex particles. This effect is used in the latex fixation test for the determination of the presence of rheumatoid factor in patient sera.

IgM Fragments

In a manner analogous to that used with IgG, IgM can be enzymatically fragmented with the help of papain as well as with pepsin (Figure 4–7). Papain attacks the molecule just above the aminoterminal disulfide bonds that hold the two H chains together on each of the five branches, yielding ten monovalent Fabμ pieces and a large Fcμ piece (which is devoid of antibody activity). Mild pepsin treatment yields bivalent F(ab′)$_2$μ pieces, but, as with IgG, no Fc piece. More prolonged pepsin treatment yields monovalent pieces equivalent to Fabμ. Isolated H and L chains can be obtained chemically in the same way as with IgG (pages 49–51).

Immunoglobulin D

IgD as a distinct class of human immunoglobulins was first discovered as a myeloma protein (Chapter 17). With the help of antisera made against that unique protein, it could be determined that immunoglobulins of that class are also present in normal adult human serum in rather small amounts (approximately 3 mg/100 ml). Its rate of synthesis is about 30 mg per day (for a human of 70 kg), and its half-life is approximately three days. IgD occurs principally (75%) intravascularly. Electrophoretically it migrates between γ and β globulin (Figure 4–2). The molecular weight of IgD is approximately 187,000, and its sedimentation coefficient is about 7 S.

The structure of IgD is similar to that of IgG (Figures 4–1 and 4–3), except that the δ chains have a higher molecular mass (71,000 daltons). The carbohydrate content of IgD is about 12%. The two δ chains are linked together by only one disulfide bond. There appear to be two IgD subclasses, Ja and La (Table 4–1). IgD H chains have four C domains.

The percentage of IgD-bearing B lymphocytes in the blood of newborn infants is extraordinarily high. Often the same lymphocytes that carry IgD also have IgM on the surface. IgD also occurs on the lymphocyte surface in a number of lymphoproliferative disorders. It has been speculated that IgD might be phylogenetically even more primordial than IgM, but no definitive explanation for the biologic function of IgD has as yet been proposed (Chapter 2).

Immunoglobulin E

IgE normally occurs in adult human serum in a concentration of 10 μg to 1 mg (average 100 μg) per 100 ml and thus represents up to 0.014% of the total serum protein. Electrophoretically IgE migrates as a slow β globulin. Its half-life is about three days and its carbohydrate content about 12%. The molecular weight of IgE is about 187,000 and that of its H (ε) chains approximately 71,000. IgE was discovered in reagin-rich sera from patients with atopic allergies and was characterized as a new immunoglobulin, the H chains of which are distinct from γ, α, μ, and δ chains. IgE H chains have four C domains.

IgE-type immunoglobulins comprise the reaginic antibodies. IgE does not pass the placenta, nor does it fix complement or rheumatoid factor. IgE antibodies give Prausnitz-Küstner reactions (Chapter 11). They are *homocytotropic*; i.e., they sensitize human mast cells and leukocytes (in particular basophils) and cause a release of histamine. IgE antibodies lose their sensitizing ability, but not their antibody activity, after heating at 56° C. Some of the IgE antibodies are in all probability formed locally in the respiratory and gastrointestinal tracts; they play a major role in the allergic diseases of these organs. In allergic individuals the serum IgE levels may be increased ten times or more. IgE may function in the organism's defense against infection, especially parasitic (Chapter 16).

Homologous Globulins

Urinary Immunoglobulin Fragments

In the urine of normal subjects immunoglobulin fragments of a molecular weight from 10,000 to 35,000 occur in small amounts. After drastic concentration of the urinary proteins, the antibody activity as well as the H and L chain classes of these fragments can be determined.

Some patients with multiple myeloma or Waldenström's macroglobulinemia (Chapter 17) produce fairly large quantities of L chains, which generally are present in the serum as dimers and which, owing to their relatively low molecular weight (approximately 42,000), are also found in urine. These proteins are called, after their discoverer, Bence Jones proteins. Fragments of the H chains of patient monoclonal proteins are also generally present in the urine in low concentrations. In some cases of monoclonal hyperimmunoglobulinemias, excess amounts of only H chains are produced and find their way into the urine. These cases are called H chain disease, or, more precisely, γ chain, α chain, or μ chain disease (Chapter 17). Even in the nephrotic syndrome and other nephropathies the occurrence of intact immunoglobulins is extremely rare. Indeed, urinary proteins of any origin seldom have a molecular weight greater than 70,000.

β_2 Microglobulin

A small globulin, first isolated from urine by Berggård and Bearn in 1968, is present in small amounts in normal serum, urine, and cerebrospinal fluid and is named β_2 microglobulin (β_2m). It has an amino acid sequence that shows a significant degree of similarity with the amino acid sequence of all three constant domains of IgG1. The similarities in amino acid sequence between β_2m and the IgG C-domains are about half as frequent as the similarities the three domains have with one another. Thus, although an undeniable homology exists between β_2m and the constant immunoglobulin domains, anti-β_2m antisera do not cross-react with immunoglobulin C domains.

A strong association exists between β_2m and molecules of the major histocompatibility (HLA) antigens on the lymphocyte membrane. Immunochemical evidence suggests that the antigenic determinants of β_2m and HLA comprise two chains of the total histocompatibility antigen.

β_2m is found on the outer membranes of platelets, polymorphonuclear granulocytes and lymphocytes. T lymphocytes contain more than B lymphocytes. Lymphocytes, cultured in vitro, synthesize β_2m. Its concentration in human serum and urine is elevated among patients with various neoplasms (Chapter 24) and nephropathies (Chapter 19). The molecular weight of β_2m is 11,600 (about the size of a single immunoglobulin domain); it is a rather symmetrically shaped globular polypeptide with no free sulfhydryl groups and no carbohydrate.

Amyloid Proteins

Although in all probability the majority of the protein constituents of amyloid (extracellular deposition of insoluble protein, accompanying a number of neoplastic and other diseases) are not related to immunoglobulins, in a number of cases the presence of proteins strongly akin to immunoglobulin L chains in amyloid deposits has been reported (Chapter 17).

Ontogeny of the Immunoglobulins

Although the human fetus starts to synthesize immunoglobulins at about the twentieth week of gestation, this immunoglobulin production is, in the absence of antenatal infection (see discussion of IgM), negligible in quantity. The newborn depends entirely on its protection against infections during the early postnatal period on his stock of maternal IgG, received through the placenta. Thus, at birth he starts out endowed with a normal, adult level of IgG and exceedingly small amounts of the other immunoglobulins (Figure 4–4). The initial stock of maternal IgG is, however, not renewable and, owing to the normal catabolism of IgG (with a half-life of 23 days), in a few months little of it is left. At about two months of age, the lowest level of immunoglobulin is reached. However, by then the infant has been exposed to a variety of antigenic stimuli and has responded with a brisk synthesis of mainly IgM and IgG antibodies. At the age of four months the infant's IgM concentration reaches and often even surpasses adult levels and the concentration of his own IgG attains about one-third the normal adult level, which he then gradually attains by the age of five years. By that age his IgM concentration has leveled off to normal. IgA levels keep increasing at a slower rate, and normal concentrations are attained by adulthood (Figure 4–4).

Bibliography

Berggård, I., and Bearn, A. G.: Isolation and properties of a low molecular weight β_2-globulin occurring in human biological fluids. *J. Biol. Chem.*, **243**:4095–4103, 1968.

Chesebro, B.; Bloth, B.; and Svehag, S. E.: Ultrastructure of normal and pathological IgM immunoglobulins. *J. Exp. Med.*, **127**:399–400, 1968.

Dorrington, K. J., and Mihaesco, C.: Subunit structure of human γM-globulins. *Immunochemistry*, **7**:651–60, 1970.

Edberg, S. C.; Bronson, P. M.; and van Oss, C. J.: The valency of IgM and IgG rabbit anti-dextran antibody as a function of the size of the dextran molecule. *Immunochemistry*, **9**:273–88, 1972.

Edelman, G. M.: The covalent structure of a human γG immunoglobulin. XI. Functional implications, *Biochemistry*, **9**:3197–3204, 1970.

Fahey, J. L.: Antibodies and immunoglobulins. I. Structure and function. *J.A.M.A.*, **194**:71–74, 1965. II. Normal development and changes in disease. *Ibid.*, **194**:255–58, 1965.

Frangione, B.; Milstein, C.; and Pink, J. R. L.: Structural studies of immunoglobulin G. *Nature*, **221**:145–48, 1969.

Gally, J. A.: Structure of immunoglobulins. In Sela, M. (ed.): *The Antigens*, Vol. 1. Academic Press, New York, 1973, pp. 161–298.

Greenwalt, T. J.; van Oss, C. J.; and Steane, E. A.: Use of a tannic acid-caffeine concentration procedure for detecting urinary proteins and hemagglutinins. *Am. J. Clin. Pathol.*, **49**:472–80, 1968.

Grey, H. M.; Abel, C. A.; Yount, W. J.; and Kunkel, H. G.: A subclass of human γA-globulins (γA2) which lacks the disulfide bonds linking heavy and light chains. *J. Exp. Med.*, **128**:1223–36, 1968.

Grubb, R.: *The Genetic Markers of Human Immunoglobulins.* Springer Verlag, Inc., New York, 1970.

Ishizaka, K., and Dayton, D. H.: *The Biological Role of the Immunoglobulin E System.* U.S. Dept. of H.E.W., N.I.H. Bethesda, Md., 1973.

Mestecky, J., and Lawton, A. R.: *The Immunoglobulin A System.* Plenum Press, New York, 1973.

Mestecky, J.; Zikan, J.; and Butler, W. T.: Immunoglobulin M and secretory immunoglobulin A: presence of a common polypeptide chain different from light chains. *Science*, **171**:1163–65, 1971.

Nisonoff, A.; Hopper, J. E.; and Spring, S. B.: *The Antibody Molecule.* Academic Press, New York, 1975.

Poulik, M. D.: β_2-Microglobulin. In Putnam, F. W. (ed.): *The Plasma Proteins,* Vol. I. Academic Press, New York, 1975, pp. 433–54.

Tomasi, T. B.: *The Immune System of Secretions.* Prentice-Hall, Englewood Cliffs, N.J., 1976.

van Oss, C. J.; Hawking, M. K.; and Bronson, P. M.: A comparison between immunochemical and physical chemical analyses of the molecular size of urinary proteins. *Biochem. Med.*, **7**:466–72, 1973.

5

Antigen-Antibody Interactions

CAREL J. VAN OSS AND ALLAN L. GROSSBERG

Introduction and Definitions

The definition of antigens is possible only in terms of the antibodies they elicit upon their introduction into an appropriate host. Conversely, the definition of antibodies is possible only in terms of antigens (Chapter 1). Notwithstanding the circularity of these basic definitions, antigens can be characterized with great precision. Antibodies can also be precisely defined as a class of specialized proteins, the immunoglobulins, which were described in detail in Chapter 4. As a general rule, an antigen consists of material that is foreign to the host into which it is introduced.

An antigen when introduced into an appropriate host will give rise to the formation of antibodies that will specifically react with that antigen. This specificity is quite pronounced. When an antigen under a given set of circumstances induces the formation of antibodies, it is said to be immunogenic. Compounds that are not directly able to elicit the formation of antibodies to themselves but that react with antibodies exactly like antigens are called haptens.

Antigens

Apart from the fact that antigens generally have to be foreign to the host into which they are introduced, they can have a variety of different properties. Physically, they tend to be large molecules, with molecular weights of 10,000 or higher. However, some nanopeptides, with a molecular weight of approximately 1000, have been shown to be antigenic. Chemically, antigens may belong to the classes of proteins or polysaccharides or consist of combinations between these two or combinations of either of these with other chemical substances. For instance, glycoproteins, lipoproteins, lipopolysaccharides, and nucleoproteins can all be antigens. Several other types of biopolymers can be antigens, notably the teichoic acids. Pure lipids by themselves are normally not antigens, nor are pure nucleic acids, although both of these substances can, in combination with proteins or polysaccharides, be antigens. Although there is a limit of molecular weight below which biopolymers seldom are antigens, there is no upper limit in size. Antigens can be insoluble particles or parts of insoluble particles, and they frequently consist of a variety of chemically different components. In such cases, antigens can have many different antigenic aspects on one and the same particle or even on one and the same molecule; these then are called antigenic determinants (Chapter 1).

Antigenic Determinants

An antigenic determinant is that minimal chemical subunit or entity of a macromolecule or particle that can give rise to the formation of a specific antibody. Soluble as well as particulate antigens can have many antigenic determinants. They can be all different or all identical or mixed.

On soluble macromolecules as well as on insoluble particles, the most readily available antigenic determinants tend to be those that are closest to the outer surface of the molecule or particle. In complex macromolecules such as proteins, certain amino acids or groups of amino acids are more antigenically potent, such as aromatic or apolar amino acids. Great variability in amino acid composition also tends to give rise to greater antigenic potency than monotonous series of the same amino acid. On large antigenic molecules or particles many different antigenic determinants can occur so that, upon introduction into an appropriate host, they can give rise to the formation of a variety of antibodies of different specificities that can all react with them.

Haptens

Many low-molecular-weight chemical compounds have the ability to be haptens. One way in which antibodies can be elicited to haptens is by coupling such haptens to either a carrier molecule or a carrier particle and then introducing it into the appropriate host (Chapter 7). When a soluble macromolecule is used as a carrier, it is essential that that macromolecule be immunogenic in the animal in question. When insoluble particles (such as polymethylmethacrylate or polystyrene latex particles) are used as carriers for the introduction of the hapten into the animal, it is not essential that the particles be antigens to the animal. Antibodies elicited to haptens in the above-described fashion will, once formed, specifically react with the single haptens even in the absence of carrier molecules or particles.

Antibodies

All antibodies are immunoglobulins. They are found among the β and γ globulins of serum; they have been described in detail in Chapter 4. It suffices here to say that most human immunoglobulins are divalent and one is decivalent.

Certain antigens, particularly proteins, and some haptens when coupled to protein carriers can give rise to another kind of immune reaction when introduced into an animal, i.e., a cellular reaction, associated with delayed hypersensitivity, in which circulating soluble antibodies play no apparent role (Chapter 11).

Antigen-Antibody Bonds

Nature of Antigen-Antibody Bonds

Antigen-antibody bonds, highly specific though they are, are relatively weak. Covalent bonds play no role in antigen-antibody interactions. Only the lower-energy noncovalent bonds are involved. Of the weaker types of

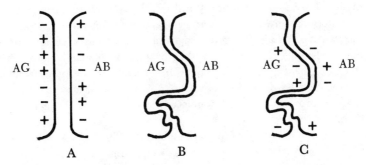

Figure 5-1. Schematic presentation of the mechanisms of antigen-antibody interactions. *A.* Case of complementarity of positively and negatively charged groups on part of the antigen (*AG*) and antibody (*AB*) molecules, resulting in Coulombic attraction. *B.* Case of complementarity of shape on part of the *AG* and *AB* molecules, permitting them to approach one another sufficiently closely to allow the short-range van der Waals–London dispersion forces to exert their attractive influence. *C.* Case of combined electrostic and spatial complementarity, resulting in both Coulombic and van der Waals–London attractions.

bonds two major ones are principally involved in antigen-antibody binding: electrostatic or Coulombic forces, on the one hand, and dispersion forces of the van der Waals–London type, on the other. Hydrogen bonds have also been implicated but it is unlikely that they often play a major role in antigen-antibody interactions. The "lock-and-key" hypothesis of Paul Ehrlich still seems, in the light of modern knowledge about antigen-antibody interactions, to describe best the most likely actual state of events. As the illustrations in Figure 5–1 show, both the electrostatic or Coulombic type of bond and the dispersion or van der Waals–London type of bond, as well as the combinations of these two types, are still best illustrated with the "lock-and-key" model of best fit.

Coulombic Type of Bonds.   These electrostatic bonds originate in the attraction between positively and negatively charged groups on the antigen and antibody molecules (Figure 5–1 *A*). The close complementarity between a positive and negative alternating series of a certain pattern on the antigen and an oppositely charged series on the antibody will obviously permit an enhanced attraction between molecules, the force (F') of which is described by the equation of Coulomb:

$$F' = \frac{Q^+ Q^-}{\varepsilon d^2} \tag{1}$$

(Q^+ and Q^- are, respectively, the positive and the negative charges in electro-static units, ε the dielectric constant of the medium, which is approximately 80 for water, and d the distance between the centers of the charged sites.)

Dispersion Forces or van der Waals–London Attraction.   Of all the weak interactions between atoms and molecules of the van der Waals type, only the van der Waals–London variety of interactions occurring between all atoms and molecules when they are brought sufficiently close together, and which are the only ones that are additive (i.e., they become stronger the bigger the molecules or particles that are being brought close together), are of particular importance in the nonelectrostatic variety of antigen-antibody interaction.

The dispersion forces are due to the universally occurring interactions between the charge fluctuation from the electron movement in one molecule and the fluctuating charge distribution of another molecule, causing the attraction between two molecules (even if neither has a permanent dipole moment). The order of magnitude of this universal attractive force (F'') between atoms or small molecules is

$$F'' = \frac{C}{d^7} \tag{2}$$

(C is a constant and d the distance between the atoms or molecules.) These forces can obviously be of importance only over extremely short distances.

But owing to the universal occurrence and the additivity of these interactions between large molecules or particles, the interacting sites of which are assumed to be reasonably flat and parallel, the free energies of attraction become, upon integration

$$\Delta F = \frac{-A}{12\pi d^2} \tag{3}$$

where A is the Hamaker constant. For antigens (subscript 1) and antibodies (subscript 2), hypothetically interacting in vacuo, $A_{12} \approx 5 \times 10^{-13}$ ergs, while the value for ΔF^{vac} would be of the order of -100 ergs/cm^2, which is about five times higher than the strongest antigen-antibody binding energies ΔF^{eq} measured by equilibrium methods (see below).

For antigens and antibodies interacting in the early, hydrated stage, in an aqueous medium, with interstitial water still present between antigenic determinant and antibody-active site, values for the applicable Hamaker constant A_{132} (3 being the subscript for water) of less than 10^{-14} ergs are found. The corresponding value for ΔF^{aq} varies between -0.01 and -1 erg/cm^2, which is generally at least an order of magnitude smaller than the binding energies ΔF^{eq} measured by equilibrium methods (see below). ΔF^{aq} reflects the free-energy change involved in the initial rapid encounter between antigenic determinants and antibody-active sites that still are wholly separated by water. As time progresses, water (which has an elevated dielectric constant) is gradually expelled from between the antigenic determinants and the antibody-active sites, thus strengthening the bonds between them. As A_{132} increases and tends toward (but never reaches) A_{12}, and as the distance d between the sites decreases and approaches a minimum, the total free-energy change strongly increases (ΔF^{aq} tends toward, but never reaches, ΔF^{vac}). The values for ΔF^{aq} and ΔF^{vac} can be derived from interfacial free-energy determinations on the surfaces of antigens and antibodies by means of contact angle measurements (see Chapter 10).

The fact that the total free-energy change ΔF^{eq} found by equilibrium methods, see equation (6), below, is larger than ΔF^{aq} means that some, but not all, interstitial water between the antibody-active site and the antigenic determinant has been squeezed out. That squeezed-out water, by becoming more randomized when changing from regularly oriented water to bulk water, also manifests itself by contributing to the increase in entropy that is frequently found to accompany antigen-antibody interactions (see below).

While these arguments pertain to van der Waals–London type interactions between antigens and antibodies, they also, at least qualitatively, apply to the Coulombic forces (F'), which in many cases contribute to antigen-antibody interactions, according to equation (1). Here also the expulsion of water between the two surfaces serves the purpose of decreasing the dielectric constant ε, as well as the distance d, thus, as Q^+ and Q^- are of opposite sign, doubly contributing to an increase in F' (and also to an increase in entropy, see above).

Figure 5–1 *B* illustrates how van der Waals–London bonds can exhibit their maximum efficiency, by bringing the antigenic and antibody-active sites as close together as is possible, by sheer shape conformation.

Finally, Figure 5–1 *C* illustrates how the electrostatic and dispersion forces can combine to give a not infrequently occurring type of antigen-antibody interaction.

Energetics of Antigen-Antibody Interactions

Thermodynamics. Arrhenius was the first to treat antigen-antibody interactions as reversible reactions:

$$Ag + Ab \rightleftharpoons AgAb \tag{4}$$

The equilibrium constant (K) of such a reaction (expressed as an association constant) is

$$K = \frac{(AgAb)}{(Ag)(Ab)} = \frac{b}{c(A_0 - b)} \tag{5}$$

where A_0 is the total concentration of antibody sites, b is the bound concentration of antigen (or antibody sites), and c is the free (unbound) concentration of antigen at equilibrium. Once the equilibrium constant has been measured (see below for the methods of measurement), the standard free-energy change $\Delta F°$ (i.e., the free energy of a reaction taking place under standard conditions of 1 molar concentration of the reagents), can be calculated:

$$\Delta F° = -RT \ln K \tag{6}$$

(R is the gas constant: 1.986×10^{-3} kcal per ° C per mole; T the absolute temperature in ° Kelvin.) Further information can be obtained by measuring K at two different temperatures, because then the enthalpy $\Delta H°$ can be calculated:

$$\frac{d \ln K}{dT} = \frac{\Delta H°}{RT^2} \tag{7}$$

allowing the calculation of the entropy $\Delta S°$ by using the van't Hoff equation:

$$\Delta F° = \Delta H° - T\Delta S^2 \tag{8}$$

$\Delta H°$ can also be obtained independently, and if K is known at the same time, both $\Delta F°$ and $\Delta S°$ can be found from those data, with the help of equations (6) and (8). The energy of interaction $\Delta F°$, found by equilibrium methods, usually expressed in kcal per mole, also may be expressed in terms of ergs/cm^2 (ΔF^{eq}, see above), provided the surface area (per molecule) of the antigen and antibody-active sites is known. For most antigen-antibody systems that surface area per site is on the order of, and not far from 200 to 400 Å².

Methods for Measuring Antigen-Antibody Interaction Parameters.

Methods for measuring the equilibrium association constant (K) of antigen-antibody interactions usually depend on the determination of free and bound forms of the antigen under conditions in which the total antibody concentration is kept constant, or is known if varied.

When the antigen is much smaller than the antibody molecules (or, particularly, when hapten-antibody interactions are studied), equilibrium dialysis with the help of a membrane that is permeable to the antigen (or hapten), and impermeable to the antibody molecules and to the antigen- (or hapten-) antibody complexes, is the method of choice.

When the antigen is soluble under conditions where the antibody molecule and the antigen-antibody complexes are insoluble (e.g., in concentrated $[NH_4]_2SO_4$ solutions) and when the antigen can be radiolabeled, usable data for obtaining K can also be derived.

All methods for determining K are faced with the fact that antibody populations are usually heterogeneous with regard to K. Exceptions are the homogeneous myeloma proteins, which bind antigens or haptens (Chapter 17). Analytic methods for determining an average value of K for a heterogeneous antibody population use a distribution function, either a gaussian error function or, more conveniently, the Sips distribution function. In the latter case, equation (5) becomes

$$K^a = \frac{b}{c^a(A_0 - b)} \quad 0 < a < 1 \tag{9}$$

where a is the Sips heterogeneity index. When analytic determinations give data fitting the above equation with $a = 1$, the antibody is homogeneous. Increasingly smaller values of a indicate increasing degrees of heterogeneity.

When using equilibrium dialysis, the numerical determination of K is best achieved by plotting a recast form of equation (9):

$$\left(\frac{b}{c}\right)^a = K^a A_0 - K^a b \tag{10}$$

If b/c is plotted against b, this equation indicates that a straight line will be obtained if $a = 1$, indicating a homogeneous antibody population; otherwise a curved line is obtained, indicating a heterogeneous antibody population. In either case, if the line is extrapolated to $b/c = O$, the resulting intercept on the b axis gives the value of A_0, since when $(b/c)^a = O$ $K^a A_0 = K^a b$. K can be determined by finding the value of b/c at which $b = A_{02}$, since then

$$(A_0/2c)^a = K^a \frac{A_0}{2}, \quad \text{or} \quad K = \frac{1}{c} \tag{11}$$

Other methods for measuring antibody combination with antigens or haptens also yield values of K. Analytic ultracentrifugation, which makes use of the fact that antigens, antibodies, and their complexes have different sedimentation velocities so that, upon separation in a gravitation field, the quantity of each can be measured, will yield K.

When one has to deal with insoluble antigens, for instance, blood group antigens on the surfaces of erythrocytes, the amounts of free and bound radiolabeled antibody can easily be obtained by simple centrifugation, to obtain K.

Fluorescence quenching has been used to quantitate the binding of haptens, which when combined with antibody cause the natural fluorescence of the protein to decrease. From the relative extent of quenching, the amount of hapten bound by a specifically purified antibody can be calculated and a value of K obtained. A similar principle can be employed in the case of haptens whose fluorescence is enhanced when they are bound to antibody. In this case, in contrast to the above, impure antibody preparations can be used and the small values of K for haptens bound weakly can be measured.

Relative values of K for both strongly and weakly bound haptens, relative to a reference hapten, can be obtained by a variety of methods. If the absolute value of K for the reference hapten is known from measurements by one of the methods described above, then absolute K values can be calculated from the relative K values. Methods employed include hapten inhibition of antibody-antigen precipitation, hapten inhibition of complement fixation, and various other competition reactions in which hapten competes with antigen for binding to antibody as, for example, in the $(NH_4)_2SO_4$ precipitation method, or with antigen (or antibody) attached to a solid absorbent.

Finally, by microcalorimetry, the standard change in enthalpy, $\Delta H°$, can be measured directly.

Some Orders of Magnitude of Antigen-Antibody Interaction Parameters. These are as follows:

K	varies from 10^3 to 10^{10}	liters/mole
$\Delta F°$	varies from -4 to -12	kcal/mole*
$\Delta H°$	varies from 0 to -10	kcal/mole
$\Delta S°$	varies from -10 to $+30$	entropy units/mole

The standard free-energy changes ($\Delta F°$) show that antigen-antibody bonds are among the weaker interactions. The enthalpy changes ($\Delta H°$) indicate that the reactions are generally exothermic. The frequent increase in entropy found as antigen-antibody complexes are formed (notwithstanding the increased "order" involved in the formation of such complexes) is

---

* Or ΔF^{eq}, depending on the surface area of the antigenic determinants and antibody-active sites (generally between 200 and 400 Å^2), varies between -3 and -17 ergs/cm^2.

Table 5-1

REPRESENTATIVE THERMODYNAMIC AND KINETIC VALUES FOR HAPTEN, ANTI-HAPTEN ANTIBODY INTERACTIONS*

Values are for the reaction:

Antibody Site (A) + Hapten $(H) \underset{k_{21}}{\overset{k_{12}}{\rightleftharpoons}}$ Site-Hapten Complex (AH); $k_{12}/k_{21} = K_A = (AHS)/(A)(H)$; $-\Delta F^\circ = RT \ln K_A$; $\Delta F^\circ = \Delta H - T\Delta S^\circ$

Antibody	Hapten	k_{12} $(M^{-1} Sec^{-1})$ $\times 10^{-8}$	k_{21} (Sec^{-1})	K_A† (M^{-1}) $\times 10^{-6}$	$-\Delta F^\circ$ (K_{cal}) $(mole^{-1})$	$-\Delta H$ (K_{cal}) $(mole^{-1})$	$-\Delta S^\circ$ $(e.u.)$ $(mole^{-1})$
Anti-p-nitrophenyl	DHNDS-NP§	1.8	760	0.6	8.0	—	—
Antidinitrophenyl	ε-N-DNP-aminocaproate	1.0	1.1	90‡	11.2	9.5	—
Antidinitrophenyl	ε-N-DNP-L-lysine	—	—	23‡	10.3	19.6	30.4
Antidinitrophenyl	2,4-dinitro-aniline	—	—	0.3‡	7.3	8.7	5.2
Anti-p-azobenzenearsonate	Terephthal-anilide-p-p'-diarsonate	—	—	0.3	7.3	0.8	-22
Anti-D-phenyl-(p-azobenzoyl-amino) acetate	D-Phenyl-[p-(p-dimethyl-aminobenzeneazo benzoylamino] acetate	—	—	0.3	7.4	7.3	-0.7
Anti-p-azophenyl-β-lactoside	p-(p-Dimethylaminobenzeneazo) phenyl-β-lactoside	—	—	0.16	7.1	9.7	8.8
Anti-SUp‖	p-(p-aminobenzeneazo)-hippurate	—	—	34	10.2	21.6	38

* From Grossberg, A. L. In Greenwalt, T. J., and Steane, E. A. (eds.): *Blood Banking, CRC Handbook Series in Clinical Laboratory Science.* CRC Press, Cleveland, 1977.

† Measured by equilibrium dialysis at 25° C, except where noted.

‡ By fluorescence quenching.

§ DHNDS-NP = 4,5 dihydroxy-3-(p-nitrophenylazo)-2,7-naphthalene disulfonate.

‖ SUp = $-(CH_2)_4NHCOCH-SCH_2CONH-$⟨phenyl⟩$-N=N-$⟨phenyl⟩$-CONHOH_2COO^-$.

73

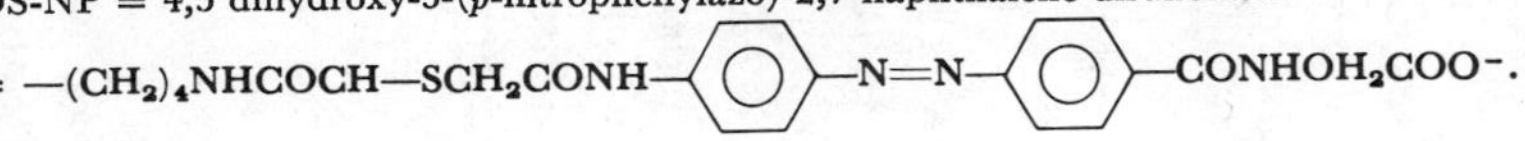

ascribed to the randomization of former water of hydration, expelled into the solution after hydrophobic interactions (see above and Table 5–1).

Specificity of Antigen-Antibody Interactions

Particularly from the work of Landsteiner, the remarkable specificity of antigen-antibody reactions has become apparent. With the appropriate antibodies as reagents, it is a relatively simple matter to distinguish between chemically closely related antigens or haptens. More details are given in Chapter 6.

For instance, antibodies elicited in rabbits to the hapten p-azotoluidine (coupled to a carrier protein for the purpose of making it immunogenic) combine more avidly with the same protein-hapten combination that gave rise to them than with the same protein coupled to m-azotoluidine, and they react even less with the protein coupled to o-azotoluidine. Another example is the fact that certain subunits of human immunoglobulins, which differ in only one amino acid (valine being substituted for leucine in position 191), can be distinguished from each other by the use of appropriate antisera to these proteins (Chapter 4).

The extraordinary specificity of immunologic reactions permits one to distinguish quite readily between similar proteins (e.g., serum albumins) from different animal species. Such a differentiation, if it were to be done chemically, would represent a major and ambitious undertaking.

Nonstoichiometry of Antigen-Antibody Interactions

As is discussed in greater detail in Chapter 6, antigens and antibodies belong to the class of complex-forming compounds. Such compounds are capable of interacting with one another in a wide range of different proportions. Antigens and antibodies, for instance, have the capability of combining under conditions of great excess of antigen as well as under conditions of great excess of antibody. It is generally only at intermediate proportions that the formed complexes will show a considerable degree of insolubility. The complexes formed at either antigen or antibody excess tend to be soluble. There is thus no stoichiometry in antigen-antibody interactions.

Valency of Antigens (or Haptens) and Antibodies

Because of the nonstoichiometry of antigen-antibody reactions, complexes can occur with general formulas ranging from Ag_nAb to $AgAb_m$. For soluble antigens and antibodies the maximum of insolubility may yield compounds of the general formula Ag_xAb_y, but the composition of such optimal precipitation complexes gives no clue as to the valency of either antigen or antibody. On the contrary, it is possible to determine the valency of antigens only in the presence of an excess of antibody and, vice versa, to determine the valency of antibodies only in the presence of an excess of antigen. The reason for this will be elaborated upon and illustrated in greater detail in Chapter 6.

With the same data that are needed to measure the equilibrium constant K, it is possible, under the proper conditions, to measure the valency of either the antigen (or hapten) or the antibody involved. For instance, under conditions of hapten excess, it is possible to measure the valency of the antibodies that combined with these haptens. By measuring the ratio (r) of the number of moles of hapten that are bound per mole of antibody at various concentrations (c) of free hapten, it is possible, by plotting r/c versus r, to find the valency of the antibody used, at $r/c = 0$ (at the intercept on the abscissa).

Dissociation of Antigen-Antibody Complexes

There are a variety of ways in which antigen-antibody complexes can be dissociated. A study of thermodynamic results shows that the formation of antigen-antibody complexes is generally exothermic so that an increase in temperature will facilitate their dissociation.

As at least part of the antigen-antibody interactions are generally due to electrostatic bonds, extremes of pH, which tend to make all proteins either negatively charged at high pH or positively charged at low pH, make them lose either their positive or their negative charges, and with that they not only lose their capacity for attracting one another but are even forced apart through the repulsion of similar charges. This method of dissociation is generally practiced at low pH (3 to 3.5). An increase of ionic strength, by the addition of salt, tends to decrease the electrostatic attraction by shielding the charges sites with counterions. Van der Waals forces can be reversed by lowering the surface tension of the liquid, and combined van der Waals and electrostatic bonds can be broken with low surface tension organic acids such as 1 M propionic acid.

Antigen-antibody complexes also generally dissociate in an excess of either antigen or antibody. Finally, antigen-antibody complexes can be dissociated by the specific (e.g., enzymatic) destruction of either antigen or antibody, thus liberating the remaining component.

In Vitro Antigen-Antibody Interactions

Over the last half-century an enormous variety of different methods have evolved for demonstrating antigen-antibody interactions *in vitro*. The most important classes of these methods will be briefly mentioned here.

Formation of Soluble Complexes

The formation of soluble antigen-antibody complexes can be demonstrated qualitatively and quantitatively in a number of ways, among them analytical ultracentrifugation and moving boundary electrophoresis, as well as gel permeation chromatography.

Precipitation

The precipitation of soluble antigens with soluble antibodies is discussed in greater detail in Chapter 6. The formation of precipitates can of course be easily followed in the test tube, but more powerful techniques now exist for studying precipitation reactions, by single or double diffusion in gels.

Agglutination

Agglutination is the destabilization of suspension of particulate antigens through cross-linking by soluble antibody molecules. When the antigen is part of an erythrocyte surface or adsorbed onto the surface of erythrocytes, this technique is frequently called hemagglutination. It is discussed in greater detail in Chapter 6.

Lysis

After interaction of certain cells, such as erythrocytes and gram-negative bacteria, with antibody, these cells will lyse through the action of complement.

The interaction of soluble antigens with certain types of antibodies gives rise to the fixation of complement. Complement-mediated lysis and complement fixation are presented in Chapter 8.

Other In Vitro Antigen-Antibody Reactions

There exists a great variety of other methods for demonstrating and measuring antigen-antibody reactions, notably those that depend on the radiolabeling of antigens and/or antibodies (Chapter 29) and those that depend on labeling antibodies with a fluorescent dye that makes them visible under ultraviolet light (Chapter 27).

Another method of studying antigen-antibody interactions is by the inhibition of a property of either antigen or antibody. A very important antigen-antibody reaction that has been studied in this manner is the toxin-antitoxin reaction, where the toxicity of the antigen is inhibited by the antibody (Chapter 26).

In Vivo Antigen-Antibody Interactions

The real importance of the reaction between antibodies and antigens *in vivo* lies, of course, in the defense of the organism against the invasion by foreign agents. All of the following mechanisms will be discussed in greater detail in Chapters 13 through 16. Only the following main classes of *in vivo* antigen-antibody interactions will be briefly mentioned here.

Agglutination of Bacteria

Antibodies that are directed to bacterial antigens can coat these microorganisms and, frequently, by cross-linking them, organize them into clumps. There is no strong indication that agglutination has any great deleterious effect on these microorganisms, but the formation of large clumps of bacteria is advantageous to the host, as it allows the disposal of several bacteria per phagocytic ingestion.

Immobilization of Bacteria and Other Parasites

Motile bacteria, whether they be motile through their own movement as is the case with spirochetes or through the movement of flagella, can be immobilized by cross-linking parts of their superstructure or of their flagella.

Inactivation of Viruses

When viruses are coated by specific antibody, this tends to inactivate their cell-penetrating power and thus reduce their pathogenicity.

Neutralization of Toxins

By interacting with bacterial and other toxins, specific antibodies frequently can neutralize their toxic activity.

Surface Recognition by Phagocytosis

Antibodies that are directed to antigenic sites on the surfaces of bacteria, viruses, or other foreign particles or molecules endow these surfaces with a more hydrophobic coating, which causes phagocytic cells to engulf the particles (Chapter 10).

Complement-Mediated Actions

As already mentioned above under the *in vitro* interactions, the interaction between antigens and certain types of antibodies can fix complement

(Chapter 8). This can give rise to the following varieties of different biologic reactions:

1. The hemolysis of erythrocytes, after interaction with specific antibodies and complement.
2. The lysis of bacteria (mainly gram-negative bacteria), after interaction with specific antibody and complement.
3. Chemotaxis; that is to say, the migration of phagocytic cells toward invading microorganisms is an important defense mechanism. The coating of microorganisms with antibody and fixation of complement increases their chemotactic ability (Chapter 10).
4. Phagocytosis of invading microorganisms, after they have been coated with specific antibody, is greatly facilitated when that antigen-antibody reaction has been instrumental in the fixation of complement (Chapter 10).
5. Other complement-mediated reactions are the formation of anaphylatoxins after antigen-antibody reactions and immune adherence, a complement-mediated mechanism for the attachment of antigen-antibody complexes to erythrocytes.

Bibliography

Arrhenius, S.: *Immunochemistry*. The Macmillan Co., New York, 1907.

Day, L. A.; Sturdevant, J. M.; and Singer, S. J.: The kinetics of the reactions between antibodies to the 2,4-dinitrophenyl group and specific haptens. *Ann. N.Y. Acad. Sci.*, **103**:611–25, 1963.

Eisen, H. N., and Siskind, G. N.: Variations in affinities of antibodies during the immune response. *Biochemistry*, **3**:996–1008, 1964.

Froese, A., and Sehon, A. H.: Kinetic and equilibrium studies of the reaction between anti-*p*-nitrophenyl antibodies and a homologous hapten. *Immunochemistry*, **2**:135–43, 1965.

Fujio, H., and Karush, F.: Antibody affinity. II. Effect of immunization interval on antihapten antibody in the rabbit. *Biochemistry*, **5**:1856–63, 1966.

Hughes-Jones, N. C.: Nature of the reaction between antigen and antibody. *Br. Med. Bull.*, **19**:171–77, 1963.

————: The estimation of the concentration and equilibrium constant of Ant-D. *Immunology*, **12**:565–71, 1967.

Kabat, E. A.: *Structural Concepts in Immunology and Immunochemistry*. Holt, Rinehart & Winston, Inc., New York, 1976.

Klotz, I.: *Energy Changes in Biochemical Reactions*. Academic Press, Inc., New York, 1967.

Landsteiner, K.: *The Specificity of Serological Reactions*. Dover Publications, Inc., New York, 1962.

Steiner, R. F., and Kitzinger, C.: Calorimetric determination of the heat of an antigen-antibody reaction. *J. Biol. Chem.*, **222**:271–84, 1956.

van Oss, C. J., and Neumann, A. W.: Comparison between antigen antibody binding energies and interfacial free energies. *Immunol. Commun.*, 6:341–54, 1977.

Visser, T. J.: On Hamaker constants: comparison between Hamaker constants and Lifshitz van der Waals constants. *Adv. Colloid Interf. Sci.*, 3:331–63, 1972.

Williams, C. A., and Chase, M. W. (eds.): *Methods in Immunology and Immunochemistry*, Vol. 3. Academic Press, Inc., New York, 1971.

6

Precipitation and Agglutination

Carel J. van Oss

Precipitation

Mechanism of Precipitation

Upon the admixture of soluble antigen with specific antiserum, antigen-antibody complexes form quite rapidly. Such antigen-antibody complexes, as already discussed in Chapter 5, can be formed at widely varying antigen/antibody ratios. Depending on the antigen/antibody ratio, the sort of antigen, and the sort of antibody used, the complexes formed will show a greater or lesser degree of insolubility. While close to the optimal antigen/antibody ratio (where neither antigen nor antibody is found in the supernatant solution), the maximum amount of precipitate is formed under conditions of antibody excess; also, in cases of pronounced antigen excess, the complexes formed give rise to little or no precipitate (Figure 6–1). At antigen/antibody proportions that are closest to the optimal ratio, the formed complexes precipitate most rapidly. Two factors play a role in the growth of these complexes into insoluble precipitates.

1. Specific cross-linking between antigen and antibody molecules and antigen-antibody complexes takes place; these grow into increasingly large entities that finally precipitate out due to their sheer size.

2. Particularly where the antigen-antibody interaction is of such a nature that upon their combination a significant number of polar groups (which, being hydrated, contribute to the solubility of proteins) is masked, the complexes formed will have a decreased solubility and will tend to aggregate into large insoluble clusters, through contact between their apolar groups.

Both these secondary mechanisms take much longer (from several hours to several days) to reach ultimate completion than the primary, rapid antigen-antibody interaction that gives rise to the initial complex formation.

Antigen-Antibody Precipitation in Tubes

The precipitation test in tubes is one of the oldest methods for obtaining quantitative information about the amount of specific antibody present in an antiserum. Much of the fundamental and pioneering work on this test was done by Heidelberger and associates. The test is generally done by adding increasing amounts of dissolved antigen to successive tubes containing a constant amount of specific antiserum. As illustrated in Figure 6–2, under conditions of great antibody excess, as well as under conditions of great excess of antigen, no precipitate appears in the tubes. At ratios close to the optimal ratio, the largest quantities of precipitate appear. The optimal ratio corresponds to the antigen/antibody ratio in that tube in which neither antibody nor antigen can be demonstrated in the supernatant solution. In practice, the largest amount of precipitate generally will be found in the tube containing a slight excess of antigen. Classically, the experiments were done with polysaccharide antigen, so that by doing a nitrogen determination with the Kjeldahl method on the washed precipitate, the amount of antibody precipitated could be expressed in micrograms of nitrogen. In this manner the total amount of specific antibody in an antiserum can be found. The habit of expressing the total amount of antibody precipitated in micrograms of antibody nitrogen has now become obsolete.

The optimal antigen/antibody ratio is generally the ratio at which soluble antigen and antibody will precipitate fastest. Particularly with certain toxin and antitoxin reactions (Chapter 26), the tube in which the precipitate appears first has been classically (and rightly) held to be the one containing the optimal antigen/antibody ratio.

The optimal ratio found can vary with a great variety of different parameters. Temperature as well as the pH and the salt concentration can play an important role. Another important factor is the manner in which antigen is added to the antibody solution: when the antigen solution is added to the antibody in several successive steps, less antigen is needed to precipitate a given amount of antibody than when all the antigen is added at once. The same effect has been described in toxin-antitoxin reactions (Danysz phenomenon).

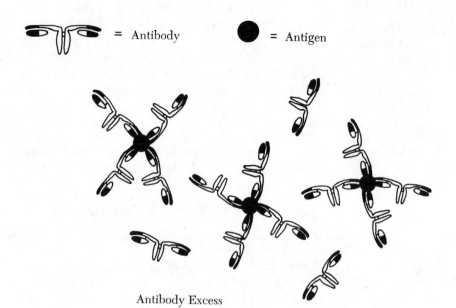

= Antibody   = Antigen

Antibody Excess

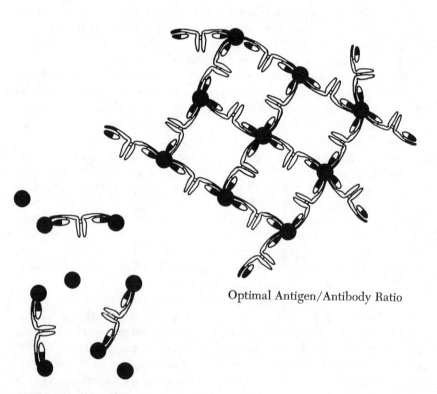

Optimal Antigen/Antibody Ratio

Antigen Excess

Figure 6-1. [*Opposite*] Schematic representation of the composition of antigen-antibody complexes. At *antibody* excess (left) free antibody occurs together with the complexes; at *antigen* excess (right) free antigen occurs together with the complexes; and only at the optimal antigen/antibody ratio (middle) neither free antibody nor free antigen is present.

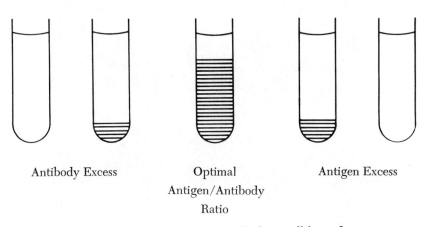

Antibody Excess   Optimal   Antigen Excess
                    Antigen/Antibody
                         Ratio

Figure 6-2. Precipitation in tubes. Under conditions of extreme *antibody* excess (far left) as well as extreme *antigen* excess (far right) the complexes formed are so small that they are entirely soluble. Under conditions of *antibody* excess (two left tubes) free antibody is present in the soluble phase, and under conditions of *antigen* excess (two right tubes) free antigen is present in the soluble phase. Only at the optimal antigen/antibody ratio (middle tube) is there neither free antigen nor free antibody in the soluble phase.

With the gel immunodiffusion test, discussed below, it has become a simple matter to determine the absence or presence of excess antibody or antigen in the supernatant of any of the tubes. It thus becomes an easy matter to ascertain on the precipitate of which tube the nitrogen determination will have to be done, if one wishes to determine the total amount of specific antibody in a given antiserum. As will be discussed in the next section, the optimal antigen/antibody ratio can also be entirely determined by the quantitative double-diffusion method.

Double-Diffusion Precipitation Methods in Gels

The remarkable specificity of antigen-antibody reactions can be aptly demonstrated when antigen-antibody precipitates are allowed to form in a gel as a result of the meeting of dissolved antigen and antibody molecules that have diffused toward one another from separate starting wells. This technique, which was first described by Ouchterlony, probably has produced more advances in our knowledge of immunology during the last two decades than any other method.

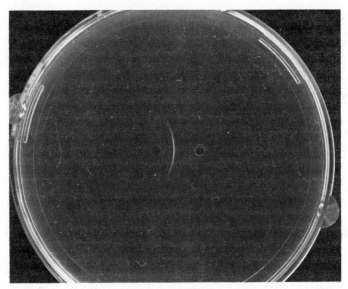

Figure 6-3. Sharp precipitate line formed by the immunodiffusion reaction between human IgM in normal human serum (left well) and rabbit antihuman IgM antiserum (right well).

Mechanism of Precipitate Line Formation.   When soluble antigen and antibody diffuse toward one another in a gel, a precipitate line forms at their place of meeting (Figure 6–3). The precipitate line actually is a thin precipitate ribbon, which seen on edge from above looks like a line. This precipitate ribbon has a peculiar property that is common to all precipitates formed in this fashion. It is a specifically impermeable barrier only to the two substances (in this case antigen and antibody) that formed it. The ribbon is entirely permeable to all other substances (e.g., to other antigens and antibodies) that have no connection with the precipitate in question. As will be shown below, this property has powerful implications for the possibility of using this method for distinguishing between qualitatively identical and nonidentical precipitating systems.

The explanation for the specific impermeability of the precipitate barrier to just the two compounds that formed it is simple. The barrier is self-repairing. As soon as a hole forms in it, some of the dissolved antigen and antibody molecules can again meet and precipitate together to plug the hole. Indeed, the specific impermeability of the barrier persists only as long as some of the forming ingredients are present in solution on either side of it. With antigen-antibody systems that form precipitates that are soluble in an excess of either antigen or antibody, the specific impermeability of the precipitate barrier remains intact only as long as the antigen and antibody on either side of it are present in equivalent concentrations. As

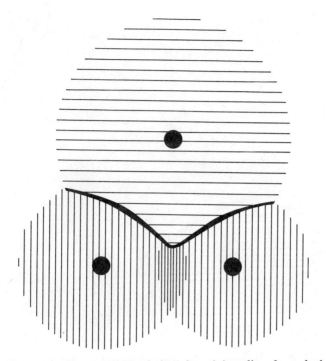

Figure 6-4. Diagram of the fusing of precipitate lines formed when two *identical* substances deposited in separate wells can *both* precipitate with a substance diffusing from the third well. (From van Oss, C. J.: Methods used in the characterization of immunoglobulins. In Greenwalt, T. J. [ed.]: *Advances in Immunogenetics.* J. B. Lippincott Co., Philadelphia, 1967, pp. 1–30.)

will be discussed later, this last consideration permits the quantitative use of the gel double-diffusion method.

Determination of Identity, Nonidentity, and Partial Identity. From the property of the specific impermeability of the precipitate barrier to the particular antigen and antibody that formed it, it follows that when two antisera (A and B) are both specific for an antigen (C), the two precipitate lines that are formed must fuse, indicating identity of the system AC and BC (Figure 6–4). When, on the other hand, two antisera (A and B) are respectively specific for two different antigens (C and D), the two precipitate systems (AC and BD, which have nothing in common) will form precipitate lines that cross one another unhindered, indicating nonidentity of those systems (Figure 6–5).

Precipitate lines form a spur (Figure 6–6 *A*) when one has, superimposed on one another, a system of identity and a system of nonidentity (Figure 6–6 *B* and *C*). Such a condition is alluded to as one of partial identity when

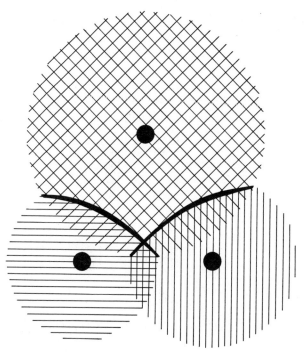

Figure 6-5. Diagram of the crossing of precipitate lines formed when each of two *different* substances deposited in separate wells precipitates with one and then the other of two substances that are both deposited in the third well. (From van Oss, C. J.: Methods used in the characterization of immunoglobulins. In Greenwalt, T. J. [ed.]: *Advances in Immunogenetics.* J. B. Lippincott Co., Philadelphia, 1967, pp. 1–30.)

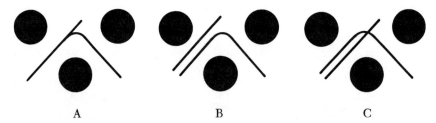

A   B   C

Figure 6-6. *A.* Diagram of spur formation in precipitate lines. This situation is best considered as the one drawn either in *B* or in *C*. In actual practice it is not always possible to decompose situation *A* into either *B* or *C*, because different antigenic determinants may reside on one and the same molecule. (From van Oss, C. J.: Methods used in the characterization of immunoglobulins. In Greenwalt, T. J. [ed.]: *Advances in Immunogenetics.* J. B. Lippincott Co., Philadelphia, 1967, pp. 1–30.)

both the identical and the nonidentical antigenic determinants are part of the same molecule.

Quantitative Double Diffusion. The fact that the precipitate line (barrier) remains intact only as long as the antigen and antibody are present on either side of it at equivalent concentrations can be used as a basis for determining the optimal antigen/antibody ratio by double diffusion in gels. When one of the dissolved reagents is present at a significantly higher concentration than the other, it can pass the precipitate band, causing it to thicken, to form several bands, or to move in the direction of the well containing the more dilute reagent. The line does not actually move but only appears to do so; in reality it dissolves in the excess reagent and reprecipitates farther on. Thus, the precipitate line remains thin, sharp, and immobile only where the reagents that formed it remain present in equivalent concentrations (Figure 6-7). With care, deviations from the optimal antigen/antibody ratio as small as 5% can be distinguished by this method, and quantities of antigen as small as 1 μg can be measured.

Remarkably enough, the place of the first formation of a precipitate line is largely independent of the initial concentrations of the antigen and antibody present in the starting wells. The place of first formation depends only on the diffusion coefficients, D_{AG} and D_{AB}, of the antigen and antibody used. If the starting wells may be considered as point sources, the place of first precipitation divides the line segment between these two point sources in the ratio $a/b = \sqrt{(D_{AG}/D_{AB})}$. Only when $D_{AG} = D_{AB}$ will the first-formed precipitate line be a straight line, bisecting the line segment between the wells. Otherwise the line will be a circle, concave toward and closest to the well containing the largest molecules, which have the smallest diffusion coefficient, with a radius $r = ab/(a - b)$.

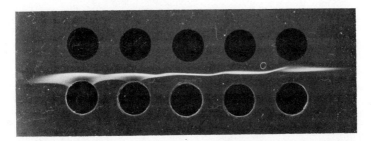

Figure 6-7. Determination by immunodiffusion of the optimal antigen/antibody ratio. In the top wells, from left to right: 0.4, 0.2, 0.1, 0.05, and 0.025% human IgG; in the bottom wells, rabbit antihuman IgG antiserum. The fineness of the line and its immobility indicate that the place of optimal antigen/antibody ratio is situated at the middle wells. Thus, the strength of the anti-IgG antibody in the antiserum used corresponds to 0.1% IgG.

Gel Precipitation Methods Independent of Diffusion. Gel precipitation methods, which depend only on molecular diffusion for bringing the reagents together, are extremely wasteful. Easily 90% of both antigen and antibody diffuse away from one another in various directions and never meet. This is one of the major causes of the low sensitivity of this type of reaction. The efficiency of the gel precipitation method, however, can be much improved if means are found for bringing a greater proportion of the reagents together. There are two ways of doing this: one is electrophoretic (counterelectrophoresis) and the other by hydrodynamic transport (rheophoresis).

COUNTERELECTROPHORESIS. This method, which is also referred to as immunoosmophoresis, crossed-over electrophoresis, electrosyneresis, and immunoelectroosmophoresis, brings antigen and antibody molecules together in an electric field. It is applicable only when the antigen and antibody have a significantly different isoelectric pH and then only by using a buffer with a pH that is intermediate between them. This method, when it can be used, is more sensitive than double diffusion and also faster. Visible precipitate lines can usually be obtained in one to two hours. It can be used for the detection of HB_S antigen (as a warning signal for the possible presence of serum hepatitis virus) in units of blood or plasma destined for transfusion.

RHEOPHORESIS. Rheophoresis, or immunorheophoresis, brings antigen and antibody together through hydrodynamic transport caused by continuous evaporation of water from the gel through a slit in the cover exactly above the spot where the precipitation reaction is to take place. If enough extra buffer is provided at the periphery, it will flow into the gel by capillary action toward the place where evaporation is taking place, thus pushing antigen and antibody together. As compared to double diffusion (with the same reagents), a threefold increase in sensitivity can be attained with this method; visible precipitate lines can usually be obtained in three to four hours. This method has been applied to unidimensional as well as to bidimensional gel precipitation, and it also has been adapted to immunoelectrophoresis; it can be used regardless of whether antigen and antibody have different isoelectric points.

Immunoelectrophoresis. The application of immunodiffusion to the identification of serum proteins by zone electrophoresis has expanded the number of recognizable serum components from six (albumin, α_1, α_2, β_1, β_2, and γ globulins) to more than 30 (Table 6-1). This method, immunoelectrophoresis, was developed in 1953. First, serum is separated into its differently charged components by means of an electric field, in an agar gel. Once the electrophoresis is completed, an antiserum to the components of the first serum is allowed to diffuse from a long trough that lies parallel to the electrophoresis pathway. Inversely, an antiserum, may first be separated into its component fractions by an electric field, after which an antigen

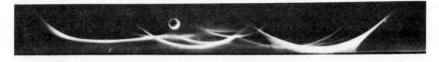

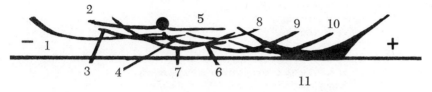

Figure 6-8. Photograph of an immunoelectropherogram of normal human serum developed with rabbit antiwhole human serum (top). The diagram (bottom) shows the principal precipitate lines that are discernible in the photograph. The main proteins that are clearly distinguishable are *1*, IgG; *2*, IgM; *3*, IgA; *4*, β_1A; *5*, α_2 macroglobulin; *6*, α_2 lipoprotein; *7*, transferrin; *8*, haptoglobin; *9*, Gc (group-specific component); *10* α_1 antitrypsin; *11*, albumin. They are listed in Table 6-1.

solution is placed in the trough). The remarkable property of nonidentical antigens to form precipitate lines that cross one another upon interaction with their respective antibodies (Figure 6-5) permits the distinction between a multitude of antigenically different but electrophoretically similar serum components that partially overlap (Figure 6-8).

As has been indicated above, in the ordinary double-diffusion reaction between two reagents originating from point sources, the precipitate line will have the shape of a circle. The same diffusion laws hold true in the configuration of immunoelectrophoresis, but the precipitate line resulting from the interaction between a homogeneous antigen (which approaches the shape of a point source) and a line-shaped antibody trough will be a parabola (see, for instance, the albumin line in Figure 6-8). With a long-drawn-out, electrophoretically heterogeneous antigen, the precipitate line resulting from the interaction of two parallel line-shaped sources will be a fairly straight line (see the IgG line in Figure 6-8). Thus, the occurrence of a sharply rounded, parabola-shaped curve in part of the normally straight IgG line is indicative of the presence of an abnormally homogeneous immunoglobulin fraction that occurs in monoclonal gammapathies such as multiple myeloma (Chapter 17).

With the help of either radioactive antigen or radioactive antibody, the presence of extremely small amounts of given antibodies or antigens can be demonstrated in immunoelectrophoresis by autoradiography; that technique is alluded to as radioimmunoelectrophoresis (Chapter 10).

Table 6-1

HUMAN SERUM PROTEINS

List of Human Serum Components Discernible by Immunoelectrophoresis of Normal Human Serum, in the Approximate Order of Decreasing Electrophoretic Mobility; see also Figures 6-8 and 6-9 C.

Tryptophan-rich prealbumin
α_1 acid glycoprotein
α_1 antitrypsin
α_1 lipoprotein
Albumin
α_1 easily precipitable glycoprotein
α_1 esterase (first component of complement)
Group-specific components (Gc-globulin)
Tryptophan-poor α_1 glycoprotein
Orosomucoid
Haptoglobins
α_1 x glycoprotein
Inter-α trypsin inhibitor
Ceruloplasmin
α_2 macroglobulin
α_2 lipoprotein
α_2 HS glycoprotein
β_2 lipoprotein
β_1A globulin (reacted third component of complement)
Transferrin
Plasminogen
β_1E globulin (fourth component of complement)
Hemopexin
β_1C globulin (unreacted third component of complement)
β_2 glycoprotein
Immunoglobulin M (IgM)
Immunoglobulin D (IgD)
Immunoglobulin E (IgE)
Immunoglobulin A (IgA)
β_2K globulin
C-reactive protein
Immunoglobulin G (γ globulin; IgG)

Single-Diffusion Precipitation Methods in Gels

Under single-diffusion precipitation methods are included those methods in which one of the reagents (generally the antiserum) is homogeneously incorporated throughout the entire gel, while the other reagent (generally the antigen) diffuses (or is forcibly electrophoresed) from a well or other starting point in the gel. Oudin was the first to apply single-diffusion precipitation, making use of gels in capillary tubes.

Radial Single Diffusion.   In radial single diffusion, antigen is allowed to diffuse from a well in a thin gel slab admixed with a fairly dilute antibody solution. The antigen, being present in relative excess compared to the antiserum, passes the precipitate it forms upon first contact with the antibody in the gel and continues to produce an ever-widening precipitate as it diffuses farther into the gel, until it is spent. At a constant antibody concentration the surface area of the precipitate formed is then directly proportional to the initial antigen concentration (Figure 6-9 *A*). If one uses various antibody concentrations in the gels, the areas of the precipitate formed are inversely proportional to the antibody concentrations used, at a constant concentration of antigen in the wells. By standardizing the antibody concentration in the gel, the method can be used for the immunochemical determination of unknown concentrations of an antigen, by comparing the areas of the precipitate discs formed with those from known concentrations of the same antigen. Provided a sufficiently long time is allowed for the precipitate to have finished growing, a plot of the *surface areas* of the precipitate discs versus the *concentrations* of antigen produces a straight line. As little as 0.01 μg of antigen can be determined with this method, and an accuracy of $\pm 2\%$ can be attained.

This method is of increasing clinical use for quantitative determinations of the levels of numerous serum protein components. It may not always be feasible to wait the required number of hours (or days) for the total completion of the radial diffusion precipitation reaction. It then is frequently the practice not to plot the areas of the precipitate discs versus the concentrations of the antigen, but rather to plot the diameters the precipitate discs have attained after a predetermined time lapse versus the logarithm of the concentrations of the antigen, in order to obtain a reasonable approach to a straight line. With this method it is particularly desirable to straddle the unknown concentration of antigen with at least two known concentrations, one of which is higher and one lower than the unknown, in order to approximate the unknown concentration by interpolation. As little as 0.15 μg of antigen can be measured this way, with an accuracy of $\pm 10\%$.

Electrophoretic Methods in Antibody-Containing Gels. Both the unidimensional and the bidimensional methods of transporting antigen electrophoretically through an antibody-containing gel are based on the same principles as the radial single-diffusion method, and the results are essentially the same. Here also, at a constant antibody concentration throughout the gel, the total surface area of precipitate attainable is proportional to the antigen concentration used.

UNIDIMENSIONAL ELECTROPHORESIS IN ANTIBODY-CONTAINING GELS. In this method, described by Laurell, various concentrations of an antigen are electrophoresed through an antibody-containing gel, from equally spaced wells as starting points, until all of the rocket-shaped precipitates have stopped growing. The antigen concentrations are then proportional to the surface area under the precipitate lines (Figure 6-9 *B*). This method has been used with as little as 0.5 μg of antigen and an accuracy of better than $\pm 2\%$ can be attained.

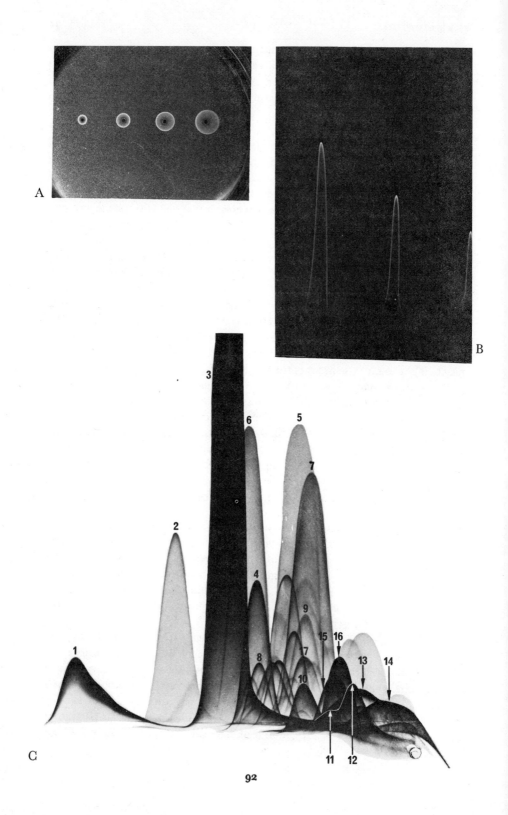

A

B

C

BIDIMENSIONAL ELECTROPHORESIS IN ANTIBODY-CONTAINING GELS. This method, also described by Laurell, is best comparable to immunoelectrophoresis. The second, double-diffusion step is replaced by a second electrophoretic transport, in a direction perpendicular to the first electrophoresis, of the initial electrophoretically separated fractions into an antibody-containing gel. This result in a series of mountain-shaped precipitate peaks, the surface area of each of which is proportional to the concentration of the antigen that formed it (Figure 6-9 C). This method allows the quantitative estimation of the principal immunoelectrophoretically distinguishable serum fractions in whole sera and other antigen mixtures.

Agglutination

Agglutination is a process that differs fundamentally from precipitation (Table 6-2). Instead of the precipitation of soluble molecules, agglutination is the aggregation of already insoluble particles or cells into larger clumps.

Figure 6-9. [*Opposite*] *A.* Radial single-diffusion titrations (Mancini plate). The agar in the plate contained a uniform solution of rabbit antihuman IgG antiserum (diluted 1/20). The wells contained, from right to left: 1.1%, 0.55%, 0.225%, and 0.1125% human IgG. The diffusion was allowed to proceed until the precipitate discs stopped growing; a plot of their surface areas versus the initial IgG concentration yields a straight line.

B. Unidimensional electrophoresis in a (1:10 diluted) rabbit antihuman serum transferrin antiserum-containing gel. The wells contained, from left to right: 0.1%, 0.05%, and 0.025% human serum transferrin. After completion of the electrophoresis in the gel (the anode was at the top), the surface area of the rockets was proportional to the initial concentrations of the human serum transferrin in the wells. The *heights* of the rockets, when plotted against the concentrations, lie on a straight line.

C. Bidimensional electrophoresis in a rabbit antiwhole human serum-containing gel. After the first electrophoresis of whole human serum (parallel to the bottom of the gel with the anode to the right), the second electrophoresis (anode at top) is done in the antiserum-containing gel. The surface areas of the rockets are proportional to the initial concentrations of the various proteins present in the serum. Apart from the fixed albumin (*1*), used as a standard, other proteins visible are *2*, prealbumin; *3*, albumin; *4*, α_1 lipoprotein; *5*, α_2 HS glycoprotein (HS after Heremans and Schmid); *6*, α_1 antitrypsin globulin; *7*, haptoglobin; *8*, α_1 easily precipitable glycoprotein; *9*, Gc (group-specific components) globulin; *10*, α_2 macroglobulin; *11*, β1-A (C3); *12*, β1-C (C3); *13*, IgA; *14*, IgM; *15*, hemopexin; *16*, transferrin; *17*, β lipoprotein. Most of these proteins are also listed in Table 6-1. (Courtesy of Medical and Biological Instrumentation Limited, Ashford, England.)

Table 6-2

DIFFERENCES BETWEEN PRECIPITATION AND AGGLUTINATION

	Precipitation	Agglutination
Physical state of the antigens	Antigens are *dissolved molecules*	Antigen are (or are part of or are attached to) *insoluble particles* that are in relatively stable suspension
Size of the antigens	From $\sim 10^3$ to $> 10^6$ or from 10 to $> 10^3$ Å	From 10^3 to 10^6 Å
Mechanism	Formation of antigen-antibody complexes, often of a decreased solubility owing to the mutual masking of some of their polar groups; in time both through further specific cross-linking and through aspecific interactions between apolar groups, these complexes grow into large precipitate entities, visible with the naked eye	Formation of large lattices through the cross-linking of many antigen particles by specific antibodies; these lattices are generally visible with the naked eye as clumps, whose sheer size causes them to sediment readily
Sensitivity	Generally not sensitive for the demonstration of less than 10^{-4} to 10^{-6} gm antibody	Sensitive for the demonstration of as little as 10^{-5} to 10^{-8} gm of antibody
Reaction time	Often long, from several hours to several days	Short reaction time, from a few minutes to a few hours at the most
Optimal type of antibodies	Most efficient with bivalent antibodies	Most efficient with decavalent antibodies
Possibility for the reaction to occur in gels	Possible	Possible in gels only in exceptional cases and when the particle size of the antigens can be made very small

Agglutination was first observed with bacterial cells that clumped together upon the addition of a serum from an animal that had been injected with these bacteria. Subsequently one of the principal applications has become the agglutination of erythrocytes by specific antibodies to antigens that are part of, or are attached to, the red cells; this method is often called hemagglutination, although that term is also used for the agglutination of red cells by viruses. Microscopically small inert particles, such as bentonite or polystyrene latex particles, which can be coated with various antigens, are now much used for agglutination.

Much less antigen is needed for obtaining a visible reaction in agglutination than in precipitation. This is largely due to the fact that in agglutination the antigenic molecules need only be part of the surface of a relatively small number of fairly large particles, whereas in precipitation the dissolved antigen molecules are initially distributed through the entire liquid, subsequently to give rise to visible precipitate particles, each consisting of large numbers of antigen molecules that are homogeneously spread through-out the entire particle. For instance, in order to obtain visible agglutination (or precipitation) in 1 ml of liquid, at least 1 mg of particulate matter of an average particle diameter of 100 μm should be present. For agglutination with red cells as particulate carriers, this involves 1 mg of red cells plus not more than 1 μg of the actual antigen attached to the surface of the red cells, and about 1 μg of antibody then suffices for agglutination. In precipitation, on the other hand, this may involve as much as 0.5 mg of antigen and 0.5 mg of antibody, or 500 times as much.

Mechanism of Agglutination

Mechanism of Cross-Linking.   The first step in agglutination is the linking together of different particles or cells by antibody molecules that specifically attach to the antigenic determinants on the surface of the particles or cells. It is used to realize the great disparity in size between the cells that are to be agglutinated and the immunoglobulins that cross-link them. When a cell (a red cell, for instance) is imagined to be enlarged to about the size of this book, the dimensions of the biggest type of antibody, the deca-valent immunoglobulin M (IgM), would be entirely comprised within a lower case "o," and divalent antibodies of the immunoglobulin G (IgG) class would be the size of the commas printed on this page. It is thus readily understandable why the somewhat large IgM, with ten binding sites, is a much more powerful agglutinator of these relatively enormous cells than the smaller IgG, with only two binding sites. Indeed, in quite a few cases (dependent on the spacing, the number, and the avidity of the antigenic sites on a cell surface), IgG-type antibodies are incapable of cross-linking and thus of agglutinating the cells. For that reason and also because of an erroneous older supposition that this incapacity was due to their mono-valency, such nonagglutinating antibodies were, and sometimes still are, alluded to as "incomplete" antibodies. These antibodies, which would be more justly termed "nonagglutinating" antibodies, are capable of specific binding to the antigenic sites on the cells; they are, under given circum-stances, unable to cross-link the cells and they thus tend to attach with both valencies to the same cell. With concentrated antisera, containing high levels of IgG-type antibodies, the antigenic sites on the cells may become so totally occupied with such "monogamously" binding antibodies that the available IgM-type antibodies, finding no more free antigenic sites, are incapable of cross-linking the cells. In such cases the IgG-type antibodies are called "blocking" antibodies. Upon dilution of the antiserum this blocking or "prozone" phenomenon generally disappears. When dilution of the antiserum is continued, an ultimate concentration of antibody is reached at which too few specific immunoglobulin molecules are present to achieve agglutination. The final dilution at which agglutination can just be demonstrated is a semiquantitative measure of the antibody content of a

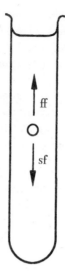

Figure 6-10. Representation of the forces competing in the sedimentation of particles suspended in a liquid. The force tending to make the particle sediment downward (sf) is the function of the density difference and of the particle's volume and is thus proportional to the third power of its radius. The force acting against the sedimentation is the friction force (ff), which is directly proportional to the particle's radius. Thus, the larger the particle, the stronger its tendency to sediment (other factors being equal).

serum; it is generally expressed as the reciprocal of that dilution and called the "titer" of the antiserum (i.e., if a 640-fold dilution of an antiserum is the last one that still yields measurable agglutination, the antibody in the antiserum is said to have a titer of 640). There are a number of direct and indirect methods (see pages 98–103) for obtaining agglutination even with IgG-type antibodies.

Mechanism of Sedimentation. The force that causes a particle or cell, which is heavier than water, to sediment is proportional to the weight of the particle and thus, for a given particle density, proportional to the third power of its radius. On the other hand, the *friction force*, which counteracts sedimentation, is proportional to the particle's radius (Figure 6-10). Big particles will, therefore, sediment readily, whereas small particles are more strongly subjected to friction forces that delay their sedimentation (Table 6-3).

Apart from their smallness, there is one other factor that may delay or even prevent sedimentation; this is the electrostatic repulsion between particles or cells that all have the same electric surface or "zeta" potential. Most cells are somewhat negatively charged and thus will repel one another to a certain extent. Enzymatic intervention (e.g., the destruction of acid groups in cell-wall polysaccharides or proteins), resulting in a decrease in

Table 6-3
SEDIMENTATION RATES OF PARTICLES OF VARIOUS SIZES

Sort of Particle*	Radius of Particle	Approximate Sedimentation Rate
Visible agglutinates	50 μm	2 cm/minute
Large cells or small agglutinates	5 μm	1 cm/hour
Small cells	0.5 μm	2 cm/week
Subcellular particles	0.05 μm	1 cm/year

* For all particles a density $\simeq 1.05$ is assumed.

cellular surface charge, tends to facilitate agglutination. Total neutralization of the negative charge of cells with positively charged polymers (such as Polybrene®) induces complex coacervation, and thus strongly facilitates agglutination and sedimentation.

Visualization of Agglutination. Agglutination can be practiced in tubes or on slides and it can be visualized with the naked eye or under the microscope. When cell-wall material can be reduced to a sufficiently small particle size to migrate into an open-pored gel, agglutination by gel double diffusion is even possible, with all its advantages with respect to the determination of identity, partial identity, and nonidentity (see discussion in the first part of this chapter).

AGGLUTINATION IN TUBES. The method still used in most agglutination tests is agglutination in tubes. Generally, constant volumes of a standardized cell or particle suspension are added to constant volumes of antiserum in increasing serial dilution. After an appropriate time lapse, during which the reaction has come to completion, the tubes are either visually inspected when large visible agglutinates are formed (see Table 6-2), or they are inspected after a few minutes of centrifugation at 1000 to 5000 × g. In both cases it is of some importance to be able to distinguish between cells or particles that have sedimented singly and those that were sedimented after agglutination. The general rule should here be kept in mind that simple sedimentation gives rise to closely packed masses of cells or particles that settle as compact buttons at the very bottom of the tubes, whereas agglutinates are loosely knit, open networks that settle as fluffy aggregates around the entire curved lower part of the tubes.

AGGLUTINATION ON SLIDES. This method has the advantage of being faster and of requiring smaller volumes of reagents than agglutination in tubes; the one drawback is that it is even less quantitative than the tube method. Generally one drop of appropriately diluted antiserum is mixed with one drop of a standardized cell or particle suspension on a glass slide. When the slide is viewed against a dark background, with side lighting, the formation of coarse agglutinates can usually be seen within minutes. Instead of glass slides, cardboard charts are often used in hemagglutination tests for routine blood-grouping purposes; after the agglutination has been performed, the chart can be dried and kept as a permanent record of the individual's blood group.

MICROSCOPIC VISUALIZATION OF AGGLUTINATION. In some cases only fairly small agglutinates are formed, which are not readily visible with the naked eye. Such agglutinates can then easily be distinguished under the microscope, at enlargements of $50 \times$ or $100 \times$. Normally, the entire tube in which the agglutination has occurred is placed under the microscope. The slide method is of course equally well suited for microscopic observation.

Hemagglutination

Active Hemagglutination. Active hemagglutination is the agglutination of red cells by antibodies specifically directed to antigens that are part of the red cell surface.

DIRECT ACTIVE HEMAGGLUTINATION. The great bulk of all the blood-grouping work is done by this method. As mentioned above, IgG antibodies are frequently incapable of achieving hemagglutination. Nevertheless, by physical or biochemical interference, hemagglutination can be obtained even with IgG-type antibodies. In the presence of high concentrations of high-molecular-weight substances such as bovine serum albumin (10 to 20%), or high concentrations of dextran, polyvinyl pyrrolidone, guaiacol, or other natural or synthetic polymers, agglutination with IgG-type antibodies becomes possible. The mechanism of this action is complex.

1. Many polymers, possibly owing to their colloid-osmotic pressure, cause erythrocytes to change their biconcave shape to a hollow, hemispheric, cup-shaped stomatocytic one, which allows the cells to approach one another over a larger portion of their surface area and thus to form stacks of cells, or "rouleaux."
2. An increase in colloid-osmotic pressure, caused by the high concentration of extracellular polymers, decreases the chemical potential of the inter-cellular water, and thus allows the cells to approach one another more closely.
3. The generally rather asymmetric high-molecular-weight polymers can cause cell aggregation by cross-linking cells through polymer bridging.
4. Some long-chained polymers, such as dextran, tend to cause spiculation in erythrocytes (probably through polymer bridging between different sites of attachment on the same cell). Spiculation (see Figure 6-11 for spiculation caused by anti-A antibodies) aids in allowing the cells to approach one another more closely in many places (see below).
5. Soluble polymers in high concentrations tend, by binding much water themselves, to decrease the degree of hydration of the antigenic determin-ants on the cell surface, which facilitates antigen-antibody binding (see Chapter 5).

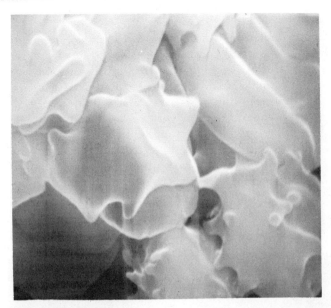

Figure 6-11. Group A_1, D-positive cells, agglutinated at room temperature in saline by an immune anti-A serum. Strong spiculation occurs. (From van Oss, C. J., and Mohn, J. F.: Scanning electron microscopy of red cell agglutination. *Vox Sanguinis*, **19**:432–43, 1970. By permission of S. Karger, Basel.)

6. As polymers of neutral electrical surface charge as well as strongly negatively charged polymers appear to be equally effective as hemagglutination-enhancing agents, the importance of their influence on the "zeta" potential of the cells is, at best, only slight. (For the influence of positively charged polymers, see above.)

Treatment of the red cells with proteolytic enzymes such as papain also can be highly effective in making agglutination by IgG-class antibodies possible. Figure 6-12 shows the drastic influence papain has on the red cell surface, involving stomatocytic changes (which allow the cells to approach one another over a larger surface area), as well as irregular extrusions (which permit a closer approach in more places). Papain also causes a reduction in the electric surface charge of the cells (see above).

All other methods for making hemagglutination with IgG-type antibodies possible tend, in one way or another, to bring the red cells closer together, which gives the specific IgG-type antibodies a chance to cross-link them. Once the mechanism for bringing them close together has been discontinued, only those cells that are actually cross-linked by specific antibodies will stay together. Means of bringing the cells closer together temporarily are shaking, centrifuging, aggregating by means of positively charged polyelectrolytes (e.g., Polybrene®, see above), or aggregating media of very

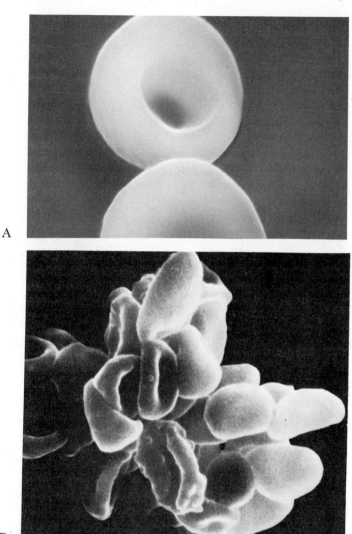

A

B

Figure 6-12. Scanning electron micrograph of red cells. *A.* Normal red cells. *B.* Red cells after treatment with papain. Strong changes in the surfaces of the cells are visible. (From van Oss, C. J., and Mohn, J. F.: Scanning electron microscopy of red cell agglutination. *Vox Sanguinis,* **19**:432–43, 1970. By permission of S. Karger, Basel.)

low ionic strength where the isotonic salt is being replaced by isotonic sugar, caused by cross-linking through the insolubilization of adsorbed euglobulins, principally IgM (Chapter 4).

By using finely divided fragments of red cell stromata, Milgrom has demonstrated that the hemagglutination reaction can take place in gels, so that

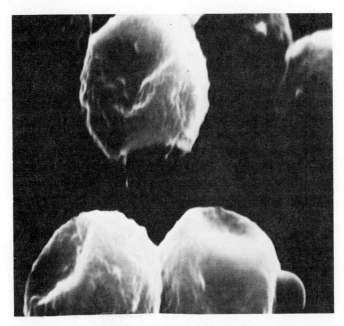

Figure 6-13. Group A_1, D-positive cells agglutinated in saline by an "incomplete" anti-D serum. The cells, although agglutinated, remain otherwise unchanged (compare with Figure 6-12 *A*). (From van Oss, C. J., and Mohn, J. F.: Scanning electron microscopy of red cell agglutination. *Vox Sanguinis*, **19**:432–43, 1970. By permission of S. Karger, Basel.)

the double-diffusion technique (see above) can be utilized, which simplifies the recognition of identity and nonidentity among blood group antigenic determinants.

The influence of antibodies of different specificities on the red cells can be considerable. Anti-A and anti-B blood group antibodies, for instance, caused the red cells to become strongly crenated or even spiculated (Figure 6-11), whereas anti-D(Rh_0) antibodies leave the red cells essentially unchanged (Figure 6-13). This tends to explain why even IgG anti-A antibodies can agglutinate group A cells, because the strong spiculation not only allows parts of the cells to approach one another much more closely, but it will also locally decrease the effective electric charge near the tips of the spicules. This also explains why IgG-type anti-D (Dh_0) antibodies are incapable of agglutinating group D (Rh_0) cells.

INDIRECT ACTIVE HEMAGGLUTINATION. In many cases where IgG-type antibodies can specifically bind to given antigenic determinants on the red cell surface without achieving agglutination, the indirect method of agglutination is used. In that method an antiserum to IgG is employed. After the red cells have been specifically coated with IgG antibodies, the rabbit anti-IgG antibodies are capable of cross-linking the red cells and

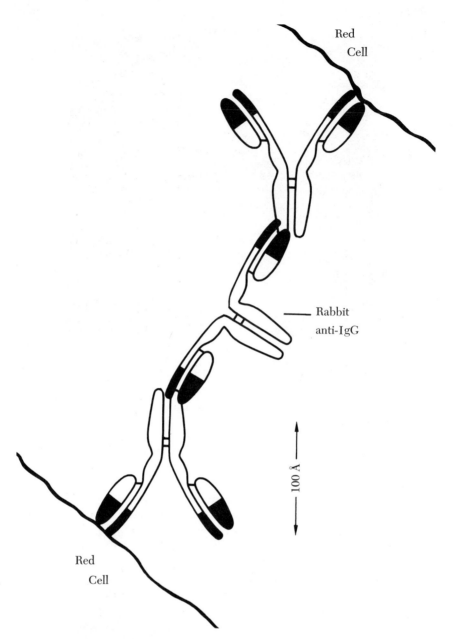

Figure 6-14. Diagram of the cross-linking of two red cells with the help of an anti-IgG antibody attached to the Fc pieces (Chapter 4) of each specific IgG-type antibody. The specific antibodies alone are incapable of bridging the distance between the two red cells and thus could not effect agglutination by themselves. It should be realized that, although only a small part of each red cell has been indicated here, their diameter is some 500 times the length of an IgG molecule.

thus cause agglutination. The reason why these anti-IgG antibodies can cross-link the red cells, while the initial specific IgG-type antibodies could not, lies mainly in their capacity of just providing the extra length, together with the specifically bound IgG molecules, to form the bridge between the two red cells (Figure 6-14). This test, which is also called the Coombs' test after the first author of the paper in which it was described, is a powerful tool in showing "incomplete" or "blocking" antibodies.

AUTOMATED HEMAGGLUTINATION. Automated tests are used more and more in clinical medicine, and a number of methods have been developed for the use of hemagglutination in automated machines. Agglutination is generally determined in one of two ways: (1) the cells and/or the agglutinates can be electronically counted with the help of a counter; (2) with the help of a T-shaped tube, the single cells can be separated from the agglutinated cells, after which the single cells are lysed. The quantity of hemoglobin thus released indicates, by difference with the total quantity of hemoglobin present in the initial sample, which proportion of the cells had been agglutinated and thus had not been lysed because they were removed.

Passive Hemagglutination. Passive hemagglutination is the agglutination of red cells by antibodies specifically directed to soluble antigens that have been previously adsorbed or otherwise attached to the red cell surface.

DIRECT PASSIVE HEMAGGLUTINATION. Most soluble polysaccharide antigens easily adsorb onto the red cell surface. Protein antigens do not spontaneously attach to red cells but will do so after the red cells have undergone ten minutes of treatment at $37°$ C with 0.005% tannic acid; tanned red cells form a much-used carrier for protein antigens. Tanned-cell hemagglutination is often used for the demonstration of antibodies to thyroglobulin. Protein antigens can also be chemically coupled to red cells by diazotization.

INDIRECT PASSIVE HEMAGGLUTINATION. This is the same method as the one mentioned above but it works indirectly, by means of an antiserum to IgG antibodies, in all such cases where IgG-type antibodies will not directly agglutinate the coated red cells.

INHIBITION OF PASSIVE HEMAGGLUTINATION. In certain systems it is more feasible to demonstrate the presence of soluble antigens through their interaction with antibodies directed to them; the more antibody has been bound, the less any residual antibody can agglutinate red cells coated with a given antigen and the higher its titer.

MIXED AGGLUTINATION. Mixed agglutination is a technique for demonstrating the presence of cell-surface antigens of a given type of cell, with the help of (sensitized) indicator red cells and antibodies that can cross-link both sensitized cell types.

Other Agglutination Methods

Bacterial Agglutination. Agglutination of bacteria as a test for the demonstration of the presence of bacterial antibodies in sera was, as

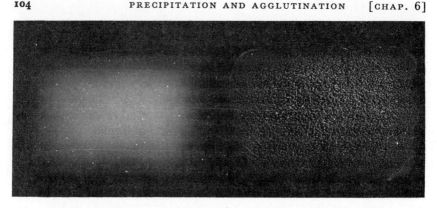

Figure 6-15. Passive agglutination of latex particles on a glass slide. Polystyrene latex particles (0.8-μm diameter), with human IgG adsorbed to their surfaces and forming a stable milky suspension (left), were agglutinated with rheumatoid factor containing serum (which is directed against human IgG) into a coarse agglomerate (right).

mentioned above, the oldest application of agglutination. The Widal test for the demonstration of typhoid and paratyphoid microorganisms as well as for the indication of typhoid and/or paratyphoid antibodies is still used. Other agglutination tests for the presence of bacterial diseases are performed with *Brucella abortus, Francisella tularensis,* and *Proteus* strains.

Passive Agglutination with Latex and Other Particles. Although bentonite and other particles of mineral origin have been used for some time as inert particulate carriers of antigens for the purpose of agglutination, a great advance was made by the introduction of monodisperse (all of one size) polystyrene latex particles. They were first used for the demonstration of rheumatoid factor (i.e., IgM antibody to altered human IgG) by Singer. Antigens are generally aspecifically adsorbed to the surface of the polystyrene beads, which have a uniform diameter of 0.8 μm (particles with a diameter of 0.25 μm are also used). Addition of specific antibody then transforms the latex (=milk) from a milky white liquid to a coarse suspension of visible granules (Figure 6-15). Latex "fixation" tests can be done in test tubes, but are more generally done on slides. Latex test kits are available for tests for rheumatoid factor, as well as for chorionic gonadotropic hormone (pregnancy test), C-reactive protein, antistreptolysin O antibodies, and antithyroglobulin antibodies.

Quantitative Agglutination Methods. SERUM AGGLUTININ DETERMINATION. This method is principally used for quantitative determinations of the agglutinin content of antibacterial sera. The method consists of incubating bacteria with the antiserum and then, after thorough washing, determining the difference in nitrogen content between bacteria that were agglutinated by antibody and the same number of bacteria that remained unreacted, as a control. Because this method depends on the measurement of small differences in nitrogen content between two fairly large total amounts of nitrogen, its accuracy is rather limited.

AGGLUTINATION WITH RADIOACTIVE ANTIBODIES. When specific agglutinins are tagged by chemically coupling them with a radioactive tracer, the amount of radioactivity adhering to the cells they agglutinated (under conditions of excess antibody) is a measure of the number of specific antibodies the antigenic determinants on the cells can accommodate. For instance, the number of antigenic determinants per red cell of various blood group specificities have been determined in this manner. For D (Rh-positive) cells it has been found that they contain above 10,300 antigenic determinants per cell when they are homozygous (DD) and 6400 antigenic determinants when they are heterozygous (Dd). On A cells the number of group A antigenic determinants is much higher: approximately 1,000,000 per A_1 cell. The considerable difference in number between blood group A and D antigenic determinants is most likely one of the reasons for the different effects anti-A and anti-D (Rh_0) antibodies have on the shape of the red cells (Figures 6-11 and 6-13).

Bibliography

Coombs, R. R. A.; Mourant, A. E.; and Race, R. R.: A new test for the detection of weak and "incomplete" Rh agglutinins. *Br. J. Exp. Pathol.*, **26**:255–66, 1945.

Fahey, J. L., and McKelvey, E. M.: Quantitative determination of serum immunoglobulins in antibody-agar plates. *J. Immunol.*, **94**:84–90, 1965.

Grabar, P., and Burtin, P. (eds.): *Immuno-electrophoretic Analysis*. Elsevier Publishing Co., New York, 1964.

Haber, J., and Rose, N.: Comparative studies of indirect hemagglutination. *Int. Arch. Allergy*, **34**:303–11, 1968.

Heidelberger, M.: *Lectures in Immunochemistry*. Academic Press, Inc., New York, 1956.

Kabat, E. A., and Mayer, M. M.: *Experimental Immunochemistry*, 2nd ed. Charles C Thomas, Publisher, Springfield, Ill., 1961.

Laurell, C. B.: Antigen-antibody crossed electrophoresis. *Anal. Biochem.*, **10**:358–61, 1965.

———: Quantitative estimation of proteins by electrophoresis in agarose gel containing antibodies. *Ibid.*, **15**:45–52, 1966.

Mancini, G.; Carbonara, A. O.; and Heremans, J. F.: Immunochemical quantitation of antigens by single radial immunodiffusion. *Immunochemistry*, **2**:235–54, 1965.

Milgrom, F.; Kano, K.; Barron, A. L.; and Witebsky, E.: Mixed agglutination in tissue culture. *J. Immunol.*, **92**:8–16, 1964.

Milgrom, F., and Loza, U.: Agglutination of particulate antigens in agar gel. *J. Immunol.*, **98**:102, 1967.

Ouchterlony, Ö.: *Handbook of Immunodiffusion and Immunoelectrophoresis.* Ann Arbor Science Publishers, Ann Arbor, Mich., 1968.

Prince, A. M., and Burke, K.: Serum hepatitis antigen (SH): rapid detection by high voltage immunoelectroosmophoresis. *Science,* **169**:593–95, 1970.

Schultze, H. E., and Heremans, J. F.: *Molecular Biology of Human Proteins,* Vol. 1. Elsevier Publishing Co., New York, 1966.

Singer, J. M.: The latex fixation test on rheumatic diseases. *Am. J. Med.,* **31**:766–79, 1961.

van Oss, C. J.: Methods used in the characterization of immunoglobulins. In Greenwalt, T. J. (ed.): *Advances in Immunogenetics.* J. B. Lippincott Co., Philadelphia, 1967, pp. 1–30.

van Oss, C. J., and Bronson, P. M.: Immunorheophoresis. *Immunochemistry,* **6**:775–78, 1969.

van Oss, C. J., and Mohn, J. F.: Scanning electron microscopy of red cell agglutination. *Vox Sanguinis,* **19**:432–43, 1970.

van Oss, C. J.; Mohn, J. F.; and Cunningham, R. K.: Influence of various physicochemical factors on hemagglutination. *Vox Sanguinis,* **34**:351–61, 1978.

Williams, C. A., and Chase, M. W. (eds.): *Methods in Immunology and Immunochemistry,* Vol. 3. Academic Press, Inc., New York, 1971.

7

Structural Basis of Antigen and Antibody Specificity

DAVID PRESSMAN AND ALLAN L. GROSSBERG

Introduction

The most striking feature of an antibody molecule is its great selectivity: the ability to combine most strongly with the structure that elicited its formation, less strongly with even closely related structures, and poorly with more distantly related structures. This selectivity of reaction is called specificity because antibodies can distinguish between antigenic structures by these gradations in their strength of binding. The gradations in strength of binding imply that differences in specificity are not reflected by all-or-none reactions. There is weaker binding of closely related structures, and the extent of this cross-reaction depends entirely on the difference in the structures of the two related molecules and the ability of the antibody to recognize this difference as described in this chapter.

Structural Features of Importance for Antigen-Antibody Combination

The most precise information about the nature of combination and the nature of specificity of the antigen-antibody interaction comes from studies of antigens composed of proteins combined with small groups, haptens, of known configurations. When a simple substance of known configuration is coupled to protein and injected, antibodies are formed that are directed against the hapten group, as shown by the fact that these antibodies will react in standard tests with an unrelated protein if it carries the hapten. The reaction must be through the hapten and antihapten antibody because the unrelated carrier protein can be shown to be nonreactive with the antibodies being tested. The hapten itself, without being coupled to protein, reacts with these antibodies, as shown by its ability to inherit precipitation of the antigen-antibody system, or by dialysis equilibrium experiments that show that the simple hapten is bound to antibody.

Antibodies can be against either charged or uncharged haptens. When antibodies are against charged haptens, the charge appears to play an important role in the combination. Antibodies have been formed against negatively and positively charged haptens, e.g., against the benzoate group and against the trimethylphenylammonium group. Antibodies can be against uncharged groups such as carbohydrate residues, hydrocarbon residues, and halogens as well as against charged groups. In each case, the antibody shows a close complementary fit against the grouping involved.

The structural features of importance can be evaluated by a study of the interaction of these antibodies with other haptens of known configuration related to the original one.

Closeness of Fit

As an example, antibodies against the *p*-azobenzoate group appear to fit closely around the van der Waals outline of the group (Figure 7-1). Benzoate ion itself combines well with this antibody. If a chlorine atom is substituted for a hydrogen atom in the para position, the hapten combines even more strongly than the unsubstituted benzoate. Apparently the chlorine atom fits into the position occupied by the azo group of the immunizing hapten, is accommodated by this antibody, and provides increased interaction energy relative to the hydrogen atom. When the chlorine atom replaces a hydrogen atom ortho to the carboxylate group, the fit of antibody around the hydrogen group is so close that the larger size of the chlorine atom interferes with the combination. When the chlorine atom is in the meta position, there is some interference in the combination. Investigations of this nature show the very close fit of the antibody around the benzoate group.

As for the other structural features, the benzene ring plays an important role in the combination with anti-*p*-azobenzoate antibody. Replacement of a benzene ring by a methyl group to give acetate reduces the binding energy to a very low level. Displacement of the benzene ring by about 1.5 Å by inserting a methylene group to give phenylacetate displaces it from its complementary position with respect to the carboxyl, and combination does not take place. Similarly, replacement of the benzene ring by

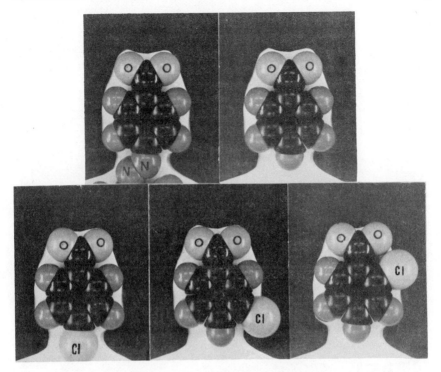

Figure 7-1. Effect on fit of substitution of azobenzoate and benzoate into combining region of anti-*p*-benzoate antibody. A chloro group is accommodated in the para position but not in the ortho and meta positions because of steric hindrance.

cyclohexane, which is somewhat thicker and does not have the polarizability of the benzene ring, causes a large decrease in combination energy. The benzene ring in proper orientation is important in many hapten systems.

Antibodies against some haptens appear to fit more closely than do antibodies against other haptens. For example, antibodies against the *p*-axophenyltrimethylammonium group and the *p*-(*p*'-azophenylazo)-phenyl-arsonate ion seem to fit less closely around the haptens than do antibodies against the *p*-azobenzenearsonate, *p*-azobenzoate, and *p*-(*p*-azophenylazo)-benzoate antigens. This is shown in Table 7-1, where metamethyl and orthomethyl substituents do not interfere with combination with the former antibodies but only with combination with the latter. Indeed, α-naphthyl derivatives show increased combination with the former, whereas decreased combination is observed with the latter, indicating that some antibodies can accommodate large substituents on one side, but others cannot. The increase, where observed, is probably due to increased van der Waals attraction of the naphthalene for the antibody or perhaps to water displacement.

Table 7-1
Closeness of Fit in Various para-Azohapten Systems

Hapten-Specific Antibody	Hapten[a]					
	(ring) *	(ring)–CH_3 *	(ring)–CH_3 *	(ring)–CH_3 *	(fused rings) *	(fused rings) *
	Relative Binding Constants					
$N{=}N$–(ring)–$N(CH_3)_3{}^+$	1.0	1.45	0.86	1.05	2.0	...
$N{=}N$–(ring)–AsO_3H^-	1.0	2.7	1.1	1.0	2.9	3.9
$N{=}N$–(ring)–AsO_3H^-	1.0	1.9	0.78	0.21	0.52	6.0
$N{=}N$–(ring)–$C{\overset{O}{=}}O^-$	1.0	1.8	0.21	0.03	0.03	1.98
$N{=}N$–(ring)–$C{\overset{O}{=}}O^-$	1.0	3.0	0.66	0.08	0.18	10.0

[a] The asterisk (*) represents $N(CH_3)_3{}^+$, AsO_3H^-, or COO^-, depending on the antibody system used.

Charge

When the antibody is directed against a charged group, the presence of the charge on the hapten is important for combination. Thus, antibody against benzoate shows essentially no combination with the nitrobenzene group in which the charged carboxylate of benzoate is replaced by an uncharged nitro group even though both groups have the same size. Specificity for the nature of the charged group is shown by the fact that if the carboxylate is replaced by the charged groups sulfonate or arsonate, there is essentially no combination, apparently because these charged groups are not accommodated by the antibody directed against the carboxylate grouping. The reason is not necessarily that the groups are too large, because the converse systems do not give good combination; i.e., benzoate does not combine well with antibenzenesulfonate or antibenzenearsonate antibodies.

When there are two charged groups on the hapten and they are close together, such as the two carboxylate groups in the orthophthalate group, two charges on a cross-reacting hapten are required for strong combination to occur. A single charge as in o-nitrobenzoate is insufficient. In this system, the energy contribution of the charge interaction is so large that the rest of the structure of the hapten is of lesser importance. Thus substituents on the ring are more easily accommodated.

If the haptenic group is not charged, other types of forces become important and additively give a comparable amount of energy of interaction.

Configuration and Conformation

Antibody directed against one optical isomer usually does not fit the antipode. Since the antibody fits the hapten in a complementary manner, as a glove fits a hand, the change from the D to the L configuration interferes much more with combination than a change in the size of the group, just as a right hand will fit into a right-hand glove, even of an incorrect size, much better than into a left-hand glove of correct size.

Another factor that can affect fit is the degree of flexibility of the hapten. If the hapten group is an extended chain, the antibody may be directed against a particular preferred orientation. This appears to be the situation with the azosuccinanilate group; this group seems to exist in a coiled configuration in aqueous solution, since antibodies directed against it combine well with succinanilate ion and also with the cis-maleanilate ion but combine only poorly with the trans-fumaranilate ion. Such cyclization of succinanilate could be stabilized by hydrogen bond formation between the carboxylate and the NH group (Figure 7-2) or perhaps between the carboxylate and the positive end of the carbonyl dipole. Benzoyl propionate seems to exist in the coiled configuration also. It combines well with antibody against the succinanilate ion, and antibody prepared against the p-azobenzoyl propionate group combines better with the cis-maleanilate ion than with the trans-fumaranilate ion.

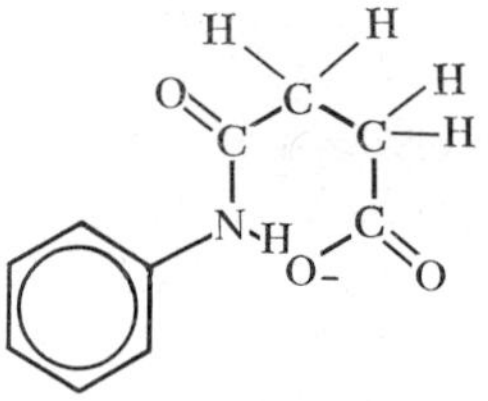

Succinanilate (coiled form)

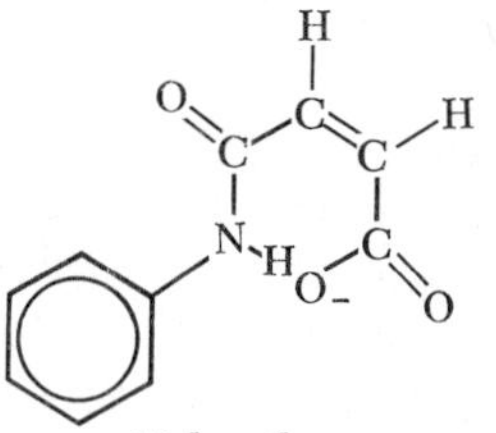

Maleanilate

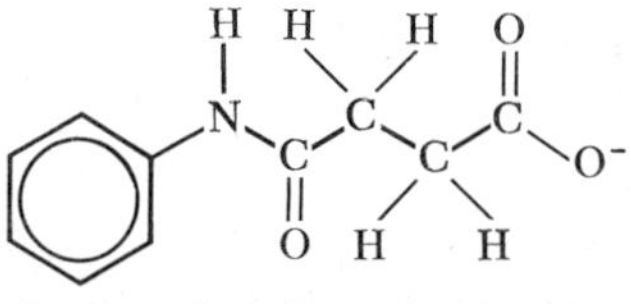

Succinanilate (extended form)

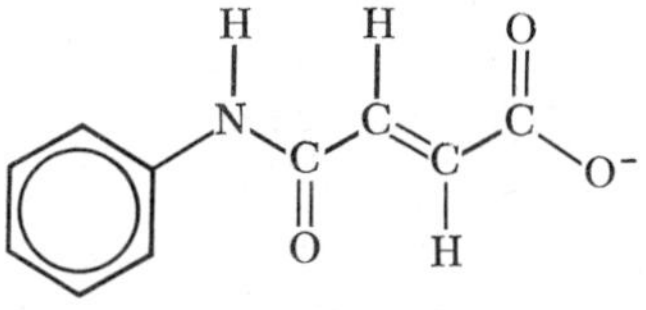

Fumaranilate

Figure 7-2. Extended and coiled forms of succinanilate compared with fumaranilate and maleanilate.

Another example of configurational factors is shown by antibody to the 4-azophthalate ion. Although the carboxylate group of a benzoate ion is coplanar with the benzene ring, this cannot be the situation for the carboxyl groups of a phthalate ion. In the phthalate ion, the carboxylates are tilted with respect to each other (Figure 7-3). This is reflected in the ability of the antibody to combine with the *o*-sulfobenzoate group, although benzene sulfonate does not combine with anti-*p*-azobenzoate antibodies. The accommodation of a sulfonate in place of a carboxylate by antiphthalate antibody may well be due to the fact that the antibody is directed against a much thicker charged region due to the tilting of the groups of the phthalate system, whereas the antibody is directed against the flat carboxylate group in the benzoate and cannot accommodate the sulfonate group.

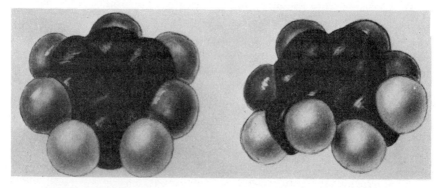

Figure 7-3. Coplanar configuration of carboxylate and benzene ring in benzoate and tilted orientation in phthalate.

Hydration

Another factor that affects fit is hydration of the molecule, since water of hydration can act sterically as a substituent on the molecule. The nitrogen of the pyridine ring is hydrated in aqueous solution. This water of hydration is a factor in the reaction with antibody. Antibodies against the o-, m-, and p-azobenzoate ions and p-(p-azobenzeneazo)-benzoate ion react with the pyridine carboxylate ions, picolinate, nicotinate, and isonicotinate as though there were a large substituent (water) on the ring in the position occupied by the nitrogen atom. The various quinoline carboxylate ions also combine with these antibodies as though there were a large substituent on the ring corresponding to the position of the nitrogen group. These results are consistent with hydration of the ring nitrogen atom. In the combination of antibody against the 4-azophthalate ion with pyridine dicarboxylate and with pyrazine dicarboxylate, the relative combining constant are 0.20 and 0.05, indicating increasing steric interference due to hydration of one- and two-ring nitrogen atoms.

Pyridine retains its water of hydration when antibodies are formed against the 3-azopyridine group. This is indicated by a region in the antibody site that can accommodate large substituents on haptens in which a benzene ring is substituted for the pyridine group. The size of this region is sufficient to accommodate large groups, such as iodo.

Hydration is not limited to the nitrogen atom, but it is probably an important factor with all the various groupings that either are charged or form hydrogen bonds. It may well be that structures written for many physiologically active substances that neglect the water of hydration are grossly incorrect with respect to their effective steric configurations.

These factors of fit and energy of reaction for the combining regions of antigens and antibodies are general factors concerned in any biologic interaction, e.g., that between enzyme and substrate.

Heterogeneity of Antibodies

Although antibodies act as though they were formed against the antigen as a template, all antibodies directed against a particular antigenic group are not necessarily identical. Antibody activity has been shown to be associated with different classes of immunoglobulin (Chapter 4). However, even antibodies of one immunoglobulin class directed against a particular antigenic group do not all have an identical combining region. A variety of different kinds of combining regions can bind one particular antigenic group. Thus, in the case of antibodies to the p-azobenzoate group (Figure 7-4), the combining regions can be directed in a large number of ways complementary to the surface of the benzoate group. All of these will react

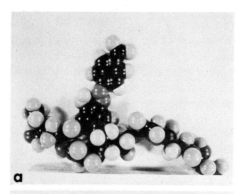

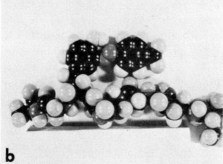

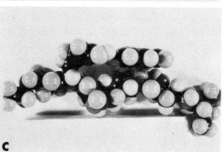

Figure 7-4. Different orientations of a haptenic group with respect to the surface of the antigen molecule. The representation is of a *p*-azobenzoate group (*a*) when extended from the surface of the carrier protein; (*b*) lying on its side; and (*c*) lying on its face.

with the benzoate group, although perhaps with different orientations of the benzoate and with different strengths of combination.

The fit of the antibody around the hapten cannot be perfect in that the extent of complementariness is limited by the ability of the polypeptide chains of the antibody to orient closely around the antigenic structures. This, in turn, depends on the flexibility of the polypeptide backbone and side-chain groups of the antibody molecule. The atoms of the antibody combining region are of the same size as the atoms composing the antigen, they occupy space, and are bound to other atoms. Thus, the degree to which a close complementary fit can occur is limited (Figure 7-5).

Individual animals appear to produce antibodies of relatively restricted heterogeneity against a given determinant. Thus, each individual rabbit

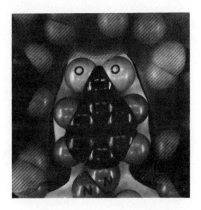

Figure 7-5. Representation of the combining region of an anti-*p*-azobenzoate antibody, indicating atoms of which the antibody is composed. Note the limitations of fit.

seems to produce only a few kinds of antibody molecules against the benzoate group. Indeed, some rabbits have been found to produce only one kind of antibenzoate antibody for extended periods of time (up to one year). This seems to be due to the stimulation of only one clone of antibody-producing cells and the concomitant shutting off of other potential antibody-producing cells.

Antibodies to Macromolecules: Groups Against Which Antibodies Are Formed

In the case of large molecules such as the proteins, there are apparently many different regions on the molecule against which antibodies are formed. Individual antibody molecules react with the protein, but each reacts with only one type of region. Cross-reactions of an antiserum formed against one protein with a closely related protein are apparently due to the reaction of some of the antibodies with similar regions on both proteins. The same antiserum may contain antibodies that do not react with the second protein. These are apparently formed against groupings present only on the first protein. A classic example of this type of phenomenon is the cross-reaction of antibodies prepared in rabbits against hen egg albumin. Some of the antibodies show extensive reaction with duck egg albumin, but other antibodies react only with hen albumin. The extent of cross-reaction has been particularly well studied in the case of serum albumins from several species. In general, the albumins of phylogenically related species have more antigenic groups in common than do the albumins of more distant species.

In the case of some protein molecules, it has been possible to split the protein into pieces and show that different fragments react with different groups of antibodies or that antibodies directed against individual fragments react with the intact protein; such has been the case with bovine serum albumin, rabbit γ globulin, horse myoglobulin, insulin, and silk fibroin. Indeed, structures of active fragments of the last three are known. In addition, synthetic polypeptides have been useful in studying the nature of groups that are antigenic.

In the case of polysaccharides, small structural units are repeated many times within the same molecule. Consequently, the number of different antigenic groups against which antibodies are directed may be fewer than formerly believed.

Chemical Nature of the Combining Region of Antibody

Most of this information has been obtained from studies of the effect of chemical alteration of antibody on its activity. Such studies are carried out by reacting antibody with a reagent that is known to react with a particular chemical group. Loss of activity indicates an effect in the binding site. However, even if the antibody is inactivated by reaction with a particular reagent, it must be proved that the loss of activity is caused by a reaction in the binding site and not by chemical alteration of the antibody molecule elsewhere, followed by a change in the general structure of the protein, which, in turn, disrupts the site. Moreover, although reagents are available that react predominantly with certain groups or amino acid residues, at least some reaction usually takes place with other residues. Therefore, it is important to demonstrate just which residue is attacked and to relate the attack of the particular residue to the loss of antibody activity.

Much information about the chemical composition of antibody sites has been obtained with five different antibodies: those directed against the p-azobenzenearsonate group (anti-R_p antibody), the p-azobenzoate group (anti-X_p antibody), the 3-azopyridine group (anti-P_3 antibody), the p-azophenyltrimethylammonium group (anti-A_p antibody), and the phosphorylcholine group (anti-PC antibody). In addition, ligand-binding sites of the myeloma proteins that bind phosphorylcholine have been studied. Information is thus available about antibodies against two negative groups, a neutral group, a positively charged group, and a group containing both a negative and a positive charge.

The combining regions of antibodies directed against different haptens necessarily differ since they have different specificities. Beside differences in complementary configuration, antibody directed against a positively charged group such as a p-azophenyltrimethylammonium group is different from antibody formed against the negatively charged p-azobenzoate group. In this instance, the difference in charge contributes to the specificity, since charge interaction is an important part of antibody-antigen combination. The antibody directed against the positively charged group has a negative charge in the combining region, and the antibody against a negative group has a positive charge in the combining region. The presence of these charges has been shown by the demonstration that the combining region with a negative charge attracts inorganic cations nonspecifically, whereas the region with a positive charge attracts anions. Antibody-combining regions to an uncharged group do not attract either type of ion preferentially.

The negative charge in the combining region of antibody directed to the positive charge on a hapten must necessarily be a carboxylate group. This has been proved to be the case. When such antibodies are treated with diazoacetamide, which is known to esterify carboxylate ions, the ability of the antibody to bind hapten is lost. The greater the degree of reaction, the greater the number of carboxyl groups esterified and the greater the loss of activity. Binding activity can be recovered by exposure of the esterified antibody to alkali, which hydrolyzes the ester, liberating the charged carboxylate group and activating the antibody site. Antibodies against negatively charged haptens are not affected by esterification, indicating that there is no carboxyl group in their combining regions. Other evidence of a negative charge in the combining region of the antipositive ion antibody is the fact that the antibody combines ten times as strongly with a hapten containing the trimethylammonium group as with one that contains a tertiary butyl group in its place. The tertiary butyl group has the same size and configuration as the trimethylammonium group but lacks the charge. Calculations based on energy supplied by charge interaction indicate that there must be a negative charge in the combining site close by, within 3 Å of closest approach.

The positive charge in the combining region of antibodies against a negative group could be contributed by an amino group such as the ε-amino of lysine or the α-amino at the end of a polypeptide chain, or by the guanidinium group of arginine. In the case of antibodies against the negatively charged benzoate, benzenesulfonate, and phthalate groups, it appears that the amino group plays a rather limited role, and the positive charge is probably due mainly to a guanidinium residue. On the other hand, amino groups appear to be more important in sites of antibodies against benzenearsonate than in antibenzoate antibodies but still not as important as the guanidinium groups. The contribution of amino groups has been shown by modifying the amino groups with maleic anhydride or N-carboxy-DL-alanine under conditions for which the tyrosines are not modified. The antibody lost a significant proportion but not all of its combining sites. The loss of sites could be prevented by the presence of specific hapten during maleylation and could be reversed by hydrolytic removal of the maleate group. Some antibenzenearsonate antibody molecules are affected by maleylation. The rest are inactivated by treatment with glyoxal or with 2,3-butanedione, reagents that modify the guanidinium groups irreversibly.

Antibodies or myeloma proteins that bind the phosphorylcholine group, which contains both a negatively charged phosphoryl group and a positively charged quaternary ammonium group, have been shown by the above methods to have specific binding sites that contain both the complementary positively charged guanidinium group and the negatively charged carboxyl group.

The nonpolar forces are probably contributed through the amino acids with a large hydrocarbon component such as phenylalanine, alanine, leucine, and isoleucine.

The tyrosine residue seems to be particularly important in the antibody-combining region. The antibodies of several antihapten antibodies contain a tyrosyl residue, as shown by various chemical reactions such as iodination and acetylation and by the fact that peptides isolated from the combining region of antibodies contain tyrosine. However, it is implicated to differing extents.

Relation of Antibody Sites to the Subunit Structure of the Antibody Molecule

The combining site of the antibody has been shown to lie in the Fab fragment, which includes both a light and part of a heavy chain (Chapter 4). Current evidence indicates that the antibody site in IgG globulin is formed from portions of both chains. It is likely, however, that the relative contributions of the two chains vary, depending on the particular antigenic determinant involved, the kinds of IgG globulin protein that make up the heterogeneous antibody preparations studied, and the animal species whose IgG globulin is considered.

There is evidence that both the heavy and light chains contribute to the binding site. Either chain, separated from the other, is able to combine with hapten, albeit much more weakly than when the chains are together as a unit in the original antibody. The heavy chain seems to combine more strongly than the light chain in the case of the rabbit antibodies thus far studied. Indeed, in order to show the binding by the isolated light chain directly, it was necessary to resort to the technique of fluorescence enhancement in which the hapten, when combined with antibody, becomes fluorescent so that a small amount of binding can be measured in the presence of a large amount of free hapten. Other evidence has come from virus inactivation studies and from chemical alteration studies.

X-ray crystallographic determination of the three-dimensional structure of Fab fragments of ligand-binding myeloma proteins has contributed information concerning the contribution of light and heavy chains to a binding site. These studies indicate that residues making up the combining site residue in the variable regions of both the heavy and light chains (Chapter 4). The residues involved appear to be located in the so-called hypervariable positions on these chains, i.e., the positions at which there is much greater variability in representation of individual amino acids than in other positions when sequences are compared for a large number of different light or heavy chains.

Confirmation of these results for induced antibodies will require isolation and identification of peptides from the site or from nearby. Experiments to this end have involved the paired-label iodination of tyrosyl residues in antibody sites and affinity-labeling techniques.

In general, isolated light chains and heavy chains from different IgG molecules will combine to give hybrid IgG molecules. However, in the case of the recombination of light and heavy chains from antibody there is a preferential combination of heavy and light chains with the correct alignment to give molecules with intact combining sites.

Bibliography

Cohen, S., and Porter, R. R.: Structure and biological activity of immunoglobulins. *Adv. Immunol.*, **4**:287–349, 1964.

Crumpton, M. J., and Wilkinson, J. M.: The immunological activity of some of the chymotryptic peptides of sperm-whale myoglobin. *Biochem. J.*, **94**:545–56, 1965.

Freedman, M. H.; Grossberg, A. L.; and Pressman, D.: The effects of complete modification of amino groups on the antibody activity of antihapten antibodies: reversible inactivation with maleic anhydride. *Biochemistry*, **7**:1941–50, 1968.

———: Evidence for ammonium and guanidinium groups in the combining sites of anti-*p*-azobenzenearsonate antibodies—separation of two different populations of antibody molecules. *J. Biol. Chem.*, **243**:6186–95, 1968.

Grossberg, A. L.; Krausz, L. M.; Rendina, L.; and Pressman, D.: The presence of arginyl residues and carboxylate groups in the phosphorylcholine-binding site of mouse myeloma protein, HOPC 8. *J. Immunol.*, **113**:1807–14, 1974.

Grossberg, A. L., and Pressman, D.: Nature of the combining site of antibody against a hapten bearing a positive charge. *J. Am. Chem. Soc.*, **82**:5478–82, 1960.

———: Modification of arginine in the active sites of antibodies. *Biochemistry*, **7**:272–79, 1968.

Grossberg, A. L.; Radzimski, G.; and Pressman, D.: Effect of iodination on the active site of several antihapten antibodies. *Biochemistry*, **1**:391–401, 1962.

Grossberg, A. L.; Roholt, O. A.; and Pressman, D.: Identification of heavy chain tyrosine 33 in the binding site of myeloma protein McPC 603 by paired label iodination. *J. Immunol.*, **116**:1596–1600, 1976.

Hooker, S. B., and Boyd, W. C.: The existence of antigenic determinants of diverse specificity in a single protein. III. Further notes on crystalline hen- and duck-ovalbumins. *J. Immunol.*, **30**:40–49, 1936.

Klostergaard, J.; Grossberg, A. L.; Krausz, L. M.; and Pressman, D.: Absence of lysine from the DNP-lysine binding site of protein 315; designation of lysine 52 of the heavy chain as a peripheral residue. *Immunochemistry*, **14**:37–44, 1977.

Landsteiner, K., and van der Scheer, J.: Serological studies on azoproteins: antigens containing azocomponents with aliphatic side chains. *J. Exp. Med.*, **59**:751–80, 1934.

Nisonoff, A., and Pressman, D.: The annular nitrogen of pyridine as a determinant of immunologic specificity. *J. Am. Chem. Soc.*, **79**:5565–75, 1957.

Pressman, D., and Grossberg, A. L.: *The Structural Basis of Antibody Specificity*. W. A. Benjamin, Inc., Menlo Park, Calif., 1968.

Pressman, D.; Roholt, O. A.; and Grossberg, A. L.: Chemical and structural differences between antibodies capable of binding a particular hapten group: evidence for limited heterogeneity. *Ann. N.Y. Acad. Sci.*, **169**:65–71, 1970.

Segal, D. M.; Padlan, E. A.; Cohen, G. H.; Silverton, E. W.; Davies, D. R.; Rudikoff, S.; and Potter, M.: The structure of McPC-603 Fab and its hapten complex. *Progr. Immunol.*, **2**:93, 1974, Brent, L., and Holborow, J. (eds.).

Sela, M.: Immunological studies with synthetic polypeptides. *Adv. Immunol.*, **5**:29–129, 1966.

Tiselius, A., and Kabat, E. A.: An electrophoretic study of immune sera and purified antibody preparation. *J. Exp. Med.*, **69**:119–27, 1939.

Weigle, W. O.: Immunochemical properties of the cross-reactions between anti-BSA and heterologous albumins. *J. Immunol.*, **87**:599–607, 1961.

8

Complement and Lysis

MANFRED M. MAYER

The Complement System

A major element in the system of humoral immunity is "complement," which refers to a group of proteins in blood serum and other body fluids that plays an important role as a mediator of both immune and allergic reactions when working together with antibodies or other factors (Chapter 1). The discoverers of complement thought that this agent merely helped antibody kill invading microorganisms, but the attack on invading cells is actually mediated by complement itself, and antibody itself identifies the invading cell as a foreign organism and activates the attack by complement. Thus, antibodies serve as information molecules that give the alarm when foreign cells invade the body. Actually, the alarm is not sounded by antibody as such but by the antigen-antibody complexes that are formed when antibodies combine with foreign antigens on the cell surface. Once activated, the intricately linked proteins, which make up the complement system, set into motion a series of processes that destroy the foreign cell.

Activation of the complement system poses a serious threat not only to invading microorganisms but also to the host's own cells. This self-destructive activity is reduced by various mechanisms that limit the dangerous potential of complement. One of these limitations results from spontaneous decay of activated complement components. Another entails interference by inhibitors in blood serum and other body fluids. The host's body is also protected because antibody fixes complement on the surface of the invading cell, thus directing the noxious activities of complement primarily against the foreign invader. However, the control of complement is not perfect and, sometimes, damage may be done to the host's own cells. Immunity is, therefore, a double-edged sword. When an immune process acts against the host's own cells, the result disrupts normal body system and processes. Such disruptions are known as allergic or hypersensitive reactions (Chapters 18 and 19).

There are 11 proteins in the complement system, all designated by the letter C and by number: C1, C2, C3, and so on up to C9. Complement factor C1 is actually made up of three subunits designated C1q, C1r, and C1s, which are held together by noncovalent bonds involving calcium ion. The numbers of the complement proteins indicate the sequence in which they react, with the exception of C4, which reacts between C1 and C2. This exception occurs because numbers were assigned before the reaction sequence was fully understood.

As the study of complement has progressed, it became evident that the 11 proteins of the complement system are subunits of three macromolecular assemblies, namely: (1) the C1q,r,s macromolecule, which is responsible for recognition of the foreign invader and for giving the alarm; (2) and $\overline{\text{C4b,2a,}}$ $\overline{\text{3b}}$ enzyme, which activates the assembly of the cytolytic attack element; and (3) the cytolytic attack element itself, which comprises complement proteins C5b through C9. Thus, what we find in blood serum or in other body fluids are only the building blocks from which each of these elements of the complement system is assembled once the activation signal has been given (Figure 8-1).

Recognition and Alarm Element: C1q, r, s

The recognition unit of the complement system is C1q. This molecule is able to combine with antigen-antibody complexes through receptors in the Fc segment of the antibody molecule. When antibody molecules combine with antigens, they change shape and this event may mobilize receptors in the Fc region that bind C1q. A reaction involving tryptophan residues in the Fc segment then activates C1q. In turn, this leads to activation of C1s to the enzymatic state designated $\overline{\text{C1s}}$ (the bar indicates the activated state). It has been found that the C1r subunit plays the role of an intermediate agent between C1q and C1s in the process of activation.

Only IgM and several subclasses of IgG have the capacity to bind and activate the C1q,r,s assembly. IgA, which is present in saliva and other secretions, and immunoglobulin IgE, a prominent mediator of allergic reactions, do not fix and activate C1q,r,s. Presumably, their Fc regions lack the receptors necessary for interaction with C1q. In the case of IgM, a single molecule of antibody on the surface of a cell is able to bind and activate

C1q,r,s, but in the case of IgG, two adjacent molecules are required for such binding. Since antibodies reactive with a cell scatter at random over its surface, the probability of two IgG molecules occupying adjacent sites is small and, therefore, it is necessary to add a large number of IgG antibody molecules to each cell to create one receptor site for C1q,r,s. In the case of the sheep erythrocyte, as many as 800 IgG antibody molecules per cell may be needed.

Much work has been done on the properties of C1q,r,s and the nature of the enzymatic action of $\overline{C1s}$. During the early days of complement research many believed that this enzyme acts on a component of the cell surface. However, this is not true. Instead, the enzymatic activity is directed against two of the other components of the complement system, namely, C4 and C2. This discovery, a turning point in complement research, opened the way to the recognition that activation of the complement system sets off a cascade of successive enzymatic reactions through which the various biologic activities of complement are generated.

Assembly of the $\overline{C4b,2a,3b}$ Enzyme

The assembly of this enzyme is initiated when $\overline{C1s}$ attacks the complement protein C4 and cleaves it into a large fragment, C4b, and a small fragment, C4a. The process of cleavage exposes a chemical group on C4b through which this fragment can combine with a receptor on cell surfaces. However, the binding site on C4b has a short life and, consequently, only a small proportion of the many C4b fragments that are produced become bound to a cell surface. The other C4b fragments, having lost their binding groups, remain in an inactive state in the fluid phase.

The next step involves adsorption of complement protein C2 to the cell-bound C4b. This reaction is promoted by magnesium salts. Following its adsorption, the C2 molecule is cleaved by a neighboring $\overline{C1s}$ molecule into two large fragments. One, C2a, becomes bound to C4b, yielding the complex $\overline{C4b,2a}$, which is an active enzyme as indicated by the symbol. The C2a subunit contributes the active site of the enzyme. The natural substrate of $\overline{C4b,2a}$ is complement protein C3.

The recognition that $\overline{C4b,2a}$ has the capacity to cleave complement protein C3 represents another discovery of major importance. One of its most interesting aspects concerns the fact that C3a and C3b, the products of cleavage of complement protein C3, possess biologic activities that play an important role in immune and allergic processes. The small fragment, C3a, molecular weight about 9000, can cause the release of histamine from cells that store this substance (basophilic leukocytes, mast cells, and platelets). The histamine increases the permeability of the blood capillaries, which enables white blood cells to penetrate into tissues in which an infectious or allergic process is underway. Thus, C3a mediates inflammation.

The larger fragment, C3b (molecular weight about 181,000), has a chemical group through which it is able to bind covalently to receptor groups on cell surfaces. However, the binding group of C3b has a short life and, consequently, only some of the many C3b molecules generated by $\overline{\text{C4b,2a}}$ become bound to the cell surface. The remainder, having lost their binding group through decay, remain in the fluid phase in an inactive state. The C3b fragments that combine with the cell surface bestow the property of immune adherence. Thus, cells carrying C3b tend to adhere to leukocytes or other cells. Immune adherence promotes phagocytosis (Chapter 10) and, consequently, the cell-bound C3b fragments contribute to defense against infection by microbes. Those C3b fragments that become bound in the proper spatial orientation adjacent to the $\overline{\text{C4b,2a}}$ enzyme become part of this complex thus converting it to the state $\overline{\text{C4b,2a,3b}}$. This trimolecular complex is another enzyme, as the symbol indicates; its substrate is complement protein C5.

Formation of the Cytolytic Attack Element: C5b–9

$\overline{\text{C4b,2a,3b}}$ cleaves complement protein C5 into two unequal fragments. The small fragments, C5a, molecular weight about 17,500, is a chemotactic factor. Like C3a, it has the capacity to mediate release of histamine from cells that store this chemical. The large fragment, C5b, molecular weight about 189,000, plays a cardinal role in the initiation of the cytolytic action of the terminal complement components. C5b is extremely short-lived and decays to an inactive form, $C5b^d$. Complement protein C6, which has the capacity to combine reversibly with C5b, serves to stabilize C5b in its activated state; i.e., C6 prevents decay to $C5b^d$. Therefore, in experimental studies of the cytolytic attack system, the C5b,6 complex is commonly used to initiate the membrane attack by the terminal components.

The C5b,6 complex can be prepared by elution from EAC1-6 (i.e., erythrocytes carrying antibody and complement proteins C1 to C6). However, since the preparation of EAC1-6 is quite laborious and the yield of C5b,6 by this procedure is poor, it is preferable to use a method in which certain pathologic human sera (e.g., sera from rheumatoid arthritis patients) are incubated briefly with yeast cell mannan (zymosan). This leads to generation of C5b,6 via the alternative pathway (see below). C5b,6 can be eluted readily from the zymosan particles. Purified C5b,6 is stable and can be stored over extended periods of time.

The cytolytic sequence is started by formation of the C5b,6,7 complex from C5b,6 and C7. Freshly formed C5b,6,7 has the capacity to combine with plain erythrocytes (i.e., red cells not carrying antibody and complement components) and to prepare them for lysis by C8 and C9. C5b,6,7 is highly labile in the fluid phase and quickly loses its capacity to combine with erythrocytes. On the other hand, the product of its reaction with erythrocytes, designated EC5b,6,7, is stable (Figure 8-1). The experimental method

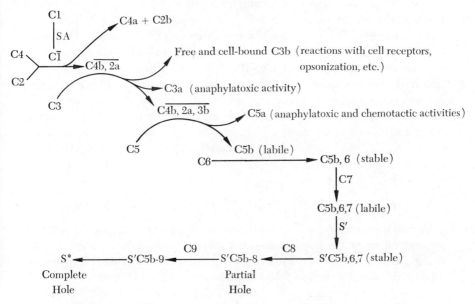

Figure 8-1. Schematic representation of the reaction sequence of the complement system. The symbols S and S′ represent sites on the cell membrane, A represents antibody, and C1, C2, C3, through C9 stand for the complement proteins. The bar over certain numbers, such as C$\overline{1}$, indicates an active enzyme. C4a, C4b, C2a, and C2b are fragments of C4 and C2, respectively. C3a and C5a are polypeptide fragments that mediate release of histamine from cells carrying this chemical and are designated anaphylatoxins. The C5a fragment also possesses chemotactic activity. The cell-bound C3b conveys the property of immune adherence to cells or immune complexes carrying this fragment and thus opsonizes them, i.e., renders them susceptible to phagocytosis (Chapter 10). The C$\overline{4b,2a,3b}$ enzyme activates C5 by cleavage, and the resulting C5b fragment combines with C6 and C7 to yield the trimolecular C5b,6,7 complex, which then becomes embedded in the phospholipid moiety of the cell membrane at a site designated S′. C5b,6,7 complexes that fail to combine with S′ lose their membrane reactivity, but the decayed C5b,6,7 still exhibits chemotaxis. At the C8 stage, cells begin to leak, as indicated by the designation "partial hole." C9 accelerates leakage greatly, thus producing the complete hole designated S*. The following are molecular weight estimates for the human complement proteins: C1—about 1 million; C1q—410,000; C1r—190,000; C1s—86,000; C2—98,000; C2a—72,000; C2b—32,000; C3—190,000; C3a—9000; C3b—181,000; C4—204,000; C5—206,000; C5a—17,500; C6—128,000; C7—121,000; C8—153,000; C9—79,000. Estimates for guinea pig complement are C2—130,000; C3—179,000; C4—180,000; C5—180,000; C6—130,000; C7—130,000; C8—150,000; C9—78,000.

known as the "reactive lysis" system was designed to minimize the decay of C5b,6,7 in the fluid phase by arranging for its formation in the presence of the target erythrocytes.

The nascent C5b,6,7 complex can react also with certain bacteria and with liposomes to yield the intermediates BC5b,6,7 and LC5b,6,7, respectively. On treatment with C8 and C9, BC5b,6,7 are killed and LC5b,6,7 are rendered leaky with respect to their aqueous contents. These liposome experiments, as well as numerous other studies with vesicular or planar lipid bilayers, indicate that the cytolytic attack by the terminal complement components, C5b-9, is directed against the lipid bilayer of membranes. Therefore, the mechanism of cytolytic attack by C5b-9 must be viewed in relation to the structure and properties of the lipid bilayer.

Fluidity of the Phospholipid Bilayer of Cell Membranes

Recent advances in studies of cell membrane structure have led to a better understanding of the possible mode of attack by the C5b-9 complex. The major components of cell membranes are lipids, proteins, and carbohydrates. The fundamental structure of the membrane is a double layer of phospholipid, in which the hydrophilic heads of the phospholipid molecules point outward toward the aqueous phase and the hydrophobic tails point inward. Compounds soluble in lipid, such as sterols, may float in the hydrophobic region of this bilayer. Some of the protein molecules are bound to the hydrophilic regions of the bilayer. Others are embedded partially in the bilayer, and some protein molecules penetrate the entire width of the bilayer. Carbohydrate molecules, being hydrophilic, would not be expected to penetrate into the interior of the phospholipid bilayer; they are probably oriented toward the aqueous phase. A crucial element of this model of membrane structure is that the phospholipid bilayer behaves like a viscous fluid, provided the temperature is not too low. Individual phospholipid molecules move rapidly within each of the leaves of the bilayer. As a consequence of the fluid state of the membrane lipids, the proteins of the cell membrane are also free to move laterally in the phospholipid domain, at least in the case of cells such as lymphocytes. With other cells, like erythrocytes, the proteins occupy fixed positions. This is not due to lack of fluidity of the phospholipid bilayer but can be attributed to linkage of the proteins in a rigid structural framework.

Donnan Effect

When cells are attacked by complement, they swell until the cell membrane ruptures explosively and the contents of the cell spill. The cause of the swelling is the Donnan effect, a physicochemical phenomenon observed with semipermeable membranes that pass small molecules or ions such as water and common salts, but do not pass large molecules, such as proteins or nucleic acids. When such a membrane comes into contact with a solution of protein, salt, and water on one side and a solution of salt and water on the other side, salt and water flow through the pores of the membrane toward the protein side.

Living cells contain protein and other macromolecules and, hence, would be subject to the Donnan effect if their membranes behaved like the artificial semipermeable membranes just described. In fact, cell membranes do not behave this way. They have transport mechanisms that actively move various substances across the membrane barrier. However, when a cell membrane is damaged by complement, it behaves like a semipermeable membrane with respect to the fact that salt and water, and other small molecules, readily flow across it. The simplest explanation for this change would be that complement makes holes in the membrane large enough to permit salt and water and other small molecules to pass, but too small to allow macromolecules, such as protein and nucleic acids, to leave the cell.

One-Hit Theory

In developing a plausible model for the cytolytic attack mechanism, one must consider the restriction imposed by the one-hit theory (Figure 8-2). This theory was developed during the 1950s from kinetic and statistical studies. When initially formulated, and until the mid-1960s, it was the accepted interpretation of this theory that a single lesion in the membrane of a cell actually suffices for lysis. However, this view became questionable when it was learned that $\overline{C1}$ produces $\overline{C4b,2a}$ complexes enzymatically, and that on reaction with C3b these are converted to $\overline{C4b,2a,3b}$, which produces C5b,6,7 complexes. Thus, a single $\overline{C1}$ can generate a series of sites carrying $\overline{C4b,2a}$ and, in turn, after conversion to $\overline{C4b,2a,3b}$, each of these can generate a series of sites in the phospholipid bilayer of the cell membrane where C5b,6,7 complexes have become embedded. In light of the discovery of these two stages of enzymatic amplification, it could no longer be assumed, a priori, that the concordance of the C1, C4, and C2 reactions with the one-hit theory necessarily indicates a single membrane lesion to be sufficient for lysis of a cell. This issue was reopened in connection with studies of the C9 reaction. Since this is the last step in the reaction sequence, the preceding amplification effects in the enzymatic action of $\overline{C1}$ and $\overline{C4b,2a,3b}$ play no part. Also, there is no evidence that an amplifying reaction giving rise to multiple membrane lesions takes place after the C9 reaction. Accordingly, the reaction of guinea pig C9 with EAC1-8 prepared with guinea pig complement components conforms to the one-hit theory, and production of a single hole in the cell membrane by the cytolytic attack element C5b-9 is sufficient for lysis of a cell.

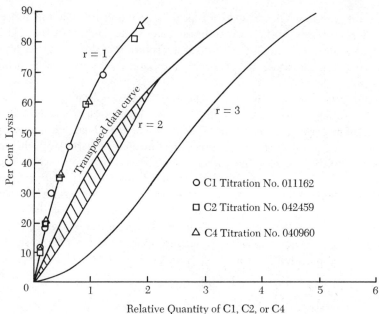

Figure 8-2. Experimental test of the one-hit theory. Comparison of C1, C2, and C4 titration curves with theoretic response curves calculated from the binomial probability distribution for threshold values of r = 1, r = 2, r = 3. The relative quantities of C1, C2, and C4, plotted on the abscissa, were adjusted factorially in order to superimpose the experimental curves upon one another. For the purpose of visual discrimination, the line through the data is also shown in a transposed position so as to superimpose its upper segment on that of the r = 2 curve. The stippled part outlines the area in which experimental measurements must discriminate between a fit with an r = 1 or r = 2 model.

Formation of a Transmembrane Channel by C5b–9

Since a single membrane lesion suffices for lysis of a cell, theoretic studies of membrane damage by complement have been restricted to those mechanisms that produce a focal lesion. Also, since the attack by complement is directed against the lipid bilayer of cell membranes, this lesion is situated in the lipid moiety of biomembranes. Two hypothetic models for the generation of such a focal lesion have been considered.

The first of these postulates production of a leaky patch, either by direct enzymatic attack on membrane lipids or by enzymatic generation of a detergent substance. In effect, such a leaky patch would be a transient hole in the fluid bilayer of the membrane that could persist only as long as enzymatic action continues.

There are clear indications that the enzymatic splitting of membrane phospholipids does not play a role in the attack by complement on membranes. For example, complement causes release of a water-soluble marker from liposomes made up of lecithin analogs that are not susceptible to attack by phospholipases. Furthermore, it has been found that planar bilayers made of oxidized cholesterol are susceptible to attack by C5b-9. These observations eliminate the possibility of direct enzymatic damage to the membrane by phospholipases, as well as the possibility of indirect damage through enzymatic production of a phospholipid derivative, such as lysolecithin, that perturbs the bilayer structure. This leaves us with only one method for production of a leaky patch, namely, by generation of a membrane active substance through enzymatic interaction among the terminal complement proteins themselves. This type of mechanism would require one terminal complement protein sufficient to supply substrate for generation of the 10^8–10^9 molecules of detergent substance that are usually required for lysis of a single erythrocyte. Obviously, it is unlikely that this requirement could be met.

The second hypothesis, termed the doughnut model (Figure 8-3), describes a stable transmembrane channel through which water and solutes of low molecular weight can pass between the interior of the cell and the extracellular environment. The late-acting complement proteins, C5b-9, represent the most probable source of the structural components of the transmembrane channel. Presumably, this is formed by insertion of polypeptide chains from the terminal complement components into the phospho-

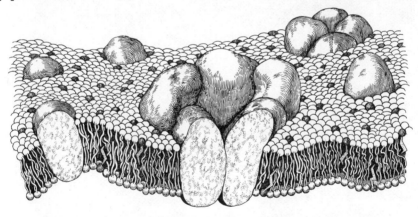

Figure 8-3. Artist's conception of a cell membrane showing a cytolic complement doughnut in the foreground. The cross-sectional view in the foreground reveals the bilayer structure of the membrane. The flexible hydrophobic tails of the phospholipid molecules and the rigid hydrophobic portion of sterol molecules are shown. The hydrophilic heads of the phospholipids are shown on top as white circles, and the sterols are drawn as black circles. Membrane proteins are shown floating in the lipid matrix. The multiunit structure of membrane proteins near the upper right-hand corner depicts "a transport pore" through which small molecules or ions may enter or leave the cell in a controlled manner.

lipid bilayer of the membrane. In the case of cells, but not liposomes, the channel would give rise to net uptake of salt and water due to the Donnan effect, resulting in swelling and rupture of the cells.

A growing body of information supports this insertion hypothesis. Specifically, the information of the transmembrane channel by C5b-9 involves at least three successive steps. In the first step, polypeptide chains from the C5b and C7 subunits of the nascent C5b,6,7 complex become partially inserted in the lipid bilayer. In the second step, C8 reacts with the inserted C5b,6,7 and extrudes a polypeptide chain that also becomes inserted. In the third step, C9 reacts with the partially inserted C5b-8 complex, and this leads to insertion of a polypeptide chain from C9 into the membrane, thus completing assembly of the channel.

The evidence for these concepts comes from four distinct experimental approaches, namely: (1) enzymatic stripping experiments, (2) elution experiments, (3) electrical conductance measurements of planar bilayer membranes that have been treated with the terminal complement com-

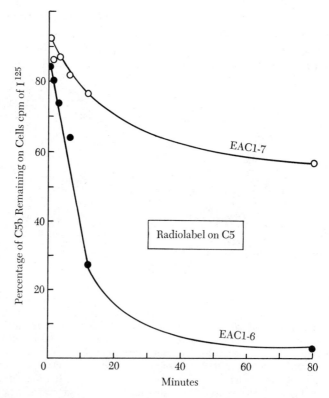

Figure 8-4. Kinetics of tryptic removal of ^{125}I from EAC1-6 or EAC1-7 carrying ^{125}I-C5b. Digestion at 27° C; ionic strength 0.074.

ponents, and (4) experiments on the generation of hydrophobic regions during activation of complement.

For example, enzymatic stripping experiments have shown that tryptic digestion of EAC1-7, carrying either ^{125}I-C5 or ^{125}I-C7, removes only about half of the radioiodine associated with C5 or C7. Similarly, tryptic or chymotryptic digestion of EAC1-8 and EAC1-9, prepared with either ^{125}I-C8 or ^{125}I-C9, releases only 9 to 19% of the cell-bound radioactivity. Thus, these complement proteins behave in part like integral membrane proteins. On the other hand, in the case of the EAC1-6 intermediate, radiolabeled C5 can be removed completely, which indicates that at this stage of the reaction sequence, C5 behaves like a peripheral membrane protein. It is believed that the process of insertion starts at the C7 stage of the reaction sequence (Figure 8-4), i.e., that the nascent C5b,6,7 becomes inserted in the membrane. This interpretation is supported by elution experiments that indicate that radiolabeled C5 can be eluted readily from EAC1-6 but not from EAC1-7. Elution experiments have also shown that neither C5 nor C9 can be eluted from EAC1-9. In the case of C9, the inserted polypeptide chain has a molecular weight of 18,000, which corresponds to one-fourth of the native C9 molecule.

Support for the insertion hypothesis has also come from experiments in which electrical conductivity across planar lecithin bilayer membranes was

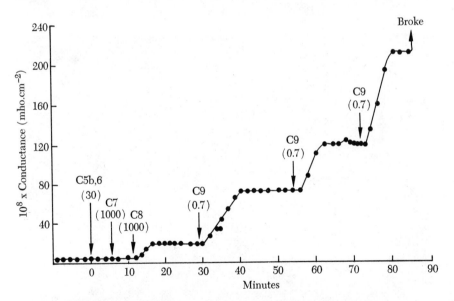

Figure 8-5. Sequential action of complement components on a planar lipid bilayer made of lecithin. The vertical arrows mark the time of each protein addition. The total number of units of activity added in each instance is given in parentheses. A small but significant increase of ion flow is seen after addition of C8. Following addition of C9, ion flow increases markedly.

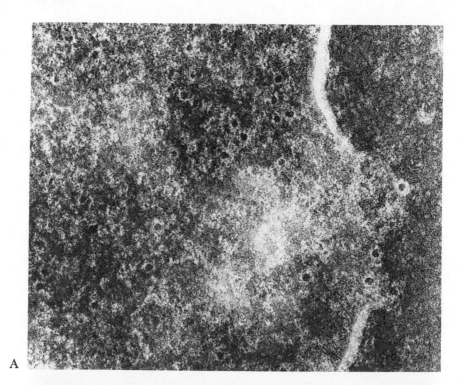

A

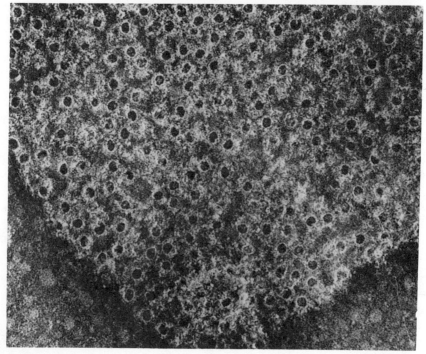

B

measured. When such membranes are treated with C5b,6 plus C7, C8, and C9, a large increase in conductivity is observed (Figure 8-5). The characteristics of this process are in accord with the hypotheses that the terminal complement components form a transmembrane channel. In similar experiments, terminal complement components produced substantial conductivity increments in membranes made from oxidized cholesterol. This rules out the possibility that the membrane attack by complement involves hydrolysis of phospholipids.

Presumably, the process of insertion of polypeptide chains is a consequence of extrusion of hydrophobic polypeptide regions from the interior of the terminal complement proteins. Thus, the reaction of C7 with the C5b,6 complex triggers a conformational change that causes extrusion of peptides from C5b and C7. Similarly, the reaction of C8 with the C5b,6,7 complex is believed to trigger a conformational change in the C8 molecule that causes extrusion of a hydrophobic polypeptide from its interior. A similar process also occurs on reaction of C9 with the C5b-8 complex. These ideas are supported by the observation that activated complement removes phospholipid from the surface of *Escherichia coli* or liposomes.

If the extrusion of these hydrophobic domains occurs in the immediate vicinity of a lipid bilayer, it is reasonable to assume that insertion will occur. On the other hand, if a lipid bilayer is not accessible nearby, the extruded hydrophobic polypeptides will probably undergo aggregation. This would lead to loss of membrane reactivity and hemolytic capacity. These observations and the associated hypothesis suggest that the process of insertion and transmembrane channel formation by the terminal complement components is a complex series of reactions in which individual complement proteins react with one another and with membrane lipids so that the multiunit structure of the transmembrane channel is assembled within the lipid bilayer of the cell membrane.

Complement Lesion Seen by Electron Microscopy

Electron micrographs of cell membranes that have been attacked by complement actually show crater-like lesions in the membrane (Figure 8-6). Each of these characteristic lesions has a light ring with a dark central portion. The ring appears to be a raised surface and the dark center appears

Figure 8-6. (*Opposite*) Complement lesions seen by electron microscopy with negative staining (× 374,000). Micrograph showing a sheep erythrocyte membrane treated with anti-Forssman antibody and guinea pig complement. The lesions have an internal diameter between 8.5 and 9.5 nm. *B.* Micrograph showing a human erythrocyte membrane treated with anti-I antibody and human complement. The internal diameter of the lesions is between 10 and 11 nm. (Courtesy of Robert R. Dourmashkin of the Clinical Research Center at Harrow, Middlesex, England.)

as a depression in the membrane. Alternatively, the light ring may be a hydrophobic region and the dark center, a hydrophilic area. The lesions are uniform in size. Those produced in red blood cells by guinea pig complement range between 8.5 and 9.5 nanometers internal diameter; those produced by human complement range between 10 and 11 nanometers. Complement from each species seems to produce lesions of a characteristic size.

However, the lesions seen by electron microscopy are not necessarily holes. Rather, they appear to be structures that are characteristic of the membrane attack by complement. This is evident from the free ring-shaped structures observed by electron microscopy of liposomes treated with complement (Figure 8-7). The free rings have probably become detached from membranes, together with lipid. A profile view of a complement lesion associated with the lipid bilayer of a liposome is shown in Figure 8-8. In this context, it should be noted that assembly of the C5b-9 complex in the aqueous phase,

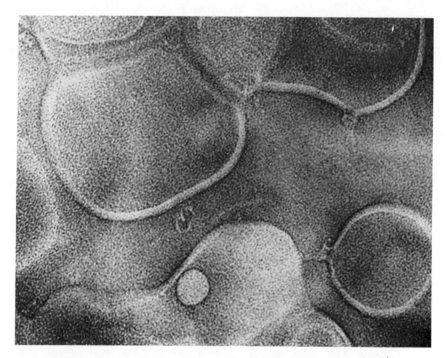

Figure 8-7. Lesions made by complement in liposomes. The liposomes (large circular shapes) in this electron micrograph were prepared from sphingomyelin and cholesterol. These lipids form concentric bilayers that enclose water and ions. When the trimolecular complex C5b,6,7, as well as C8 and C9, is added to the liposomes, lesions form in the bilayer. Detached lesions in this micrograph indicate that once the lesions are formed, they are relatively stable. Other lesions appear on the surface of liposomes.

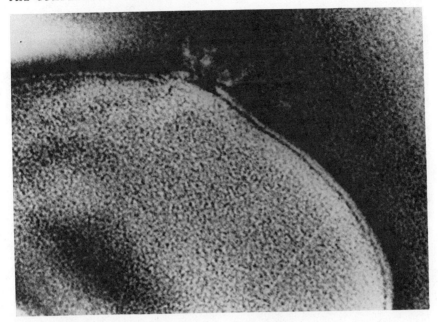

Figure 8-8. Complement lesion in profile. A funnel-shaped complement lesion in a liposome prepared from lecithin (about 10 or 11 nanometers thick) with a hollow core appears hydrophilic because it is penetrated by the stain.

i.e., in the absence of a lipid bilayer, does not yield structures such as those shown in Figures 8-6, 8-7, and 8-8.

In studies with cultured lymphocytes, the susceptibility to lysis by complement is restricted to the resting stage. Nevertheless, the characteristic complement lesions have been observed at all stages of the cell cycle. Cell membranes may undergo cyclic changes that affect susceptibility to damage by the membrane attack element C5b-9. This could be due to changes in accessibility of the phospholipid bilayer of the cell membrane. The presence of the characteristic lesion does not necessarily indicate a hole. Conversely, however, a hole through the membrane, when formed, probably is directly associated with the lesion.

The freeze-fracture technique of electron microscopy, in which a frozen membrane is cleaved along the plane of its bilayer, thus exposing the interior of the membrane, has also produced evidence that the terminal complement components form transmembrane channels. Sheep erythrocytes treated with antibody and complement showed globular doughnut-shaped aggregates made of several units not found in similar cells treated with antibody alone (Figures 8-9 and 8-10). What is of cardinal importance and what was first demonstrated is that complement lesions actually penetrate the lipid bilayer.

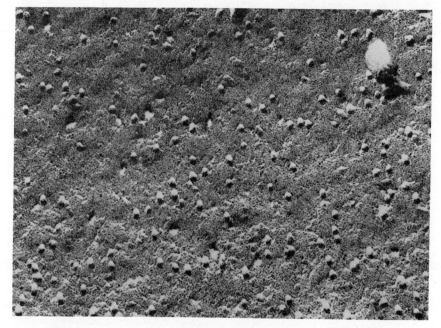

Figure 8-9.   Electron micrograph of freeze-fractured membrane of sheep red blood cell treated only with antibody (× 210,000). The fracture takes place between the two leaves of the lipid bilayer of the membrane. The interior of the membrane is visible. The protein globules penetrating the membrane are normal in size, shape, and distribution.

Alternative Pathway

The incubation of normal blood serum with microbial cells, certain microbial polysaccharides (such as zymosan, a carbohydrate of the yeast-cell membrane, or endotoxic lipopolysaccharide from gram-negative bacteria), certain kinds of immune complexes, or a factor from cobra venom activates the complement system by a route that bypasses antibody C1, C4, and C2. When this pathway was discovered in the early 1950s, it was thought to involve a single agent called properdin. Later it was learned that this alternative pathway of complement activation is a complex enzyme system that becomes activated on incubation with microbial cells or other agents. The alternative pathway comprises two closely related enzymes that activate C3 and C5, respectively, by cleavage. Both enzymes are multiunit complexes and correspond in their respective functions to the C4b,2a and C4b,2a,3b complexes of the classical pathway. They can be distinguished from these classical enzymes by insusceptibility to inhibition with anti-C2. Since there is no C4 requirement, the alternative pathway is operative in C4-deficient guinea pig serum.

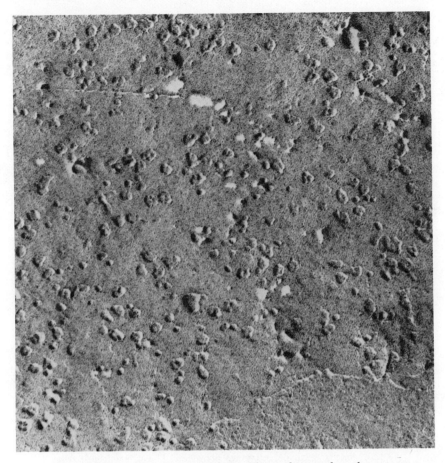

Figure 8-10. Electron micrograph of freeze-fractured erythrocyte membrane treated with antibody and complement (× 226,000). The interior aspect of the exterior leaflet of the membrane contains large doughnut-shaped aggregates of globules.

Both alternative pathway enzymes contain two subunits that are essential, namely, Bb, a fragment of factor B, and C3b; other subunits perform an accessory function (Figure 8-11). The catalytic subunit in both alternative pathway enzymes is Bb. This is derived from factor B (also called C3PA or C3 proactivator, or GBG, for glycine-rich β glycoprotein). This factor can be regarded as the counterpart of C2 in the corresponding complement enzymes. The activation of factor B by cleavage is mediated by a serine esterase of molecular weight 22,000, designated factor $\overline{D}$ or C3Pase or GBGase, which is present normally in blood. The activation of B by cleavage takes place after this factor has become complexed with C3b in the presence of Mg^{++}. The resulting C3-cleaving enzyme of the alternative pathway thus has the composition $\overline{C3b,Bb}$.

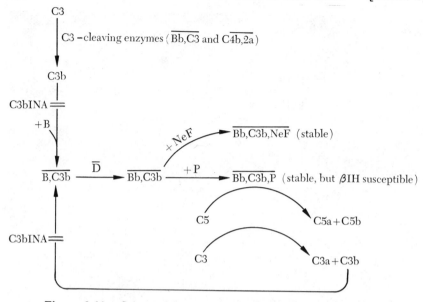

Figure 8-11.   Schematic representation of the alternative pathway. This route of complement activation is mediated by two closely related enzymes that cleave C3 and C5. Each enzyme is made up of the subunits Bb, C3b, and P. The Bb subunit supplies the catalytic center, C3b furnishes binding site, and P is a stabilizer. C3b is initially supplied by the complex $\overline{Bb,C3}$, which is present normally in blood. $\overline{C4b,2a}$ can also supply C3b. Under normal physiologic conditions assembly of the properdin system enzymes is blocked by C3bINA, the C3b inactivator. However, on the surface of certain microbes and on certain immune aggregates, the controlling function of C3bINA is circumvented and assembly of the alternative pathway enzymes proceeds. The alternative pathway generates the same biologically active fragments and complexes that are produced by the classic pathway, namely C3a, C3b, C5a, and C5b, which then react with the late-acting complement proteins to form the C5b-9 complex. The molecular weight estimates for the human proteins are B—100,000; D—23,000; P—184,000. The estimates for the guinea pig proteins are B—100,000; D—22,000.

The difference between the properdin system enzymes that cleave C3 and C5, respectively, derives from the number of molecules of C3b involved. Thus, a single C3b molecule in association with Bb suffices for cleavage of C3, whereas one or more additional C3b molecules are required for cleavage of C5.

The formation of the alternative pathway enzymes requires a source of C3b. Their formation is dependent on an enzyme that cleaves C3 to the fragments C3a and C3b. Actually, continuous slow cleavage of C3 occurs in blood and generates these fragments. The enzyme probably responsible for this is a complex of B and C3 that has become activated by $\overline{D}$ to the form $\overline{Bb,C3}$. This enzyme cleaves C3 much more slowly than the alternative pathway enzyme proper ($\overline{Bb,C3b}$) and differs structurally from the latter since it contains the subunit C3 rather than C3b.

Small amounts of $\overline{C4b,2a}$ may be generated by immune complexes. For example, an invading microorganism may combine with traces of complement-fixing antibody to generate $\overline{C4b,2a}$. Thus, the alternative pathway may be initiated by a specific reaction as well as by the nonspecific route represented by the enzyme $\overline{Bb,C3}$. (Conversely, the classical pathway can be initiated nonspecifically by substances that react with C1q without the benefit of antibody.)

However, under normal physiologic conditions the production of a small quantity of C3b per se does not initiate the alternative pathway since the C3b fragment is destroyed by a control protein, the C3b inactivator, which cleaves it to fragments designated C3c and C3d. In order to understand the role of the C3b inactivator it is helpful to distinguish between activation of the alternative pathway in the fluid phase, e.g., in blood, and activation in the local microenvironment on the surface of a microorganism. Generalized activation of the alternative pathway in blood is seen when C3b inactivator is lacking or deficient, as in the case of certain genetic disorders, or when it is artificially manipulated, for example, when specific antibody neutralizes it. Generalized activation can also be produced by addition of a factor from cobra venom to blood serum. Cobra factor is an analog of C3b that is resistant to the C3b inactivator. The cobra factor is useful as an agent for inactivating complement *in vivo* or *in vitro*.

On the other hand, on the surface of certain microorganisms, on certain microbial polysaccharides, or on certain kinds of immune complexes, activation and assembly of the alternative pathway enzymes do proceed, despite the C3b inactivator. Presumably, conditions on these agents are such that the control action of the C3b inactivator is impeded or circumvented. The reason for this is not understood. An additional factor may be involved. However, the C3b subunit in the enzymic complex $\overline{Bb,C3b}$ is resistant to the C3b inactivator. In any case, whatever is responsible for impeding the C3b inactivator, conditions in the local microenvironment are such that the active enzyme $\overline{Bb,C3b}$ can be assembled and, once it has been formed, the control action of the C3b inactivator is inoperative.

In this context the alternative pathway is an autocatalytic system because its enzymatic activity produces C3b, one of its subunits. As a consequence, when the control action of the C3b inactivator is abrogated, formation of enzyme and consequent cleavage will proceed until the supply of factors B and C3 becomes exhausted. This happens in patients who suffer from a genetic defect involving the C3b inactivator.

At this point it becomes necessary to consider another property of the enzyme $\overline{Bb,C3b}$, namely, the tendency of its subunits to dissociate from one another. When this happens, the C3b subunit becomes susceptible to the

C3b inactivator. As a consequence, the lifetime of $\overline{\text{Bb,C3b}}$ is quite short. This decay is prevented by two proteins that have the capacity to stabilize $\overline{\text{Bb,C3b}}$; i.e., these proteins prevent dissociation into the subunits. The first of these factors is properdin, a basic protein that complexes with $\overline{\text{Bb,C3b}}$ and stabilizes this enzyme. Thus, the stable form of the C3-cleaving enzyme of the alternative pathway is actually a complex of three subunits, namely, $\overline{\text{P,Bb,C3b}}$. Another stabilizer, called NeF, which stands for "nephritic factor," is found in the blood of patients with certain forms of nephritis (Chapter 19). Like properdin, it promotes enzymatic activity of the alternative pathway through stabilization of $\overline{\text{Bb, C3b}}$. Another control factor that participates in regulating the alternative pathway is a protein, $\beta 1H$. This factor promotes breakdown of the complex $\overline{\text{P, Bb,C3b}}$, but not the complex stabilized by NeF.

Activation of the alternative pathway produces all of the biologically active fragments and complexes that are generated by the classic pathway, including the C5b-9 membrane attack system. Hence, the alternative pathway is believed to play an important role in immune defense against microbial infection, especially during the early phases when substantial quantities of specific complement-fixing antibodies have not yet been formed. This protective effect is attributable primarily to the opsonizing action of cell-bound C3b (see below). In addition, the histamine-releasing action of C3a and C5a, as well as the chemotactic activity of C5a, promotes the migration of leukocytes to infected tissue. Generation of the inflammatory products of the complement system via the alternative pathway may play a role in some allergic processes (Chapter 14).

Biologic Activities of Complement

Although the early investigations of complement were concerned mostly with the bactericidal and hemolytic activities, its possible involvement in other immunologic processes was suspected. As detailed information on the cascade of enzymatic reactions involving the early complement components became available, these suspicions were confirmed. Apart from mediating cell attack, complement is involved in the release of histamine, the production of chemotactic factors, the phenomenon of immune adherence, and the modification of blood coagulation. These activities are an important part of the inflammatory response, which plays a central role in immune (Chapter 19) and allergic (Chapter 14) reactions.

Bactericidal Action of Complement

Cells other than erythrocytes are attacked by complement. With respect to infectious disease it is of interest that many bacteria, notably those classified as gram negative, are killed by complement; indeed, some are disintegrated in the process (Chapter 13). Because bacteria have a cell wall surrounding their cytoplasmic membrane, the bactericidal reaction is more complicated than lysis of animal cells. Blood serum contains the enzyme lysozyme, which attacks the glycopeptide responsible for the rigidity of the bacterial cell wall. The attack by lysozyme dissolves the rigid layer of the wall. Lysozyme and complement act synergistically in the attack on bacterial cells. To what extent this attack plays a role in the process of defense against microbial infection is not well understood. Complement participates in the destruction of bacterial cells, but it appears that *in vivo* its bactericidal action may be overshadowed by the phagocytosis of bacterial cells.

Histamine-Releasing, Chemotactic, and Adherence Activities of Complement

As noted in an earlier section, the C3a and C5a fragments cause the release of histamine from cells that store this substance. The histamine increases the permeability of the blood capillaries, which enables leukocytes to penetrate into tissues where an infectious or allergic process is underway. With respect to chemotaxis, both C5a and the C5b,6,7 complex possess this property; they cause certain leukocytes to migrate toward the site from which they are diffusing and thus to accumulate at loci where immune reactions are under way. Another important biologic activity is immune adherence due to deposition of C3b (Figure 8-12). Cells or particles carrying C3b tend to adhere to leukocytes and to other cells. In this way, immune adherence promotes phagocytosis. C3b has also been implicated as a factor in the antibody response to thymus-dependent antigens.

Promotion of Phagocytosis by Complement

Phagocytosis (Chapter 10) is a prime mechanism of defense against bacterial infections. It has been known since the 1930s that antibody and complement render bacteria more susceptible to phagocytosis, a process called opsonization. Pathogenic bacteria are often resistant to phagocytosis unless they are treated with antibody and complement.

The manner in which complement mediates opsonization was not known until the 1950s when the binding of C3b on cell surfaces produced immune adherence. In addition, the movement of phagocytic cells toward the infectious agent is facilitated by the increase of vascular permeability due to the histamine-releasing activity of the C3a and C5a fragments. A directional element is provided by the chemotactic action of the C5a fragment and the C5b,6,7 complex.

Studies of the protective role of complement have been made in mice infected with pneumococci. Quantitative and kinetic comparisons of pneumococcal infection in normal mice with that in genetically C5-deficient

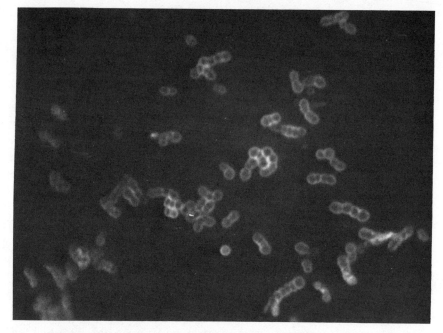

Figure 8-12. Photomicrograph showing deposition of C3b on the surface of pneumococci treated with fresh normal guinea pig serum. Deposition of C3b is due to activation of the properdin pathway. C3b is made visible by staining with fluorescent rabbit antibody to purified guinea pig C3. Pneumococci coated with C3b are readily ingested by phagocytes.

mice have shown that the rate as well as extent of defense against this infection is enhanced by complement protein C5 (Figure 8-13). Mice artificially depleted of C3 by treatment with a factor from cobra venom are more susceptible to infection with pneumococci than untreated mice of the same strain (Table 8-1). Patients with certain defects related to C3 exhibit a pronounced susceptibility to pus-producing bacterial infections. The opsonic action of C3b appears to be especially important in the early stages of infection when sufficient antibody is not yet available and when activation of complement depends on the properdin pathway.

Immune Complex Diseases

In general, when immune complexes form in an organ or a tissue, the complement system will be activated at that site, through the classic pathway, the properdin pathway, or both. The biologically active complement fragments and complexes can become involved in reactions that damage the host's cells, and these pathogenic processes can result in the development of disorders that are called immune complex diseases (Chapter 19). For

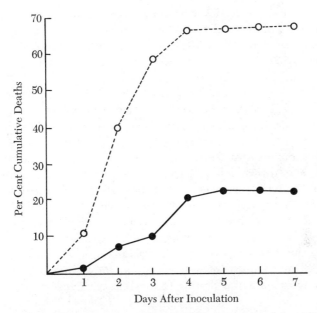

Figure 8-13. The role of C5 in antipneumococcal defense. This graph combines a large set of data obtained with doses of pneumococci ranging from 5.0×10^5 to 1.3×10^8. The comparative combined cumulative deaths occurring at all dose levels are shown in normal mice (●) and in genetically C5-deficient mice (○) that were inoculated intraperitoneally with type III pneumococci of moderate virulence.

example, in some forms of nephritis, complement damages the basement membrane of the kidney, resulting in the escape of protein from the blood into the urine. The disease disseminated lupus erythematosus belongs to the category of immune complex diseases; its symptoms include nephritis, visceral lesions, and skin eruptions. The pathogenic processes observed in rheumatoid arthritis also involve immune complexes. Another immune

Table 8-1

NUMBER OF PNEUMOCOCCI REQUIRED TO KILL 50% OF MICE*

Experiment Number	Normal Mice	Mice Depleted of C3 with Cobra Venom Factor
1	$10^{7.8}$	$10^{6.3}$
2	$10^{7.8}$	$10^{5.9}$
3	$10^{7.6}$	$10^{6.0}$

* The role of C3 in antipneumococcal defense is illustrated in these experiments by Jerry A. Winkelstein and Hyun S. Shin of Johns Hopkins University School of Medicine. Mice were treated with a cobra venom factor to deplete C3. Two hours later they were injected intraperitoneally with a strain of type III pneumococci of moderate virulence. In the C3-depleted mice the lethal dose of pneumococci is small and indicates impairment of the defense mechanism.

complex disease is serum sickness, which may develop after inoculation of large amounts of antitoxin from horses or other animals for the treatment of diphtheria or tetanus. In this disease the host makes antibody against the foreign antitoxin and, consequently, immune complexes are formed that activate the complement system.

How is complement involved in such diseases? As we have seen, the histamine released by the C3a and C5a fragments changes the permeability of the blood vessels near the site of complement activation. The chemotactic property of the C5a fragment and the C5b,6,7 complex promotes migration of leukocytes into the area. Furthermore, the C3b fragment binds to immune complexes, and this action promotes the ingestion of the complexes by phagocytes. In turn, phagocytosis (Chapter 10) is followed by release of lysosomal enzymes that damage the surrounding cells and tissues. The membrane-damaging capacity of the terminal complement components, C5b-9, may contribute to cell damage in the immediate vicinity. A further element in this series of events is the acceleration of blood clotting by activation of the complement system. This action results from the complement-mediated release of a clotting factor from platelets.

Complement and Anaphylaxis

Anaphylaxis (Chapter 18) is a type of hypersensitivity reaction that may occur following repeated exposure to an antigenic substance. Its symptoms are caused by the release of histamine and some other chemicals from certain cells. These chemicals cause local or general disturbances, the nature of which varies in different animal species. For example, in the guinea pig, the most striking effect is the contraction of smooth muscle producing bronchospasm.

In man, insect stings, inoculation with certain drugs, inhalation of antigenic materials, or the ingestion of some foods may cause anaphylaxis. It can be serious and may even cause death.

It has been suspected for a long time that complement might be involved in the production of anaphylaxis. This view comes from the discovery more than 60 years ago that treatment of serum with certain substances, notably bacterial polysaccharides or lipopolysaccharides, i.e., substances that activate the properdin system, causes the formation of toxic substances so that injection of the treated serum into an animal produces symptoms that resemble those of anaphylaxis. Therefore, the term "anaphylatoxin" was coined to describe the toxic substance generated by treatment of the serum with the bacterial polysaccharides. The nature of anaphylatoxin became clear when it was discovered that activation of the complement system via the properdin pathway leads to cleavage of C3 and C5, with resultant production of the polypeptide fragments C3a and C5a, which display histamine-releasing and, hence, anaphylatoxic activity. Consequently, these fragments are now referred to as anaphylatoxins.

However, the role of these anaphylatoxins in the production of anaphylaxis is quite uncertain. It is known that anaphylactic reactions, such as those observed in hay fever, are produced by a different mechanism involving antibodies belonging to the IgE class of immunoglobulin. The possible role of the anaphylatoxins in anaphylaxis has been investigated extensively in experiments involving production of local anaphylaxis with antibody from a different animal species. These studies introduce an artifactual element due to the use of heterologous antibody and, therefore, are not directly relevant to anaphylaxis induced by the animal's own antibody. However, they serve to demonstrate that activation of the complement system by immune complexes, with consequent production of C3a and C5a, can produce local anaphylactic events. As noted already, these contribute to phagocytic defense and immune complex disease.

Effect of Complement on Blood Coagulation

Although a relation between these systems has long been suspected, clear evidence has become available only recently. The polysaccharide inulin, as well as lipopolysaccharide from gram-negative bacteria, which have the capacity to activate complement via the properdin pathway, has accelerated the clotting reaction. This occurs by way of complement-mediated release of a clotting factor from platelets.

Genetic Deficiencies of Complement

Genetic deficiencies of certain complement components in humans and animals have been studied extensively in attempts to define the biologic role of complement (Chapter 17). Deficiency of C2 has been studied in man. Deficiencies of C4, C5, and C6 have been found in guinea pigs, mice, and rabbits, respectively.

Guinea pigs lacking C4 are in good health, presumably because of the protective role of the properdin pathway in providing resistance to bacterial infection. However, they exhibit some abnormalities. For example, under certain experimental conditions, their phagocytic mechanism does not function properly, as revealed by failure to clear antibody-coated isologous erythrocytes from the blood. Also, the antibody response of these guinea pigs to protein antigens is defective. This may be related to other experiments that suggest that C3b-mediated immune adherence may be a factor in the activation of antibody-forming lymphocytes.

C5-deficient mice also appear healthy, though, in appropriately designed experiments, their resistance to pneumococcal infection was found impaired. These animals are also less resistant to a common pathogen for mice related to the bacillus that causes diphtheria in man.

Complement and Graft Rejection

Under certain conditions participation of complement in the process of allograft rejection has been observed (Chapter 23). For example, C5-deficient mice reject skin grafts more slowly than their normal counterparts. Impairment of skin graft rejection has also been noted in studies with rabbits lacking C6. These observations suggest that complement plays a role in graft rejection in addition to the cellular immune mechanisms that are as yet poorly defined. Renal allograft rejection in man is accompanied by decline of C2 titer. Changes of C3 have been reported also.

Summary

Complement is a complex enzymatic reaction system that may be activated directly by antigen-antibody complexes or indirectly, via the alternative pathway, by certain polysaccharides from microbial cells, or by other agents. The proteins that make up the complement system function in three distinct phases, namely, the recognition and alarm element C1q,r,s, the $\overline{\text{C4b,2a,3b}}$ enzyme, and the cytolytic attack element C5b-9. The $\overline{\text{P,Bb, C3b}}$ enzymes of the alternative pathway serve the C3- and C5-cleaving functions of $\overline{\text{C4b,2a}}$ and $\overline{\text{C4b,2a,3b}}$ of the classic pathway. The complement proteins found in blood serum are the building blocks from which these elements are assembled following activation. The activation reactions involve enzymatic cleavage of some of the complement components. Several of the resulting fragments mediate biologic activities such as histamine release, chemotaxis, and opsonization.

The most significant defensive function of complement appears to be the promotion of phagocytosis of microorganisms, especially gram-positive bacteria. This effect is particularly important during the early stages of the infectious process when significant antibody synthesis has not yet developed and when activation of the complement system is mediated via the alternative pathway. Complement also plays a major role in the pathogenesis of immune complex diseases. Thus, on the one hand, the complement system aids immune protection, while on the other, it contributes to allergic and autoimmune disorders.

Bibliography

Müller-Eberhard, H. J.: Complement. *Annu. Rev. Biochem.* **44**:697, 1975.
Vogt, W.: Activation, activities and pharmacologically active products of complement. *Pharmacol. Rev.*, **26**:126, 1974.

9

Cell-Mediated Cytotoxicity

ROBERT H. SWANBORG AND NOEL R. ROSE

Introduction

Some of the most important immune reactions, such as the destruction of tissue grafts and tumors, are due to the direct effect of cells, especially lymphocytes. The mechanisms through which the lymphocytes mediate these immune phenomena are not entirely clear, but it is likely that several are involved, including both the production of soluble mediators and the direct interactions between lymphocytes and the target tissue cells. With respect to the latter mechanisms, several *in vitro* models have been developed that show that immune lymphocytes are capable of destroying target cells directly, without the apparent involvement of soluble mediators. The lysis of target cells by immune cells is referred to as cell-mediated cytotoxicity (Figure 9-1).

Several methods have been devised to study cell-mediated cytotoxicity *in vitro*. They include the microcytotoxicity assay in which effector lymphocytes are added to monolayer cultures of target cells bearing the relevant antigen against which the effector cells are immunized or sensitized. Obviously this method is useful only in systems in which the target cells can be grown on monolayers. After incubation for 48 to 72 hours the cells can be examined microscopically, and cytotoxicity is evidenced by the destruction of the

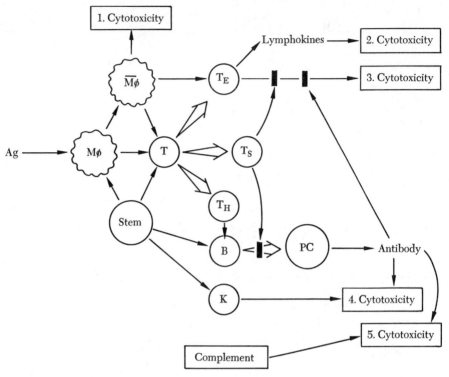

Figure 9-1. Mechanisms of cytotoxicity (compare with Figure 1-2, page 9). Cytotoxic effects may be exerted by (*1*) activated macrophages, (*2*) cytotoxic lymphokines, (*3*) effector T cells, (*4*) antibody and K cells, (*5*) antibody and complement. Ag = antigen; $M\phi$ = macrophage; $\overline{M\phi}$ = activated macrophage; T = T cell; T_E = effector T cell; T_S = suppressor T cell; T_H = helper T cell; B = B cell; K = K cell; PC = plasma cell.

monolayer. A drawback to this method is the possibility of nonimmunologic damage to the monolayer by factors such as enzymes released from dying cells in the culture. Moreover, quantitation is difficult since evaluation of monolayer damage is subjective.

The second procedure for detecting cytotoxicity involves the measurement of release of radioactive markers from labeled target cells in the presence of appropriate effector cells. Although several isotopes have been employed in this method, radioactive chromium (^{51}Cr) has been found to be particularly useful for labeling target cells. For example, the target cells can be labeled by incubation in nutrient medium with inorganic ^{51}Cr (usually in the form of $Na^{51}CrO_4$); the ^{51}Cr binds to proteins and other constituents of the cells. The release of label into the supernatant provides a sensitive and reproducible index of cell damage. It is, of course, important to select a target cell that takes up and retains ^{51}Cr. Thus, one must make sure in advance that spontaneous release levels are well below 2% per hour. Moreover, the target

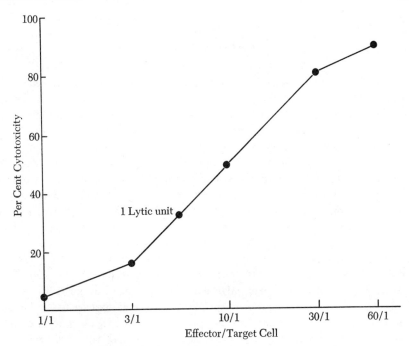

Figure 9-2. Relationship between cytotoxicity and concentration of effector lymphocytes, assayed after four-hour incubation at 37° C. Per cent of cytotoxicity is equivalent to the per cent of specific ^{51}Cr released into the supernatant after subtracting spontaneous release.

cell membrane must be susceptible to effector cell damage, as reflected by specific release of ^{51}Cr. An advantage to the use of ^{51}Cr over other radio-active isotopes is that released label is generally not reutilized by other target cells in the system. A variety of target cells have been successfully employed in this procedure, and there is no requirement that the cells grow on mono-layers. Indeed, target cells in suspension appear to be more susceptible to effector cell lysis than are cell monolayers, presumably owing to increased target cell–effector cell contact.

Release of radioactive label into the supernatant is proportional to the percentage of cytotoxicity and gives a relative estimate of the frequency of cytotoxic cells in the effector cell population. In this procedure the percentage of lysis is linear with respect to the logarithm of the effector cell concentration (Figure 9-2). Cerottini and Brunner have defined the number of effector lymphocytes necessary to obtain 33% cytotoxicity (i.e., lysis) as 1 lytic unit.

Several cell types have been observed to function as effector cells in cell-mediated cytotoxicity including T lymphocytes, thymus-independent lym-phocytes, which are referred to as "null" or killer (K) cells, and, in certain circumstances, monocytes and macrophages. In some parasitic infections eosinophils have been implicated as the effector cell.

T Cell Cytotoxicity

In this system the sensitized T lymphocytes interact directly with the target cell bearing the corresponding antigenic determinants. Destruction is carried out without antibody or complement. Indeed, antibody may actually inhibit T cell-dependent cytotoxicity. Close contact between the T effector cell and the target cell is required.

Evidence that the effector cell in this system is a T lymphocyte is derived from several types of experiments. For example, T cell-dependent cytotoxicity can be abrogated by treating the effector cell population with anti-θ serum plus complement in studies carried out in the mouse, whereas anti-B cell or anti-plasma-cell sera are not effective in preventing cytotoxicity. Moreover, removal of B cells on anti-immunoglobulin immunoadsorbent columns does not interfere with the cytotoxic response. Cytotoxic T cells are produced in mice and rats following tissue transplantation and also following immunization of animals with certain kinds of tumor cells.

In the mouse, the progenitor of the cytotoxic T cell appears to be a small lymphocyte that can be found in the spleen, lymph node, peripheral blood, thoracic duct, and thymus but is not usually found in the bone marrow. Cytotoxic cells can be detected three to four days after a tissue graft is placed. The early cytotoxic effector cell is a lymphoblast that is found in the peritoneal exudate fluid, blood, thoracic duct, spleen, and lymph node, in decreasing order of frequency, but not in the thymus. Later, another cytotoxic cell with the appearance of a small lymphocyte can be found. Moreover, cytotoxic T cells can be elicited *in vitro* provided macrophages are present in the cell population. Recently it has been found that 2-mercaptoethanol can replace the requirement for macrophages in production of cytotoxic T cells *in vitro*.

As mentioned above, close contact between the cytotoxic T cell and the target cell is required for killing to occur. Dosage studies suggest that one cytotoxic T cell is capable of killing more than one target cell. The reaction is temperature dependent, proceeding most efficiently at 37° C. Although cytotoxicity fails to occur at 4° C, contact between effector cell and target cell can be observed at that temperature. This observation suggests that cell contact is not sufficient for target cell destruction, and that the cytotoxic T cell must be both viable and metabolically active in order to effect cytotoxicity. In support of this hypothesis are the findings that cytotoxic actions of T cells are impaired by inhibitors of RNA or protein synthesis but not by irradiation. The finding that cytotoxicity is also inhibited by the chelating agent EDTA suggests that divalent cations are required in the cytotoxic process.

With respect to the specificity of T cell-mediated cytotoxicity, it has been established that immune T cells lyse target cells with the corresponding histocompatibility antigen on their surface but have no effect on unrelated target cells included in the same culture. This finding shows that soluble mediators are not involved in the cytotoxic process unless, of course, they are relatively short-range mediators that act at the surface of the contact between the cytotoxic T cell and the target cell.

K Cell Cytotoxicity

It has been determined by Perlmann and his colleagues that lymphocytes from normal donors in the presence of immune serum are capable of exerting cytotoxic effects on target cells to which the antibodies are directed. This antibody-dependent, cell-mediated cytotoxicity, referred to as K cell lysis, can be seen in heterologous systems, for example, in which normal human lymphocytes are capable of lysing chicken red blood cells coated with rabbit antichicken red blood cell IgG antibodies. Moreover, K cell lysis can also be observed within the same species in the human, mouse, and rat.

Evidence that the effector cell is not a T cell comes from the finding that K cell cytotoxicity is not impaired if the effector cell population is treated with anti-θ serum plus complement, and from the finding that K cell cytotoxicity does occur in hosts that are deficient in T cells, for example, in thymectomized rats. The K cells can be removed on anti-Ig immuno-adsorbent columns but not on anti-Ig Fab columns. The latter finding suggests that the K cell is not an immunoglobulin-positive cell but probably bears an Fc receptor. Therefore, the K cell appears to be an Fc receptor-bearing Ig-negative cell. In rats, K cells can be found in the peritoneal exudate, spleen, and blood, in decreasing frequency, but not in the thoracic duct or thymus.

K cell cytotoxicity is induced by antibodies of the IgG class that are specific for the target cell. The antibodies must possess intact Fc regions, which serve to attract the K cells through interaction with their Fc receptors. Thus antibody provides the link between target cell and effector cell and also provides specificity for the system. Very few antibody molecules are needed for K cell cytotoxicity, probably in the order of a few hundred molecules/target cell. Frequently, antiserum dilutions of 10^{-5} to 10^{-7} are effective, illustrating the high sensitivity of the system. Moreover, excess antibody inhibits cytotoxicity as does aggregated immunoglobulin or antigen-antibody complexes in which the antigen is unrelated. The mechanism of this inhibition is presumably the blocking of the Fc receptor of the K cell. In the human, K cell cytotoxicity requires IgG antibody. With few exceptions IgM-class antibody does not mediate K cell cytotoxicity but may actually inhibit ^{51}Cr release. Complement is not involved in this phenomenon.

With respect to the mechanism of K cell cytotoxicity, close contact between the effector cell and the target cell is required. Studies by scanning electron microscopy with a plaque assay revealed that the K cell develops

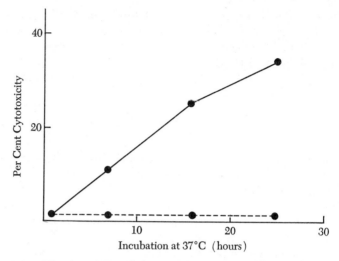

Figure 9-3. Kinetics of K cell cytotoxicity. Per cent of specific
^{51}Cr release (expressed as per cent of cytotoxicity with increasing
time of incubation at 37° C). Target cells: chicken erythrocytes;
effector cells; purified human lymphocytes. Antibody: rabbit antichicken erythrocyte IgG fraction. The effector/target cell ratio was
25/1. Solid line: antibody. Broken line: normal rabbit serum.

uropods that attach to the target cell and ultimately lyse the latter. The K
cell is then free to lyse other target cells. When lymphocytes are responsible
for antibody-dependent, cell-mediated cytotoxicity, lysis (Chapter 8) cannot
be equated with phagocytosis (Chapter 10). However, since other cell types,
e.g., macrophages and monocytes, also bear Fc receptors, they are sometimes
capable of functioning as effector cells. In the case of cytotoxicity mediated
by macrophages, phagocytosis may accompany lysis. Specific chromium
release can be seen within one hour and increases in linear fashion if the
effector cell is a true lymphocytic K cell (Figure 9-3). In the case of macro-
phage- or monocyte-mediated cytotoxicity, lysis exhibits a rapid onset and
stops in a few hours. In immune reactions to animal parasites like schistosomes, eosinophils have been reported to act as antibody-dependent killer
cells.

The K cell must be viable and metabolically active, although protein
synthesis may not be required for cytotoxicity. Despite the observation that
monocytes and macrophages sometimes exert effector function, the finding
that purified lymphocyte preparations ($>98\%$ lymphocytes) are highly
active rules out the possibility that K cell cytotoxicity is due only to these
contaminating cells in the effector cell population.

The specificity of K cell cytotoxicity is due entirely to the antibody
involved. The K cells can even be of heterologous origin. Studies with mixed
populations of target cells, i.e., mixtures of target cells bearing different

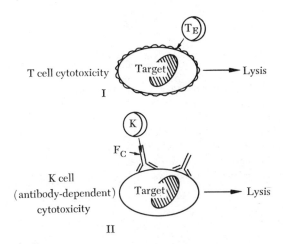

Figure 9-4. Schematic representation of effector/target cell interactions leading to cell-mediated cytotoxicity. The cytotoxic T cell (*I*) presumably recognizes a complementary antigenic determinant on the target cell membrane. In contrast, the K cell (*II*) interacts with the Fc fragment of an antibody molecule that has bound to a determinant on the target cell.

surface antigenic determinants, reveal that target cell lysis is confined to cells bearing an antigen corresponding to the specificity of the antibody present. Such studies also tend to exclude the involvement of long-range soluble mediators in the cytotoxic process.

Summary

Living target cells are susceptible to the action of lymphocytes and occasionally other cells. As illustrated schematically in Figure 9-4, at least two mechanisms of lymphocyte-mediated target cell killing are known. Sensitized T cells are capable of interacting directly, presumably by virtue of membrane receptors for antigen, with relevant target cells (Figure 9-4 *A*). On the other hand, nonimmune Fc receptor-bearing lymphocytes (K cells) have the capacity to interact with the Fc fragment of IgG antibody bound immunologically to target cell-bound antigenic determinants (Figure 9-4 *B*). The result of both cell-cell interactions is lysis of the target cell (assuming it is susceptible to lysis). Although T cell and K cell cytotoxicities have been shown operative *in vitro* in numerous immune systems (including allograft and tumor rejection and experimental autoimmune disease), their role in immunologic tissue destruction *in vivo* is not yet clear.

Bibliography

Biberfeld, P.; Wahlin, B.; Perlmann, P.; and Biberfeld, G.: A plaque technique for assay and characterization of antibody-dependent cytotoxic effector (K) cells. *Scand. J. Immunol.*, **4**:859, 1975.

Cerottini, J.-C., and Brunner, K. T.: Cell-mediated cytotoxicity, allograft rejection, and tumor immunity. *Adv. Immunol.*, **18**:67, 1974.

Perlmann, P.: Cellular immunity: antibody-dependent cytotoxicity. In Bach, F. H., and Good, R. A. (eds.): *Clinical Immunobiology*. Academic Press, New York, 1976, pp. 107–32.

10

Phagocytosis

CAREL J. VAN OSS

Introduction

Phagocytosis is the ingestion of particles by single cells. Phagocytosis by circulating and fixed white cells is the organism's most important means of defense against invading matter. Phylogenetically phagocytosis is the oldest and most fundamental defense mechanism; it plays a predominant role in the defense against foreign invaders in all animal species. Among the most primitive forms of animal life (e.g., among amebae), phagocytosis is one of the principal means of ingesting food; this application of phagocytosis antedates its evolvement into a defense mechanism among the more advanced multicellular animals.

The mammalian phagocytic defense consists of the polymorphonuclear phagocytic system, the first line of defense, comprising the circulating polymorphonuclear leukocytes, also called granulocytes, and the mononuclear phagocytic system, the second line of defense, comprising the circulating monocytes as well as the free and the fixed macrophages, also known as the reticuloendothelial system.

The inactivation, removal, and disposal of all invading microorganisms are done by phagocytes, often aided by antibodies and complement. Antibodies and complement (Chapter 8) rarely suffice to inactivate microorganisms, and they are entirely incapable of effecting their removal and disposal. Phagocytes, on the other hand, readily eliminate many microorganisms and other particles that happen to be foreign, but they are incapable of discrimination between foreign and nonforeign objects without the help of antibodies. The recognition of foreign particles and organisms is done by specific antibodies, which then, with the help of various complement factors, give chemical signals to the phagocytes, causing them to move to the scene by chemotaxis. Antibodies, frequently with the help of complement, also effect changes on the surface of the recognized particles, thus enhancing their palatability for the phagocytes, a process called opsonization.

Phagocytosis was first described by Metchnikoff in 1887. For many years a heated scientific controversy persisted concerning the question of whether the defense against invading organisms is based on humoral or on cellular mechanisms. This controversy has cooled in recent times, thanks to the growing realization of the different but equally indispensable and collaborative roles of both humoral and cellular activities.

Polymorphonuclear Phagocytic System

The polymorphonuclear leukocytes, or granulocytes, are phagocytes that are in constant peripheral circulation. In the blood of a normal adult human they number approximately 2.5×10^{10} (or about 1/1000 the number of circulating red cells), whereas in the bone marrow there is, in addition, a reserve of 2.5×10^{12} granulocytes or their immediate precursors. Granulocytes, once released into the bloodstream, are expendable end cells, with a half-life of only a few days. They can penetrate by diapedesis (see below) into the tissues, where they have a half-life of only a few hours. Granulocytes are called neutrophils, eosinophils, and heterophils (or acidophils and basophils), according to the staining properties of their cytoplasmic granules. The vast majority of them are neutrophils; they normally represent about two-thirds of the total white cell count, the rest being mainly lymphocytes. Figure 10-1 *A* represents a human neutrophil with its typical nuclear lobes and multiple cytoplasmic granules, which are round or oblong homogeneous structures, many of them lysosomes, whereas the numerous small dots are glycogen deposits. Eosinophils (acidophils) occur in fairly small numbers (about 3% of the total white cell count). They are avidly attracted to antigen-antibody complexes in the blood, which they readily phagocytize. They also seem to play some role in hypersensitivity reactions, the precise mechanism of which is not yet clear. Basophils, which normally represent only about 0.3% of the total white cell count, contain granules that are rich in histamine and heparin; they seem to play a role in IgE-mediated hypersensitivity reactions (Chapter 4).

Phagocytes of the polymorphonuclear system represent in the truest sense

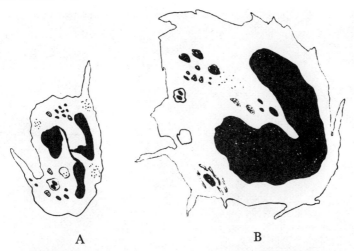

A   B

Figure 10-1. Schematic representation of a polymorphonuclear granulocyte (neutrophil) (*A*) and a macrophage (*B*). In *A* the typical multilobar nucleus is visible, as well as the cytoplasmic granules; the small dots indicate glycogen deposits. In *B* much the same processes are visible, but the nucleus is more of one piece and kidney shaped. The macrophage is a significantly larger cell than the granulocyte. Typical for both cells (and for all phagocytic cells) are pseudopods and other protruberances; see also Figure 10-2.

the organism's first line of defense against invading particles. Even in the realm of the mononuclear phagocytic system (RES) the granulocytes are indispensable for the policing of bacteria in the vascular beds. In the absence of granulocytes, bacteremia and death ensue rapidly.

Mononuclear Phagocytic System

The mononuclear phagocytic system comprises both the mobile and the fixed highly phagocytic cells of the reticuloendothelial system (RES). Since the concept of the RES as a description of all highly phagocytic mononuclear cells is open to criticism and lacks precision, the term "mononuclear phagocytic sytem" is now increasingly preferred. This system comprises, in the order of increasing phagocytic capacity, the:

Promonocytes (in the bone marrow), which give rise to the:
Monocytes (in the peripheral blood), which in turn give rise to the:
Macrophages (free and fixed), in the following tissues:
  Bone marrow (macrophages, sinusoidal lining cells)
  Bone tissue (osteoclasts)
  Liver (Kupffer cells)

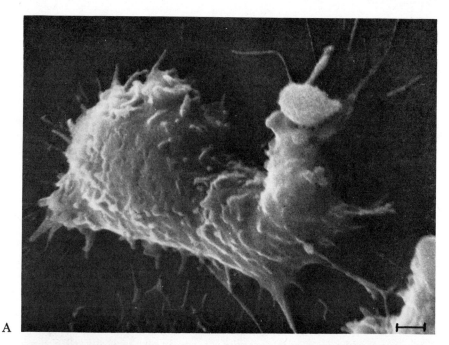

A

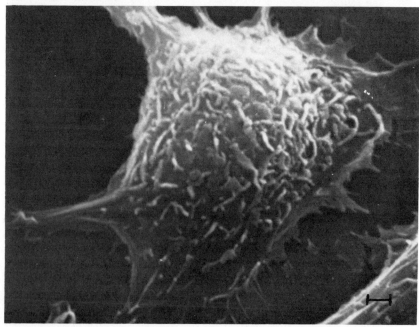

B

Figure 10-2. Scanning electron micrographs of human polymorphonuclear granulocytes (*A*) and guinea pig macrophages (*B*).
The bars indicate a length of 1 μm.

Lung (alveolar macrophages)
Lymph nodes (free and fixed macrophages)
Medullary tissue of the intestinal Peyer's patches (macrophages)
Nervous system (microglial cells)
Serous cavity (peritoneal macrophages)
Spleen (free and fixed macrophages, sinusoidal lining cells)

In peripheral blood among adults there are normally up to 2×10^9 monocytes in circulation. They give rise to daughter cells, which can leave the bloodstream and populate the various tissues enumerated above as macrophages.

Macrophages

Macrophages are considerably larger than granulocytes and have a single, often kidney-shaped nucleus (Figure 10-1). The macrophages of the mononuclear phagocytic system form the second line of defense against invading particles.

Contrary to polymorphonuclear phagocytes, many macrophages will continue to divide. They can also fuse into multinucleate giant cells, which serve to dispose of the larger foreign bodies. Invasions that give rise to protracted intervention by macrophages, with accumulation of epithelioid cells, can give rise to granulomata, e.g., in tuberculosis or in *Listeria monocytogenes* infections.

Inflammation

In inflammation the participating macrophages can be divided into three groups: (1) the recent arrivals from the circulation; (2) a somewhat self-propagating population, which nevertheless mainly depends on continued immigration of fresh macrophages; and (3) an almost totally self-sustaining population that is largely independent of renewed macrophage influx. Corticosteroids and cytostatic agents, such as cyclophosphamide and particularly 6-mercaptopurine, are strongly anti-inflammatory because they cause a rapid reduction in the number of fast-reproducing but short-lived peripheral monocytes, thus cutting off the influx of fresh macrophages. In contrast, agents that act directly on already existing macrophages, such as antimacrophage antiserum, have very little effect on inflammation.

Macrophage Activation

Macrophages can be "activated" by substances emitted by delayed-hypersensitivity-type lymphocytes when the latter are stimulated with specific antigen (Chapter 11). Activated macrophages adhere more strongly to glass and phagocytize more avidly than do unactivated macrophages.

They also develop more lysosomal granules and show an accelerated bactericidal activity. Macrophages thus play a collaborative role in the delayed hypersensitivity type of antimicrobial defense (Chapter 11), although the specific antigen recognition aspect entirely resides in the other partner: the committed lymphocytes.

Macrophages and Antibody Formation

The role of macrophages in antibody formation is also collaborative. Macrophages themselves are incapable of antibody synthesis, and they are devoid of any specific antigen recognition mechanism. Macrophages are, however, prone to be present near sites where antibody-forming cells are active. The main function of macrophages is the removal and disposal of antigen. However, macrophages and/or the closely related dendritic cells, by means of their "sticky" cell surface, can play an auxiliary role in the formation of those antibodies for which "helper T lymphocytes" are also required, in "presenting" many (generally proteinaceous) antigen molecules in a regular array to the antibody-forming B lymphocytes (Chapter 3).

Phagocytosis

Phagocytosis of foreign particles comprises a number of quite separate steps and activities in which the particles that are to be phagocytized and the phagocytic cells each play an important role. The two systems, of circulating polymorphonuclear phagocytes and of free and fixed macrophages, continuously police the peripheral and the lymphatic circulation as well as the respiratory and gastrointestinal tracts and strive to safeguard these from foreign particles. However, granulocytes as well as macrophages also need (and have) a mechanism for seeking out invasive agents that have sequestered themselves in more remote locations. Phagocytes also need a mechanism for distinguishing between self and nonself. The mechanisms of all these aspects of phagocytosis are described here, to begin with the signal (warning that there is a foreign particle to be phagocytized in a given location) followed by the pursuit (the locomotion of the phagocyte toward the foreign particle), the surface recognition (including the opsonization of the particle that is to be phagocytized), the engulfment, and finally the destruction of the invader, which is the ultimate aim of the whole operation.

The Signal

Once the surface of a foreign particle has bound specific antibodies, which then react with complement factors C1, C4, C2, C3, C5, relatively low-molecular-weight pieces of some of these complement components (notably of C3a and C5a) diffuse out from the center of the reaction, establishing a concentration gradient of these chemotactic factors (Chapter 8). Granulocytes are attracted by these chemotactic factors and tend to propel themselves upstream into their concentration gradient. This process is called chemotaxis. Monocytes are less influenced by this chemotactic system and tend to move to the scene at a much later stage, probably under the influence of another chemotactic system, the precise nature of which still remains to be established.

Sensitized lymphocytes exhibiting delayed hypersensitivity (Chapter 11) are stimulated by their specific antigen to produce a lymphokine that is chemotactic for monocytes and macrophages.

Local tissue injury can also cause migration to the scene of phagocytes in the absence of immunologic involvement. The causative chemotactic factors in these cases appear to be prostaglandins.

The Pursuit

After the phagocyte has "noticed" the chemotactic signal, it will start moving in the direction of increasing concentration of the chemotactic factor. This movement occurs in a typical ameboid fashion, by slowly striding forward with the help of continuously evolving and retracting pseudopodic processes, coupled with considerable protoplasmic streaming. The phagocytes, on their way to the chemotactic signal, move through the walls of blood venules, a process called diapedesis. Granulocytes as well as monocytes and macrophages pass the cells that form the walls of the blood vessels through their intracellular junctions (contrary to the locomotive habits of lymphocytes, which preferentially pass straight through the cell membranes). Cellular locomotion and diapedesis are energy-requiring processes. At low and high glucose levels as well as at high ethanol levels, diapedesis of phagocytes is decreased.

Surface Recognition

Surface Properties. Although the decision of whether or not a particle is going to be phagocytized is solely linked to the particle's surface properties, nothing so sophisticated as actual recognition by the phagocyte of foreignness of the particle is involved. Only physical properties determine whether a particle can be engulfed by a phagocyte: the interfacial tension between the surface of the particle and water must be higher than the interfacial tension between the surface of the phagocyte and water; in other words, the particle must be more hydrophobic than the phagocyte in order to become engulfed by it. A practical way of determining the interfacial tensions between cells and water is by measuring the contact angle made by a drop of saline water, placed on a flat monolayer of cells, with that monolayer. This contact angle is a measure of the interfacial tension between the cell surface and its surrounding medium.

Most nonpathogenic bacteria are more hydrophobic than phagocytes and are thus spontaneously engulfed. There are also pathogenic microorganisms (e.g., *Mycobacterium tuberculosis, Listeria monocytogenes*) that are quite hydrophobic. These organisms are readily phagocytized; their pathogenicity is based on their resistance to the subsequent, digestive action of the phagocytes (see below).

Bacteria that are more hydrophilic than phagocytes (mainly the ones that are provided with a slimy hydrophilic capsule) undergo little phagocytosis and thus are generally quite pathogenic (e.g., *Streptococcus pneumoniae, Klebsiella pneumoniae*). However, specific anticapsular antibody raises the interfacial tension of encapsulated bacteria to a higher level than that of phagocytes, which then makes phagocytosis possible. Complement (C3b) increases the interfacial tension and the phagocytosis of antibody-sensitized bacteria even further. Complement alone, in the absence of specific antibody, usually has no significant influence on either the interfacial tension or the phagocytosis of bacteria. In other words, phagocytes do not distinguish between self and nonself, but just between particles that are more hydrophilic or more hydrophobic than themselves.

The relatively low interfacial tension of phagocytes, which causes them spontaneously to adhere to and to engulf most particulate materials, also is the cause of the unique property of phagocytic cells readily to adhere to flat surfaces of greater hydrophobicity, such as glass. Much use is made of this phenomenon for the preparation of monolayers of phagocytes on glass slides, with the automatic exclusion of all other, nonadhering cells, and also for the selective removal of phagocytic cells from leukocyte preparations or from whole blood, by adsorbing them on glass or nylon beads or fibers.

The mechanism of "surface phagocytosis," by which encapsulated bacteria can be phagocytized at an early stage of the infection, before anticapsular antibodies have had time to form in demonstrable quantities, is not based on interfacial tension differences but rather on the roughness of the surrounding surfaces, which literally offer "footholds" for the pseudopodic process of the phagocytes so that the phagocytes can trap the microorganisms against tissue surfaces or between other leukocytes or gaps in adjacent fibrin clots. The precise mechanism of surface phagocytosis has not yet been elucidated, but some recognition principle must be involved, possibly based on small amounts of preexisting "natural" antibodies or on weakly cross-reacting antibodies (Chapter 5), and complement (Chapter 8).

Opsonization.   Opsonization of bacteria and other particles ("rendering them more palatable") is done by a variety of hitherto not clearly defined substances (opsonins) that are present in normal fresh plasma. There are heat-stable and heat-labile opsonins (the latter are destroyed by heating for 20 to 30 minutes at 56° C). It has now become obvious that the heat-stable opsonins are nothing but antibodies, and possibly also to some extent aspecifically adsorbed immunoglobulins, of the IgG class. And the heat-labile opsonins are principally the collective complement components C1, C4, C2, C3 (giving rise to the hydrophobic C3b) (Chapter 8), which need prior triggering by the antigen-antibody interaction (Chapter 5) between surface antigens and the heat-stable opsonins. The specificity of the self-vs.-nonself recognition of the phagocytes is thus entirely related to the specific antibodies, and the first four complement factors play a secondary, reinforcing role. The heat-stable opsonizing component that increases the interfacial tension (and the hydrophobicity) of bacterial surfaces is situated in the Fc part (Chapter 4) of the immunoglobulins involved. (The Fab part, which contains the antibody specificity, is of course needed for the specific binding of the immunoglobulin to the antigen, but it is inactive as an opsonin when deprived of the Fc part.) The tail end of the Fc part represents the most prominent hydrophobic component of the IgG molecule. Nevertheless, single intact IgG molecules, notwithstanding the hydrophobic Fc tails, do not become phagocytized, whereas large antigen-antibody complexes with many Fc tails on their periphery become engulfed. The explanation of that phenomenon lies in the fact that a single IgG molecule has too high a kinetic energy per square centimeter of hydrophobic surface area to become engulfed. However, antigen-antibody complexes with three or more IgG molecules at their periphery have a low enough kinetic energy per area of attachment for phagocytosis to become possible in the absence of complement. In the presence of complement it is possible for complexes with just two closely spaced IgG molecules to become phagocytized. One IgM molecule per complex should suffice to cause its phagocytosis, after having combined with complement. The known experimental data conform closely to these calculations.

IgA plays no direct role in opsonization, and the roles, if any, of IgD and IgE in opsonization are as yet unknown. The lack of opsonizing power of IgA may be of biologic importance. IgA-class antibodies do not increase the hydrophobicity of particles above the point where they would become readily phagocytized. This would tend to segregate IgA virus complexes extracellularly, which helps explain the importance of secretory IgA in the antiviral defense of the upper respiratory tract. There are probably still other, not yet characterized, opsonizing plasma components.

Ingestion and Digestion

Once contact is made with a particle, the surface of which is more hydrophobic than the surface of the phagocyte itself, engulfment usually ensues, starting with a deep invagination of the outside of the phagocyte's cell membrane, which ultimately envelops the particle entirely in a tangential phagocytic vacuole. The vacuole then migrates into the phagocyte, and its membrane soon fuses with the membrane of one or more leukocytic granules (or lysosomes). These granules contain a large variety of hydrolases, which are thus brought in contact with the ingested particle, within the confines of the pouch formed by the fused membranes of the phagocytic vacuole and the granules.

The ingested particle then becomes exposed to the whole array of hydrolases (including glucuronidase, lipases, nucleases, peroxydases, phosphatases, proteases, and, in the case of neutrophils, the bactericidal substances lysozyme and phagocytin), quickly resulting in the death and destruction of most bacteria. Cytoplasmic destruction of the phagocyte itself is avoided because the entire digestive process takes place within the vacuolic-lysosomal pouch. The fusing of the granules with the vacuole and the subsequent decrease in optical density of the granular content, due to the liquefying effect of their enzymatic activity, give rise to a visual impression of "degranulation." The entire process generally results in the irreversible inactivation of most bacteria within about 15 minutes. Some microorganisms (e.g., *Mycobacterium tuberculosis*; Chapter 13), however, resist these bactericidal onslaughts for considerable lengths of time; this is one of the principal mechanisms for their pathogenicity.

The digestive step of phagocytosis requires metabolic energy; this is principally derived from glycolysis. Hence, extremely low glucose concentrations have been found to impair phagocytosis. High glucose concentrations also cause a decrease in phagocytosis, but high ethanol levels (although they have some influence of diapedesis, see above) have no influence on the phagocytic act. The type of decrease in phagocytic activity caused by hyperglycemic glucose levels (which tend to render phagocytic cells more spheric, and thus less capable of making contact with foreign particles) probably is closely connected with the decreased resistance to bacterial infections that is common among inadequately controlled diabetics.

Measurement of Phagocytosis

There is a variety of methods for the quantitative study of phagocytosis, *in vitro* as well as *in vivo*. The particles used vary greatly, from India ink (carbon particles with a diameter of about 250 Å, frequently coated with gelatin), polystyrene latex particles, and emulsions of lipid droplets, to aggregated bovine serum albumin and various bacteria. Generally the phagocytosis characteristics of any given particle are governed only by its surface. Different particles coated with the same substance are phagocytized to the same extent, whereas identical particles, when coated with different substances, are phagocytized differently. The explanation for this phenomenon can be found in the preceding section.

In Vitro *Measurements*

In vitro measurements are either done in small glass or plastic chambers or in excised perfused organs of animals (e.g., for the study of particle clearances in liver or spleen). For measurements in small chambers one generally makes use of the fact that only phagocytes (granulocytes and mono-cytes as well as macrophages) adhere to glass surfaces, so that it is quite simple to study the phagocytosis of particles by monolayers of phagocytes, under various conditions and subject to different additives. With the help of chambers, divided into a particle and a phagocyte compartment by a microporous membrane of such a pore size that phagocytes can penetrate them only with a certain degree of difficulty, chemotaxis studies can be done. The sources of circulating phagocytes for *in vitro* studies are generally animal or human peripheral granulocytes, and animal peritoneal or alveolar macrophages.

In Vivo *Measurements*

Most *in vivo* phagocytosis studies are done for the measurement of clearance rates of particles, injected intravenously in animals. In these cases the numbers of particles still in circulation compared to the number initially injected, at any given moment, are plotted against time and clearance rates. Constants can be derived from the curves obtained under a variety of circumstances. Injection of high doses of particles can give rise to blockade of the animal's fixed phagocytes, so that the animal cannot for some time afterward bring about a decrease in concentration of further injected particles of the same type, although a blockade with one type of particle does not necessarily influence the clearance of other types of particles. This blockade is most likely due to the temporary exhaustion of a given plasma opsonin (see above). Clearance studies can also be done *in vitro*, with perfused isolated organs (see above).

Bibliography

Brogan, T. D.: Mechanisms of phagocytosis in human polymorphonuclear leuco-cytes. *Immunology*, **10**:137–48, 1966.

Downey, R. J.: Functions of granulocytes in infectious diseases. In Dunlop, R. M., and Moon, H. W. (eds.): *Resistance to Infectious Disease*. Saskatoon Modern Press, Saskatoon, 1970, pp. 195–216.

Hirsch, J. G.: Phagocytosis. *Annu. Rev. Microbiol.*, **19**:339–50, 1965.

Malawista, S. E., and Bodel, P. T.: The dissociation by colchicine of phagocytosis from increased oxygen consumption in human leukocytes. *J. Clin. Invest.*, **46**:786–96, 1967.

Metchnikoff, E.: *Lectures on the Comparative Pathology of Inflammation*. Dover Publi-cations, Inc., New York, 1968.

Murphy, P.: *The Neutrophil*. Plenum, New York, 1976.

Quie, P. G.: Bactericidal function of polymorphonuclear leucocytes. *Arch. Environ. Health*, **19**:849, 1969.

Quie, P. G.; Messner, R. P.; and Williams, R. C.: Phagocytosis in subacute bacterial endocarditis: localization of the primary opsonic site to Fc fragment. *J. Exp. Med.*, **128**:553–70, 1968.

Stuart, A. E.: *The Reticuloendothelial System.* E. & S. Livingstone, Ltd., London, 1970.

van Furth, R. (ed.): *Mononuclear Phagocytes.* Blackwell Scientific Publications, Ltd., Oxford, 1970.

van Oss, C. J.: Influence of glucose levels on the *in vitro* phagocytosis of bacteria by human neutrophils. *Infect. Immun.*, **4**:54–59, 1971.

van Oss, C. J.: Phagocytosis as a surface phenomenon. *Annu. Rev. Microbiol.*, **32**:19–39, 1978.

van Oss, C. J.; Gillman, C. F.; and Neumann, A. W.: *Phagocytic Engulfment and Cell Adhesiveness.* Marcel Dekker, Inc., New York, 1975.

Wood, W. B.; Smith, M. R.; and Watson, B.: Studies on the mechanism of recovery in pneumococcal pneumonia. *J. Exp. Med.*, **84**:387–402, 1946.

11

Delayed Hypersensitivity

STANLEY COHEN AND ROBERT T. McCLUSKEY

Introduction

The immunologic responses defined as "immediate hypersensitivity reactions" (Chapter 18) are mediated by antibodies of various immunoglobulin classes. The interaction of antigen with an appropriate antibody modifies that antibody and leads to the exposure of new reactive sites. This central event triggers the set of reactions that lead to the particular biologic effect. In the case of both anaphylaxis (Chapter 18) and the Arthus reaction (Chapter 18), as well as complement-dependent cell lysis (Chapter 8), these reactions involve the release of various nonantibody mediator substances. In the case of delayed hypersensitivity, there is an analogous process in which various mediator substances produce an immunologic reaction. In the delayed response, however, the initial triggering event involves the interaction of antigen with an antibody-like receptor on the surface of a sensitized lymphocyte rather than the interaction of antigen with preformed antibody. In this chapter we examine the mechanisms involved in this reaction in detail. In subsequent chapters the relationship of this form of immunologic reactivity to autoimmunity (Chapter 25), transplantation (Chapter 22), and the response to infectious agents (Chapters 13–16) will be considered.

Definition

Delayed hypersensitivity is a form of immunologic response that is mediated by sensitized lymphoid cells rather than antibody. It is characterized by a slowly evolving inflammatory reaction at the site of injection of antigen into a previously sensitized individual. The reaction reaches maximal size in 24 to 48 hours and is composed predominantly of lymphocytes and macrophages. The usual site of challenge is the skin, but the reaction may also be elicited in other locations such as the cornea, the bladder mucosa, or the joint surfaces. In the skin, the gross appearance is a raised, erythematous, indurated lump; the most familiar example is a positive tuberculin reaction in man. Microscopically, in man and in the guinea pig, the reaction has a rather typical appearance and is composed predominantly of lymphocytes and macrophages. Since in routine histologic sections it is not always possible to distinguish between lymphocytes and macrophages, they are usually collectively referred to as "mononuclear" cells. In other species, the reaction may take on a more pleomorphic appearance. In the mouse, for example, the reaction is rich in neutrophils. Even in the guinea pig, appropriate experimental manipulation can result in delayed-type reactions characterized by either eosinophil or basophil infiltration.

Although the delayed reaction is not dependent on circulating antibody, it may occur in the presence of such antibody. In this situation, the response to local injection of antigen is complex; other forms of immunologic response such as the Arthus reaction or anaphylaxis may be superimposed on the delayed reaction, and this leads to a pleomorphic histologic appearance (Chapter 18).

Delayed hypersensitivity is exhibited to varying degrees in different species and is especially pronounced in man and the guinea pig. Most experimental data are derived from studies utilizing the guinea pig.

Requirements for Induction and Elicitation of Delayed Hypersensitivity

It was long believed that delayed hypersensitivity occurred only in response to antigens of microorganisms, but it is now known that this type of reactivity may develop toward purified proteins or simple chemicals (haptens) conjugated to proteins (carriers) (Chapter 5). Moreover, under certain circumstances, the direct cutaneous application of various low-molecular-weight substances with reactive chemical groups can produce a similar response. The latter phenomenon, known as "contact sensitivity," is essentially a delayed hypersensitivity response in which the chemical becomes conjugated *in vivo* to certain proteins of the host itself.

In general, intradermal injections of antigen are most effective in the induction of delayed hypersensitivity, and intravenous injections are least effective. In fact, intravenous administration of antigen can sometimes prevent induction of delayed hypersensitivity by subsequent intradermal administration of antigen. This can happen even though antibody production is not altered. For this reason, the phenomenon is known as "partial tolerance" or "immune deviation." This state can also be produced by injecting relatively small amounts of antigen.

Delayed hypersensitivity may be produced most readily when the antigen is incorporated into an adjuvant. When ovalbumin is injected into foci of tuberculous infection in the guinea pig, delayed hypersensitivity is more likely to develop than if ovalbumin is injected into normal animals. Mixtures of ovalbumin with the wax isolated from mycobacteria are effective in producing delayed hypersensitivity. The most effective method of producing delayed reactivity is by means of emulsification of an aqueous solution of antigen with Freund's complete adjuvant, which consists of mineral oil, a surfactant, and killed mycobacteria.

If mycobacteria are not present, the mixture is known as "incomplete Freund's adjuvant." The reactivity resulting from immunization with incomplete adjuvant is more transient than when complete adjuvant is used. The skin reactions, though grossly similar to those elicitable after immunization with complete Freund's adjuvant, have a somewhat different histologic appearance and are characterized by the presence of basophils as well as mononuclear cells in the infiltrate. The reactivity following incomplete Freund's adjuvant is referred to as Jones-Mote sensitivity.

Although adjuvants enhance the formation of a delayed response, they are not indispensable. Sensitivity can be produced by the injection of small amounts of protein in saline or by the injection of antigen-antibody complexes prepared in excess of antibody.

As stated previously, delayed hypersensitivity may be produced by an antigen that consists of a simple hapten conjugated to a protein carrier. If, for example, guinea pigs are immunized with dinitrophenylated bovine γ globulin (DNP-BGG) and are skin-tested with that antigen one week later, they exhibit strong delayed reactions. If they are tested with the same hapten coupled with an unrelated protein such as ovalbumin, delayed reactions are usually not observed. Conversely, a skin test with an unrelated hapten such as o-chlorobenzoyl chloride (OCBC) conjugated to the original protein usually gives a positive reaction. This phenomenon is known as "carrier specificity." It is quite different from the situation for reactions mediated by antibody, such as the Arthus reaction or anaphylaxis (Chapter 18) in which the haptenic group per se is the important determinant for reactivity (hapten specificity).

Although haptens are capable of combining with preformed antibody, they are not in themselves immunogenic. It is only when they are conjugated to a protein (or other) carrier that they are capable of inducing an immune response (Chapter 5). Thus, the carrier specificity involved in eliciting a delayed reaction suggests that the triggering antigen must be immunogenic even though the animal has already been immunized. This requirement was demonstrated directly with the aid of synthetic polypeptides. For this purpose, dinitrophenylated polylysine molecules of various sizes were studied. The smallest antigen capable of inducing either antibody formation or delayed hypersensitivity was a single DNP molecule conjugated to a polylysine molecule containing seven lysine residues. The antibody response was directed in large measure against the DNP determinant, and, as expected, even DNP conjugated to a single lysine was capable of combining with the antibody so formed. Similarly, molecules containing fewer than seven lysines were capable of eliciting Arthus or anaphylactic reactions, both of which are mediated by antibodies (Chapter 18). On the other hand, a molecule containing a minimum of seven lysines was required to elicit a delayed reaction. In other words, a wholly immunogenic molecule is required for the expression of delayed hypersensitivity.

This distinction between delayed hypersensitivity and antibody-mediated reactions (Chapter 3) is quite important. It shows that the triggering event for the delayed reaction must involve recognition mechanisms similar to those involved in antibody induction. The requirement for immunogenicity is not surprising in view of the fact that the initial step in the delayed reaction involves the interaction of antigen with a receptor on an immunocompetent cell rather than with antibody. A similar antigen-receptor reaction is the stimulus for antibody induction.

Lymph Node Changes in Delayed Hypersensitivity

Lymphocytes that populate lymphoid tissue are derived from precursors in the bone marrow (Chapter 3). Those lymphocytes that come under thymic influence at some stage prior to this colonization are called T cells; others that do not are called B cells. The T cells, for the most part, are found in the paracortical areas of lymph nodes adjacent to the medulla and outside of follicles. It is known as the thymic-dependent zone of the lymph node. When an animal is immunized in a manner designed to induce delayed hypersensitivity, the earliest change is an increase in large pyroninophilic cells (immunoblasts) in these thymic-dependent areas. The immunoblasts contain many ribosomes but little endoplasmic reticulum and no demonstrable immunoglobulins. Animals in which these immunoblasts are labeled with tritiated thymidine show accumulation of labeled small mononuclear cells as the immunoblasts diminish in number after the fourth day, suggesting that the former are derived from the latter. These small mononuclear cells are lymphocytes that contain lysosomes. This cellular transformation reaches a maximum approximately four days following immunization. If animals are immunized so as to develop contact sensitivity in the absence of antibody formation, germinal center formation and plasma cell accumulation are not conspicuous features of the lymph node reaction.

Passive Transfer of Delayed Hypersensitivity

Contact sensitivity can be transferred by means of peritoneal exudate cells from immunized to nonimmunized guinea pigs. Similar transfer in the case of tuberculin sensitivity can be effected using lymph nodes, spleen, and peritoneal exudate cells. Since these early observations, numerous investigators have shown that passive transfer of delayed sensitivity is possible with living mononuclear cells from a variety of sources in several species, including man. In contrast, attempts by numerous investigators to transfer delayed sensitivity with serum have been unsuccessful or inconsistent.

The success of transfer depends on the source of the cells, the species, and the sensitivity of the donor, but in any case, large numbers of cells (several hundred million) are required. Furthermore, even with the use of large numbers of cells from highly sensitized donors, transfer is not always successful. When cells are injected intravenously, there is no latent period before the appearance of a reaction of delayed sensitivity in the recipient. In contrast, anaphylactic antibodies cannot be detected for at least two days following transfer of cells from animals with both delayed and anaphylactic sensitivity (Chapter 18). Transferred delayed sensitivity usually lasts only several days in the recipient; its termination appears to depend on the destruction of the donor cells by the homograft reaction, which is discussed in Chapter 22. When an inbred strain is used, transferred sensitivity persists indefinitely. Further, in inbred animals, sensitivity can be transferred with a relatively small number of cells, in which case it becomes apparent only during the second or third week after transfer. Transfer cannot be achieved between species and is not always successful between two different strains of inbred guinea pigs.

The immediate appearance of delayed sensitivity in the recipient and its rapid disappearance (except in inbred strains) indicated that transfer is not due to active sensitization.

The best available evidence indicates that in experimental animals intact living cells are required for transfer of delayed sensitivity. Treatment of the cells with mitomycin C, or actinomycin, which arrests the synthesis of RNA, abolishes their capacity to effect transfer. Although sporadic reports of successful transfer of delayed sensitivity in animals with subcellular fractions, or "transfer factors," have appeared in the literature, these observations have not been confirmed. Such "transfers" may be the result of nonspecific inflammatory reactions. As will be discussed below, the situation is somewhat different in man.

Cellular Components of the Delayed Reaction

In the skin, the most intense infiltrate is seen in the lower part of the dermis, especially just above the muscle layer. In this location, many of the inflammatory cells are found adjacent to small blood vessels. A large, diffuse infiltrate is also present in the upper dermis. Only small numbers of mononuclear cells may be found within the epidermis. In contact reactions, on the other hand, where the antigen is topically applied, the infiltrate is mainly confined to the upper dermis and epidermis. Epidermal necrosis is much more common in contact reactions than in delayed reactions elicited by intradermal injection.

In all delayed reactions neutrophil infiltration may be seen. Eosinophils are not present in a "pure" delayed reaction. However, they may be seen in situations where antibody is present, or where antigen is reinjected into a site at which a delayed reaction had previously been elicited. This latter phenomenon is known as the "retest" reaction. It begins about two hours after injection of antigen and becomes maximal approximately eight hours later. The mechanism by which eosinophils accumulate in the reaction is not clear. However, recent studies have shown that the interaction of preformed immune complexes with a factor derived from the lymphocytes of donors with delayed hypersensitivity leads to the generation of a chemotactic factor for eosinophils *in vitro*. The material is highly effective when injected into normal guinea pig skin, and this suggests that it might play a role in the retest reaction.

As stated previously, basophils may be conspicuous if the animal has previously been immunized with incomplete Freund's adjuvant.

Nature and Origin of Mononuclear Cells

Most of the information concerning the nature of the mononuclear cells that accumulate in delayed reactions has come from histochemical and radioautographic studies, since these cells cannot be readily identified on morphologic grounds even with the aid of electron microscopy. It is known from such studies that most of the cells in the infiltrate are young macrophages that have emigrated from the circulation. These cells are derived from precursors in the bone marrow and migrate to the dermis through venules at the site of reaction. In most situations, lymphocytes are in the minority in delayed hypersensitivity reactions, although they are always present in significant numbers.

Until recently it was thought that the mononuclear cells comprising the infiltrate of delayed reactions represented sensitized cells possessing some sort of immunologic specificity directed toward the antigen, and some mechanism served to attract such cells to the reaction site. However, only a small number of the infiltrating cells are specifically sensitized cells; moreover, these cells do not specifically accumulate at the reaction site. As was stated previously, the delayed reaction can be transferred by mononuclear cells from a sensitized donor. When the donor cells were labeled with tritiated thymidine and a transfer study was carried out, small numbers of labeled cells were found in reactions in the recipient. Conversely, when the recipients and not the donors were injected with tritiated thymidine prior to transfer, the great majority of cells in the reaction site were labeled. These experiments show that most of the cells were of recipient origin and were, therefore, not sensitized cells.

The bulk of the experimental evidence favors the view that there is no specific accumulation of sensitized cells at a delayed reaction. In general, the experimental design has involved the use of two donors sensitized to different antigens, one contributing a set of labeled cells and the other a set of unlabeled cells to the recipient. In most of these studies, if the recipient was skin-tested with the two antigens at different skin sites, no difference in the number of labeled cells at each site was noted. On the basis of such findings and other considerations, it must be presumed that the reaction is mediated by contact between antigen and a small number of specifically sensitized lymphocytes that arrive randomly at the reaction site.

Effectors of Delayed Reactions

The population of sensitized lymphocytes that mediate delayed hypersensitivity are able to produce a variety of nonantibody effector substances when stimulated by antigen (Table 11-1). These are collectively known as "lymphokines" (Chapter 1). For the most part, lymphokine activity has been evaluated in *in vitro* systems.

Early experiments demonstrated that peripheral leukocytes or spleen cells from tuberculin-sensitive guinea pigs were damaged *in vitro* by exposure to tuberculin. The damage was manifested by inhibition of cell migration in tissue culture, as well as by cell death. Since that report, many investigations of the *in vitro* effects of antigens on cells from animals with delayed hypersensitivity have been conducted. For example, the effects of antigen on washed guinea pig peritoneal exudate cells cultivated in capillary tubes were studied. Normally, migration of cells from the end of the tube occurred, with the formation of a mass of cells readily visible at 24 hours. When cells were taken from guinea pigs with tuberculin sensitivity or pure delayed sensitivity to purified proteins, inhibition of cell migration was observed in

Table 11-1

SOME LYMPHOCYTE PRODUCTS AND THEIR PROPERTIES

Factor	Biologic Activity
1. Eosinophil chemotactin	Attracts eosinophils following interaction with immune complexes
2. Interferon	Antimicrobial activity
3. Lymphotoxin	Kills various nucleated target cells
4. Lymphocyte chemotactin	Attracts other lymphocytes
5. Macrophage activation factor	Enhances macrophage motility and phagocytosis
6. Macrophage chemotactin	Attracts macrophages
7. Migration inhibition factor	Prevents macrophage migration *in vitro*
8. Mitogenic factor	Causes blast transformation in lymphocytes
9. Neutrophil chemotactin	Attracts neutrophils
10. Skin reactive factor	Produces inflammatory reaction in skin
11. Transfer factor	Passive transfer of delayed hypersensitivity in man

the presence of specific antigen. In experiments using hapten-protein conjugates, the phenomenon had the same carrier specificity as delayed reactions *in vivo*. That the inhibition of migration was not due to the presence of conventional antibody, either absorbed on the cells or produced in the system, was shown by the failure of addition of antibody to a culture of normal cells to reproduce the effect. Furthermore, cells from guinea pigs immunized by intravenous injection, which showed circulating antibody but not delayed sensitivity, did not exhibit the phenomenon. However, peritoneal cells from guinea pigs that exhibited both delayed sensitivity and circulating antibodies did show this effect.

Experiments were then performed to analyze the respective roles of lymphocytes and macrophages in the specific inhibition of migration of peritoneal cells by antigen. When a preparation of macrophages presumably devoid of lymphocytes was used, the cells migrated normally despite the presence of antigen; on the other hand, the addition of lymphocytes from sensitive animals resulted in the inhibition of migration of macrophages obtained from normal animals in the presence of antigen. It, therefore, appears that upon contact with specific antigen, sensitized lymphocytes release a material that reacts with the macrophages to prevent migration. In support of this concept, the culture fluid taken after 24 hours of incubation of sensitized lymphocytes with antigen inhibits the migration of normal macrophages. The active material appears to be synthesized after contact of the cell with the antigen, since it is not released when the lymphocytes are incubated in the presence of puromycin (a drug that interferes with protein synthesis). The exact nature of this material is not known, but it appears that the activity resides in a nondialyzable protein fraction with a molecular weight close to that of albumin. Therefore, it cannot be conventional antibody. This substance has been called "migration inhibition factor" or MIF and was one of the first lymphokines to be described.

When the effects of antigen on cells from tuberculin-sensitive animals or man are judged in suspensions of isolated cells rather than in capillary tubes or explant cultures, the results are somewhat different. With suspensions, there occurs initially death of some cells followed in a few days by proliferation. Recent experiments have established that lymphoid cells from sensitized animals can be transformed and stimulated to divide *in vitro* by specific antigen, as shown by an increase in nucleic acid synthesis accompanied by appearance of "blast" forms and a mitotic response. Cells obtained from animals with circulating antibody but without delayed sensitivity do not respond in this fashion. Further, in studies using hapten protein conjugates, his *in vitro* effect had the same specificity as delayed reactions. In addition, it appears that the stimulated cells release cytotoxic substances, because syngeneic fibroblasts are killed when they are incubated with lymph node cells of animals having delayed sensitivity in presence of the specific antigen. This situation is analogous to the capillary tube migration experiments in which cells from nonimmunized animals are affected by material released from a few sensitized cells.

Some of these phenomena are due to direct effects of antigen on lymphocytes or of activated lymphocytes on other cell types. Similar effects, however, have been shown to be mediated by soluble factors produced by the activated lymphocytes. Examples of such lymphokines are "blastogenic factor" and "cytotoxic factor." There are many other known lymphokines including a class of substances that are chemotactic for a variety of inflammatory cell types.

In addition to these factors, there is a lymphocyte product that to date has been unequivocally demonstrated only in man. This substance, discovered by Lawrence, is known as "transfer factor." Transfer of delayed hypersensitivity in man can be accomplished not only with intact living lymphocytes but with killed cells or cell extracts. Transfer factor is the responsible substance and can be extracted from peripheral lymphocytes by lysis or by freezing and thawing. It can also be released from cells during incubation *in vitro* in the presence of the antigen: the released factor remains effective in spite of its contact with antigen. The cells are left apparently intact but are no longer able to effect transfer. Although transfer factor, or killed cells, are injected locally, they confer a general state of sensitivity in the recipient. After transfer, reactivity becomes apparent within a few hours, as indicated by the flareup of negative skin sites injected with the antigen a few days previously; maximal reactivity, however, is reached only after a few days. The state of reactivity appears to last months or years, and sequential transfers have been successful; i.e., cells from one recipient have been able to transfer sensitivity to a second recipient. This suggests that the factor passes from one cell to another, is self-replicating, or rapidly induces a state of active sensitization. It is not known whether circulating antibody against the relevant antigen is produced in the recipients.

Transfer factor is effective in transferring sensitivity to a variety of antigens, such as tuberculin, diphtheria toxoid, and coccidioidin. Transfer of sensitivity to artificial antigens has also been achieved by the use of killed leukocytes. This is particularly important, since it is highly unlikely that the responsible antigenic determinants could have been encountered by the recipient before. The activity of transfer factor is not affected by DNase, RNase, or trypsin; it is stable for at least several days at room temperature and several months at low temperature; it is dialyzable, and gel filtration indicates that it has a molecular weight lower than 10,000.

The precise nature and mode of action of transfer factor are unknown. It is certainly one of the major riddles in the problem of delayed hypersensitivity in man. It does not appear to represent antibody, since it cannot be neutralized by antigen *in vitro* and often leads to long-lasting sensitization in the recipient. It does not act like antigen, since it creates a state of sensitivity in the recipient immediately after contact. The mechanism by which transfer factor passively confers sensitivity remains obscure.

In Vivo Significance of Lymphokine Production

The elaboration of many, if not all, of the lymphokines is correlated with the state of delayed hypersensitivity of the lymphocyte donor. For this reason, assays for such factors, most notably MIF, are considered to represent *in vitro* models of delayed hypersensitivity. Moreover, it is assumed that the expression of delayed hypersensitivity *in vivo* requires the participation of various lymphokines. Evidence supporting this latter contention is of relatively recent origin; however, inflammatory reactions have been produced in guinea pig skin by the intradermal injection of lymphocytes cultured in the presence of the specific antigen supernatants. This "skin-reactive factor" produced lesions that resembled delayed reactions early in their evolution. Such studies are not entirely satisfactory because of the essentially non-specific nature of the inflammatory exudate in delayed hypersensitivity reactions. An alternate approach was an unsuccessful attempt to passively transfer tuberculin or contact sensitivity by implanting sensitized lymphocytes in micropore chambers into normal guinea pigs. This failure, however, may have been related to barriers to free diffusion of soluble mediator and/or antigen in the test system, which involved the subcutaneous implantation of chambers containing cells but no antigen. Also, these studies made no attempt to purify the cell populations used for transfer. Donor macrophages were present with the lymphocytes in the chambers, and they may have absorbed sufficient amounts of mediator substance to prevent the reaction outside the chamber. In any case, with the exception of transfer factor in man, no *in vivo* extracellular mediator of delayed hypersensitivity in the skin appears to have been documented. Instead, evidence for a lymphokine-dependent mechanism in delayed hypersensitivity *in vivo* comes from experiments involving the "macrophage disappearance reaction" (MDR).

The intraperitoneal injection of antigen into guinea pigs with delayed hypersensitivity bearing preexisting glycogen-induced peritoneal exudates leads to a marked reduction in the macrophage content of these exudates. This provides several lines of evidence that this "macrophage disappearance reaction" is a manifestation of delayed hypersensitivity. Purified populations of small lymphocytes could passively transfer the MDR to nonimmunized recipients. The reaction could be transferred when the donor lymphocytes were contained within micropore chambers, and supernatants from cultures of antigen-stimulated sensitized lymphocytes were almost as effective as intact cells in eliciting the MDR. It was concluded that soluble products of antigen-activated lymphocytes could modify the *in vivo* behavior of macrophages in at least one reaction associated with delayed hypersensitivity.

Further evidence for *in vivo* lymphokine activity comes from studies in which skin sites of delayed reactors were homogenized and the aqueous eluates tested for various activities. Such eluates had strong chemotactic activity for macrophages, and the chemotactic agent was similar to substances previously isolated from supernatants of antigen-stimulated lymphocyte cultures.

It is also possible to detect MIF in serum of delayed hypersensitive experimental animals, provided that they have received an intravenous injection of specific antigen within four to six hours. In addition, serum MIF can be detected in patients with certain disorders such as lymphoproliferative diseases (Hodgkin's disease, chronic lymphatic leukemia, Sezary syndrome) and sarcoidosis.

Desensitization

As stated previously, systemic administration of antigen alone prior to footpad injection of antigen in complete Freund's adjuvant can lead to the development of partial tolerance with respect to delayed hypersensitivity without diminution of antibody formation. Moreover, even after delayed reactivity has been established, intravenous injection of antigen may lead to temporary loss of delayed reactivity. This process is known as "desensitization."

A single intravenous injection of 1 to 2 mg of antigen will suffice to desensitize guinea pigs to purified proteins by the previous injection of immune complexes. The state of desensitization typically lasts for several days and is somewhat more prolonged if very large doses of antigen are used.

It is also possible to desensitize *in vitro* in a transfer system by preincubating the sensitized lymphoid cells with antigen prior to transfer. The mechanism of this reaction is not clear but is probably related either to the blocking of antigen-combining sites on the cells prior to their arrival at the skin site or to antigen-triggered release of mediator substances *in vitro* with subsequent "exhaustion" prior to transfer. In any case, it is clear that desensitization, both *in vitro* and *in vivo*, is a consequence of the interaction between sensitized cells and antigen.

Another mechanism for desensitization that has recently been described involves the intravenous administration of large amounts of exogenous MIF-containing materials. This apparently involves preemption of effector macrophages (and other cells) systemically so that they are not available at the local reaction site. This mode of desensitization may have clinical significance, since those patients shown to have MIF in their serum after desensitization demonstrate anergy with respect to skin testing.

Lymphocytes Involved in the Delayed Response

It is well established that the immune response is dependent on the interaction of several cell types, including T cells and B cells. A variety of observations (1) on birds, where there is especially sharp dissociation between the two lymphoid systems; (2) on neonatally thymectomized mammals; and (3) on immunologic deficiency states in man have all provided indirect evidence that delayed hypersensitivity is mediated by T cells. For example, neonatal thymectomy in the rat leads to a decrease in the capacity of the animal to develop delayed sensitivity and, to a lesser extent, antibody production. The capacity of thymectomized rats to exhibit delayed reactions following passive transfer of cells from sensitized donors is unimpaired. The reduction in the development of delayed sensitivity has been attributed to the lymphopenia that occurs following thymectomy. Suppression of delayed reactivity has also been described in neonatally thymectomized mice. In guinea pigs, neonatal thymectomy does not prevent the induction of contact sensitivity, but the guinea pig is more immunologically mature at birth than animals of other species.

In birds there are two central lymphoid organs, the thymus and the bursa (Chapter 3). Neonatal thymectomy depresses hypersensitivity, whereas neonatal bursectomy suppresses antibody formation. Although it has been suggested that there is a bursal equivalent in mammals, possibly the gut-associated lymphoid tissue, the evidence for this is scanty. The recent description of a marker on T cells of mice (θ antigen) has allowed more direct studies of the relationship of these cells to delayed hypersensitivity. Most of these studies involved the specific destruction of cells carrying this marker by the use of anti-θ antibody and complement. Such treatment suppresses reactions involving contact sensitivity, *in vitro* reactivity to non-specific lymphocyte-stimulating agents such as phytohemagglutinin, graft-vs.-host reactions, lymphocyte cytotoxic reactions, graft rejection, and the mixed lymphocyte reaction. All of these reactivities are correlated with delayed hypersensitivity. Thus, the evidence that delayed hypersensitivity is mediated by T cells is convincing. Nevertheless, there are few studies in the literature showing *directly* that any of the various lymphokines, the putative mediators of delayed hypersensitivity, are produced by T cells. However, mouse lymphocytes may be divided into two populations on the basis of whether or not they possess complement receptors on their surface. Convincing evidence has been presented that these populations correspond to B cells and T cells. The "complement receptor lymphocytes" (CRL) correspond to B cells and the "noncomplement receptor lymphocytes" (NCRL) correspond to T cells. A similar functional distinction between populations of lymphocytes has been found in the guinea pig. In this species, the NCRL could mediate the MDR, whereas the CRL could not. Since the MDR is mediated by a lymphokine, one can surmise that a lymphocyte population that corresponds to T cells can generate lymphokine activity *in vivo*.

More recently, it has been demonstrated directly that purified populations of T cells can respond to specific antigen stimulation with MIF production. Surprisingly, B cells could also make MIF provided they were stimulated with a B cell mitogen. The capacity of B cells to make MIF and other lymphokines has now been confirmed in many laboratories. In general, T cells can respond to either specific antigens or T cell mitogens. B cells can respond to B cell mitogens. In one report, B cells appeared to respond to specific antigen as well, but subsequent studies suggest that this might have been due to the antigenic stimulation of small numbers of contaminating T cells, which then made a mitogenic factor (one of the known lymphokines) and triggered the B cells.

Lymphokines and Cell Interactions

Many of the lymphokines participate in reactions in which lymphocytes modify the behavior of other cell types. The best-known example is MIF, which inhibits the migration of macrophages on glass surfaces. Two factors that are distinct from MIF have recently been described as chemotactic agents for neutrophils and macrophages. Also, one lymphokine is chemotactic for eosinophils. This factor has a unique requirement for interaction with preformed immune complexes in order to generate biologic activity. Lymphocytes from delayed hypersensitive guinea pigs are cultured in the presence of specific antigen under conditions that result in optimal MIF activity. The supernatants from such cultures are incubated with preformed antigen-antibody complexes. The resulting reaction leads to the generation of potent and specific eosinophil chemotactic activity. The material, although generated *in vitro*, had both *in vitro* and *in vivo* activity.

Several other examples of cellular interactions mediated by lymphokines are known. As mentioned above, one mitogenic factor stimulates other lymphocytes. A lymphokine chemotactic for lymphocytes has also been discovered. In addition, several studies suggest other lymphokine-mediated phenomena involving multiple cell types. Thus, there is a lymphocyte-dependent mechanism for histamine release by platelets. Also, certain reactions of cellular immunity are characterized by extensive basophil infiltrations; this suggests that lymphocytes might produce a factor that is chemotactic for these cells. Of the agents listed above, the chemotactic factors appear to be of greatest biologic interest, because there seem to be factors specific for each of the cells that participate in inflammatory reactions.

Effects of Drugs on Delayed Hypersensitivity

Guinea pigs treated for three weeks with cortisone (2 mg daily) following immunization failed to exhibit delayed sensitivity to tuberculin. However, peritoneal exudate cells of these animals were able to transfer tuberculin sensitivity to normal recipients. In addition, cortisone, when given shortly before testing, inhibited tuberculin reactions in rabbits. Cortisone has also diminished or abolished contact reactivity, even though cortisone-treated animals can serve as donors in transfer reactions. In view of these considerations and in view of the known anti-inflammatory effect of cortisone, it seems that its capacity to suppress delayed sensitivity is primarily due to an anti-inflammatory action.

Nitrogen mustard administration leads to neutrophil depletion. As might be expected, this drug has no effect on tuberculin reactivity.

Treatment with the chemical 48/80, before skin testing previously immunized animals, inhibits contact reactivity. This surprising result, which awaits confirmation, suggests that materials released from mast cells may participate in the mediation of the delayed reaction perhaps by increasing vascular permeability locally. However, the increase in permeability observed in delayed hypersensitivity cannot be inhibited by antihistamines injected at the time of testing.

Finally, the administration of heparin or warfarin shortly before a skin test depressed the intensity of tuberculin contact reactions. The suppressive effect is not due to an action on complement (Chapter 8). The mechanism of action of anticoagulants is not known, although the fact that two unrelated anticoagulant agents exert a comparable effect suggests that at least one aspect of the delayed reaction is related in some manner to the coagulation mechanism. A likely possibility is that permeability factors operative in delayed hypersensitivity might be chemically related to certain members of the clotting sequence.

Depression of Delayed Sensitivity in Disease

Impairment or absence of delayed sensitivity is commonly observed in diseases characterized by thymic aplasia, i.e., either in the Swiss type of agammaglobulinemia or in the other forms of developmental failure of the thymus associated with normal immunoglobulins; in contrast, delayed sensitivity is frequently unimpaired in the usual form of agammaglobulinemia, which is not associated with thymic abnormalities (Chapter 17). Depression or absence of delayed hypersensitivity has been considered a hallmark of ataxia-telangiectasia, a hereditary neurooculocutaneous disease. The immunologic abnormalities of this disease have been attributed to a failure of thymic development.

Patients with certain diseases, such as Hodgkin's disease, Boeck's sarcoid, and Sjögren's syndrome, may also show a loss of delayed hypersensitivity. In Hodgkin's disease, this depression can be seen in many patients as a loss of previously established sensitivity and can be shown in a high percentage of patients by their inability to become sensitized. This effect is not a consequence of massive lymph node involvement and is much more common than in any other form of neoplastic disease. Delayed sensitivity may sometimes reappear when the disease becomes quiescent. Although the matter is not entirely settled, recent observations suggest that the capacity to form circulating antibodies is unimpaired. The anergy of Hodgkin's disease may be due to an abnormal response of lymphocytes to antigen since lymphocytes from patients with Hodgkin's disease show a strikingly depressed mitotic response to phytohemagglutinin, *in vitro* or when lymphocytes of histoincompatible individuals are mixed in the same culture (mixed lymphocyte culture MLC). A similar abnormal response of lymphocytes to phytohemagglutinin has also been observed in Boeck's sarcoid and Sjögren's syndrome. However, it seems unlikely that the failure of lymphocytes to respond could be the entire explanation for the impairment of delayed sensitivity in Hodgkin's disease, since it is not possible to transfer delayed sensitivity to Hodgkin's patients using cells from sensitized normal individuals. Another possibility is the mechanism already discussed in a previous section that involves the suppression of reactivity caused by the presence of circulating lymphokines (page 178).

Depression of delayed sensitivity is also observed in chronic lymphatic leukemia, multiple myeloma, and lepromatous leprosy. In these diseases, in contrast to Hodgkin's disease and sarcoidosis, the capacity to develop hypersensitivity to new antigens appears to be more markedly impaired than the delayed response to previously encountered antigens. Transfer of delayed sensitivity was successfully carried out in chronic lymphatic leukemia and multiple myeloma.

Tuberculin sensitivity may temporarily disappear during the course of some infectious diseases; the best-known example of this phenomenon, which was mentioned by von Pirquet in 1911, is the lack of reactivity observed during measles. This loss of reactivity does not depend on the rash, since it can be observed during the incubation period of the disease and is also seen after measles vaccination. Depression of delayed hypersensitivity may also occur in uremia.

Summary

The delayed hypersensitivity reaction consists of a slowly evolving mononuclear inflammatory infiltrate at the site of injection of antigen into an appropriately immunized individual. The cells for the most part are nonspecific macrophages and lymphocytes that accumulate as a consequence of the interaction of antigen with small numbers of specifically sensitized, thymus-derived lymphocytes (T cells) that arrive randomly at the reaction site. The interaction of antigens with antibody-like cellular receptors leads to anatomic and functional alterations of these sensitized cells, and ultimately to the synthesis and release of certain effector substances known as lymphokines. The various lymphokines are thought to be the direct mediators of the delayed reaction. For example, chemotactic substances are produced that attract macrophages, lymphocytes, neutrophils, and in some circumstances eosinophils. Another substance, migration inhibition factor (MIF), probably serves to immobilize macrophages at the reaction site. Other lymphokines activate macrophages and make them more phagocytic. In some situations, where the antigenic stimulus comes from an invading cell, whether microorganism, neoplasm, or transplant, cytotoxic lymphokines may play a role as well.

The delayed hypersensitivity reaction, like the many reactions of immediate hypersensitivity, consists of a chain of events in which the activity of one cell type modifies or induces the activity of another. The outcome of this sequence of changes may be beneficial or harmful to the individual, depending on the given clinical or experimental setting.

Bibliography

Cohen, S.: The role of cell-mediated immunity in the induction of inflammatory responses. *Am. J. Pathol.*, **88**:502–28, 1977.

McCluskey, R. T., and Cohen, S.: *Mechanisms of Cell-Mediated Immunity*. John Wiley & Sons, Inc., New York, 1974.

12

Immunologic Unresponsiveness

FELIX MILGROM AND
WOLFGANG MÜLLER-RUCHHOLTZ

Introduction

The concept of immunologic tolerance was advanced by Burnet and Fenner in 1949. They were concerned with the explanation of the fact that autologous, "self" components of the vertebrate organism are eliminated without immune response, and they assumed that all antigens encountered in early development stages are recognized as "self" and, as a consequence, do not elicit immune responses. Accordingly, self-recognition is acquired early in ontogenesis and is not inherited (Figure 12-1). Furthermore, Burnet and Fenner postulated that foreign antigens presented in the early stages of development will be treated by the body like "self" components; i.e., they will induce a state of immunologic unresponsiveness or acquired immunologic tolerance.

Our discussion will involve tolerance to transplantation antigens and tolerance to chemically defined antigens. Previously, the latter was often referred to as immunologic paralysis, but there is no reason to treat these two forms of tolerance separately.

183

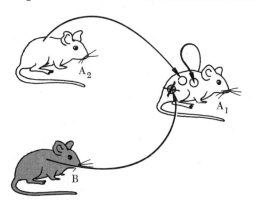

Figure 12-1. Physiologic tolerance is limited to self-structures.
$A_1 \rightarrow A_1$: autogeneic skin graft:
accepted.
$A_2 \rightarrow A_1$: syngeneic skin graft
(from an identical twin
or another animal of
the same inbred strain):
accepted.
$B \rightarrow A_1$: allogeneic skin graft:
rejected.

Naturally Occurring Tolerance

Silent Virus Infection

In the 1930s, Traub described infection with lymphocytic choriomeningitis
(LCM) virus in a mouse colony at the Rockefeller Institute. When mice
were infected by intrauterine transmission, a normal survival time resulted
even though they harbored the virus, as evidenced by overt infection and
severe disease of normal adult mice injected with organs from members of
the asymptomatic colony. Thus, an apparently asymptomatic carrier state
was developed. At that time, Traub could find no antibodies in these mice.
Burnet postulated that by not responding to the virus, the mice lived with it
in "peaceful coexistence."

Chimerism

In 1945, Owen studied blood groups in nonidentical cattle twins. In
hemolysis tests, he found that such twins frequently have two erythrocyte
populations, a finding that agreed with the already known fact that the
blood in cattle twins is exchanged through placental anastomoses. Burnet
and Fenner stressed the case of persisting chimerism (presence of cells
derived from different zygotes) in these twins and considered this to be a
consequence of the exchange of hemopoietic precursor cells and the acquisition of mutual immunologic tolerance by the twins. In 1951, Medawar and
his associates exchanged skin transplants between such dizygotic cattle twins
and found that the grafts were usually accepted, whereas grafts exchanged
between siblings from different pregnancies were rejected. Chimerism in
sheep has also been described, although it occurs infrequently. The results of
these studies were quite similar to those observed in cattle.

Human chimerism seldom occurs. The first case, Mrs. McK., was described
by Dunsford and his associates in 1953. On examining her blood groups,

these investigators noted a mixture of A_1 and O erythrocytes. They suspected chimerism and learned that Mrs. McK. had had a twin brother who died at the age of three months. Mrs. McK. herself was of blood group O, as evidenced by secretion of H but not A blood group substance. The A_1 cells apparently originated from her twin brother. Following separation of the O from the A_1 erythrocytes, further blood group differences were found between these two cell populations. Subsequently, several more human chimeras were described. The proportion of the twin's erythrocytes varied considerably. In Mrs. McK., 40% of the red blood cells were of her twin's origin. It is quite obvious that in all O-A chimeras, the formation of anti-A is suppressed.

Experimental Tolerance

Tolerance to Chemically Defined Antigens

The early descriptions of experimental tolerance (paralysis) date from the 1920s and pertain to chemicals. Frei, and later Sulzberger, found that intravenous injection of neoarsphenamine in man or guinea pig prevented the development of skin hypersensitivity to this drug. Chase found in 1946 that oral administration of simple chemicals to guinea pig interfered with skin sensitization to these chemicals.

In the 1940s, Felton and his associates described unresponsiveness of mice to pneumococcal polysaccharides, which are antigenic for this species. By a single injection of 100 to 1000 times more polysaccharide than its immunizing dose, paralysis was elicited and the mice failed to develop immunity when injected with whole pneumococci. The paralysis was specific for the given strain of pneumococci. It was long lasting because the antigens remained in mice for long periods of time, probably due to lack of depolymerases for these polysaccharides.

Studies in the 1950s contributed further important information indicating that tolerance can also be induced against easily metabolized antigens, such as serum proteins. Newborn rabbits injected repeatedly with bovine serum albumin showed specific unresponsiveness to this protein. Dixon and Maurer succeeded in inducing unresponsiveness even in adult rabbits by daily infusions of large volumes of human plasma. In most cases, however, the tolerance lasted only about as long as the foreign proteins were detectable in the host. These authors were the first who attempted to make adult animals more prone to the development of tolerance by instituting immuno-suppression during antigen administration. They showed that irradiated adult rabbits developed a long-lasting specific unresponsiveness to xeno-geneic serum proteins, comparable to that inducible in newborn rabbits.

In 1959, Schwartz and Dameshek introduced cytotoxic drugs that had been used in cancer chemotherapy. They demonstrated that adult rabbits, after simultaneous treatment with 6-mercaptopurine and human serum albumin, became specifically tolerant to this protein. The term "drug-induced tolerance" was coined, and among the many drugs studied, the alkylating agent cyclophosphamide proved to be especially effective.

In the early 1960s, Dresser discovered that the state of aggregation of proteins is of great importance for their immunogenicity. High-speed centrifugation of bovine gamma globulin yielded a soluble preparation in the supernatant, which was "tolerogenic" rather than immunogenic for mice. It was concluded that the physical state of aggregation confers an "adjuvanticity" that is necessary to induce sensitization. It has been proposed that aggregated, but not disaggregated, gamma globulin adheres readily to macrophages that present this antigen to lymphocytes in a way that initiates antibody formation. Studies on disaggregated gamma globulin showed that in various strains of mice, there are great differences in the readiness with which unresponsiveness is elicited. Some evidence suggested that the induction of tolerance may be under genetic control similar to the induction of immunity.

Transplantation Tolerance

First reports on transplantation tolerance were published in 1953 by Billingham, Brent, and Medawar. Intrauterine injections of embryos of mouse strain CBA with allogeneic cell suspensions of strain A origin resulted in the spectacular finding that the injected CBA mice "tolerated" skin grafted in adulthood for more than one year. Later, Medawar's group replaced intrauterine injections of fetuses by intravenous injections of newborn mice with allogeneic cells. Also, the same group of investigators elicited tolerance in chickens injected in embryonal life with homologous blood (Figure 12-2).

About the same time, a group of Czech investigators led by Hašek developed a technique of embryonal parabiosis in avian species by bringing

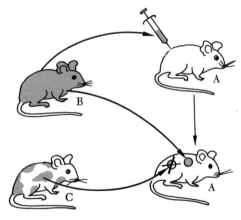

Figure 12-2. Experimentally induced tolerance to foreign structures is specific.

1. Inducing treatment. Adequate systemic application of a proper dose of B antigen to A.

2. Subsequent test protocol. Selectively, a B graft is accepted by A; a C graft is readily rejected.

together chorioallantoic membranes of the two partners. The membranes developed vascular anastomoses and the embryos exchanged blood. Parabiosis was "naturally" terminated at hatching. Grafts exchanged between the partners in adulthood were accepted; the procedure resulted in mutual tolerance reminiscent of that observed in cattle twins. Hašek and his colleagues also succeeded in eliciting tolerance by injecting allogeneic cells into a vein exposed on the chorioallantoic membrane.

The following definition was presented by Medawar's group in 1956: "Tolerance represents a specific and systemic failure of the mechanism of immunological response which is brought about by exposing embryos or very young animals to antigenic stimuli, i.e., to stimuli which would have caused older animals to become sensitive or immune. It is due to primary central failure of the mechanism of immunological reaction, and not to some intercession at a peripheral level." The immaturity of the animal was stressed. A concept of "critical period" was postulated, during which exposure to antigens induces tolerance but not immunity. An explanation of immunologic tolerance was offered in terms of the clonal selection theory postulating that introduction of an antigen in early stages of development results in the elimination of the clones of cells committed to the given antigen.

The theory of "critical period" was consistent with the classic immunologic beliefs in immunologic immaturity of fetal and newborn animals. These beliefs, however, proved to be incorrect. Transplantation immunity was successfully induced in fetal animals by injection of very small doses of allogeneic cells, less than that required for tolerance. Moreover, a group of investigators at the University of Minnesota led by Good induced tolerance in adult mice by injecting large doses of allogeneic cells. In many instances, however, in order to achieve tolerance in adults, one would have to inject such large amounts of cells that this is not feasible.

Medawar's revised interpretation stated in the mid-1960s that a tolerant animal has no cells responding to the tolerated antigens; i.e., the animal has a "central failure" of response. Cells, which are newly differentiated from stem cells and have the potential to respond to the given antigen, give up this potential or die in the presence of an excess of this antigen. In the embryo or newborn, the predominant cell population is immature and uncommitted; therefore, tolerance is easily induced but sensitization can be established only with difficulty. On the other hand, most cells in the adult are mature and committed and, therefore, sensitization can be achieved readily but tolerance is difficult to establish since committed cells must be destroyed.

Kinetics of Tolerance

Obviously, as seen from the above discussion, immunologic tolerance is a state of specific, antigen-induced unresponsiveness. Mitchison discussed tolerance considering nonimmunogenic, weakly immunogenic, and strongly immunogenic antigens. Nonimmunogenic antigens are those which evoke unresponsiveness in adult animals if injected without adjuvant. For example, injection of bovine gamma globulin in a nonaggregated state would elicit unresponsiveness in mice at doses that engender immune response in the presence of adjuvant. Bovine serum albumin is a weak antigen in mice. If injected in small quantities without adjuvant, it elicits unresponsiveness (low-dose tolerance); larger doses induce immunity; still larger doses again evoke unresponsiveness (high-dose tolerance). Finally, strong antigens, such as most proteins, result in immunity unless injected in doses so high that they induce paralysis.

The induction phase of tolerance could be studied by cell transfer experiments. In these experiments, sublethally irradiated mice or rats served as recipients of syngeneic lymphoid cells. Depending on the antigen and species of the experimental animal, unresponsiveness was established by transfer of donor cells obtained a few days or even a few hours after the inducing injection of the antigen, but never by transfer of cells obtained immediately after the injection of the antigen. The period of time between injection of antigen and acquisition of tolerance-transferring capacity by lymphoid cells should be considered as the lag phase in induction of unresponsiveness.

Other transfer experiments have been performed, primarily by Weigle and his associates, using separated T and B cells from tolerant or normal mice syngeneic with irradiated recipients. Thereafter, the recipients received immunogenic injections of the antigen, human gamma globulin (which is T cell dependent). Recipients of normal T cells plus tolerant B cells or tolerant T cells plus normal B cells were tolerant, as were recipients of tolerant T and B cells. Only animals that receive normal T and B cells were capable of responding to the antigen.

Further studies showed different kinetics and different antigen dose requirements for induction of tolerance of T and B cells. T cells became tolerant more quickly and at a much lower antigen concentration than B cells. Also, tolerance persisted longer in T cells than in B cells. The low-dose tolerance discussed by Mitchison (see above) was T cell tolerance with reactive B lymphocytes, whereas the high-dose tolerance involved both T and B cells. In some situations, innate tolerance is limited to T cells. This may be the case with homologous and autologous thyroglobulin. If altered thyroglobulin is injected, T lymphocytes reactive against the altered constituents of the molecule become activated. Thus, thyroglobulin can now be presented by T cells. As a consequence, autoantibodies to native configurations of thyroglobulin are formed (Chapter 25).

Information on the kinetics of recovery from tolerance also has been provided by experiments on cell transfer to irradiated recipients. Spleen cells from unresponsive animals will transfer the unresponsive state only for a limited period of time (a few weeks). Thereafter, even though the donor still is tolerant, the cells behave as normal cells. The explanation for this phenomenon is that the amount of antigen persisting in the donor suffices to maintain the state of unresponsiveness even though the cells have started to recover from tolerance. On the other hand, the concentration of antigen in the recipient does not suffice to produce a similar effect. This explanation, reflecting a generally accepted rule, is in agreement with the finding that animals that show long-lasting transplantation tolerance after embryonal or neonatal injection of allogeneic cells are chimeras. Termination of chimerism by injection of proper cytotoxic antiserum is followed by termination of tolerance.

Mechanisms of Tolerance

There is now general agreement that the term "tolerance" does not cover a single state of specific unresponsiveness brought about by a single mechanism. Additional information obtained during the last six years also indicates that we cannot explain all experimental findings by some "central failure."

Functional unresponsiveness may be based not only on nonreactivity (i.e., the absence of specifically reactive cells) but also on some kind of altered reactivity (i.e., an effect of a specifically suppressive mechanism). Even within one animal, these alternatives are mutually exclusive only at one given time. At a different time, the same functional state might be achieved by a different mechanism. This becomes understandable when one considers that all potentially responsive clones are renewed throughout life from undetermined hemopoietic stem cells.

Clonal Abortion or Inactivation

As pointed out above, the original reasoning of Burnet and Medawar was based on the assumption of antigen-mediated elimination or inactivation of potentially reactive cells. Any *in vitro* test with sera or lymphocytes of a specifically nonreactive animal would fail to demonstrate any activity. This negative phenomenon would not be transferable to reactive syngeneic recipients; i.e., it would not be of an "infectious" type (Figure 12-3). On the other hand, adoptive transfer of lymphocytes from a normally reactive donor should reconstitute the responsiveness.

For "central tolerance" to major transplantation antigens, lack or inactivity of specifically reactive T cells is the one absolute requirement. The existence of such a deficit is supported by numerous reports that showed that rats and mice made tolerant by neonatal inoculation of a high number of foreign cells have no lymphocytes capable of eliciting specific graft-vs.-host reaction (Chapter 23) or mixed lymphocyte reaction (Chapter 22). Neither do they have lymphocytes capable of suppressing normally reactive lymphocytes *in vitro* or *in vivo*.

This is not in contradiction to recent findings in allophenic (tetraparental) mice, which are obtained by fusion of mouse embryos at the blastomere

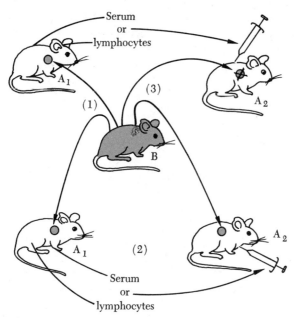

Figure 12-3. Mechanisms of tolerance: central failure vs. specific suppression Test procedure: (1) demonstration of tolerance in A_1, (2) transfer experiment, (3) testing for tolerance in A_2. Central failure, i.e., specific nonreactivity of A_1 to B, cannot be transferred to a reactive syngeneic recipient A_2. Specific suppression, i.e., "infectious tolerance," can be transferred by humoral antibodies or by suppressor lymphocytes.

stage of 8 to 16 cells and which differ from F_1 hybrids in that they contain separate cells from each embryo. Hellström and his associates found that lymph node cells from allophenic mice are cytotoxic against cultured fibroblasts of one parental strain. However, it is known that only some of these animals are detectably chimeric in their immune system and that the degree of chimerism may vary markedly. Some fused embryo may provide only a secluded tissue of one parent (similar to a teratoma), and thus the requirements of disseminated cellular chimerism, providing steady antigen exposure sufficient for clonal abortion or inactivation, may not be fulfilled.

In adults, drug-induced tolerance has been interpreted as a stimulate-and-kill mechanism: antigen-reactive cells are stimulated by the administration of antigen, and these metabolically activated and proliferating cells become especially susceptible to the cytotoxic agent. However, alternative possibilities (see below) are not excluded. Inactivation, rather than elimination, is suggested for B lymphocytes following the binding of certain polymeric T-independent antigens. Nossal and Pike have recently studied the behavior of murine B cells placed in tissue culture with T cell-independent antigens, and subsequently assessed them for immune competence after transfer into syngeneic hosts. An antigen concentration as low as 2.5×10^{-8} M was effective in preventing maturation of B lymphocytes. Klaus and Humphrey have shown that a simple hapten coupled to pneumococcal polysaccharide can block the resynthesis of surface receptor immunoglobulin, presumably by cross-linking and inhibition of antigen clearance from the cell surface. These authors have further shown that primed B cells, $B\gamma$, have a lower tolerance threshold for such T-independent antigens than $B\mu$ cells, presumably because of their higher avidity for the antigen. This is in contrast to easily degradable protein antigens, which elicit tolerance in immunized animals with considerable difficulty.

As a general rule, it is much easier to induce tolerance in the newborn than in the adult animal, and most examples of neonatally induced tolerance are probably based on specific nonreactivity. In contrast the majority of examples of experimental models of tolerance to transplantation antigens in adult animals are probably based on suppressive mechanisms.

Humoral Blocking Factors

Passive administration of specific IgG antibody may prevent primary active production of antibodies to the given antigen, although this does not yet imply lasting tolerance. Moreover, sustained antibody formation may mediate a functionally specific unresponsiveness by suppressing other immune reactions, such as cytotoxic T cell functions (Chapter 9).

Specific prevention of sensitization was observed at the beginning of this century. Immunization with toxin-antitoxin mixtures in excess of passively administered antitoxin resulted in the suppression of formation of antitoxic antibodies (Chapter 26). In the 1950s, Uhr demonstrated suppression of antibody formation by injecting guinea pigs with complexes consisting of egg albumin, bovine gamma globulin, or bovine serum albumin and their corresponding antibodies. Antibodies injected simultaneously with antigen would interfere with further active formation of antibodies. IgG, but not IgM, antibodies of homologous and heterologous species origin were suppressive.

During the last 12 years, fascinating studies on suppression of the antibody response to human blood group antigen Rh_0 were carried out. First experiments conducted on Rh-negative male volunteers showed that injection of anti-Rh serum prevented responsiveness to subsequently administered Rh-positive erythrocytes. Again, IgG antibodies were responsible for suppression. Thereafter, Rh-negative women, within 48 to 72 hours after delivery of an Rh-positive baby, were injected with IgG fraction of anti-Rh serum. This prevented, in most instances, the Rh sensitization that follows a breakthrough of fetal erythrocytes into the maternal circulation during delivery. Antibodies may interfere with the afferent limb of sensitization in that they wall off the antigenic determinants on red blood cells, which are then eliminated by the liver rather than by the spleen. This does not induce lasting suppression and, therefore, the procedure has to be repeated following another Rh-incompatible pregnancy.

Other important studies on antibody-mediated suppression relate to transplantation (Chapter 22) and tumor antigens (Chapter 24). In the 1930s, Cassey and his associates noted that, following the injection of killed and preserved allogeneic Brown-Pearce carcinoma cells into rabbits, subsequent grafts of live tumor grew more vigorously. These authors introduced the descriptive term "immunologic enhancement." Kaliss, in 1956, was the first to show that enhancement of the growth of such tumors in mice can be transferred to normal animals by serum from immunized animals. The tumors in these investigations were allogeneic and, therefore, preferentially induced a response to transplantation antigens rather than to tumor-specific antigens as would be the case in experiments with syngeneic tumors. Thus, in these instances, humoral transplantation antibodies protected the tumors from rejection by cell-mediated transplantation immunity and enabled their growth. Studies on antibody-mediated enhancement of syngeneic tumors will be discussed in Chapter 24.

The protection of normal allogeneic tissues from rejection was also investigated. Hellström and his associates used the classic model of Medawar and his coworkers of tolerance induced in neonatal CBA mice by injections of A spleen cells. *In vitro* experiments showed that lymph node cells from functionally tolerant mice exerted cytotoxic effects on A fibroblast cultures and that the serum of such animals could specifically suppress cytotoxicity of CBA lymphocytes to A fibroblasts. Similar findings have been reported by others and seem to contradict the clonal inactivation hypothesis even in the tolerance elicited in newborn. However, Brent and his coworkers showed that by increasing the number of allogeneic cells used for induction of neonatal tolerance, a "shift" appears to take place from suppression to nonreactivity.

In vivo studies on antibody-mediated suppression revealed several limitations in the efficiency of this mechanism. Antibody-mediated suppression of the rejection of skin grafts differing from the recipient in minor histocompatibility antigens could be established with success. On the other hand, similar experiments with skin allografts differing in antigens determined by major histocompatibility loci were, by and large, unsuccessful unless some additional measures were employed (see below). Experiments using renal allografts have been much more successful than those carried out with skin. However, in donor-recipient combinations differing in major histocompatibility antigens, success was achieved only by reducing the incompatibility barrier, as when parental rats were grafted with semiallogeneic F_1 hybrid kidneys. There were also a few clinical trials of antibody-mediated suppression with human renal grafts, but thus far, encouraging results have not been achieved.

Additional short-term immunosuppression with cytotoxic drugs and especially with antilymphocyte serum has resulted in much stronger specific suppression in several experiments on adult rodents. Even skin grafted across a major histoincompatibility barrier has been shown to survive for extended periods of time.

Once formed or passively administered, suppressive antibodies have apparently acted in an immunoregulatory fashion on the afferent, central, or efferent levels, alternatives that are by no means mutually exclusive. The first possibility, a masking of antigenic determinants, has been discussed above. The efferent mechanism may consist of interference by antibodies or antigen-antibody complexes with the interaction of sensitized lymphocytes and target cells, which prevents killing of these cells (Chapter 9). The complexes may block the lymphocytes through free antigenic sites and the target cells through free antibody-combining sites.

Central interference could mean that the "blocking" antibodies inhibit the production of other (e.g., cytotoxic) antibodies and interfere with the sensitization of T helper and/or killer lymphocytes. Some evidence for this mechanism comes from experiments on preincubation of mouse spleen cells with 7 S antibody, which led to a marked reduction of the ability of the treated spleen cells to produce this specific antibody in culture. Hildemann showed that murine IgG_2 antibodies may inhibit the formation of cell-mediated immunity. Several experiments suggested that this interference may be on the "macrophage level." The handling of antigen could be inhibited by binding the Fc portion of the IgG antibody to the surface of these cells. It certainly is a question of semantics whether the action of macrophages should be considered an afferent or central activity of the immune apparatus.

Another truly central mechanism may be based on the effects of anti-idiotype antibodies, i.e., antibodies against the unique configuration of the combining site of a specific antibody molecule or of a specifically reactive lymphocyte. The possibility that such antibodies are involved in immunologic suppression must be considered. After *in vitro* exposure of the lymphocytes to relevant anti-idiotype sera, selective abrogation of the graft-vs.-host reaction (Chapter 23) as well as specific inhibition of the mixed lymphocyte reaction (Chapter 22) and cell-mediated cytotoxicity (Chapter 9) was shown.

Suppressor Cells

Immunologic tolerance based on a specific suppressive mechanism, which may be transferred passively to another animal, has been referred to as "infectious tolerance." Since 1970, it has become more and more obvious that this may be achieved not only by the transfer of antibodies, but also by the transfer of lymphocytes. Significantly, in the donors of such lymphocytes, unresponsiveness could not be abrogated by infusion of lymphocytes from normally reactive syngeneic animals, indicating that the underlying mechanism was not a central failure.

The suppressive effects of T lymphocytes were observed by Gershon and Kondo in studies on tolerance of mice to sheep erythrocytes. Thymectomized, lethally irradiated and bone-marrow-reconstituted CBA mice developed substantial degrees of unresponsiveness following repeated injections of sheep erythrocytes only if small numbers of thymus cells had been supplied prior to the tolerizing injections. Transfer of lymphocytes from these mice suppressed the normal cooperation between T and B cells in repopulated secondary hosts. The authors concluded that this effect was produced by "tolerized" suppressor T cells.

This type of finding has since been described in several experimental models, including those of unresponsiveness to transplantation antigens. Brent and his coworkers have established long-lasting, strain-specific unresponsiveness to H-2-incompatible skin allografts by pretreatment of recipient mice with crude liver extract from the strain of the graft donor combined with a dose of *Bordetella pertussis* vaccine and a short course of antilymphocytic serum. Lymphocytes of these mice, bearing healthy grafts many months after transplantation, showed normal or nearly normal *in vitro* reactivity to the donor strain antigens, as indicated by mixed lymphocyte reactions (Chapter 22) and cell-mediated cytotoxicity (Chapter 9) assays. Spleen cells, however, were capable of transferring the *in vivo* unresponsiveness.

With regard to neonatally induced tolerance, the case for suppressor cells is less clear at present. Some seemingly convincing experiments have not been reproducible thus far. Therefore, the working hypothesis has been proposed that clonal deletion may affect the less mature cells, and suppression may affect those cells that have already acquired peripheral T cell properties. Indeed, most of the publications have identified suppressor cells as T lymphocytes regulating T cell cooperation with other T cells and with B cells, but there is also an indication that B cells may inhibit the generation of reactive T cells. Recent evidence from experiments on mice indicates that the phenotype of suppressor cells, as determined by cell-surface antigenic markers (Ly antigens), is different from that of helper cells.

At present, little is known about the mechanism through which suppressor cells may work. Specifically suppressive, soluble products of T cells that are distinct from, but antigenically related to, immunoglobulins have been described recently. These products may also arm other cells, such as macrophages, for suppressive activity. Their possible relationship to anti-idiotype antibodies (see above) remains to be elucidated.

Summary

As has been discussed in the foregoing chapter, the classic concept of tolerance, advanced by Burnet and Medawar, could not be substantiated in many experimental models and had to be broadened continuously during the last two decades.

Looking at the phenomena from another, teleologic point of view, one should have expected a multiplicity of mechanisms for specific unresponsiveness. For any highly developed macroorganism requiring an immune apparatus to survive microbial attacks and to control aberrant cells, it is absolutely vital to prevent any major immunologic aggression against the

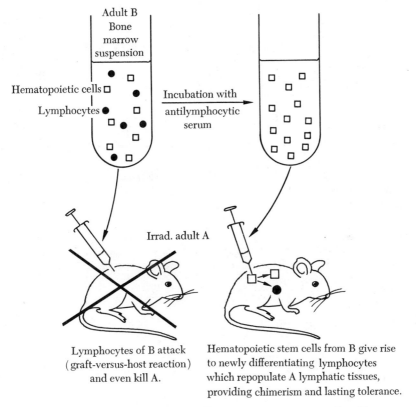

Figure 12-4. Repopulation with hematopoietic stem cells of irradiated animal.

body's normal constituents, i.e., autoaggression. Considering the importance of this regulatory discrimination, it is understandable that nature seems to prefer to rely on more than just one mechanism. The suppression mechanisms may provide backup systems to protect against autoaggression by immunocompetent cells that have managed to escape the deletion or inactivation mechanism.

Whichever mechanism is operating in a given situation in a given individual, it appears to be developed by those cells representing the lymphatic offspring of undetermined hematopoietic stem cells. There is good recent evidence that transplantation of these stem cells, even into strongly allogeneic surrounding (recipients), gives rise to lymphoid offspring that may easily become tolerant to these surroundings. Undetermined stem cells exist in bone marrow throughout life, providing a source of cells in the adult, which could be manipulated promisingly. For a variety of reasons, manipulation to achieve specific unresponsiveness in the adult is of great interest in clinical medicine, especially in the transplantation of tissues and organs and in the restitution of self-tolerance in autoimmune diseases (Figure 12-4).

Bibliography

Dresser, D. W. (ed.): Immunological tolerance. *Br. Med. Bull.*, **32**:99–184, 1976.

Fitch, F. W.: Selective suppression of immune responses. *Prog. Allergy*, **19**:195–244, 1975.

Howard, J. G., and Mitchison, N. A.: Immunological tolerance. *Prog. Allergy*, **18**:43–96, 1975.

Katz, D. H., and Benacerraf, B. (eds.): *Immunological Tolerance*. Academic Press, New York, 1974.

Müller-Ruchholtz, W.; Wottge, H.-U.; and Müller-Hermelink, H. K.: Bone marrow transplantation in rats across strong histocompatibility barriers by selective elimination of lymphoid cells in donor marrow. *Transplant. Proc.*, **8**:537–41, 1976.

Nossal, G. J. V., and Pike, B. L.: Single cell studies on the antibody-forming potential of fractionated, hapten B cells. *Immunology*, **30**:189–202, 1976.

Weigle, W. O.: Immunological unresponsiveness. *Adv. Immunol.*, **16**:61–122, 1973.

UNIT II

Clinical Immunology

13

Immunology of Bacterial Diseases

Erwin Neter

Introduction

Bacterial infection results in an immune response of the host, provided that the antigen reaches the cells of the immune apparatus, the host has immunologic competence, and the antigen does not elicit unresponsiveness (tolerance). This immune response may be documented either by the appearance of circulating antibodies (humoral immunity) (Chapter 4) and/ or by the emergence of immunologically committed cells operative in the phenomenon of delayed hypersensitivity (cellular immunity) (Chapter 11). Since a single strain or species of bacteria produces a large variety of antigenic substances, antibodies of different specificities are engendered. Often, it is a particular antigen that has proved to be of singular importance in applied immunology.

The immune response of the host to bacterial antigens may result in immunity (specific resistance) to, or prompt recovery from, the particular infection. This immune response, then, is protective in nature. Bacteria elicit responses to many other antigens that are not pathogenetic. Antibodies directed against these antigens usually do not affect the course of the disease nor do they provide immunity. Nonetheless, they are important, for documentation of these immune responses is being widely used for diagnostic purposes. Under unusual circumstances, antibodies or delayed hyper-sensitivity directed against bacterial antigens may result in immunologic cell injury.

It is the aim of this chapter to discuss, largely on the basis of suitable examples, the immunology of bacterial diseases under two major headings: (1) bacterial antigens and (2) host responses to bacterial antigens. The latter topic includes serodiagnosis (the use of antisera for the identification) of bacterial pathogens, immunologic diagnosis of bacterial diseases, as well as immunity to, and immunization against, bacterial pathogens. Only brief reference will be made to the topics of serodiagnosis and immunization, since they are the subjects of Chapter 26. Finally, a few comments will be offered on bacterial antigens in the diagnosis of immune deficiencies and on bacterial antigens as adjuvants of the immune response.

Bacterial Antigens

Structural Antigens

Although primitive, in the system of plants, bacteria, nonetheless, are enormously complex both in structure and in function. Many of the substances making up discernible structures of the bacterial cell are antigenic in nature, as are metabolically important products, such as enzymes and toxins. Fortunately, only a relatively limited number of antigens produced by various human pathogens are of importance from the medical point of view.

The major structures of bacterial cells, including flagella, fimbriae, capsules, and cell walls, are made up of antigenic molecules. For the purposes of illustration, the presently known facts regarding the typhoid bacillus (*Salmonella typhi*) are briefly summarized. Motile strains of this pathogen produce a protein, referred to as flagellin, that is the building block of the flagella of this microorganism. This protein has been studied in detail regarding both its function of locomotion and its antigenic characteristics. Flagellin is extraordinarily immunogenic in suitable hosts, as little as 1 nanogram engendering antibodies upon intravenous injection. Of interest is the fact that certain alterations of the molecule yield a tolerance-inducing product. It has been known for more than half a century that antibodies against the flagella produced by patients with typhoid fever caused immobilization of the organism and agglutination of bacteria through flagella-antibody-flagella complexes. Whereas in *Salmonella typhi* the flagellar protein occurs only in a single phase, representing antigen d, in other salmonellae two different H antigens are produced. The two antigenically different H antigens represent phases 1 and 2. Their identification is required for determination of the particular serotype, as may be seen from data on selected *Salmonella* serotypes shown in Table 13-1.

Table 13-1
ANTIGENIC COMPOSITION OF *Salmonella typhi*
AND OTHER *Salmonella* SEROTYPES*

| Serotypes | O Antigens | Groups | H Antigens | |
			PHASE 1	PHASE 2
Salmonella typhi	9, 12, Vi	D_1	d	—
Salmonella ndolo†	9, 12	D_1	d	1, 5
Salmonella enteritidis†	1 9, 12	D_1	g, m	—
Salmonella dublin†	1, 9, 12	D_1	g, p	—
Salmonella typhimurium†	1, 4, 5, 12	B	i	1, 2
Salmonella paratyphi B†	1, 4, 5, 12	B	b	1, 2
Salmonella paratyphi C†	6, 7 (Vi)	C_1	c	1, 5

* Adapted from Edwards, P. R., and Ewing, W. H.: *Identification of Enterobacteriaceae*, 3rd ed. Burgess Publishing Co., Minneapolis, 1972, p. 233.

† Also referred to as *S. enteritidis* ser Ndolo, Enteritidis, Dublin, Typhimurium, Paratyphi B, and bioser Paratyphi C, respectively.

In addition to flagella, certain strains of enterobacteriaceae have hairlike appendages, referred to as fimbriae. These structures consist of protein, contribute to attachment of the bacteria to certain animal host cells, and are operative in the transfer of genetic information between bacterial cells. Genetically these fimbriae are host determined. In contrast, similar structures, the so-called pili (sex pili), also operative in the transfer of genetic information, are under plasmid control.

Surface and Cell-Wall Antigens

Intensive studies on the chemical and immunologic makeup of the cell wall have been carried out. A surface antigen, resembling bacterial capsules of other microorganisms, is an acidic polymer, a highly immunogenic substance. This antigen is referred to as Vi antigen. The name was derived on the basis of the assumption that this antigen contributes to the virulence of this microorganism, an assumption that has been shown to be not entirely correct. The Vi antigen has some properties of unusual interest to immunologists. It has been known for many years that its presence on the surface of typhoid bacilli, and of certain other enterobacteriaceae as well, interferes with bacterial agglutination by antibodies directed against the O antigen of the cell wall. This inhibition of agglutination is not due to the blocking of the O antigen determinant, for the bacteria do absorb the corresponding O antibodies. Rather, the inhibition of agglutination is due to alteration of the surface charge, which interferes with the second, nonspecific phase of the agglutination reaction. Proof of this interpretation is incisively provided by the demonstration that erythrocytes to which both Vi and O antigens are attached are agglutinated by Vi antibodies but not by O antibodies, and, since complement-mediated hemolysis is not dependent upon agglutination, hemolysis induced by O antibodies is not affected by the simultaneous presence of the Vi antigen on the surface of the red blood cells. It is important to emphasize that interference by Vi antigen (and of the related K antigens of other enteric bacteria) is abolished by heating of the bacterial suspension. It is for this reason that in the diagnostic laboratory heated suspensions are used for the identification of O antigens by O antisera, whenever it is suspected that interfering surface antigens are present. In addition to *Salmonella typhi*, a few other salmonellae produce Vi antigen. It is of considerable interest to note that Vi antigen also functions as a receptor for certain bacteriophages. K antigens of enteric bacteria are surface antigens akin to the Vi antigen. Current information indicates that the amount of K antigen produced by various strains of *Escherichia coli* may be related to the pathogenic potential of the microorganism, for example, in the development of pyelonephritis as a complication of infection of the lower urinary tract or in the pathogenesis of meningitis. The identification of K and O antigens of a given serotype does not necessarily imply that the two antigenic determinants are located on two distinct molecules.

The major antigenic portion of the cell wall is comprised of macromolecules consisting of lipid, polysaccharide, and protein. Aside from being the major building blocks of the cell wall of *Salmonella typhi* and of other enterobacteriaceae, this complex accounts for serologic specificity and for endotoxicity as well. The polysaccharide components carry the important O (somatic) antigenic determinants, and the lipid A of the lipopolysaccharide complex accounts, in part at least, for endotoxicity. The structure of this lipopolysaccharide complex, as visualized at the present time, is shown in Figure 13-1.

The O antigen of the typhoid bacillus contains two major antigenic determinants, referred to as antigens 9 and 12. Repeating side chains of sugars are responsible for O specificity. In the case of the typhoid bacillus it is tyvelose, an unusual 7-carbon sugar (3,6-dideoxy-D-mannose), that is the immunodominant determinant for antigen 9. Similar side chains of varied chemical composition account for the O specificity of other groups of the genus *Salmonella* and of serogroups or serotypes of other entero-

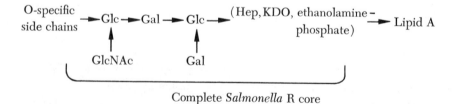

Complete *Salmonella* R core

Figure 13-1. General structure of *Salmonella* lipopolysaccharides depicted schematically. Hep, L-glycero-D-manno-heptose. (From Schmidt, G.; Fromme, I.; and Mayer, H.: Immunochemical studies on core lipopolysaccharides of Enterobacteriaceae of different genera. *Eur. J. Biochem.*, **14**:357–66, 1970.)

bacteriaceae. A few illustrative examples are shown in Table 13-1. It must be emphasized that these sugar molecules alone act as haptens, and that the antigen becomes fully immunogenic if present as part of a larger molecule. Certain changes in O-antigen composition of salmonellae are due to bacteriophage infection, resulting in lysogenic conversion. For example, following phage infection, *Salmonella anatum* becomes *Salmonella newington*, and O antigens 2, 10 become O antigens 3,15. O antigens of various enteric bacteria show numerous cross-reactions, because of shared antigenic determinants, as discussed below.

The lipopolysaccharide complex of gram-negative bacteria produces a variety of pathologic changes in susceptible hosts, collectively referred to as endotoxicity. The alterations produced by these endotoxins include the Sanarelli and Shwartzman reactions, enhanced reactivity to epinephrine, fever, activation of complement via the alternate pathway, alteration of metabolism, leukopenia followed by leukocytosis, stimulation of B cells, increased susceptibility or resistance to infection, and lethality. In addition, and of particular interest to immunologists, is the adjuvancy of these endotoxins, enhancing the immune response to unrelated antigens in a variety of hosts. Under certain circumstances, the identical endotoxins may also suppress the antibody response.

A change from S (smooth) to R (rough) forms results in the elimination of the O-antigenic determinants and the emergence of the R antigen. Different R antigens have been described among the enteric bacteria. Chemically, they consist of a core polysaccharide and lipid A. It is the core polysaccharide that accounts for the serologic specificity of the R antigen, and it is the lipid A that is responsible for endotoxicity. Thus, endotoxicity does not depend on the S or virulent phase of the strain. The R lipopolysaccharides also function as receptor sites for certain bacteriophages.

It is of interest to point out that the protein components of the complete O antigens may function as bacteriocins, substances of bacterial origin that cause killing of other bacterial cells, and that antibodies directed against the bacteriocins inhibit this cidal action.

Recent investigations have revealed that lipid A, which plays a major, albeit not exclusive, role in endotoxicity, is antigenic, and that lipid A antibodies may affect its biologic activity.

Although not listed in Table 13-1, polynucleotides of bacteria are potential immunogens, and antibodies have been identified that react with bacterial DNA, such as that of *Escherichia coli*, *Clostridium perfringens*, and *Micrococcus lysodeikticus*.

Bacterial Toxins

From the medical point of view, it is these three structural (Vi, O, and H) antigens that are of prime importance, although *Salmonella typhi* produces many other antigenic products. At the other extreme of a long list of human pathogens are microorganisms that produce a single soluble antigen that is of major clinical significance. *Clostridium botulinum, Clostridium tetani,* and *Corynebacterium diphtheriae* are representatives of pathogens that cause human disease only because of the production of powerful toxins (Chapter 1). Structural antigens do not play a significant role in these host-parasite relationships. In fact, botulism may be acquired without contact or ingestion of the microorganisms themselves, since the highly toxic protein is produced *in vitro,* is not destroyed in the stomach, and is absorbed from the gastrointestinal tract. This toxin is extraordinarily effective; a minimal lethal dose for man is 10 μg and for the mouse 0.01 μg! Toxins of similar biologic activity but of different antigenic specificity are produced by *Clostridium botulinum,* necessitating the availability of several specific antitoxins as prophylactic and therapeutic agents. The presently available evidence indicates that these immunologically distinct toxins, though different in their toxicity to various animal species, cause the toxic effects through a seemingly identical mechanism, namely, the blocking of acetylcholine release from demyelinated ends of cholinergic motor nerves. These facts clearly illustrate the relevance today of the original concept of Paul Ehrlich regarding toxins, namely, the existence of a molecular structure accounting for toxicity (toxophore group) and of a different part of the molecule carrying the antigenic determinant (haptophore group).

In 1951, Freeman made the remarkable discovery that the production of diphtheria toxin is dependent on bacteriophage infection of *Corynebacterium diphtheriae.* Infection results in modification of the bacterial genome, the so-called lysogenic conversion. Thus, the formation of the pathogenetically singularly important toxin is, in fact, due to a viral infection of the bacterial cell. It is of interest to note that the production of the erythrogenic toxin of group A hemolytic streptococci, responsible for the rash of scarlet fever, of certain enterotoxins of *Escherichia coli,* and of staphylococcal penicillinase, is also due to plasmids or episomes.

Biologic Significance of Bacterial Antigens

For the discussion of the relationship between bacterial antigens and disease, *Streptococcus pyogenes* (group A hemolytic streptococcus) has been selected. This pathogen produced a large number of antigen of biologic and clinical significance. Among these antigens are structural antigens, notably the M protein and C polysaccharide cell-wall antigens. The former confers type specificity and the latter group specificity to the strains. It is of particular importance to emphasize that immunity to hemolytic streptococcal infection is solely type specific, owing to antibodies against the M protein antigen. There exist some 50 or more different serotypes. It is not surprising, therefore, that infection with this pathogen seemingly does not confer immunity to recurrent disease, since the host remains susceptible to other serotypes of hemolytic streptococci. The information on type-specific immunity is also compatible with the epidemiology of poststreptococcal disease. It has been known for many years that rheumatic fever is apt to recur, unless antibiotic prophylaxis is practiced. Recurrences are initiated by repeated attacks of streptococcal infection. It is the capacity of any type of group A streptococci to set in motion the events leading to the development of acute rheumatic fever that is the basis for the frequency of recurrences. In contrast, glomerulonephritis, another poststreptococcal disease, is triggered by only a few types of group A hemolytic streptococci, such as type 12, which stimulates type-specific immunity. Thus, recurrences of glomerulonephritis are extraordinarily rare, and antibiotic prophylaxis is not indicated.

In addition to these structural antigens, group A hemolytic streptococci produce a fairly large number of other antigenic products (Table 13-2). One of these antigens is the erythrogenic toxin responsible for certain features of scarlet fever, notably of the rash. The production of this toxin is dependent on the presence of a plasmid, an extranuclear DNA molecule. Streptokinase and streptodornase also engender delayed hypersensitivity (Chapter 11), and these antigens are being used to assess the capacity of "cellular immunity" in patients with suspected immune deficiency diseases (Chapter 17).

Whereas antibodies to the protein antigens are protective against *Streptococcus pyogenes* infection, polysaccharide antibodies account for immunity against *Haemophilus influenzae* and *Streptococcus pneumoniae*. These pathogens produce capsular antigens, polysaccharide in nature, that account for type specificity and are incisively related to the virulence of the strains. Accordingly, type-specific antibodies are protective, and their presence is related to the epidemiology of these infections. An excellent example is the epidemiology of *Haemophilus influenzae* type b meningitis. Susceptibility clearly is related to the absence of either passively transferred or actively produced type-specific antibodies of the IgG class. Since many adults are immune, the newborn infant usually is protected by the passively acquired antibodies for a period of several weeks to a few months. Silent infection accounts for increasing immunity with advancing age. Thus, *Haemophilus influenzae* type b meningitis is most prevalent between the ages of three months and two years.

Delayed Hypersensitivity to Bacterial Antigens

Tuberculous infection evokes a particular type of hypersensitivity, as first described by Robert Koch and—in the form of the tuberculin skin test—by von Pirquet in 1907. It was not until four decades later that its nature was clearly established. The tuberculin test—and delayed hypersensitivity to other antigens—is due not to humoral antibodies but to cellular immunity (Chapter 11). Immunologically specific lymphocytes rather than circulating immunoglobulins are responsible for this specific reaction. In fact, the tuberculin reaction has become the prototype reaction for this type of allergy. Tuberculoproteins of *Mycobacteria*, brucellergen of *Brucellae*, and streptokinase of streptococci are among bacterial antigens evoking delayed

Table 13-2

Antigens of Selected Bacterial Pathogens
and Their Clinical Relevance

Microorganisms	Antigens	Clinical Relevance
Streptococcus pneumoniae	Capsular polysaccharide antigens	Type specific, protective
	Cell-wall polysaccharide (C substance)	Species specific, reacts with C-reactive protein
	M protein antigens	Type specific, not protective
	Pneumolysin	Toxic, hemolytic
Streptococcus pyogenes	M protein antigen (cell wall)	Type specific, protective
	C polysaccharide antigen (cell wall	Group specific, nonprotective
	T and R protein antigens (cell wall)	Not related to virulence
	Glycerol teichoic acid	Antigen common to other gram-positive bacteria
	Erythrogenic toxins	Related to scarlet fever
	Streptolysin O	Hemolytic; antistreptolysin O of diagnostic significance
	Diphosphopyridine nucleotidase	Leukocytotoxic
	Streptokinases (A and B)	Activates plasminogen
	Deoxyribonucleases (A, B, C, and D)	Depolymerizes extracellular DNA
	Hyaluronidase	"Spreading factor"
	Proteinase	Biologic role uncertain
	Heterogenetic antigen	Reacting with heart muscle
Salmonella typhi	O somatic (lipopolysaccharide) cell-wall antigen	Group specificity (*Salmonella* group D)
	Vi acidic polymer surface antigen	Inhibitor of O agglutination; partly related to virulence
	H flagellar antigen	Type specific, nonprotective antigen
Escherichia coli, enteropathogenic	K surface antigen	Inhibitor of O agglutination, virulence factor (?)
	O somatic (lipopolysaccharide) cell-wall antigen	Type specific
	Lipid A	Antibodies cross-react with lipid A of other enterobacteriaceae
	H flagellar antigen	
	Fimbriae (protein) in certain strains	Related to interaction with host cells and to conjugation
	Enterotoxin	Toxin responsible for enterotoxicity
Haemophilus influenzae	Capsular polysaccharide antigens (type b: polyribosephosphate)	Type specific, protective
Clostridium botulium	Protein exotoxins	Pathogenetic product, protective, type specific (A to E)

Table 13-2—*continued*

Microorganisms	Antigens	Clinical Relevance
Mycobacterium tuberculosis	Protein (tuberculoprotein)	Delayed hypersensitivity
	Polysaccharide (tuberculo-polysaccharide)	Not protective
	Phosphatides	—
	Numerous other antigens (some 20 proteins, 10 polysaccharides, and 4 lipids)	
	RNA fraction (Tb antigen?)	(Informational?)
	Cord factor (trehalose-6,6′-dimycolate)	Adjuvant

reaction. *In vitro* tests for delayed hypersensitivity, such as inhibition of macrophage migration, have become available in recent years.

Cross-Reacting (*Heterophilic or Heterogenetic*) Antigens

During the past decades the major efforts toward identification of bacterial antigens were directed to those antigens that characterize either species, serogroups, or serotypes, or account for pathogenicity. Indeed, this information is of particular import with regard to (1) classification and identification; (2) mechanisms of pathogenicity, (3) epidemiology of bacterial infections, and (4) immunization, both active and passive. It is understandable, therefore, that less attention has been paid to antigens that are shared by various bacterial serotypes, species, genera, or families, and to those antigens that are common to bacteria, high plants, and/or animals. However, such cross-reactions must be kept in mind at all times by the diagnostic microbiologist. Examples of such shared antigens were discussed by Landsteiner in his classic volume, *The Specificity of Serological Reactions*, and summarized in Chapter 21. Numerous other examples have been identified since that time. Cross-reacting antigens are common, and only a few examples are cited for illustrative purposes. Some of these cross-reacting antigens have been discovered accidentally or even on the basis of mistaken assumptions or interpretations. Thus, the chance isolation of a strain of *Proteus* from a patient with rickettsial infection led Weil and Felix to the discovery of a useful diagnostic test, named in their honor. The test is based on a shared antigen and not, as erroneously assumed, on the etiologic role of *Proteus* in rickettsial disease. Cross-reactions are particularly numerous among polysaccharides of enterobacteriaceae. Suffice it to mention that *Salmonella adelaide* (O antigen 35), *Escherichia coli* (O antigen 111), and *Salmonella arizonae* (O antigen 20) share an antigenic determinant. Vi antigen of identical specificity, consisting of N-acetyl-D-galactosamine uronic acid, is produced not only by *Salmonella typhi* but also by *Citrobacter ballerup* and certain strains of *Escherichia coli.*

Cardiolipin, a diphosphatidylglycerol, is the hapten utilized in serologic tests for syphilis. This antigen is present not only in animal tissues, such as beef heart, but also in plants and spirochetes. *Haemophilus influenzae* type b produces a type-specific polysaccharide that strongly cross-reacts with the specific soluble substance of pneumococcus type 6 and an antigen of *Escherichia coli* O75. Because of the existence of these rather numerous cross-reactions, serologic identification of any microorganism usually is not sufficient for its characterization without regard to morphology, growth requirements, biochemical activities, and so on. Immunodiffusion tests (Chapter 6) lend themselves particularly well to the demonstration of such cross-reacting antigens, when a given antiserum is placed in the center well and various cultures in the outer wells.

Recently, two antigens have been discovered by serendipity, one produced by gram-positive and the other by certain gram-negative bacteria. The former antigen is formed by streptococci, staphylococci, *Listeria*, and certain anaerobic bacilli; chemically, it is a teichoic acid. The latter antigen is produced by *Escherichia, Klebsiella, Salmonella, Shigella, Proteus,* and *Serratia.* Production of this antigen by pigmented *Serratia* and failure of production by pigmented *Flavobacterium* is in accord with the classification of these organisms, illustrating that the presence of such common, heterogenetic antigens may be utilized as one of many indicators for classification.

Antigens shared by bacteria and various animals include the Forssman antigen and moieties of blood group specificity. Among bacteria producing Forssman antigen are certain strains of *Shigella dysenteriae, Pasteurella, Streptococcus pneumoniae* (C substance), and *Bacillus anthracis.* Blood group substances of A and B specificities are produced by numerous bacteria, notably enterobacteriaceae. Seeding of *Escherichia coli* O86 with B activity to germ-free chickens leads to the production of B antibodies, strongly suggesting that the development of "natural" blood group antibodies may be due to the antigenic stimulus provided by the environment, such as the microbial flora.

From the medical point of view, these common, shared, or heterogenetic antigens may have significance regarding both serodiagnosis of pathogens as well as pathogenesis and prevention of bacterial infection. A few illustrative examples may be cited. A single antiserum against the common antigen of enterobacteriaceae has been used successfully for the detection of gram-negative enteric bacteria in kidney tissue by the fluorescent antibody (FA) technique in connection with studies on the pathogenesis of pyelonephritis. This serologic diagnosis otherwise would have required the use of more than 100 antisera against the group-specific O antigens. A certain serogroup of *Escherichia coli*, namely, serogroup O14, shares an antigenic determinant with a tissue antigen present in the colon. Thus, it is conceivable that antibodies engendered by this microorganism—and others sharing the same antigen—may play a role in the pathogenesis of ulcerative colitis through cell injury by bacterial antibody and complement. Streptococci share an antigen with heart muscle and probably play a significant role in the pathogenesis of rheumatic fever; also, a cell-membrane antigen of strepto-cocci sensitizes animals to skin homografts. Thus, the immune response of the host to these and other heterogenetic antigens may contribute to the development of immunologic injury. On the other hand, immunization with a single antigen shared by various species of bacteria may engender immunity. Various enterobacteriaceae share such a common antigen, and antibodies against this determinant promote phagocytosis (opsonization) of different microorganisms having this antigenic determinant on their surface (Chapter 10). Experimentally, both active immunization with this common antigen and passive immunization with the corresponding antibody afford protection to rabbits against experimental pyelonephritis.

From the foregoing sections it is evident that bacterial antigens may be proteins, polysaccharides, lipids, or nucleic acids. Isolated products may act as haptens and yet, when present in the bacterial cell, as immunogens. For example, the polysaccharides of pneumococci act as haptens in the rabbit, but the pneumococci themselves readily engender the corresponding poly-saccharide antibodies. A given substance may act as a hapten in one animal species and as an immunogen in another. To illustrate, pneumococcal polysaccharides are fully immunogenic in mouse and man, but not in the rabbit.

Nonantibody Reactions Between Bacterial Antigens and Immunoglobulins

As outlined in Chapter 5, the reaction between an antigen and the corresponding antibody refers to the interaction between the antigenic determinant and the Fab portion of the immunoglobulin. It is the comple-mentariness of the two molecules that is associated with extraordinary specificity. An unusual antigen has been isolated from staphylococci that reacts with immunoglobulins on a different basis. This antigen, referred to as antigen A, reacts with the Fc portion of immunoglobulins, a reaction that must be clearly differentiated from a true antigen-antibody reaction. Nonetheless, such interaction may have biologic significance, particularly since antigen A is a structural component of the cell wall, and immuno-globulin molecules become attached to the surface of the cells, presumably altering the pathogenic potential of the microorganisms. Antigen A has proved to be a valuable reagent for identification of antibodies. Similarly, the pneumococcal C substance has attained clinical importance, not as an important pneumococcal antigen, but rather as an indicator for the presence of C-reactive protein. The latter is present in the serum of patients with acute infections and certain other diseases. Thus, the test for C-reactive protein is used as a nonspecific indicator of certain pathologic processes. C-reactive protein is *not* an antibody, and its reaction with the C substance does not represent an antigen-antibody reaction.

Host Response to Bacterial Antigens

Significance and Applications

Appropriate contact with bacterial antigens leads to one or more characteristic immune responses of the host. These responses include the following: (1) production of circulating antibodies of one or more classes of immunoglobulins, such as IgG and IgM (Chapter 4); (2) production of secretory antibodies, notably IgA, such as those of the intestinal and respiratory tracts (Chapter 4); and/or (3) emergence of specifically committed cells responsible for delayed hypersensitivity and cellular immunity (Chapter 11).

Diagnostically, antibodies are used for the identification of bacterial antigens when dealing with unknown microorganisms in the clinical laboratory; alternatively, their production by the host is utilized for the immunologic diagnosis of bacterial infections or the determination of host susceptibility and immunity. The other major utilization of antibodies relates to immunization.

The immune response may be either protective, pathogenetic, or indifferent for the particular host. In fact, so far as our present knowledge indicated, antibodies to bacterial antigens often do not significantly affect the course of bacterial infections and host susceptibility. Other antibodies are uniquely protective. For example, antitoxins against the toxins of diphtheria, tetanus, and botulinus bacilli, when present in adequate titers, unquestionably provide protection against these diseases. Similarly, antibodies against the type-specific polysaccharides of pneumococci, *Haemophilus influenzae*, and other bacteria provide protection, as do antibodies against certain type-specific proteins, such as those of streptococci. Immunity to certain infectious diseases, notably tuberculosis, brucellosis, and salmonellosis, is due to cellular rather than humoral immune responses. In all likelihood, immunologically committed lymphocytes, though as yet inadequately understood mechanisms, endow certain phagocytes with increased bacteriacidal activity, and it is the intracellular destruction of viable bacteria that contributes to increased resistance to infection. Thus, the initiation of the process and its recall are immunologically specific; the final result, namely, intracellular killing, is nonspecific in nature. Finally, under certain circumstances, an immune response may, in fact, be responsible for certain pathogenic processes. As pointed out above, an immune response to a certain streptococcal antigen, which cross-reacts with cardiac muscle, is involved in the pathogenesis of rheumatic fever.

Serologic and Immunologic Procedures

Numerous methods are being used for the identification of bacterial antigens by antisera of known specificity and for the demonstration of the immune response of the host with known antigens. Practical considerations of reliability, sensitivity, simplicity, and cost have influenced, to a large extent, the use of one or another serologic procedure in the diagnostic laboratories. Examples of various serologic procedures to problems of diagnosis are presented in Table 13-3 and include the following. The direct and indirect fluorescent antibody (FA) tests are useful for the serologic identification of group A streptococci (*Streptococcus pyogenes*), certain serogroups of enteropathogenic *Escherichia coli*, *Bordetella pertussis*, and other pathogens as well. One of the obvious advantages of the FA technique is its speed, since results usually are obtained within a few hours.

The precipitation test and its various modifications, including gel diffusion and capsular swelling tests, are widely used, for example, in the serodiagnosis of syphilis by means of the VDRL reagent, identification of certain bacterial toxins, such as diphtheria toxin, demonstration of capsular antigens in body fluids, and serogrouping of hemolytic streptococci according

Table 13-3
EXAMPLES OF SEROLOGIC AND IMMUNOLOGIC METHODS
FOR THE DIAGNOSIS OF BACTERIAL INFECTION

Methods	Examples of Tests
I. *In vitro* Methods	
1. Fluorescent antibody test	Serodiagnosis of pathogens, e.g., *Streptococcus pyogenes*, enteropathogenic *E. coli*
2. Precipitation	VDRL test, gel diffusion, titration of diphtheria toxin, *Streptococcus* grouping
Capsular swelling	Neufeld test
3. Agglutination	
Bacterial	Widal, Weil-Felix tests
Passive hemagglutination	Titration of polysaccharide antibodies
Tanned cell hemagglutination	Titration of protein antibodies
Latex, bentonite agglutination	Titration of bacterial antibodies
4. Toxin neutralization	ASO test
5. Immobilization	*Treponema* test
6. Lysis, killing	*Vibrio cholerae* lysis, titration of batericidins against bacteria
Passive hemolysis	Titration of antibodies to bacterial polysaccharides
7. Complement fixation	Wassermann test
8. Opsonization	Enhanced phagocytosis of bacteria, e.g., of *Staphylococcus*
9. Immune adherence	Titration of bacterial antibodies
II. *In vivo* Methods	
1. Immediate-type hypersensitivity	Detection of pneumococcal antibodies
2. Delayed-type hypersensitivity	Tuberculin, brucellergen tests

to Lancefield. The Neufeld (capsular swelling) test represents precipitation within, and visualization of, an enlarged capsule. Various forms of agglutination procedures are widely used, both for the identification of bacterial pathogens, such as salmonellae, shigellae, enteropathogenic *Escherichia coli*, *Bordetella pertussis*, and *Francisella tularensis*, as well as for the identification and titration of the respective antibodies. Attachment of bacterial antigens to inert particles or carriers, such as red blood cells or latex and bentonite particles, makes agglutination tests possible for the titration of the corresponding antibodies. The sensitivity of certain agglutination tests can be enhanced by the use of suitable antiglobulin (Coombs') sera.

The toxin neutralization test is based on the fact that the *in vivo* or *in vitro* effects of toxins on animals or cells are specifically abolished, thus making possible the titration of antitoxins. A good example of such a test is the antistreptolysin O test; inhibition of hemolysis is the result of antitoxin action.

Antibodies directed against certain components of motile microorganisms inhibit motility. The *Treponema* immobilization test represents application of this phenomenon.

In the presence of complement, certain bacterial antibodies produce lysis and/or killing of the respective microorganisms (Chapter 8). Lysis of *Vibrio cholerae* and the killing of various enterobacteriaceae are examples. The above-mentioned passive hemagglutination test can be modified to a passive hemolysis test by the use of suitable erythrocytes (sheep) and the addition of complement. A satisfactory explanation is not available for the observation that with the identical bacterial antigen, antibody, and complement system, sheep cells are readily lysed and human erythrocytes are not.

As discussed in Chapter 8, certain antibodies in the presence of antigen and complement cause complement fixation. For many years, this test has found application for the titration of antibodies of various specificities. The classic Wassermann test represents an excellent example of this methodology.

Antibodies against certain bacterial pathogens can be titrated on the basis of their capacity to increase phagocytosis by leukocytes (opsonization). Enhanced phagocytosis plays a significant role in host defense (see Chapter 10).

Finally, attention is called to the immune adherence reaction. Certain microorganisms, in the presence of the corresponding antibody and complement, adhere to cells, such as erythrocytes of certain animal species or platelets. This highly sensitive test has been used for the titration of *Salmonella typhi* and *Treponema pallidum* antibodies.

Hypersensitivity and Bacterial Antigens

For the detection of immediate-type hypersensitivity (Chapter 18) to bacterial antigen, skin tests may be employed. With the appearance of pneumococcal antibodies in the circulation during pneumococcal infection, an inflammatory response takes place at the site of antigen administration. Similarly, a reaction occurs in subjects with delayed-type hypersensitivity upon local administration of tuberculin, brucellergen, and streptokinase-dornase. Attention is called to the fact that certain *in vitro* tests are now available for the demonstration of delayed-type hypersensitivity (Chapter 11).

Serodiagnosis of Bacteria and Their Products

Antisera of known specificity and titer are widely used for the identification of bacterial antigens and thus for the diagnosis of the particular microorganism. Examples are presented in Table 13-3. Antigenic analysis of microorganisms thus supplements other basic information for identification, namely, morphology, staining characteristics, growth requirements, and biochemical activities. With suitable antisera, unknown microorganisms are identified as representative of a given species, such as *Salmonella typhi, Francisella tularensis, Bordetella pertussis, Corynebacterium diphtheriae, Clostridium tetani,* and *Treponema pallidum.* Often, group- and type-specific antigens allow the recognition of serogroups and serotypes, such as the Lancefield groups of hemolytic streptococci, the 75-odd pneumococcal types, numerous serogroups and serotypes of enterobacteriaceae (including more than 1300 *Salmonella* serotypes), several types of *Neisseria meningitidis,* and antigenically different toxins of *Clostridium botulinum.*

Immunologic Diagnosis of Bacterial Infections

The subject of serodiagnosis is presented elsewhere (Chapter 26). For this reason only a few comments are made here regarding some applications of fundamental principles of immunology. Immunologic diagnosis can be accomplished either by the identification and titration of bacterial antibodies in serum (and in the future in certain secretions) *in vitro,* by the documentation of the presence of such antibodies through *in vivo* tests, or by the demonstration of specific allergic reactions of either the immediate or delayed types.

The immunologic diagnosis of certain bacterial infections has been a routine procedure for many years, such as the Widal test for the diagnosis of typhoid fever, the Weil-Felix test for rickettsial infections, and the Wassermann test for syphilis. Some of these serologic procedures have been improved and expanded, for example, by the introduction of various methods for identifying antibodies directed against the antigen of *Treponema pallidum* for the specific diagnosis of syphilis.

A probable diagnosis often can be made of the basis of the examination of a single serum specimen, provided that the titer of the antibodies is sufficiently high and the test rather specific. Interpretation of the results must be related to the titers of antibodies of identical or similar specificity present in the serum of healthy subjects or individuals without the particular infection. Such "natural" antibodies are commonly found in human and animal sera; the titers of these antibodies often vary with age and between different population groups. For these reasons, the documentation of a significant increase in the titers of antibodies is often more informative and indicative of current or recent infection.

The immunologic approach to the diagnosis of bacterial infections is particularly helpful in diseases that, under natural conditions, last for at least a week, because under these circumstances diagnostic problems may still exist and antibody production can be expected to have occurred. When it becomes desirable to examine two consecutive serum specimens, the assumption is frequently made that these blood samples must be obtained at least a week apart. This is not always correct. When the first blood specimen is taken on the fifth day of the illness and the appearance of circulating antibodies to the infecting microorganism requires approximately seven days, then it follows that the second blood specimen may be taken two or three days after the first sample. Thus, an immunologic diagnosis may be made more rapidly than generally practiced. Indeed, under these circumstances we have shown a significant and reproducible increase in antibody titers within 48 and even within 24 hours.

Documentation of a specific antibody response is particularly helpful when a suspected pathogen is isolated from the respiratory or intestinal tracts, in order to differentiate recent infection from the carrier state. During an acute infection an increase in the antibody titer is to be expected, whereas a significant change in antibody titer is less likely to occur during a prolonged carrier state. Further, demonstration of an immune response to two isolates from the intestinal, respiratory, or urinary tracts, or from wounds, provides support for the assumption of a double or mixed infection.

Another advantage of the immunologic approach to the diagnosis of certain bacterial infections is that a suspected pathogen may no longer be present at the time of the examination or cannot be isolated for technical reasons, including the presence of antibiotics, and yet antibody levels are maintained for weeks.

Placental Transfer of Bacterial Antibodies

Information on the placental transfer of various classes of immunoglobulins has found an important application in the diagnosis of fetal infections. Of the major immunoglobulins, IgG is readily transferred from the mother to the newborn child, the blood levels in the cord blood being essentially identical to those of the mother or even slightly higher. In contrast, the levels of IgM antibodies in cord blood usually are less than 20 mg/100 ml, compared to levels of around 120 mg/100 ml in the serum of adults. For this reason, when infection of the fetus results in the production of IgM antibodies, the cord blood levels exceed normal values. Determination of these levels, then, can be used as a screening procedure for the diagnosis of fetal infection. Syphilis, cytomegalovirus infection, toxoplasmosis, and rubella are among fetal infections leading to IgM antibody production.

Documentation of a decrease in the titers of antibodies is of diagnostic value in the newborn infant. When (IgG) antibodies have been acquired passively in the absence of fetal infection, a continuously decreasing titer of antibodies is expected, whereas an increase is indicative of active disease.

Local Immune Response

In localized infections, such as cholera and shigellosis, antibodies are produced at the site of infection and are present in the intestinal contents. These antibodies have been referred to as coproantibodies. They may appear prior to those found in the circulation. Local production of antibodies is a rather general phenomenon, and antibodies against certain pathogens are protective. Among these antibodies in secretions IgA antibodies are of major importance. The biologic importance of secretory IgA antibodies is illustrated by the fact that such antibodies may prevent attachment of bacteria to the mucous membrane and thus inhibit penetration and initiation of bacterial disease. Even cellular immunity can be elicited as a local immune response.

In Vivo *Tests for Presence of Bacterial Antibodies*

The presence of certain circulating antibodies can be determined also by appropriate *in vivo* procedures. Best known is the Schick test. In this test, diphtheria toxin injected intradermally produces a discernible skin reaction, unless diphtheria antitoxin in adequate amounts is present in the circulation. Thus, a negative Schick test indicates immunity and a positive test susceptibility to this infection. Conversely, the presence of circulating antibodies may be determined by a positive rather than a negative skin reaction. It was shown, many years ago, that injection of type-specific pneumococcal polysaccharides causes a rapidly developing (30 to 60 minutes) wheal-and-erythema reaction in human subjects only if type-specific circulating antibodies are present. Thus, this reaction develops with the appearance of these antibodies in subjects with pneumococcal pneumonia at the time of crisis and recovery. In view of the fact that active immunization with type-specific polysaccharides has attracted renewed interest, these observations are of both theoretic and practical significance.

Delayed Hypersensitivity

All the above approaches are based on the demonstration of humoral antibodies. A specific immunologic response of the host to certain pathogens may result in the development of specific, delayed hypersensitivity (Chapter 11), akin to cellular immunity. The tuberculin test has served for many years as the prototype of delayed hypersensitivity. Individuals infected with *Mycobacterium tuberculosis* react to tuberculin or PPD in a specific and characteristic manner, the reaction developing after 18 to 24 hours and reaching an optimum at around 48 hours. This form of allergy can be demonstrated for many years after the onset of the original infection. From a diagnostic point of view, the tuberculin test has been used to exclude the presence of tuberculosis in subjects with negative reactions, particularly in populations with a low incidence of tuberculosis. Conversely, in infants and young children a positive tuberculin test is usually diagnostic. Even more important for the diagnosis of current tuberculosis is the documented conversion of a negative to a positive test within several weeks or a few months. On occasion, conversion can be detected when a negative tuberculin skin test (read at 48 hours) becomes positive several days or even a few weeks later. This series of events is due to the facts that enough of the antigen remains *in situ* and that immunologically committed cells responsible for delayed hypersensitivity are emerging during this period. It is of both practical and theoretic interest to note that delayed hypersensitivity may be suppressed during and following measles and even following immunization with attenuated measles virus vaccine. Anergy may be present also during overwhelming tuberculous infection. It has become evident that various members of the genus *Mycobacterium* produce products of different immunologic reactivity. Through the use of these various tuberculins, tentative differentiation of tuberculosis from infection due to other mycobacteria, the so-called atypical mycobacteria, can be made.

Delayed hypersensitivity develops during other bacterial infections as well, for example, during brucellosis. Again, a positive brucellergen test indicates only that infection has occurred in the past and not necessarily that it is active at the time of the test. Streptokinase-dornase includes two products that are operative in delayed hypersensitivity and used diagnostically to identify immunologic deficiency. Delayed hypersensitivity to diphtheria toxoid may also develop following active immunization with this antigen.

Remarkable progress has been made during the past few years in our understanding of the basic principles of delayed hypersensitivity. A transfer factor has been isolated from leukocytes of subjects with delayed hypersensitivity to tuberculin or to other antigens. This factor is capable of inducing prompt and prolonged (months to a few years) delayed hypersensitivity in previously nonreactive subjects. Information derived from experimental animals on the *in vitro* demonstration of delayed hypersensitivity is being applied to man by means of the macrophage migration inhibition test, utilizing human peripheral blood lymphocytes and guinea pig peritoneal macrophages as indicators. Delayed hypersensitivity can be documented even in certain subjects with negative skin tests due to drug- or disease-induced hyporeactivity.

Immunity to Bacterial Infections

Active Immunity

It has been known for centuries that certain infections result in solid and long-lasting immunity. With other infections, immunity does not develop, as is evident from the frequency of either recurrences or chronicity of the infection. However, it is also clear that recurrence of an infection does not always preclude the existence of immunity, since the latter may be type specific rather than species specific. It is for this reason that *Streptococcus pyogenes* infections frequently recur, although not by the identical serotype.

In only a few of the many bacterial infections is the information on active immunity convincing and unequivocal and the mechanism of immunity clearly identified. Needless to say, such information is of crucial importance in attempts to reproduce natural immunity by artificial means. In diphtheria, tetanus, and other bacterial diseases due to a single antigenic toxin, antitoxin in adequate levels is clearly protective. Protection may also occur when a secondary (recall) immune response takes place during the early phases of the incubation period. The mechanism of immunity to type-specific polysaccharides, such as those produced by pneumococci and *Haemophilus influenzae*, and to type-specific protein antigens, such as the products of group A hemolytic streptococci, is protective, and an adequate level of the corresponding antibodies in the circulation produces significant immunity.

Although this factor was considered decades ago, it is only recently that solid evidence has emerged on the role of the local immune response as a protective mechanism. Antibodies in human secretions, usually of the IgA secretory class, have been found in the respiratory, intestinal, and urinary tracts. Information on the antibody specificity to various bacterial species is as yet incomplete. In patients with cholera the predominant class of these immunoglobulins is IgA. Recent information suggests that such secretory cholera antibodies may be protective by interfering with the attachment of the pathogen, *Vibrio cholerae*, to the intestinal mucosa and by inhibiting the growth of these microorganisms at this site. In this connection, it is of interest to point out the immunologic role of Peyer's patches; in the rabbit, at least, this tissue is a rich source of precursors of IgA-producing immunocytes. These findings are of particular importance as the basis for the development of effective vaccines.

Circulating antibodies and immunoglobulins in secretions do not play a significant role in immunity to certain intracellular bacterial pathogens, such as *Mycobacterium tuberculosis*, brucellae, *Listeria monocytogenes*, and salmonellae. It is cellular immunity rather than humoral antibodies that accounts for protection. Largely through the research of Mackaness, a better understanding of the fundamental aspects of cellular immunity has become possible. The antigenic stimulus results in the appearance of immunologically committed lymphocytes, which, probably through molecular mediators, activate macrophages, resulting in enhanced antimicrobial activity. The immunologically committed lymphocytes, therefore, are not effector cells. Initiation of the process is immunologically specific; the end result, however, is not specific in nature. The activated macrophages, when compared to nonactivated cells, are more heavily endowed with mitochondria and lysosomes and exhibit greater phagocytic as well as bactericidal activity. The cellular immunity can be recalled specifically by the original antigen. The immunologically committed lymphocyte transfers cellular immunity. Recently, an *in vitro* model of cellular immunity in the guinea pig has become available.

Active immunity develops following either overt or subclinical infection, and it is because of the existence of clinically inapparent infection that the immunizing agent frequently is not identified. In addition, cross-reacting antigens may, in fact, elicit the immune response. At the present time, information on the stimulation of the immune response by cross-reacting antigens and on its role in clinical immunity is inadequately explored.

Artificial active immunization has been in use for many decades. When the resulting immunity is solid and long-lasting, proof of the efficacy of the vaccine readily emerges even without a double-blind controlled study. Such was the case with tetanus immunization during World War II, when this infection was almost entirely prevented in the immunized but not in the nonimmunized soldiers. When the immunity is of limited degree and duration, controlled studies are indispensable. Thus, typhoid vaccine was used widely for decades since its first introduction by Wright in 1897, and yet its efficacy, although suspected, was not established until field trials with appropriate controls were begun by the World Health Organization in 1954.

For reasons that are not entirely clear, the degree and the duration of the immune response, including antibody production, immunologic memory, and cellular immunity, elicited by various bacterial immunogens differ strikingly. From a practical point of view it is important to emphasize that adequate primary immunization with tetanus toxoid engenders long-lasting immunologic memory, and that secondary antibody production can be elicited even some two decades after primary immunization, thus protecting the individual from the development of this serious illness when exposure to tetanus bacilli is suspected.

Since the topic of artificial active immunization is covered in Chapter 26, it suffices to call attention to the following trends that have emerged from the fundamental knowledge of immunology. First, the route of administration of a given immunogen, as conceived decades ago by Besredka, may have profound effects on the development of clinically effective immunity. For this reason aerosol and oral immunizations are being explored more intensively than in the past. For example, a live streptomycin-dependent vaccine of *Salmonella typhi* provides protection when given by· mouth to human volunteers. From these considerations it is also evident that the determination of the titer of circulating antibodies may be inadequate. Rather, it is important to learn of the kind and amounts of locally produced antibodies. Even cellular immunity (Chapter 11) may be elicited by local administration of antigen. In addition to enteric infections, such as entero-pathogenic *Escherichia coli* enteritis, shigellosis, and cholera, these considera-tions may apply to respiratory diseases as well, for example, to pertussis. Second, recent observations strongly suggest the use of certain mutants for active immunization, similar to the previously established employment of BCG. In these efforts attention is being paid both to the immunogenicity and to the lack of virulence of the immunizing strains. To illustrate some of the approaches presently being explored, reference is made to studies on oral immunization against shigellosis. Based on a far better understanding of the pathogenesis of this infection than previously available and on advances in genetics that make possible the development of hybrids between a pathogenic *Shigella* and a nonpathogenic *Escherichia coli* (K12), an attenu-ated strain given by mouth afforded significant immunity to monkeys against experimental infection. Similarly, protection against experimental salmonel-losis can be induced by the administration of epimeraseless mutants of *Salmonella typhimurium*. Third, and perhaps most important, is the information that certain RNA preparations of bacteria and of cells of immunized animals induce cellular and/or humoral immunity. Youmans and Youmans have shown that the capacity of bacterial RNA to induce immunity to tubercu-losis is related to its structure and is maximal when RNA is either double stranded or double helical, or has a highly organized structure. The mode of action of these RNA preparations has not been fully elucidated. One important question relates to the possible presence of antigenic determinants in the RNA preparations. Such preparations do not necessarily contain fragments of the antigen needed to stimulate the secondary response. The resulting immunity is not due to delayed hypersensitivity. Such immunogens have been developed in the laboratory for protection against tuberculosis, salmonellosis, and staphylococcal infection. It remains to be seen whether these basic studies will find practical application in the foreseeable future. Fourth, the identification of the transfer factor responsible for delayed-type hypersensitivity offers the opportunity for replacement therapy in subjects with impaired cellular immunity. Certainly, these investigations focus attention on a mechanism of inducing an immune response other than that by the antigen (immunogen) itself.

Passive Immunity

In man, passive immunity occurs naturally only in the newborn or young infant, either because of transplacental acquisition of antibodies or because of the ingestion of antibodies present in colostrum and mother's milk.

In man, IgG is transferred quantitatively and may be present even in somewhat higher concentrations in the blood of the newborn infant than in that of the mother. In contrast, IgM and IgA are not transferred. In cattle, no antibodies are transferred to the fetus. The newborn calf, for protection against otherwise fatal bacterial infection, is protected by the ingestion of antibody-containing colostrum, and these antibodies are, in fact, absorbed from the gastrointestinal tract. In the newborn infant, antibodies present in colostrum remain localized within the gastrointestinal tract and do not reach the bloodstream in significant amounts. However, it must not be assumed that such colostral antibodies are of no value to the newborn, for they may have a protective effect against infection originating from the gastrointestinal tract. Indeed, it is the impression of clinicians that in breast-fed infants enteropathogenic *Escherichia coli* enteritis is less common and, if it occurs, less severe than in bottle-fed newborns. The passive transfer of IgG results in immunity of the newborn against certain bacterial infections, such as diphtheria, tetanus, and *Haemophilus influenzae* infection. Obviously, this protection is acquired by the newborn only if the mother has the respective antibodies in adequate titers. In addition to providing protection against certain infections, the presence of passively acquired IgG antibodies plays a role also by temporary interference with active immunization.

Artificial passive immunization has been used effectively ever since the introduction of diphtheria antitoxin. The principle has been applied subsequently to the treatment and prevention of a variety of bacterial infections, such as tetanus, botulism, *Haemophilus influenzae* meningitis, pertussis, and pneumococcal infections. With the advent of modern chemotherapy, notably of antibiotic treatment, serum prophylaxis and serum therapy have become much less important. When there is an indication for the administration of antibodies, it is preferable to employ immunoglobulins of human rather than animal origin. At the present time, both pertussis and tetanus immunoglobulins of human origin are available.

Bacterial Antigens, Antibodies, and Immunologic Injury

Immunologic injury may develop on the basis of immune response to bacterial antigens under certain circumstances. For example, excessive delayed hypersensitivity (Chapter 11) may unfavorably influence the course of tuberculous infection. Attachment of bacterial antigens to cells may produce immunologic injury provided that the corresponding bacterial antibodies as well as complement are present. This model has been investigated in detail in experimental animals, utilizing the reinfusion of the animal's own cells after the attachment of a given bacterial antigen. In the absence of the corresponding bacterial antibody, cell survival is normal; in its presence, hemolysis develops *in vivo*. Finally, attention has been called to the possible role of cross-reacting antigens. An immune response of the host to the microbial antigen may, under certain circumstances, lead to injury of those cells that share the antigenic determinant (Chapter 25).

Immune Deficiency Diseases

Resistance to, and recovery from, certain bacterial infections depend, in part, on the integrity of the immune apparatus of the host. It is not surprising, therefore, that deficiencies in this system can be associated with unusually frequent and particularly serious infections. Since the original description by Bruton of agammaglobulinemia, these deficiency syndromes have been studied in great detail and have contributed materially to our understanding of the function of the various components of the immune apparatus, as discussed in Chapter 17. Only brief reference is made to the various bacteriologic tests used in the diagnosis of these immune deficiency diseases.

1. Circulating, humoral antibodies
    a. *In vitro* determination, for example, titration of diphtheria and tetanus antitoxins. Other tests used are *Salmonella* H and O antibody determinations, the former largely identifying IgG and the latter IgM antibodies.
    b. *In vivo* tests, such as the Schick test, measuring a minimally effective antitoxin level.
2. Cell-mediated immunity (delayed hypersensitivity) (Chapter 11) to bacterial antigens, as measured by means of the tuberculin and streptokinase-dornase skin tests.
3. Secondary reactions, such as phagocytosis (Chapter 10). In this procedure the uptake of various microorganisms can be determined indicative of the ability of the cells to phagocytize and of the presence or absence of opsonins. In addition, it is often important to measure the bactericidal activity of phagocytes by determining the death rates of ingested organisms.

Bacterial Adjuvants

The immunogenicity of antigens can be enhanced by a variety of measures, including aggregation of the antigen and the admixture of various substances, the adjuvants. The latter have been used for some five decades to enhance antibody response, to analyze the various components of the immune apparatus, to study immunosuppression, to produce experimental autoimmune diseases, and—in the practice of medicine—to fortify such immunogens as diphtheria and tetanus toxoids. Among the adjuvants are bacteria and certain bacterial products, and brief reference to adjuvants is made in this chapter. The complete Freund's adjuvant, so widely used in experimental studies, contains mycobacterial cells. The endotoxins of gram-negative bacilli (lipopolysaccharides) are highly effective adjuvants. Of other bacteria, species, *Bordetella pertussis* and *Corynebacterium parvum* are rather unique in their adjuvanticity. The mode of action of various bacterial adjuvants has not yet been completely elucidated; changes in antigen distribution, antigen uptake, alteration of cell metabolism (cyclic AMP), attraction of cells to areas of antigen deposit—all may play a role in enhancing an immune response and termination of unresponsiveness (tolerance).

Bibliography

Ackroyd, J. F. (ed.): *Immunological Methods*. F. A. Davis Co., Philadelphia, 1964.

Alexander, J. W., and Good, R.: *Fundamentals of Clinical Immunology*. W. B. Saunders, Philadelphia, 1977.

Barber, H. R. K.: *Immunobiology for the Clinician*. John Wiley & Sons, Inc., Somerset, N.J., 1976.

Bellanti, J. A., and Schlegel, R. J.: The diagnosis of immune deficiency diseases. *Pediatr. Clin. North Am.*, **18**:49–72, 1971.

Bennett, C. W.: *Clinical Serology*. Charles C Thomas, Publisher, Springfield, Ill., 1971.

Bergsma, D.; Good, R. A.; Finstad, J.; Paul, N. W. (eds.): *Immunodeficiency in Man and Animals*. Sinauer Associates, Inc., Sunderland, Mass., 1976.

Brambell, F. W. R.: *The Transmission of Passive Immunity from Mother to Young*. American Elsevier Publishing Co., Inc., New York, 1970.

Carpenter, P. L.: *Immunology and Serology*. W. B. Saunders Co., Philadelphia, 1965.

Davis, B. D.; Dulbecco, R.; Eisen, H. N.; Ginsberg, H. S.; and Wood, W. B., Jr. (eds.): *Microbiology*, 2nd ed. Harper & Row, Publishers, New York, 1975.

Davis, B. D., and Warren, L. (eds.): *The Specificity of Cell Surfaces*. Prentice-Hall, Inc., Englewood Cliffs, N.J., 1967.

Dayton, D. H., Jr.; Small, P. A., Jr.; Chanock, R. M.; Kaufman, H. E.; and Tomasi, T. B., Jr. (eds.): *The Secretory Immunologic System*. U.S. Government Printing Office, Washington, D.C., 1971.

Freedman, S. O.: *Clinical Immunology*, 2nd ed. Harper & Row, Publishers, New York, 1976.

Friedman, H. (ed.): Immunological tolerance to microbial antigens. *Ann. N.Y. Acad. Sci.*, **181**, 1971.

Fudenberg, H. H.; Stites, D. P.; Caldwell, J. L.; and Wells, J. V. (eds.): *Basic and Clinical Immunology*. Lange Medical Publications, Los Altos, Calif., 1976.

Gell, P. G. H., and Coombs, R. R. A. (eds.): *Clinical Aspects of Immunology*, 3rd ed. Blackwell Scientific Publications, Ltd., Oxford, 1975.

Haynard, A. R.: *Immunodeficiency*. Williams & Wilkins, Baltimore, 1977.

Kwapinski, J. B. G. (ed.): *Analytical Serology of Microorganisms*, Vol. 2. Interscience Publishers, New York, 1969.

Landsteiner, K.: *The Specificity of Serological Reactions.* Harvard University Press, Cambridge, Mass., 1945.

Lawrence, H. S.: Transfer factor and cellular immune deficiency disease. *N. Engl. J. Med.*, **283**:411, 1970.

Lüderitz, O.; Jann, K.; and Wheat, R.: Somatic and capsular antigens of gramnegative bacteria. In Florkin, M., and Stotz, E. H. (eds.): *Comprehensive Biochemistry*, Vol. 26A. Elsevier Publishing Co., Amsterdam, 1968, pp. 105–228.

Mackaness, G. B.: Cellular immunity. *Ann Inst. Pasteur (Paris)*, **120**:428–37, 1971.

Merler, E. (ed.): *Immunoglobulins.* National Academy of Sciences, Washington, D.C., 1970.

Michael, J. G.: Natural antibodies. *Curr. Top. Microbiol.*, **48**:43, 1969.

Mudd, S. (ed.): *Infectious Agents and Host Reactions.* W. B. Saunders Co., Philadelphia, 1970.

Neter, E.: The immune response of the host: an aid to etiology, pathogenesis, diagnosis, and epidemiology of bacterial infections. *Yale J. Biol. Med.*, **44**:241–46, 1971.

Neter, E., and Milgrom, F. (eds.): *The Immune System and Infectious Diseases.* S. Karger, Basel, 1975.

Nowotny, A. (ed.): *Cellular Antigens.* Springer-Verlag, New York, 1972.

Parish, H. J., and Cannon, D. A.: *Antisera, Toxoids, Vaccines and Tuberculins in Prophylaxis and Treatment.* Williams & Wilkins Co., Baltimore, 1962.

Park, B. H., and Good, R. A.: *Principles of Modern Immunology.* Lea & Febiger, Philadelphia, 1974.

Rose, N. R., and Friedman, H. (eds.): *Manual of Clinical Immunology.* American Society for Microbiology, Washington, D.C., 1976.

Solomon, J. B.: *Foetal and Neonatal Immunology.* American Elsevier Publishing Co., Inc., New York, 1971.

Task Force on Immunology and Disease: *Immunology, Its Role in Disease and Health.* U.S. Government Printing Office, Washington, D.C., 1976.

Thaler, M. S.; Klausner, R. D.; and Cohen, H. J.: *Medical Immunology.* J. B. Lippincott, Philadelphia, 1977.

Weiser, R. S.; Myrvik, Q. N.; and Pearsall, N. N.: *Fundamentals of Immunology.* Lea & Febiger, Philadelphia, 1969.

Wilson, G. S., and Miles, A. A.: *Topley and Wilson's Principles of Bacteriology and Immunity*, 6th ed. Williams & Wilkins Co., Baltimore, 1975.

14

Immunology of Mycotic Diseases

JOSEPH H. KITE, JR.

Introduction

Fungi (yeasts and molds) have unique characteristics that need to be considered in attempts to apply immunologic principles to their detection and identification or to evaluate the treatment and prognosis of the human disease produced. Mycotic diseases of man are conveniently grouped according to three major sites of infection—cutaneous, subcutaneous, or systemic. Some fungi are dimorphic, i.e., occurring as one morphologic form at body temperature (usually yeast cells) and appearing as another form (usually mycelium) on culture at room temperature. Frequently fungi produce characteristic asexual spores that permit morphologic identification microscopically. Further characterization is aided by biochemical (especially fermentation and assimilation tests) and by immunologic reactions. The inoculation of laboratory animals is often possible but usually not required for identification.

Confirmation of the isolated microorganism as the causative agent of the disease may be complicated by the fact that some infections may be caused by organisms that are endogenous (i.e., living as part of the normal flora of the host), whereas others are clearly exogenous. Infection by an oral endogenous organism such as *Actinomyces israelii* may occur following pyremia or tooth extraction with tissue damage. *Candida albicans* occurring normally on the skin and mucous membranes may be able to multiply and cause disease following suppression of normal flora with broad-spectrum antibiotics. Occasionally, organisms usually thought to be saprophytes (e.g., *Torula glabrata*) may cause systemic infection following debilitating diseases, such as tuberculosis or diabetes, or after the use of steroids that result in a lowering of the immune response. Mycotic infections are good imitators of the clinical signs of other diseases (Chapter 17). This has led frequently to difficulty in diagnosis and delay in treatment.

Sometimes the fungus may be intracellular in location, such as *Histoplasma capsulatum*, which is a parasite of the mononuclear phagocytic system. Therefore, it may be less accessible to the action of the immune system of the host. Other fungi produce superficial infections, such as the dermatophytes, and their antigenic products may not reach the antibody-producing cells of the body to stimulate them adequately. Some fungi are highly infectious (over 90% of individuals in an endemic area being infected), but host defense mechanisms are excellent and only a few exposed individuals will show clinical signs or develop disease. Such organisms of high infectivity but low pathogenicity include *Histoplasma capsulatum* and *Coccidioides immitis*. A subclinical infection may lead to the development of a delayed hypersensitivity skin reaction (Chapter 11), serving merely to demonstrate present or past contact with the organism. The development of immunity may occur concomitantly with hypersensitivity and evidence most frequently suggests the possibility of a cellular immune reaction rather than a role of humoral antibody, although the mechanisms are not clearly established.

The virulence of a yeast such as *Cryptococcus neoformans* is partially dependent upon a polysaccharide capsule. Macrophages and neutrophils are able to phagocytize (Chapter 10) and destroy the yeast, but this process is inhibited by very small amounts of cryptococcal polysaccharide. Heat-stable components of serum facilitate attachment of cryptococci, whereas heat-labile opsonins are necessary for maximal initial rates of phagocytosis. The most important function of the heat-stable components of serum appear to be in triggering the ingestion of attached yeast. Several types of peripheral blood leukocytes, excluding T cells, can also kill *C. neoformans* by a nonphagocytic mechanism, namely, antibody-dependent fungicidal activity. The size of the capsule of *C. neoformans* is not the entire explanation for its virulence. When cells are cultivated in appropriate media so as to have large or small capsules and then are inoculated intravenously into mice, virulence is characteristic of the isolate and is not affected by the size of the capsule of the cells in the inoculum.

Resistance to infection of fungi may be due to some mechanism other than immunity. The dermatophytes characteristically invade the superficial layers of the skin but do not invade the deeper layers. Invasion usually stops where there are viable cells. There may be inhibiting factors in the serum that prevent further growth rather than a deficiency of nutrients.

Table 14-1
HUMAN DISEASES CAUSED BY FUNGI AND FUNGI-LIKE BACTERIA*

Cutaneous (Skin, Hair, Nails)	Subcutaneous	Systemic (Disseminated)
A. Superficial mucoses	A. Chromomycosis	A. Fungi-like bacteria
1. Tinea versicolor	1. *Fonsecaea* (*Hormodendrum*)	1. Actinomycosis
Malassezia furfur	*pedrosoi*	*Actinomyces israelii*
2. Tinea nigra	2. *Fonsecaea* (*Hormodendrum*)	2. Nocardiosis
Cladosporium	*compactum*	*Nocardia asteroides*
werneckii		
3. Piedra	3. *Philophora verrucosa*	B. Yeast fungi
Black	4. *Cladosporium carrionii*	1. Candidiasis
Piedraia hortai		*Candida albicans*
White	B. Sporotrichosis	2. Geotrichosis
Trichosporon	*Sporothrix schenckii*—	*Geotrichum candidum*
cutaeum (*beigelii*)	dimorphic	
B. Dermatophytoses	C. Mycetoma	3. Cryptococcosis
1. Microsporum group	1. Eumycotic	*Cryptococcus*
	(maduromycosis)	*neoformans*
M. audouinii	a. Yellowish-white	
M. canis	granules	C. Dimorphic fungi
M. gypseum	*Allescheria boydii*	1. Histoplasmosis
2. Epidermophyton	*Cephalosporium sp.*	*Histoplasma*
group	b. Black granules	*capsulatum*
E. floccosum	*Madurella grisea*	2. Blastomycosis
3. Trichophyton group	*Madurella*	*Blastomyces*
T. mentagro-	*mycetomi*	*dermatitidis*
phytes	*Phialophora*	(N. American)
T. rubrum } ecto-thrix	*jeanselmei*	B. (*Paracoccidioides*)
T. verru-	2. Actinomycotic	*brasiliensis*
cosum	a. Yellowish-white	(S. American)
T. tonsu-	granules	3. Sporotrichosis
rans } endo-thrix	*Nocardia asteroides*	*Sporothrix schenckii*
T. viola-	*N. brasiliensis*	4. Coccidioidomycosis
ceum	*N. caviae*	*Coccidioides immitis*
T. schoenleinii—	*N.* (*Streptomyces*)	D. Mold fungi
favic	*madurae*	1. Aseptate mycelium
T. concentricum—	*Streptomyces*	a. Phycomycosis
skin only	*somaliensis*	(zygomycosis)
		Rhizopus sp.
		Mucor sp.
		2. Septate mycelium
		a. Aspergillosis
		Aspergillus
		fumigatus
		A. flavus

* This table is not intended as a complete list of fungi pathogenic for man but as a review of the more important microorganisms divided according to their major sites of proliferation.

Serologic techniques have been used to detect antigen in tissues or clinical specimens or to detect antibodies in patient serum. Intracutaneous skin tests for delayed hypersensitivity (Chapter 11) can be performed with the appropriate extract of fungal antigens. Sometimes these tests are prognostic as well as diagnostic.

Immunosuppression may arise as a consequence of disease (hematopoietic or lymphoreticular malignancies) or the administration of corticosteroids and other drugs as therapy for homograft rejection or malignant diseases. The result of immunosuppression may be a higher-than-normal incidence of invasive fungal infections such as candidiasis, aspergillosis, mucormycosis and cryptococcosis. *Candida,* normally a superficial colonizer, may invade the gastrointestinal, respiratory, or urinary tract. *Aspergillus* and *Mucor* species may cause hemorrhagic or necrotizing pneumonias and secondarily spread to the brain. *Cryptococcus* may infect the meninges in the appropriate host.

More than 75% of fungal infections following immunosuppression are caused by *Candida, Aspergillus,* and *Phycomycetes,* and the incidence of infection with each of these three pathogens is increasing. Cryptococcosis occurs more frequently than expected in the compromised host. Histoplasmosis may also be more frequent in immunosuppressed patients, and sporotrichosis and coccidioidomycosis, although not more common, may present an atypical appearance or cause more severe infections than observed in the immuno-competent host.

In addition to barriers of nonspecific immunity, the high incidence in the normal population of immunologic skin reactions to *Candida* antigens suggests that a specific acquired immunity may also be required for keeping the fungus on a commensal level. However, a few relatively minor defects in either the nonspecific or specific protective mechanisms may alter it in favor of the fungus, which then becomes parasitic.

This chapter will limit presentation to those fungus diseases pathogenic for man, where significant information is available and where immunologic tests are of value. A list of some fungus diseases and their causative agents is found in Table 14-1.

Serologic Reactions

Detection of Antigen in Tissues and Clinical Specimens

The fluorescent antibody technique, using labeled antiserum specific to fungal antigens, has the advantage of being rapid and selective in detecting these antigens in pus, exudates, tissue impression smears, spinal fluid specimens, and cultures. Tests with sputum and tissue sections are more difficult but may be improved with adequate enzymatic and chemical digestion, thereby permitting better interaction between antigen and anti-body. Fungi detected by this procedure include *Blastomyces dermatitidis,*

CRYPTO CSF CRYPTO CSF CRYPTO CSF
1:10   1:100   1:1000

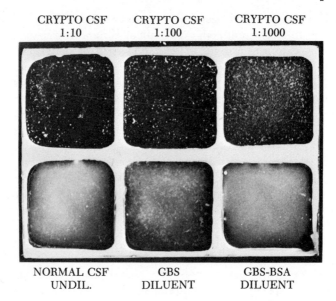

NORMAL CSF GBS   GBS-BSA
UNDIL.   DILUENT DILUENT

Figure 14-1. Latex fixation slide agglutination test for detection of cryptococcal antigen in body fluids. Lower row contains negative controls, undiluted and diluted normal cerebrospinal fluid (CSF); upper row, tenfold dilutions of positive spinal fluid, with reactions of 4+, 4+, and 2+, left to right. (From Hazen, E. L.; Gordon, M. A.; and Reed, F. C.: *Laboratory Identification of Pathogenic Fungi Simplified.* Charles C Thomas, Publisher, Springfield, Ill., 1970.)

Candida species, *Coccidioides immitis, Cryptococcus neoformans, Histoplasma capsulatum, Paracoccidioides brasiliensis,* and *Sporothrix schenckii.*

Immunofluorescence (Chapter 27) enables a more rapid diagnosis in sporotrichosis where it is difficult to detect organisms in clinical material with light microscopy. The correlation between immunofluorescence and culture for detection of *S. schenckii* in lesion exudates has been over 90%.

Early in the course of cryptococcosis, serologic tests will show antibody but not antigen. As the diseases progresses, there is a rapid multiplication of yeast cells and production of large amounts of capsular antigen that neutralizes the antibody. Prior to recognition and treatment with specific chemotherapy, the increased amount of antigen may be detected by a latex fixation slide agglutination test (Figure 14-1). In this procedure rabbit antibodies to *C. neoformans* are attached to latex particles. This test is extremely sensitive and can detect 0.002 μg of capsular polysaccharide per milliliter of body fluid. It can detect antigen in serum or cerebrospinal fluid and has detected infection in several instances where the standard India ink examination was negative.

For optimal results, both the complement-fixation (Chapter 8) and latex agglutination (Chapter 6) tests should be done to detect the antigen of *Cryptococcus.* The latex antigen test is useful for anticomplementary specimens and the complement-fixation test for specimens with interfering anti-globulins as may occur in patients with rheumatoid factor.

The titer of antigen in body fluids reflects the severity of the disease, with a high titer indicating a poor prognosis. When effective chemotherapy such as amphotericin B is instituted, the antigen titer drops with clinical improvement. When the antigen has almost completely disappeared, the antibody may once again become detectable.

In localized cutaneous cryptococcosis, or in the presence of a focal pulmonary infection, antibody but not antigen generally is detectable. Therefore, in cases of suspected cryptococcosis, tests for both antigen and antibody should be done since there appears to be an inverse relationship between the two.

Detection of Circulating Antibody

Following the infection of man or animals with one of the pathogenic fungi, serum antibodies are frequently produced to the fungal antigens. A variety of serologic tests used to detect antibodies have included agglutination, precipitation, complement fixation, immunofluorescence, and neutralization. Various refinements of these tests (e.g., immunoelectroosmophoresis) have been made to improve the sensitivity, shorten testing time, and reduce the quantity of reagents.

The antigens used for testing may be prepared from any fungus culture and are generally crude and impure but useful. Antigens may be used as whole yeast cells or as ground preparations of yeast or mycelium and may be used directly in suspension or attached to erythrocytes, latex particles, charcoal particles, collodion, or ion-exchange resins.

The ability to detect antibody in serum may be reflected by several situations. In asymptomatic and mild infections, serologic tests are frequently negative. A rising titer as the disease progresses is almost diagnostic. On the other hand, a falling titer, except in a moribund patient, indicates a good prognosis.

Stimulation of antibodies by yeast cells has been more successful than the use of moldlike cultures. Thus disease in which the yeast phase exists in the body may lead to better antibody production. In the case of the dermatophytes, the infection is superficial and the antibody-producing cells of the body are not stimulated to produce sufficient antibody for detection. The nature of the antigen also influences its ability to stimulate antibodies.

In several systemic fungal diseases, precipitation and complement fixation have been the most useful serologic tests for the diagnosis and prognosis of the disease. The precipitation test is superior in recognizing the early stages, the complement-fixing test in determining the later stages, particularly dissemination (Figure 14-2). Precipitating antibodies appear early, usually in the first week of illness, and begin to decrease by the third week. A single line of precipitation (using a commercial antigen preparation) is specific and

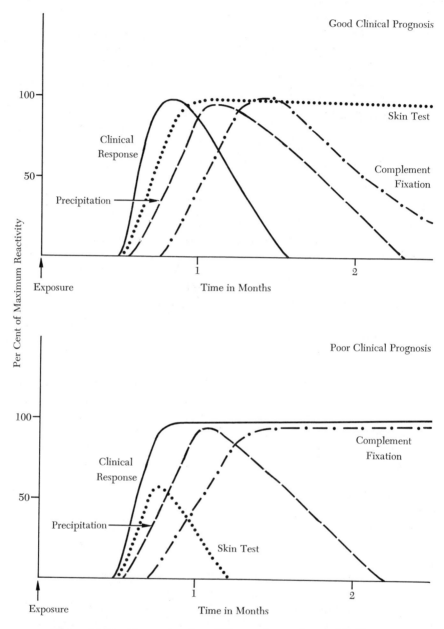

Figure 14-2. Composite view of diagnostic tests for coccidioidomycosis. A favorable clinical prognosis is indicated by a persistently positive skin test and a fall in the complement-fixation titer. A poor prognosis is indicated by a persistently high complement-fixation titer and a negative skin test.

diagnostic for active coccidioidomycosis. Complement-fixing antibodies appear in two to six weeks and serve as an excellent prognostic tool. If the complement-fixation titer drops, then the infection is usually benign and recovery is beginning. If the complement-fixing titer continues to rise and stays high, this is an indication of dissemination and the prognosis is poor.

Antibody detected by either the complement-fixation or immunodiffusion techniques appears to correlate well with infection and severity of disease. In patients with past or asymptomatic primary infection, antibodies usually are absent. This type of relationship between precipitation and complement fixation may also be found in histoplasmosis and blastomycosis. The interpretation of the skin test will be discussed on pages 234–36.

In patients with acute infections of histoplasmosis, antibody can be detected in the first few weeks of the infection by precipitation or by agglutination using histoplasmin attached to latex particles or erythrocytes.

Five precipitin bands have been shown to be present in the serum of patients. These appear at different times and follow in sequence. All sera from patients with proven histoplasmosis produce at least two bands, designated h and m. The h band appears to be specific for histoplasmosis and is not induced by skin testing with histoplasmin. The antibody responsible for the m band is present in the disease state, but also appears in healthy individuals who have had a recent positive skin test with histoplasmin. However, this antibody is not induced by the histoplasmin skin test in individuals who fail to react to histoplasmin. The c band represents an antigen that is common in *H. capsulatum*, *B. dermatitidis*, and *C. immitis* and explains the cross-reaction seen in both skin tests and serologic tests. No single human serum has been observed to have more than four bands.

Immunoelectrophoresis (Chapter 6) has been used to obtain the separation of five detectable precipitin bands (Figure 14-3). Sixty-two percent of patients with chronic histoplasmosis had antibodies to antigen 2 (corresponding to the m antigen previously described). Precipitins to antigen 3 or the h antigen were observed in 28% of patients, and their persistence beyond nine months after therapy was related to a high rate of relapse despite the fact that the sputum of the patient remained negative on culture for periods of as long as 16 months.

Part of the difficulty in the interpretation of various serologic tests is the fact that *H. capsulatum* contains a variety of antigens that induce antibodies at different rates in different patients. In addition, some types of antibodies predominate early in infection and others in the chronic form of the disease.

Precipitins tend to appear early in the infection, but this antibody is transient. It will disappear later and be replaced by a complement-fixing antibody. The interpretation of these tests is similar to that described in the case of coccidioidomycosis.

Occasionally in histoplasmosis, cross-reactions are seen with high-titer sera from patients with coccidioidomycosis but are much more common in patients with blastomycosis. A patient suspected of having histoplasmosis

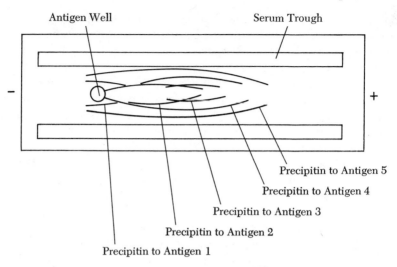

Figure 14-3. Five types of precipitin lines observed in the sera of patients with histoplasmosis when tested against histoplasmin by immunoelectrophoresis. The precipitin band to antigen 3 or the h antigen appears to have prognostic and clinical significance. (From Walter, J. E.: The significance of antibodies in chronic histoplasmosis by immunoelectrophoretic and complement fixation tests. *Am. Rev. Resp. Dis.*, **99**:50, 1969.)

should have his serum tested against histoplasnim, blastomycin, and coccidioidin. In nearly all cases, the highest titer will be with the homologous antigen.

Serologic tests for the diagnosis of blastomycosis are less reliable than for histoplasmosis and coccidioidomycosis because there appear to be several antigens shared with other fungi and because man also does not respond as readily or as vigorously to these antigens.

Antibodies to *Cryptococcus neoformans* can be detected by agglutination of formalin-killed whole yeast cells. Another test is the indirect fluorescent antibody technique in which patient serum is added to yeast cells fixed on a slide. An antihuman globulin conjugated to fluorescein isothiocyanate is then added to indicate antibody specifically attached to cellular antigen. The former test is more specific.

In aspergillosis a precipitating antibody to extracts of *Aspergillus fumigatus* may be of diagnostic value, although such precipitins have been found in some individuals having no evidence of disease.

Candida species are frequently found in the normal adult mouth and intestinal tract. Although the presence of antibodies is proof of the invasion of the body by the organism, it does not establish whether the invasion is primary or secondary. Therefore, serologic tests for *Candida* are of little diagnostic value unless a rising titer can be found on repeated tests. Since the mycelial growth phase of *C. albicans* occurs during infection, the detection by immunofluorescence (Chapter 27) of antibody to the germ tube has been reported as a more discriminating diagnostic test. There is need for more rapid detection of systemic candidiasis occurring as a complication of leukemias and lymphomas, renal transplants, and the use of prosthetic heart valves or intravenous catheters. Counterimmunoelectrophoresis (Chapter 6) employing commercial *Candida albicans* cell extract and patient serum has resulted in the formation of early precipitin lines (within two hours) without a reported loss of specificity or sensitivity. Such a procedure may be helpful for monitoring serum from patients who are immunologically compromised by immunosuppressive drugs.

Hypersensitivity

Clinical Manifestations

Several fungi that cause pathologic lesions in man may also produce hypersensitivity reactions that can be manifest clinically. Superficial infections caused by the dermatophytes may lead to the development of dermatophytids or "id" reactions, which are secondary eruptions occurring on the skin in specifically sensitized individuals as a result of the hematogenous spread of fungi or their allergenic products from a primary focus. In a patient expressing this hypersensitivity reaction, a primary fungous lesion can usually be found and fungi can be demonstrated in such a lesion. However, fungi cannot be isolated from the secondary or "id" lesion.

The fingers and hands are the most common sites of the "id" eruption, although the feet, legs, and body in general may sometimes be affected. Frequently, a series of vesicles may appear along the sides of the fingers or on the hands. These vesicles are tense, edematous, and filled with clear or cloudy fluid. The "ids" may follow irritation of the primary focus brought on by trauma or overtreatment, and disappear after clearing of the fungi from the primary lesions.

In candidiasis a similar "id" reaction may occur with the presence of *candidids*, sterile grouped vesicular lesions, which may be found over the hands and body. The diagnosis depends on the clinical characteristics of the lesions and on the demonstration of hypersensitivity in the patient.

In primary pulmonary coccidioidomycosis, approximately 4% of white males and 10% of white females develop *erythema nodosum* or *multiforme* even when the primary infection was asymptomatic. This delayed hypersensitivity reaction occurs in approximately 20% of patients with clinically diagnosed disease. These allergic reactions usually appear three days to three weeks after the termination of the febrile period. Numerous tender nodular lesions develop over the shins, but occasionally are found scattered over the arms, thighs, buttocks, and scalp. They are usually painful and after two or three days begin to fade leaving brownish pigmented areas that may persist for several weeks. In rare instances, a second crop of nodules may appear after an interval of weeks. The progressive type of the disease rarely occurs in patients who develop such allergic reactions following the primary infection.

Periodontal disease is an indolent and chronic inflammatory disease caused by the accumulation of oral bacteria in dental plaque that forms around the gingival margin. There is considerable evidence that microbial products act as antigens and initiate periodontal inflammation by activating the immune responses of the host. A direct correlation has been found between the severity of periodontal disease and the amount of lymphocyte trans- formation induced by the cell walls of oral bacteria (*Actinomyces* and certain gram-negative anaerobes) and by solubilized dental plaque.

Other fungi that are incapable of invading the body's tissues, or only occasionally do so as opportunistic pathogens, may still be the cause of significant pulmonary disorders by acting as antigenic substances. Examples of such diseases include Farmer's lung, bagassosis, mushroom picker's disease, and air-conditioner disease (Chapter 18). The inhalant involved is often "moldy" hay or grain, "moldy" extract of sugarcane fiber (bagasse), mush- room dust or compost, or dust or water from air conditioning systems.

These lung diseases occur after inhalation of thermophilic actinomycetes and fungi in vegetable dusts or animal products. Current evidence suggests that these pulmonary hypersensitivity reactions are due to a pulmonary Arthus type of reaction (Chapter 19). Antigen-antibody complexes localize in tissue with release of vasoactive amines, deposition of complement com- ponents, and attraction of neutrophils leading to release of enzymes from these cells and production of tissue injury.

Aspergillus may cause allergic rhinitis without actually invading the tissues. Patients usually have reaginic antibodies (IgE) but not precipitins (IgG) in their serum.

Detection of Hypersensitivity by Skin Tests

Superficial dermatophycoses and some of the deep mycoses produce cutaneous delayed hypersensitivity to the fungus in many patients. This can be demonstrated by positive skin reactions following intradermal inoculation of the appropriate antigen.

Type-specific antigens for skin tests that have been found of excellent value are: coccidioidin from *Coccidioides immitis*, histoplasmin from *Histoplasma capsulatum*, blastomycin from *Blastomyces dermatitidis*, and sporotrichin from *Sporothrix schenckii*.

Skin tests with antigens of the dermatophytes, *Microsporum*, *Trichophyton*, and *Epidermophyton*, vary from good to poor in their specificity. Many species give cross-reactions. Some species, such as *E. floccosum*, *M. audouini*, *T. schoenleini*, and *T. rubrum*, have little sensitizing action in comparison to other species of the same genera. The use of oidiomycin (from *Candida*) is of little diagnostic value. Since a large percentage of apparently normal individuals will give positive reactions, this merely reflects the ubiquitous nature of the organisms. However, such tests may aid the clinician since the management of the individual patient depends on whether or not he is hypersensitive to the fungus.

The nature of the skin test antigen will be discussed in the section on vaccines (pages 244–46). In essence, whole killed yeast or mycelial phase cells (crude or purified extracts of such cells) have been used for intra-cutaneous inoculation.

The skin test is performed by injecting 0.1 ml of a suitable dilution of the vaccine intracutaneously (e.g., 1:100 dilution of a commercial standardized coccidioidin or histoplasmin). The vaccine may also be injected by jet injection or by the tine test. In the latter test the vaccine is injected with four triangular prongs or tines, 2 mm long and 4 mm apart, projecting from a stainless steel disc. Both these methods are more rapid than the intra-cutaneous skin test, but slightly less sensitive.

Reaction to intracutaneous tests may be immediate, with "wheal-like" reactions occurring within a few minutes, delayed for 24 or 48 hours, or even occasionally delayed as long as two weeks. The immediate reactions are difficult to interpret. Attention is directed to delayed reactions with erythema and induration of 5-mm diameter or larger.

A positive skin test is interpreted in the same manner as a positive tuberculin test, i.e., a positive test indicates past or present infection. In mild infections or in extensive or overwhelming infections, the skin test may be negative. *Coccidioides immitis*, *Histoplasma capsulatum*, and *Blastomyces dermatitidis* will produce a high degree of infectivity but frequently without clinical signs. Therefore, many positive skin tests will reflect an unrecognized encounter with the organism sometime in the past. Such hypersensitivity can be demonstrated years after lesions have healed (sporotrichosis) or after the individual has moved away from the endemic area (coccidioidomycosis).

Positive skin tests may not be indicative of actual infection of the tissues by the fungus, since the patient may be sensitive to the fungus (*Aspergillus*). Also some skin test antigens are less specific (*Aspergillus*) and may show cross-reaction with other species (of *Aspergillus*) and saprophytic fungi.

However, the skin test does have diagnostic value, when a conversion to a positive test occurs during an infection in which an earlier test was negative. In coccidioidomycosis, histoplasmosis, or blastomycosis, a persistently positive test can be prognostic as well (Figure 14-2). The time of first appearance of a positive skin test following infection has been studied. With sporotrichosis, experimental inoculation of man has demonstrated that the skin test can be positive as early as the fifth day after the appearance of the lesion. In coccidioidomycosis the skin test becomes positive in 87% of patients during the first week of clinical symptoms and in 99% after the second week of illness. In histoplasmosis the skin test may become positive four days after the onset of illness but usually during the second or third week and one to two weeks before the appearance of the positive serologic tests.

Recovery from disseminated disease often results in the gradual fall of complement-fixation (CF) titer and the reestablishment of coccidioidin sensitivity (Figure 14-2). The cause of the poor skin sensitivity during disseminated disease could be either desensitization by excessive amounts of circulating antigen or the inability of the body to react to any cutaneous stimulation. It has been postulated that the alteration of lymphocyte surface receptors during the course of the disease may lead to the formation of auto-antibodies that may block the reactivity of these cells and cause skin anergy to coccidioidin.

The specificity of the skin test is a troublesome problem. Patients sensitive to coccidioidin, histoplasmin, or blastomycin may react also to one of the other two vaccines but to a lesser degree. Therefore, it is desirable to perform skin tests with all three antigens simultaneously. Paracoccidioidin is reasonably specific at a 1:100 dilution but gives cross-reactions at 1:10 with histoplasmosis and coccidioidomycosis. Some false positive reactions may represent subclinical infections not previously recognized. Antigens of the yeast form of *S. schenckii* appear specific, and the skin test is positive in almost all cases.

The occurrence of positive skin tests without obvious infection increases with age and indicates previous sensitization. False positive tests are infrequent in children. Repeated skin tests do not result in sensitivity to coccidioidin or histoplasmin if the individual has never been in contact with the organism.

Patients with primary coccidioidomycosis and erythema nodosum usually are extremely sensitive to coccidioidin and may give a strong reaction to 0.1 ml of a 1:10,000 dilution. Also, a primary skin test with a 1:100 dilution should not be used since it may aggravate the erythema nodosum or even cause this condition to appear in a patient previously free of it. However, in disseminated coccidioidomycosis a slight reaction or no reaction may be elicited from a 1:10 dilution of coccidioidin.

Hyposensitization

Hyposensitization or desensitization is an attempt to reduce patient hypersensitivity and concomitant clinical manifestations. Repeated injections of gradually increasing amounts of vaccine or antigenic preparation of the specific fungus responsible for the disease are administered. Although considerable controversy as to the value of such therapy has developed, it has been justified in recalcitrant infections that have not responded to regular treatment. Desensitization is of little value in advanced cases where a state of anergy is present. The prognosis for cure in these cases is poor.

Skin testing should precede desensitization, and the dilution of vaccine to be used is determined roughly by the size of the wheal produced when the patient is skin-tested with the full-strength vaccine. For example, if the skin test material (blastomycin) produced an erythematous zone about 2 cm in diameter, the vaccine should be diluted 1:100; if the reaction is as large as 3 cm in diameter, a dilution of 1:1000 should be used.

One possible procedure of hyposensitization is to give three injections a week subcutaneously. Beginning with 0.1 ml, the dosage is increased by 0.1 ml at each injection until a total of 1 ml of the undiluted vaccine is reached. It is important to keep the dose below that capable of producing severe local or general reactions.

Hyposensitization has been recommended for blastomycosis, dermatomycoses, and candidiasis. Sometimes an autogenous vaccine made from the same strain infecting the patient has been used in place of a stock strain.

Immunity

Immunity Following Infection

Most of the fungi produce granulomatous diseases with histologic characteristics of tuberculosis. Suppuration, tuberculoid granuloma formation, and histiocytosis characterize the basic types of reactions that may occur in various combinations.

If an organism invades the skin and multiplies, a local inflammatory reaction occurs. As the adjacent lymphatic system becomes involved and specific antibodies are produced, the actual number of organisms in the indurated inflamed dermal lesions decreases. For this reason it is often difficult to observe organisms in the primary skin lesions infected with *Sporothrix* and *Histoplasma*. At this stage it is possible for the body to confine the organisms and destroy them, resulting in a spontaneous cure.

In sporotrichosis spontaneous recovery results in some relative immunity. A second inoculation in such an individual might produce a local lesion, as in tuberculosis, but the lymphatic spread characteristic of sporotrichosis would be prevented. A small superficial inoculation could evolve so slowly that enough immunity would develop to prevent the lymphatic spread, but this amount of immunity would not cure the primary lesion.

Spontaneous recovery without development of recognizable clinical symptoms occurs in a high percentage of individuals (80 to 90%) who have become infected with the causative organism in an endemic area. This has been especially true of coccidioidomycosis, histoplasmosis, and blastomycosis. Often it is only by the performance of a skin test that previous infection can be determined. If the disease does not disseminate during the primary infection, immunity develops and prevents dissemination even in the presence of open cavities in the lungs. Recovery appears to confer immunity to exogenous reinfection.

The immune response is affected by the route of administration, with the intranasal route less effective than the subcutaneous route in the case of *C. immitis*. Not unexpectedly, the amount of *C. neoformans*, with a predilection for the central nervous system, that is necessary to kill mice increases in the following order: intracerebrally, intravenously, and intraperitoneally.

Role of Circulating Antibody and Cell-Mediated Immunity

The role of circulating antibody in protection against fungal infections, in aiding recovery from disease, or in preventing relapse is difficult to assess. The transfer of serum antibodies from infected animals to normal animals has failed to protect them against subsequent challenge by the homologous fungus, such as *C. immitis*, *C. neoformans*, *H. capsulatum*, or *C. albicans*. This would suggest that such antibodies are not protective. However, the presence of antibodies may reflect activity of the infectious process.

Some fungi, notably *C. neoformans* and less markedly *B. dermatitidis*, are not strongly antigenic so that low levels of antibody are produced. Furthermore, circulating antibody may not be detectable early in the course of an acute illness and may be absent throughout the whole course of an overwhelming fulminating disease.

Treatment of generalized candidiasis with human serum containing agglutinins to *C. albicans* may be of help in neutralizing the excess antigenic polysaccharide fraction and has been used in conjunction with amphotericin B therapy.

On the other hand, most evidence suggests the role of a cellular immune mechanism in protection. Hypersensitivity and resistance have been closely linked in an individual's response to fungal infections. Most dermatophyte infections of the inflammatory type heal spontaneously. This correlates with a halt in the spread of infection, a spontaneous resolution of the lesion, an acquired immunity (partial) to reinoculation, and resistance to experimental infections with a small fungal inoculum. Patients with chronic dermatophytosis appear to have a relatively specific defect in delayed hypersensitivity to trichophytin, but their cell-mediated responses to other antigens may also be somewhat decreased as measured by skin tests or by stimulation of lymphocytes with a mitogen such as phytohemagglutinin.

Positive skin tests to some of the systemic diseases have been followed for their prognostic role, indicating a correlation between recovery and the development and persistence of delayed hypersensitivity (Chapter 11). Hypersensitivity responses such as erythema nodosum in coccidioidomycosis appear to be associated with a high degree of resistance to spread of the infection. Delayed hypersensitivity to coccidioidin can be passively transferred from man to man by the injection of leukocytes from a sensitive individual. Patients with nonlymphopenic hypogammaglobulinemia but a normal cellular response appear to have an adequate immunologic defense against pulmonary histoplasmosis, despite this severe deficit in humoral immunity.

An evaluation of cell-mediated immune responses in patients with deep mycotic diseases indicates a spectrum of clinical and immunologic manifestations reflecting host resistance to the parasite. Variations will be found between patients with almost normal cell-mediated immunity (Chapter 11) and others unresponsive *in vivo* to the specific antigen and showing a depression in the majority of the T cell responses.

A battery of skin tests and *in vitro* tests of patient cells and serum may need to be carried out to determine the location of the defect. Chronic mucocutaneous candidiasis contains the best-documented examples of humoral and cellular defects that may affect expression of fungous disease. Some of this information may be relevant to other fungous diseases. A better understanding of immune abnormalities is required before optimal treatment can be given to an individual patient.

Defects in Cell-Mediated Immunity

Table 14-2 outlines several possible reasons for defective resistance to candidiasis. A defect in the generation or differentiation of lymphoid stem cells would produce combined immunologic deficiency syndromes. Children born with no thymus have a defect in delayed hypersensitivity (Chapter 17) that apparently results from failure to differentiate antigen-reactive cells. More detailed consideration of some lesser abnormalities in T cell function

Table 14-2

MECHANISMS OF DEFECTIVE RESISTANCE TO CANDIDIASIS

I. Defects in cell-mediated immunity
   1. Primary defects in the thymus
   2. T cell abnormalities
   3. Defective phagocytic function
   4. Dysfunction of T-B cell interactions

II. Defects in humoral immunity
   1. Deficiency of serum antibodies to *C. albicans*
   2. Deficient secretory IgA
   3. Deficiency of complement components

III. Other factors
   1. Defective intraleukocyte killing
   2. Deficiency of candidacidal substances
   3. Presence of a factor(s) blocking sensitized lymphocytes
   4. Antibiotic therapy
   5. Drug therapy
   6. Deficiency of iron, vitamin A, or other agents
   7. Defective production of fatty acids

observed in different patients is presented in Table 14-3. In pattern I, lymphocytes can recognize antigen (*C. albicans*) and become activated to DNA synthesis. However, they do not produce active mediator, migration inhibitory factor (MIF), and for this reason probably cannot produce delayed hypersensitivity skin reactions *in vivo* since macrophages would not appear at the site of antigenic stimulus.

In pattern II, although lymphocytes were not stimulated *in vitro*, MIF was produced. However, no delayed hypersensitivity skin test occurred. If MIF is adequate and monocytes are immobilized, the latter may be defective and fail to eliminate the antigenic substance, resulting in a granuloma. In other immunologic patterns described in Table 14-3, macrophages may not be present or, if present, are effective in removing antigen so that the characteristic clinical manifestation is one of macular and scaling skin lesions.

In pattern III, a factor in serum probably combines specifically with *Candida* antigen and prevents activation of sensitized lymphocytes. Thus, there is no lymphocyte transformation and no production of MIF. The inhibitor is *Candida* specific, but there is no correlation with agglutinating or precipitating antibodies in the sera. Lymphocytes are capable of responding to other antigens *in vivo*, e.g., purified protein derivative (PPD) and dinitro-chlorobenzene (DNCB), and MIF can be produced by a mitogen, concana-valin A.

In pattern IV, no significant abnormalities are seen in cellular or humoral immunity. Several possible reasons for defective resistance are listed in Table 14-2, section III.

It is still not clear whether an immune defect always occurs prior to a fungal infection or whether in some cases the infection may actually cause the defect. Studies have been performed in patients who were in apparent good health and had no evidence of an earlier disease, cryptococcosis or coccidioidomycosis, for over one year. Lymphocytes from these patients had reduced T cell reactivity to the specific fungal antigen and less reactivity to other fungal antigens than the normal population. These findings may suggest an underlying defect, although one cannot rule out the possibility that the effects produced could persist for many months or years after an apparent cure. On the other hand, an impaired T cell function in patients with coccidioidomycosis can be reversible; thus, impairment of cell-mediated immunity may be associated with active disease. The degree of impairment of the cellular immune response in paracoccidioidomycosis is aggravated as the disease progresses. It is not known whether the basic defect is a true tolerant state to certain antigens of *P. brasiliensis* or an immune deviation affecting only some cell-mediated immune responses.

Some patients with chronic mucocutaneous candidiasis manifest a positive Schick test despite adequate immunization with diphtheria toxoid. Although these patients have IgM-neutralizing antibody to diphtheria toxin, they have no IgG-neutralizing antibody. It would appear that the T-B cell interaction fails to facilitate the IgM to IgG switch in these patients.

Table 14-3

IMMUNOLOGIC PATTERNS OF ALTERED T CELL FUNCTION IN WHICH CHRONIC MUCOCUTANEOUS CANDIDIASIS HAS APPEARED*

Immunologic Patterns	In vitro Reactions			In vivo Reactions			Cause of Defect
	Candida INHIBITORY SERUM FACTOR	ANTIGEN RECOGNITION BY LYMPHOCYTE TRANSFORMATION	PRODUCTION OF MEDIATOR MIF	DELAYED HYPERSENSITIVITY SKIN TESTS			
				Candida	PPD†	DNCB†	
I	−	+	−	−	−	−	Failure to attract macrophages due to lack of MIF
II	−	−	+	−	−	−	Failure of macrophages to remove *Candida*
III	+	−	−	−	+	+	Serum factor blocks *Candida*, preventing lymphocyte transformation and MIF release
IV	−	+	+	+	+	+	Other factors (see text)

* Adapted from Valdimarsson, H.; Higgs, J. M.; Wells, R. S.; Yamamura, M.; Hobbs, J. R.; and Holt, P. J. L.: Immune abnormalities associated with chronic mucocutaneous candidiasis. *Cell. Immunol.,* **6**: 348–61, 1973.
† MIF = macrophage migration inhibitory factor; PPD = purified protein derivative; DNCB = dinitrochlorobenzene.

Defects in Humoral Immunity

Patients with abnormalities of the B lymphocytes usually have repeated bacterial rather than fungous infections (Chapter 17). However, cases have been reported of patients with excess fungal infections. In laboratory animals, experiments indicate that both active immunization with the cell wall of *C. albicans* and passive immunization with immune serum favorably influenced the survival rate following challenge with this fungus. Therefore, humoral antibodies may play a significant role in helping to contain the infection or to lessen its severity.

Another interesting defect in humoral immunity has occurred in a patient with normal IgA synthetic capacity, but greatly diminished levels of IgA in the saliva and jejunal fluid, and failure to synthesize IgA locally at intestinal-mucosal sites. This patient also showed persistent gastrointestinal candidiasis. The basis of this disorder is thought to be a defect in the homing of IgA precursor cells to secretory sites or in the selective proliferation/differentiation of IgA cells at such sites. This finding could also be pertinent in cases of vaginal candidiasis where antibody response is mainly local and consists of secretory IgA.

The participation of complement in cutaneous lesions of chronic muco-cutaneous candidiasis has been detected by immunofluorescence. Deposits of C3 along the basement membranes suggest that intense inflammatory infiltrates occur as a consequence of complement activation (Chapter 8). Although the inflammatory infiltrates do not rid the hosts of the infecting organisms, they may prevent the organisms from invading more deeply into the skin. An alteration in complement activity has been demonstrated in three members of one family with chronic mucocutaneous candidiasis. Activity of total serum complement was decreased but no other consistent abnormality was seen. A deficiency in one or more complement components may alter the effectiveness of opsonization, phagocytosis, and killing of ingested organisms (Chapter 10).

Other Factors Important in Resistance

Although these factors are probably nonimmunologic in nature, their contribution to the total resistance of the host is sufficiently important that they should be mentioned briefly. A defect in the intraleukocyte killing of *C. albicans* has been closely linked to available intracellular myeloperoxidase (MPO) hydrogen peroxide, and a suitable halide (Chapter 17). Conditions with partial or complete lack of leukocyte candidacidal activity include hereditary MPO deficiency, chronic granulomatous diseases, MPO deficiency in association with refractory megaloblastic anemia, and the Chediak-Higashi syndrome. However, additional findings of unexplained candidacidal defects in leukocytes of patients suggest that our present knowledge of the leukocytic killing mechanism is still incomplete.

Normal human serum has an adverse effect on the development of colonies of *C. albicans*. Although the responsible factors are not fully characterized, they are not classic antibodies and may be unsaturated transferrin and sodium chloride. Another constituent, apparently a protein different from transferrin, termed the "candidacidal" substance, may also be important.

Plasma or serum factors appear to be responsible, at least in part, for impaired *in vitro* lymphocyte responses in chronic mucocutaneous candidiasis, histoplasmosis, paracoccidioidomycosis, several bacterial diseases, carcinoma, and Hodgkin's disease. The nature of these depressive factors is unknown.

The frequent and sometimes indiscriminate use of broad-spectrum antibiotics alters the microbiologic flora so that fungi, especially *Candida*, that normally would be contained by bacterial organisms can now grow and produce disease. The depression of cell-mediated and humoral immunity by various drugs, e.g., corticosteroids, will render ineffective some host mechanisms of resistance and allow proliferation of fungi.

A deficiency of iron, vitamin A, or other agents may allow the fungus to become invasive through the epithelial barrier. In some cases, a defective production of fatty acids may reduce fungicidal properties.

Finally, patients with certain other diseases or conditions, such as leukemia, diabetes mellitus, granulocytopenia, and leukopenia, may have a greater incidence of candidiasis. It is not known whether some common factor may be involved in expression of disease or reduction in host resistance.

Treatment directed only to the causative organism can be inadequate since a persisting immunologic deficiency will provide a suitable environment for an organism to grow again. Therefore, it is important to recognize a defect in cell-mediated immunity (Chapter 11) so that immunotherapy might be instituted.

Present evidence indicates that a combination of chemotherapy and immunotherapy may be advisable for the future treatment of patients with a defect in cellular immunity. Attempts at immunologic rehabilitation of patients with chronic mucocutaneous candidiasis include bone-marrow grafts, transplantation of the thymus, administration of transfer factor, and injection of circulating lymphocytes. Clinical improvement has occurred but usually lasted for only 6 to 12 months.

A patient with chronic mucocutaneous candidiasis and defective cellular immunity has been treated by transfusion with HLA identical leukocytes from a healthy brother. There was an improvement in the clinical condition and a return to normal of the immune response. He can now express delayed hypersensitivity to *Candida*, and lymphocytes can be stimulated *in vitro* to release MIF activity. Close attention to host and donor antigens is necessary to provide acceptance of donor cells and to prevent graft-vs.-host reactions (Chapter 23) in the recipient.

Dialyzable transfer factor from donors with positive skin tests to *Candida albicans* offers the advantage of not requiring living donor lymphocytes of an identical HLA type. Filtered extracts have the advantage of being free of hepatitis virus and transplantation antigens. Transfer factor may be effective for only a matter of months, but this would have value when anti-fungal drugs are not effective in recurrent or persistent infections.

In one case where transfer factor was not effective, a fetal thymus trans-plant was effective in restoring positive delayed-type skin tests. Eventually, both skin tests and *in vitro* tests became unreactive. However, transfer factor was then effective in inducing positive skin tests, suggesting that thymus-derived cells are required for acquisition of transfer factor-induced cellular immunity. The potential value of human bone marrow transplantation has been demonstrated in mice. Transplantation of normal bone marrow resulted in normal granulopoiesis and a reversal of increased susceptibility to challenge with intravenous *C. albicans*. Another advantage offered by the study of a patient's lymphocytes *in vitro* is that such techniques provide a means of monitoring the transfer of delayed hypersensitivity (Chapter 11) and thus avoiding the use of skin tests.

In studies of HLA-linked human immune-response genes, families with a high incidence of chronic cutaneous candidiasis showed an increased incidence of delayed cutaneous unresponsiveness, and positive associations were noted between HLA haplotypes and cutaneous hypersensitivity responses to a number of antigens (Chapter 22). Additional genetic studies of a group of patients with chronic oral candidiasis and no other significant clinical abnormality have led to the designation of the term "familiar chronic mucocutaneous candidiasis." It may be a genetically determined abnormality inherited as an autosomal recessive trait that results in susceptibility to *Candida* infection. A fundamental abnormality of iron metabolism may be associated with familial chronic mucocutaneous candidiasis.

Vaccines

Methods of Preparation and Nature of Antigens

Vaccines are prepared for use in skin testing (pages 234–36), for hypo-sensitization (pages 236–37), and in an attempt to prevent or treat infection (page 238). These can be prepared in the same manner, although different preparations might be preferred for some tests. At present the vaccines available are usually mixtures of antigens and represent either crude extracts or partially purified antigens. Vaccines are usually named according to the organism plus an "-in" ending, e.g., coccidioidin obtained from *Coccidioides immitis*. Vaccines may be autogenous, i.e., prepared from the same strain causing the disease, from stock strains, or purchased commer-cially. The latter are better standardized.

Antigens may be prepared from any fungus culture, but the most useful vaccines have come from *B. dermatitidis*, *P. brasiliensis*, *H. capsulatum*, *C.*

immitis, S. schenckii, C. albicans, and *C. neoformans.* When a particular fungus is dimorphic, the various antigens are frequently prepared from the tissue phase.

Vaccines are prepared by several methods. The mycelial growth (room temperature culture) may be ground with saline in a mortar with a pestle. After a uniform suspension is prepared, the organisms are killed by heating for a minimum of two hours in a water bath at 60° C. For preservation 0.5% phenol, 0.3% tricresol, or 1:10,000 thimerosal may be added. Vaccines prepared from the yeastlike form (37° C culture) of the systemic dimorphic fungi have greater specificity than those prepared from mycelium. Whole cells or ground yeast cells may be used. In addition, an extract may be prepared, such as the filtered-broth medium of the mycelium phase of *C. immitis.* Coccidioidin has also been prepared from the *in vitro* culture of spherules, the tissue phase of *C. immitis.* The latter preparation induces a stronger immunity, possibly due to heat-labile antigens either not present or present to a lesser extent in the mycelial preparation.

For serologic tests, whole or ground yeast cells have been used to detect antibodies to histoplasmosis, blastomycosis, paracoccidioidomycosis, sporotrichosis, or cryptococcosis. Ground mycelial phase has been used for detecting antibodies to coccidioidomycosis.

For skin testing, a purified polysaccharide fraction gives better results for sporotrichosis, candidiasis, and aspergillosis. Extracts containing greater amounts of protein have proved best for histoplasmosis, cryptococcosis, and nocardiosis.

From *Nocardia asteroides* a "sensitin" purified protein derivative (PPD) similar to human tuberculin PPD has been used for skin testing. Additional studies have been made with a nocardin active polypeptide (NAP-A) from *N. asteroides,* which produced positive and specific skin test reactions in guinea pigs to *N. asteroides.* Future testing may prove this to be of value in determining whether a patient is infected with tubercle bacilli or *Nocardia.*

From dermatophytes, a trichophytin or oidiomycin vaccine is available commercially, but the preparation of standardized antigens is difficult. Common antigens are shared by dermatophytes and saprophytes, and repeated stimulation with saprophytes may lead to the production of antibodies reacting with dermatophytes.

Immune Response

Vaccines have been investigated for their ability to produce immunity and thus protect an animal or man against infection, or they have been used to treat an active fungus disease by helping to produce an additional immune response that may be protective.

Coccidioidin prepared from the spherule phase of *C. immitis* has proven successful in preventing infection of mice and guinea pigs. An intramuscular injection in human volunteers has resulted in irregular dermal sensitivity and little or no serologic response. In histoplasmosis, a reinfection of endogenous origin is marked by chronicity and poor prognosis. This occurrence has suggested the desirability of developing a vaccine to be given to children in heavily endemic areas before they develop a primary infection.

Immunization with vaccines has also been used in the treatment of disease. Treatment of blastomycosis with potassium iodide is the most reliable method of therapy in both the cutaneous and the systemic forms of the disease. But patients with recent infection may have no hypersensitivity and no complement-fixing antibodies in the serum. In the absence of humoral immunity the administration of iodides may be followed by dissemination of the infection. Consequently, attempts have been made to induce antibodies by injecting undiluted vaccine. When either antibodies or a positive skin test can be demonstrated, iodide therapy can be initiated. This procedure has been recommended in the treatment of blastomycosis, sporotrichosis, and candidiasis. Cures of actinomycosis have been reported following vaccine therapy, but this may have been successful because of hyposensitization.

Bibliography

Catanzaro, A.; Spitler, L. E.; and Moser, K. M.: Cellular immune response in coccidioidomycosis. *Cell. Immunol.*, **15**:360–71, 1975.

Conant, N. F.; Smith, D. T.; Baker, R. D.; and Callaway, J. L.: *Manual of Clinical Mycology.* W. B. Saunders Co., Philadelphia, 1971.

Diamond, R. D., and Allison, A. C.: Nature of the effector cells responsible for antibody-dependent cell-mediated killing of *Cryptococcus neoformans. Infect. Immunol.*, **14**:716–20, 1976.

Emmons, C. W.; Binford, C. H.; and Utz, J. P.: *Medical Mycology*, 2nd ed. Lea & Febiger, Philadelphia, 1977.

Grappel, S. F.; Bishop, C. T.; and Blank, F.: Immunology of dermatophytes and dermatophytosis. *Bact. Rev.*, **38**:222–50, 1974.

Graybill, J. R., and Alford, R. H.: Cell-mediated immunity in cryptococcosis. *Cell. Immunol.*, **14**:12–21, 1974.

Kirkpatrick, C. H.; Ottenson, E. A.; Smith, T. K.; Wells, S. A.; and Burdick, J. F.: Reconstitution of defective cellular immunity with foetal thymus and dialysable transfer factor. Long-term studies in a patient with chronic mucocutaneous candidiasis. *Clin. Exp. Immunol.*, **23**:414–28, 1976.

Provost, T. T.; Garrettson, L. K.; Zeschke, R. H.; Rose, N. R.; and Tomasi, T. B., Jr.: Combined immune deficiency, autoantibody formation, and mucocutaneous candidiasis. *Clin. Immunol. Immunopathol.*, **1**:429–45, 1973.

Salit, I., and Hand, R.: Invasive fungal infection in the immunosuppressed host. *J. Clin. Pharmacol.*, **11**:267–76, 1975.

Sorenson, G. W., and Jones, H. E.: Immediate and delayed hypersensitivity in chronic dermatophytosis. *Arch. Dermatol.*, **112**:40–42, 1976.

Staples, P. J.; Boujar, J.; Douglas, R. G.; and Leddy, J. P.: Disseminated candidiasis in a previously healthy girl: implication of a leukocyte candidacidal defect. *Clin. Immunol. Immunopathol.*, **7**:157–67, 1977.

Valdimarsson, H.; Higgs, J. M.; Wells, R. S.; Yamamura, M.; Hobbs, J. R.; and Holt, P. J. L.: Immune abnormalities associated with chronic mucocutaneous candidiasis. *Cell. Immunol.*, **6**:348–61, 1973.

15

Immunology of Viral Diseases

ALMEN L. BARRON

Nature of Viruses

Long before the nature of viruses was understood, it was known that recovery from certain viral infections such as smallpox resulted in lasting immunity, and individuals did not contract the disease a second time following exposure. The foundation for the emergence of the two fields known today as immunology and virology was laid by the contributions of Edward Jenner. Evidence for the stimulus provided by his work will be found throughout this text. Thus, for the student of immunology, many of the basic concepts of this discipline are found in studies concerned with viral infection.

Definition and Mode of Reproduction

As more information is gained concerning viruses, a strict definition becomes increasingly difficult. Viruses are considered to be ultramicroscopic microorganisms that can reproduce themselves only within living susceptible cells. They are devoid of ribosomes, mitochondria, and other organelles found in cells. The basic structure of the virion (virus particle) is that of a core of nucleic acid surrounded by a protein coat called the capsid. The nucleic acid is of a single species, either RNA or DNA. Certain RNA viruses contain small amounts of DNA. For some viruses (e.g., poliovirus) naked nucleic acid alone is infectious. In most cases the nucleic acid contains all of the genetic information for complete replication of the virus. However, some viral genomes are deficient and require the presence of a second "helper" virus to provide the information required for synthesis of the complete virus. The capsid is composed of subunits and may be in the form of a tubular structure around the nucleic acid (helical symmetry) or an icosahedral shell (cubic symmetry). The capsid protects the nucleic acid core from the harmful effects of enzymes and environmental conditions. Some virions also possess an outer envelope that is acquired; this depends on their site of replication from modified host cell membrane material. The envelope is acquired, usually when the nucleic acid–containing capsid egresses from the outer cell membrane. In a few cases, virions contain enzymes required for some step in the process of viral replication. Viruses lack energy-synthesizing systems and the machinery necessary for the synthesis of proteins or other large molecules.

The steps involved in viral replication have been documented in biochemical detail for many viruses, and the major events may be divided somewhat simply into (1) adsorption, (2) penetration and uncoating, (3) synthesis of new viral proteins and nucleic acid, (4) assembly, and (5) release. The effect of viral replication on the host cell, the subcellular sites of viral synthesis, and the molecular events leading to the formation of new virions vary tremendously from one virus group to another. In Table 15-1 the major groups of animal viruses are shown, and their salient characteristics summarized. It is doubtful whether many new groups remain to be discovered. However, much information is still needed concerning the role of many viruses in human disease.

Pathogenesis and Cytopathology

To appreciate the events that occur during infection of the human host by a particular virus from the immunologic point of view, it is necessary to have some basic understanding of the various pathways of viral pathogenesis. A scheme is shown in Figure 15-1, which underscores some of the major principles to be considered. Respiratory tract infections caused by influenza, parainfluenza, and respiratory syncytial virus follow the simplified route of replication confined to the respiratory tract. Other viruses that also can cause respiratory disease, such as the adenoviruses and certain enteroviruses, may produce a more disseminated infection and appear in the alimentary tract as well. The viruses of the common diseases of childhood, mumps, measles, and chickenpox, follow the latter more complicated route.

Monocytes in peripheral blood and macrophages located in such tissues as the liver and spleen play an important role in response to viral infection. Mononuclear cells are frequently attracted to sites of viral infection. Thus,

Table 15-1
Major Groups of Animal Viruses*

Group	Virion			Nucleic Acid		Viruses in Group† Important to Man	
	SIZE‡	CAPSID SYMMETRY§	ENVELOPE	STRANDED-NESS‖	M.W. × 10⁶ (Daltons)	NAME	NO. SEROTYPES
DNA Viruses							
Adenovirus	70–90	C	–	D	23	Adenovirus	31
Herpesvirus	150	C	+	D	54–92	Epstein-Barr (EBV)	?
						Cytomegalovirus (CMV)	?
						Herpes simplex (HSV)	2 subtypes
						Varicella-zoster (V-Z)	1
Papovavirus	43–53	C	–	D	3–5	Human wart	?
Parvovirus (picodnavirus)	18–22	C		S	2		
Poxvirus	230 × 300	Complex	Complex coats	D	160	Variola Vaccinia	1
RNA Viruses							
Arenavirus	50–150	?	+	?	3.2	Lymphocytic choriomeningitis (LCM)	
Coronavirus	70–120	?	+	S	?	Coronavirus	3
Oncornavirus (leukovirus)	±100	?	+	S	10–13		
Myxovirus							
Orthomyxovirus	90–120	H	+	S	2–4	Influenza	3 subtypes
Paramyxovirus	150–300	H	+	S	4–8	Parainfluenza	4
						Measles	1
						Mumps	1
Metamyxovirus						Respiratory syncytial	4 subtypes
Picornavirus	20–30	C	–	S	2–2.8	Enterovirus	
						Poliovirus	3
						Echovirus	32
						Coxsackievirus	
						Group A	24
						Group B	6

Reovirus							
Reovirus	75–80	C	–	D	15		
Orbivirus#							
Rhabdovirus	70 × 175	H	+	S	3–4	Rabies	1
Togavirus (arbovirus)**	40–70	C	+	S	3	*Group A* (alphavirus)	
						Eastern equine encephalitis	1
						Western equine encephalitis	1
						Venezuelan equine encephalitis	1
	40–50	C	+	S	3	*Group B* (flavivirus)	
						Yellow fever	1
						Dengue fever	4
						St. Louis encephalitis	1
						Russian spring-summer; Powassan	1
						Other togaviruses	
	40–70	C	+	?	?	Rubella††	1
						California encephalitis	
Bunyamwera supergroup (arbovirus)**	90–100	?	+	S	?	Other groups Many	
Unclassified						Viral hepatitis type A (infectious hepatitis), HAV-hepatitis A virus	
						Viral hepatitis type B (serum hepatitis), HBV-hepatitis B virus	
						Spongiform encephalopathies: kuru, Creutzfeld-Jakob	

* Most data from Melnick, J. L.: Taxonomy of viruses, 1975, *Progr. Med. Virol.*, **19**:353–58, 1975. Courtesy of S. Karger AG, Basel.
† Selected for general medical importance and/or occurring in the U.S.
‡ Nanometer, diameter, or diameter × length.
§ C = cubic, H = helical.
‖ D = double, S = single.
Proposed name for viruses (bluetongue, etc.) that have double-stranded RNA but are distinguished from reoviruses by structural, antigenic, and biochemical differences. No human pathogens are as yet in the group.
** Classification of arboviruses is based on ecology.
†† Horzinek, M.; Maess, J.; and Laufs, R.: Studies on the substructure of togaviruses. *Arch. Gesamte Viruschforsch*, **33**:306–18, 1971.

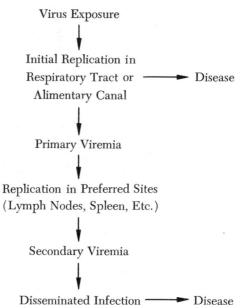

Figure 15-1.   Major pathways of pathogenesis in viral infections. (From Meyer, H. M., Jr.: The control of viral diseases. *J. Pediatr.*, **73**:653–75, 1968.)

mononuclear phagocytes are to be taken into account when considering the spread of viral diseases. Age is a factor in this regard. Macrophages from immature animals are much less efficient than those from adults. This function of mononuclear phagocytes in limiting virus spread occurs to a great extent as a result of interplay with sensitized lymphoyctes and antibodies. Viruses that are capable of growth in macrophages as well as host cells will have an advantage over those that cannot. The degree of destruction of monocytic cells will influence the outcome of the infection. Direct infection of polymorphonuclear leukocytes by influenza, mumps, or Coxsackieviruses has been shown.

In a simple way, viruses can spread in an extracellular form following maturation and release from infected host cells. Extracellular virus is more susceptible to antibody interaction than intracellular virus because of cell-antibody barrier. Certain viruses (e.g., herpesviruses) are efficiently transmitted from cell to cell. Perhaps overlooked is the fact that virus in the form of integrated genome (provirus) can be passed from parent to offspring at cell division.

Information gained by studies using cell cultures (tissue cultures) shows that the effects of different viruses on host cells are varied. Poliovirus is an example of a cytocidal virus that destroys the host cells. At the other end of the scale are those viruses, such as some myxoviruses, that cause infection without greatly affecting the architecture or activities of the cell. Viruses may affect cells by specific activity in cell division or may transform cells to malignant states.

The immunologist has more than a passing interest in the cytologic aspects of viral replication. For those viruses that mature by budding from the cell surface (e.g., paramyxoviruses), viral antigen and altered host membrane appear on the surface of the infected cell, which in turn affects the immunologic status of that cell. Such cells may stimulate the formation of humoral antibodies directed against the altered cell surface antigens. These antibodies, particularly in the presence of complement (Chapter 8), may cause cell damage. Cells may also be destroyed as a result of viral antigen-antibody reactions on their surfaces as mediated by T lymphocytes or even macrophages. Viral antigen-antibody complexes have also been shown experimentally to result in glomerulonephritis associated with immune complexes (LCM) (Chapter 19).

Viral Antigens

Immunochemical and Genetic Considerations

Even in early studies in immunology, the potency of viruses as antigens was recognized. The fact that the chemical composition of the capsid is protein and that viral antigens are uniquely distinct from antigens of the host cell contributes to their immunogenicity. In the infected host the virus replicates and thus a large amount of antigen needed for antibody response is synthesized. The transport of viral antigen to antibody-forming sites is also of significance for a favorable antibody response and is influenced by the natural pathogenesis of the virus, as outlined in Figure 15-1. A virus that remains superficially associated with the cells of the respiratory tract will have less accessibility to the immunologic apparatus than a virus that is disseminated in the host.

Viral infection results in the formation of antibodies directed against a variety of viral-associated antigens. In addition to antibodies to intact virions, the host will form antibodies to subunits of viral components and even to other macromolecules, such as enzymes, that are synthesized during viral replication. As is true for other infectious agents, many of these antibodies will not play a significant role in protective immunity but many serve as useful indicators of viral infection in diagnostic virology.

As noted in Table 15-1, many viruses exist in nature in the form of multiple serotypes, whereas others such as mumps, rabies, and measles viruses have only one. Antibodies capable of combining with a virus to render it noninfectious (neutralization, see pages 262–63) will be reactive for all isolates (strains) of a serotype in the world at all times.

The specificity of the antibodies produced against a given serotype is truly remarkable when one considers that the virions of different serotypes are of the same size, nucleic acid content, and general chemical constitution.

The surface of the virion, either capsid or envelope, is sufficiently different antigenically to stimulate the formation of antibodies that will interact with homologous virions only. The lesson taught by serotype specificity is well worth learning. If polioviruses existed in nature as 20 serotypes rather than three, it is highly unlikely that a successful vaccine against poliomyelitis could have been developed. Failure to encounter immunity in the case of the common cold may be explained, in part, by the fact that the rhinoviruses are composed of at least 100 serotypes.

Viruses as living entities have genetic characteristics that are entirely analogous to other forms of life, and indeed much of our knowledge of molecular genetics originates from studies with viruses. They have an ancestry and are capable of throwing off mutants in successive generations. Recombination and other genetic phenomena have been demonstrated. In considering immunity to virus infections, genetic stability regarding the antigenic composition of a virus becomes a problem of considerable concern. The most important culprit in manifesting genetic instability has been influenza virus, and over the years a continuous emergence of new antigenic subtypes, particularly of influenza A, has been observed. Genetic changes leading to the appearance of new antigens or other properties related to virulence of the virus are also of great importance in vaccine production (Chapter 26).

Viral Oncogenesis

Information has been available for many years that viruses are capable of tumor induction. Such viruses are called oncogenic and their tumorigenic effect on cells is termed transformation. Oncogenic viruses are found among both DNA and RNA viruses. DNA viruses that have been well studied in recent years are the papovaviruses (polyoma, SV_{40}) and the adenoviruses.

In this chapter, infection of a cell by a virus has been discussed only in terms of viral replication. Another major possibility of virus-cell interaction is encountered when viral replication does not occur, but rather the viral genome becomes associated with host genetic apparatus in the absence of synthesis of infectious virus. This phenomenon occurs during transformation of cells by DNA viruses. Transformed cells carry viral genome and continue to divide in the absence of any viral replication. However, the ability to produce infectious virus may still be retained and demonstrated many cell generations later by special techniques. Thus the stage is set for continued cell production of viral-associated antigens that are not found in the virus and continue to be synthesized in the absence of infectious virus.

Among the RNA viruses (oncornaviruses) are found the avian tumor viruses, murine leukemia, and mammary tumor virus of mice. A virus (Mason-Pfizer) has been isolated from a spontaneous mammary carcinoma in monkeys. Particles similar to these oncogenic viruses of lower animals have been observed in human milk and breast carcinoma.

The pattern of viral replication in the case of oncogenic RNA viruses is quite different. Biologically, these agents resemble myxoviruses and contain a lipoprotein envelope surrounding an internal protein capsid and viral RNA. Complete virus is formed by a budding process at the plasma membrane. The viral envelope, therefore, contains altered cells membrane as an integral component of the complete virion. RNA viruses are continuously synthesized during and after transformation with little damage to the infected cells, which are able to continue dividing. Oncornaviruses contain an RNA-directed DNA polymerase (reverse transcriptase). Complementary DNA is transcribed from viral RNA genome and the DNA integrates in the host cell genome.

As a result of transformation of cells by viruses, new antigens (neoantigens) have been demonstrated. To understand the synthesis of these new antigens, replication of the viruses involved should be considered. Biochemically, infection with the oncogenic DNA viruses results in the formation of many early proteins. These proteins do not require viral DNA synthesis for their formation nor are they generally found in the completed virions. These macromolecules are most likely enzymes required for viral synthesis. Late proteins appear that require viral DNA synthesis and are mainly structural antigens found in the intact virion.

Antigens formed in the process of transformation may be divided into those that appear intracellularly and those found on the surface of the cells. The T antigens are intracellular neoantigens located in the nucleus and have been well studied with the DNA oncogenic viruses. These antigens have been demonstrated by a variety of serologic procedures including immunofluorescence (Chapter 27), complement fixation (Chapter 8), and immunodiffusion (Chapter 6). The T antigen is virus specific and can usually be found in all tumors produced by a given virus. T antigen appears early in the replicative cycle and does not require viral DNA synthesis. T antigens of recently isolated human papovaviruses do apparently cross-react with T antigen from SV_{40} (monkey) virus.

An example of new antigens appearing on the surface of cells as a result of viral transformation is the tumor-specific transplantation antigen(s) (TSTA). This neoantigen is responsible for rejection of the tumor when it is transplanted to an appropriate recipient system (Chapter 24). TSTA (papovavirus) from cells of different species but formed by the same virus cross-react. However, the antigen appears to be virus specific. Other surface antigens have also been demonstrated on viral transformed cells by a variety of serologic procedures such as immunofluorescence and mixed agglutination. The relation of these antigens to TSTA is of great interest and the subject of many investigations.

Vaccination against malignant disease has been applied recently in protecting chickens against Marek's disease caused by an oncogenic herpesvirus.

Immunologic Resistance to Viral Infection

Humoral Immunity

Viruses, like other infectious agents, are essentially recognized as foreign invaders by the host. The immune response involves the interplay of T lymphocytes, B lymphocytes, and macrophages (Figure 15-2). These interactions result in manifestations of the humoral immune system (antibody) and/or cell-mediated immunity system. Analysis of the response involves consideration of two elements; recovery of the host from the current viral infection and subsequent immunity to further attacks by the same virus.

The antibody response observed in viral infections follows the same sequence of events as observed with any other antigenic stimulus. IgM antibodies are usually detected early in infection followed by IgG. Anamnestic response is mainly of the IgG class but IgM antibodies are also found. The role of IgG antibodies in providing lasting immunity is reasonably established.

Experimentally, antibodies play an important role in recovery from enterovirus infections. Thus, immunosuppression of adult mice can lead to fatal infections with Coxsackieviruses. Viremia can be terminated by passive administration of antibodies with subsequent protection of the animals. A similar role in recovery has been shown for infections with togaviruses (arboviruses). Virus-antibody complexes interacting with lymphocytes may play a role in recovery through the induction of lymphokines.

The importance of secretory IgA antibodies in secretions is now well accepted. These immunoglobulins are found in secretions generally as a result of local synthesis by lymphoid tissue mainly in the respiratory and intestinal tracts. Secretory IgA antibodies play a significant role in the protective layer of the mucosa, and their ability to complex is an advantage in this regard. IgA antibodies in respiratory secretions against important respiratory viruses such as influenza, parainfluenza, and adenoviruses have been readily found. In addition, their role in influencing the spread of infection by enteroviruses (polioviruses) has been demonstrated in gastrointestinal secretions.

Immunologists have been impressed by the long-term persistence of viral antibodies in certain diseases such as measles and yellow fever. Persistence of antibodies is explicable on the grounds that reexposure to virus results in abortive infection, in which the virus replicates but the infection does not progress to a stage where symptoms appear. The switchoff is apparently due to an anamnestic response resulting in rapid production of antibodies. The above explanation cannot be applied in all instances since there are examples in which individuals have been removed epidemiologically from any source of reinfection yet antibodies still persist for many years following the initial

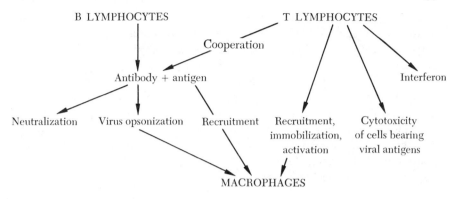

Figure 15-2. Interactions of T and B lymphocytes and macrophages in recovery from virus infections. (From Allison, A. C.: Interactions of T- and B-lymphocytes and macrophages in recovery from virus infection. *Proc. Roy. Soc. Med.*, **66**:1151–54, 1973.)

infection, e.g., yellow fever. Persistence of the virus in some form that causes a low-level stimulus for antibody formation is offered as a possible explanation for such situations. A small degree of turnover of viral synthesis over a long period of time is conceivable for such viruses as herpes simplex and adenoviruses.

The newborn child is passively protected against many viral infections prior to full maturation of his own immunologic system. Immunoglobulins of the IgG class are transported across the placenta and protect the baby against such diseases as measles, mumps, and chickenpox.

Cell-Mediated Immunity

Delayed hypersensitivity, a manifestation of the cellular immunity mechanism, is seen in a number of viral infections including measles, mumps, and smallpox. This form of hypersensitivity may be detected by a skin reaction following the intradermal injection of antigen, as in the classic tuberculin procedure.

As has been mentioned, the appearance of viral antigens on the surface of infected cells makes these cells the target of attack by alerted sensitized lymphocytes. This provides a mechanism for elimination of virus-infected cells. In addition, macrophages that actively destroy viruses may be called into play mediated by chemotactic substances elaborated by lymphocytes.

Sensitized lymphocytes responding to stimulation by appropriate antigens may produce interferon(s) (Chapter 11). Interferon(s) is a low-molecular-weight protein that is synthesized by cells as a result of stimulation by a wide variety of intracellular infectious agents and other substances, including endotoxins and synthetic polynucleotides. Once produced, it is effective in inhibiting replication of a number of different viruses and is, therefore, not virus specific. It is specific, however, for the species of cells in which it was produced and has little protective capacity for cells of other species. Interferon appears to play a major role in recovery from viral infections.

Cell-mediated immunity plays an important role in recovery from infection with herpesviruses (herpes simplex). Recovery from poxvirus infection is also highly influenced by cell-mediated immunity. It is quite difficult in this regard to delineate clearly between roles in resistance to reinfection and recovery from infection in the case of the herpesviruses because of the property of latency.

Immunopathology

Virus-antibody interactions do not always result in a favorable effect on the host and in certain instances can even result in damage. As has been mentioned, if a virus replicates by budding at the cell membrane, then antibodies directed against altered cell membrane may be destructive for cells. Also virus-antibody complexes circulating in the bloodstream may eventually localize and cause immune complex damage to organs such as the kidney (Chapter 19). Studies on lymphocytic choriomeningitis (LCM) (arenavirus) infections of mice have demonstrated these effects. In the context of these experiments the earliest explanation was based on immunologic tolerance (Chapter 22). Data have clearly shown that in the case of infection of newborn mice with LCM, an antibody response does indeed take place. In recent years, immune complexes have been associated with hepatitis B antigen (Australia antigen), immunoglobulins, and complement in periarteritis nodosa, and nephritic conditions accompanying hepatitis.

A second example where the presence of antibodies may be unfavorable is infection of infants with respiratory syncytial virus. Infants with maternal antibodies frequently develop a more severe infection than those without antibodies. The underlying mechanisms in this situation have not been completely uncovered.

The work with ectromelia (poxvirus) virus in mice shows that the lesion produced during infection is, in part, due to a delayed hypersensitivity reaction. Also, following a number of viral infections such as measles and chickenpox, patients may develop severe central nervous system manifestations described as postinfectious encephalitis. At this time infectious virus is not recovered and the histopathology resembles that observed in experimental allergic encephalitis.

Other evidence for the unfavorable role of delayed hypersensitivity is seen from data obtained by experimentation with vaccines. Immunization of children with killed measles vaccine resulted in the establishment of a delayed hypersensitivity state in addition to the formation of circulating antibodies. When these children later contracted natural measles, instead of being immune they developed a bizarre and serious form of measles.

Persistent Viral Infections

As a rule, viral infections are not associated with continuous shedding of virus over long periods of time. In respiratory infections, viruses may disappear from respiratory secretions two to three days following onset of illness. Enteroviruses are shed in the feces for several weeks following infection. When the recovery mechanisms function, viral replication is turned off. Instances of prolonged shedding even after a number of years are found in congenital infections with rubella and cytomegalovirus. Persistent infection occurs despite the presence of viral antibodies.

In addition to prolonged shedding, recurrent disease in the presence of viral antibodies is also recognized. The best examples of this phenomenon are the cold sores or fever blisters associated with infection caused by herpes simplex virus. After primary infection, the virus becomes latent, to be activated at a later time. The patient is subjected to a series of exacerbations with the formation of lesions on the lips, nose, or genitalia and periods of quiescence with no clinical manifestations.

A complete explanation for recurrent disease is not yet available. It has been proposed that cell-mediated immunity is the controlling system (Chapter 11). Alteration of T cell response would permit exacerbation of disease. Individuals suffering from recurrent disease may indeed shed infectious virus intermittently during periods of quiescence. A nonneutralizable fraction in a viral population is known in a number of viral systems. Such viral particles would be unaffected by the presence of antibodies. In addition, antibodies may vary in their capacity to neutralize viruses, and virions coated with relatively weak neutralizing antibodies may be protected from more active antibodies.

A rare disease of childhood, subacute sclerosing panencephalitis (SSPE), was linked to a persistent infection with measles virus. These studies and others mainly associated with the spongiform encephalopathies of man (kuru, Creutzfeldt-Jakob disease) as well as rather bizarre diseases of animals (scrapie, maedi-visna), have opened new vistas in virology, relating to persistent viral infections and diseases caused by the so-called "slow" viruses. In the case of scrapie and kuru, for example, immunologic responses have not been detected. On the other hand, in latent herpes simplex as well as in SSPE, humoral and cell-mediated immune responses occur.

Immunologic Defects and Immunosuppression

Frequently, useful information concerning the function of a system is obtained when nature provides the opportunity to study its impairment. Individuals with immunologic deficiency diseases provide such an opportunity when they encounter viral infections (Chapter 17).

Defects in humoral antibody have been documented for a number of disorders. In infantile sex-linked hypogammaglobulinemia (Bruton type) only humoral antibody formation is defective. The cellular immune system is apparently normal. Patients with this condition usually recover from viral infections such as herpes simplex or chickenpox without difficulty. They may also be successfully vaccinated against smallpox. Children with severe hypo-gammaglobulinemia, however, were more prone to paralytic poliomyelitis than normal children after exposure to oral vaccination. Failure to manage respiratory tract infection in patients with ataxia telangiectasia is explainable on the grounds that a deficiency in production of secretory IgA is found. Limitation of the spread of infection is impaired in patients with severe combined immunodeficiency disease (Swiss type) where cellular as well as humoral immunity is impaired. Common viral infections, such as herpes simplex and measles, are a serious threat to persons with this disorder. A high degree of susceptibility to infection with herpesviruses (herpes simplex, cytomegalovirus) has been noted in children with Wiskott-Aldrich syndrome; it involves a defect in cell-mediated immunity associated with T cells but not macrophages. As would be expected, vaccination against smallpox may have disastrous results. In cases of progressive vaccinia or vaccinia gangrenosa, which are progressive diseases following vaccination against smallpox, normal γ globulin levels are often present but delayed hypersensitivity is apparently not normal. In measles, a defect in delayed hypersensitivity may lead to giant cell pneumonia.

An alteration in response to viral infections in individuals whose immuno-logic apparatus is compromised by various forms of therapy is frequently seen. Individuals receiving immunosuppressive drugs commonly used in the treatment of certain malignant disorders may suffer severe viral infections that are normally controlled. Patients receiving immunosuppression therapy for renal transplantation are prone to viral infection, particularly cyto-megalovirus. In general, immunosuppression by chemotherapy or in conditions such as Hodgkin's disease, in which alteration of cell-mediated immunity results, leads to serious consequences involving herpesviruses (herpes simplex, varicella, cytomegalovirus).

In experimental infection of mice with vaccinia virus, pretreatment with antilymphocyte serum (ALS) was found to enhance the infectious process if the virus was administered peripherally. In contrast, treatment with ALS or even neonatal thymectomy did not alter the response to enteroviruses or arboviruses in mice. Also, ALS treatment was not observed to have any broad experimental effect when mice were inoculated intranasally with influenza virus. ALS-treated mice produced normal levels of humoral anti-bodies and interferon.

Immunosuppression with cyclophosphamide resulted in a lethal effect in adult mice normally refractive to infection with Coxsackieviruses. In LCM a pathologic role has been assigned to the immune response with regard to infection of adult mice. Administration of cyclophosphamide to adult mice infected with LCM virus resulted in a persistent nonpathologic infection. Often, immunosuppression with chemical agents does not lead to a clear-cut effect on humoral antibody or cell-mediated immune responses.

Viral Infection of Immunologic Apparatus

Viral infections generally lead to immunosuppression although stimulation has been documented. It is reasonable to predict that cells of the immunologic apparatus are themselves directly infected or altered by viruses. Certain oncornaviruses will apparently infect cells derived from either T or B lymphocytes. It is known that Epstein-Barr virus (EBV), a herpesvirus of man, can transform B lymphocytes. The herpesvirus causing Marek's disease in chickens, on the other hand, selectively replicates in T lymphocytes. A permanent depression of cell-mediated immunity has been documented following infection of mice with a herpesvirus called the "thymus agent," which causes destruction of mouse thymocytes.

The importance of macrophages in the immune response has already been discussed (Chapter 10). Viral infection of macrophages has been known for some time. Poliovirus is selectively infective for macrophages. LCM virus will infect mouse peritoneal macrophages. In the case of murine hepatitis virus (coronavirus), infection of macrophages is specific for genetically susceptible mice.

Inoculation of mice with Friend leukemia virus (oncornavirus) resulted in depression of antibody response to a variety of antigens including sheep red blood cells and Salmonella lipopolysaccharides. On the other hand, Venezuelan equine encephalitis virus produced an enhancement of antibody production to human and bovine γ globulins. Along these same lines, anaphylaxis (Chapter 18), which is mediated by humoral antibody, may also be inhibited as a result of viral infection.

Analysis of depression of antibody response by viruses has shown that IgM response is relatively unaffected and the major impact seems to be on primary IgG response. The effect may be on T helper cells required for IgG production, but this may not be the whole story.

Viral infection may directly affect cellular immunity (Chapter 17). Inhibition or delay in graft rejection is known (Chapter 23). In measles, infection often leads to a general depression of delayed hypersensitivity. The virus is capable of replication in cells of the cellular immunity system. In chickenpox, and even with poliovirus, depression of delayed hypersensitivity may also occur. Depression of blast transformation in vitro may be considered a general viral phenomenon since it occurs with a wide range of viruses.

Diagnostic Procedures

The purpose of this section is to bring to the reader's attention the major serologic procedures used in clinical virology as well as virologic research.

Many texts are available for details on technical aspects of the procedures employed, and these will not be discussed.

In the determination of viral antigen-antibody reactions, the serologic procedures applied throughout immunology are used. A few tests, such as neutralization and hemagglutination-inhibition, have some special virologic connotations, but their counterparts may be found in nonvirologic serology. Hyperimmune sera prepared in animals are used to study viral antigens, and the reader is reminded that in many instances such antigens are not found in the complete virions. Animal immune sera are particularly valuable in the identification of isolates in the clinical virology laboratory.

The detection of antibodies as a result of viral infection is of great importance and widely used for diagnosis and epidemiologic surveys. Most of these studies are performed on serum specimens, and the major classes of immunoglobulins involved are IgG and IgM. Although in some instances separation of the immunoglobulins is performed, no attempt is usually made to identify them. In serum specimens collected during the acute phase of illness, both IgM and IgG antibodies may be detected, whereas in the convalescent phase of illness, IgG is the main immunoglobulin class. Because of the complexities involved in the interpretation of the presence of antibodies in human sera, clinical virologists attempt to demonstrate some change, either rise or fall in antibody titer, during the period of the particular illness under investigation. Two specimens are routinely collected over a reasonable time interval, approximately two to three weeks, to allow detection of a change.

Generally, complement-fixing antibodies appear after neutralizing antibodies and hemagglutination-inhibiting antibodies and disappear from the serum more rapidly than either of these. This situation is frequently an aid in diagnosis. The variation in time of appearance of antibodies, as detected by these serologic methods, may be explained as being due to differences in sensitivity. Many virologists accept the premise that these antibodies are distinct and directed against different viral antigens. Antigens that are not present on the surface of the virion but are internal components or associated with other viral synthesis processes, would not elicit antibodies detected by neutralization or hemagglutination-inhibition but may stimulate complement-fixing antibodies.

Neutralization

Viral neutralization is performed by incubating an appropriate dose of virus with serum containing neutralizing antibodies. The mixture is then inoculated into a susceptible host, which may be a laboratory animal, chick embryo, or cell culture, depending on the virus. If the host remains uninfected, virus neutralization is presumed to have occurred. By this procedure an unknown virus can be identified, with the use of specific antiserum. Quantitation of antibodies in a serum specimen can also be determined for any given virus. At present, of the major immunoglobulin classes known (Chapter 4), neutralizing antibody activity has been demonstrated for IgM, IgG, and IgA. In certain instances, neutralization of virus infectivity by antibody requires complement (Chapter 8).

The mechanism of neutralization has been the subject of considerable research. Neutralization is a surface phenomenon; specific reaction occurs between intact infectious virions and their corresponding antibodies. Steric hindrance caused by the antigen-antibody mixture probably accounts for the failure of virus to adsorb to and penetrate into host cells. Virus-antibody complexes are not completely stable, and neither reagent is destroyed as a result of the interaction. In some instances, penetration of the neutralized complex has been shown, and in this situation, uncoating failure accounts for the absence of infection. Virus circulating in the bloodstream may also be coated with weak neutralizing antibodies that do not prevent infection but competitively inhibit interaction with strong neutralizing antibodies. All data collected imply that humoral antibody is effective only when the virus is extracellular. Intracellular virus appears to be protected from circulating antibody, which cannot penetrate the cell barrier and is thus incapable of neutralization. If a virus is capable of infection via the cell-to-cell route, spread of infection is possible in spite of the presence of neutralizing antibody in the bloodstream.

Hemagglutination Inhibition

Viruses that have the ability to agglutinate various species of erythrocytes can be specifically inhibited in this activity by antibody. Thus the detection of antibodies in a serum against such viruses as measles, influenza, and rubella is feasible by the *in vitro* hemagglutination-inhibition test. A major technical consideration in hemagglutination inhibition is the frequent presence in serum of nonantibody inhibitory substances capable of reacting with the virus to prevent hemagglutination. It is frequently necessary to pretreat the serum in order to remove these inhibitors.

Complement Fixation

The detection of antibodies using the classic complement-fixation test has been widely applied throughout virology. The antibodies detected by complement fixation may be directed against subvirion components, for example, or even other large molecules synthesized during the course of viral replication. Detection of antibodies by the complement-fixation test provides a useful means of determining infection with a given virus since the immunologic imprint is specific.

Other Procedures

Many other procedures are used in the study of the immunologic response to viral infections. Most techniques used have been designed for the detection of humoral antibodies or for the detection of viral antigen in infected cells and tissues. Techniques for measuring cell-mediated immunity have been refined and simplified in recent years so that they are finding increased use in the clinical laboratory.

Tests involving humoral antibody:

1. Immunofluorescence (direct, indirect)
2. Indirect hemagglutination
3. Immunodiffusion
4. Radioisotope precipitation
5. Radioimmunoassay
6. Counterimmunoelectrophoresis
7. Immunoelectron microscopy
8. Peroxidase-labeled staining

Tests involving cell-mediated immunity:

1. Delayed hypersensitivity skin test
2. Lymphocyte transformation
3. Macrophage migration inhibition
4. Lymphocyte-mediated cytotoxicity

Bibliography

Allison, A. C., and Virelizier, J. L.: Effects of viruses on immune responses. *Adv. Nephrol.*, 5:115–33, 1975.

Dick, G. (ed.): Host-virus reactions with special reference to persistent agents. *J. Clin. Pathol. (Suppl.)*, 25:1–158, 1972.

The immune response to infectious diseases. *Transplant. Rev.*, 19:3–254, 1974.

16

Immunology of Parasitic Diseases

Howard C. Goodman, Paul-Henri Lambert, and Jacques Mauel

Introduction

The impact of the parasitic and other tropical infections that continue to kill or destroy the quality of life of hundreds of millions of people in developing countries imposes a burden of such magnitude in many countries that it overwhelms attempts at health planning, perpetuates poverty and disease itself, and effectively stultifies efforts toward social and economic development. Malaria affects over two hundred million people in the world and kills one million children every year in Africa alone. Even more people are infected with other major parasitic diseases, such as schistosomiasis and filarial infections. Because of the chronicity of many parasitic diseases, with persisting parasites apparently unaffected by host immune responses, it has even been asked whether immunity to parasites existed. Immunologists, trained for the most part in countries where parasitic diseases were absent or well controlled, focused attention on problems like bacterial or viral infectious diseases or transplantation, autoimmune diseases, cancer, and the like. In the past decade, an increasing number of immunologists have taken up the study of immune responses in protozoan and metazoan models of both veterinary and human diseases. This number is still small compared to the magnitude of the public health and veterinary health problems posed by the parasitic diseases.

Immunology as a discipline makes contributions in three important areas of parasitic disease. Studies of *immunity* could lead to the development of vaccines or immunotherapy that does not now exist for human parasitic diseases. An irradiated larval vaccine is already commercially available for a nematode-caused cattle disease (*Dictyocaulus viviparus*), and attenuated vaccines are under study for two protozoan diseases of cattle (babesiosis and anaplasmosis). *Immunodiagnostic* tests, although widely used for clinical diagnosis and epidemiologic studies, are frequently nonspecific and utilize crude extracts of parasites.

Finally, *immunopathologic studies* are already yielding information about the pathogenesis of tissue damage in parasitic diseases, e.g., the renal lesion in the nephropathy associated with malaria and the liver granulomata of schistosomiasis. Few studies have been carried out to learn about possible immunopathogenetic mechanisms in the cardiac disease of American try-panosomiasis (Chagas' disease), the cardiac and central nervous system lesions of African trypanosomiasis, elephantiasis in filariasis, the eye lesions causing blindness in onchocerciasis, and so on. Even if future research discovers preventive vaccines or effective nontoxic drugs to prevent or treat these parasitic infections, millions already afflicted will develop progressive tissue lesions.

Immunity

Innate, or *natural, resistance* is responsible for the different susceptibility of different species to parasitic infections (Chapter 1).

Mechanisms of parasite survival in immune hosts are many and probably even more complex than those postulated for bacteria and viruses, which also have managed to develop means to enable long survival in immunologically competent hosts. The complicated life-cycles of parasites pose problems, and in malaria, for example, resistance to the erythrocytic stage of the parasite does not extend to the exoerythrocytic stages in man, chimpanzee, or monkey. Conversely, birds, rodents, or human beings successfully immunized against sporozoite challenge are fully susceptible to infection by erythrocytic stages of the parasite (Table 16-1).

Antigen variation is most evident in pathogenic African trypanosomes, which characteristically produce successive waves of parasitemia. The trypanosomes in each wave have a new antigenic coat and thereby are unaffected by the antibody formed in the previous wave. Less marked antigenic variation has also been described in certain malaria parasites. *Soluble circulating antigens* of parasites (exoantigens) have been detected in try-panosomiasis, malaria, and schistosomiasis, and their presence should be investigated in other parasitic diseases. Alone or in immune complexes,

Table 16-1
SOME MECHANISMS OF IMMUNE
EVASION*

Antigen variation
Soluble antigen (immune complexes)
   Blocking of antibody
   Blocking of K cells
   T or B cell tolerance
   Activation of suppressor T cells
   Immune deviation
Antigenic disguise
Intracellular location
   Within macrophages
      Nonfusion with lysosomes
      Resistance to lysosomal enzymes
   Within other cells and cysts
Production of "impedins"

---

* From Cohen, S., and Sadun, E. H. (eds.): *Immunology of Parasitic Infections.* Blackwell Scientific Publications, Ltd., Oxford; J. B. Lippincott Co., Philadelphia, 1976.

they may block immune effector mechanisms or interfere with the induction of immunity.

Antigenic disguise refers to the mechanism by which adult schistosomes are coated with host antigen and thereby evade the immune response that effectively eliminates challenge infections. *Intracellular localization* of plasmodia (red cells) and *Leishmania* and *Toxoplasma* (macrophages) shield them from circulating antibody, and from cell-mediated attack unless their antigens are expressed on the cell surface. The term "impedins" was used (Table 16-1) to cover a number of phenomena such as the generalized immunosuppressive effects noted in malaria and trypanosome infections or the specific depression of cell-mediated immunity in disseminated cutaneous leishmaniasis.

Acquired immunity to parasitic infections is rarely effective enough to completely eliminate the parasite and produce lifelong specific resistance to challenge. The best example of effective acquired immunity is in cutaneous leishmaniasis. In the USSR and the Middle East, vaccination to produce subsequent immunity is performed with an avirulent strain of *Leishmania tropica*, which produces the severe long-lasting (six to nine months) ulcer of the natural disease. This vaccination has the cosmetic advantage of developing only one lesion at the chosen site and results in a scar on the buttocks instead of a disfiguring facial scar.

Usually, immunity takes the form termed "premunition" by parasitologists: a *relative* resistance to a specific new challenge associated with persistence of the original infection. Infection of rhesus monkeys with *Schistosoma mansoni* stimulates immunity, which prevents reinfection with new cercariae, although the adult worms from the original infection remain alive and continue to produce viable eggs. This phenomenon has also been termed "concomitant immunity," after the finding in transplanted tumors that animals bearing one tumor are resistant to a second graft, although the first tumor grows progressively (Chapter 24).

Immune Effector Mechanisms

Parasites are eliminated by immune responses through the effector mechanisms, which are reviewed in Chapter 9. These involve specific humoral antibody, specifically sensitized T cells (cell-mediated immunity), and the interaction of these two mechanisms with other cells such as macrophages and mast cells. One such effector mechanism has emerged from recent studies in experimental and human schistosomiasis. In Nairobi, circulating human eosinophils have been clearly implicated as the effector cell in antibody-dependent, cell-mediated damage in an *in vitro* assay system employing ^{51}Cr-labeled schistosomula. These results are consistent with the ablation of immunity against schistosome reinfection in mice after the administration of antieosinophil serum. Reports of macrophage-mediated damage to schistosomula dependent on IgE antibodies, and adherence of mast cells to schistosomula through complement components generated by the alternative pathway, may indicate that a combination of effector mechanisms is required to eliminate effectively an organism as large and complex as a parasitic worm. Further studies will be needed to define the mechanisms relevant to protection against infection for each parasite.

Natural Resistance

Although man and animals harbor various microorganisms, they are naturally immune against most potential pathogens. This stage of resistance is generally called *innate* or *nonspecific immunity*. However, these expressions may lead to semantic confusion, and the term "natural resistance" is preferred. Not all mechanisms of natural resistance are innate, i.e., genetically determined, and they can indeed be very specific. In addition, the use of the term "immunity" might imply that these mechanisms bear a necessary relationship to those of acquired immunity discussed elsewhere (Chapter 1). By definition, natural resistance does *not* depend on the recall of immunologic mechanisms conferred by previous exposure to the microbe.

What are the characteristics that determine the capacity of a host to overcome a parasitic infection in the absence of an allergic response? Experimental data suggest two categories of mechanisms, which will be briefly discussed below: (1) an incompatibility between parasite requirements and the conditions found within a potential host, and (2) in hosts that offer a metabolic environment acceptable to parasites, the occurrence of preexisting humoral or cellular defense mechanisms perhaps related to those evoked during the course of an acquired immune response.

Host-Parasite Incompatibility

In certain cases, incompatibility between host and parasite appears to be genetically determined. For instance, mouse strains can be divided into three categories depending on the outcome of infection by *Leishmania donovani*: "acutely susceptible" strains, where infected animals tend to harbor high parasite loads for life; "acutely resistant" strains where infection fails to become established (a nonimmunologic phenomenon); and intermediate strains in which the parasite survives well at first but is rejected later by an immunologic process.

The factors that determine the fate of a parasite within tissues of a non-immune host are unknown in the majority of cases, but in the following examples, some of the factors have been identified with differing degrees of precision.

One of the best examples of incompatibility is illustrated in the resistance of West Africans to infection by *Plasmodium vivax*. The resistance appears to be linked to the absence of a proper erythrocyte receptor for the merozoite. There is good evidence that the receptor on the red cells of susceptible individuals is associated with the presence of the Duffy antigen (Fy^a or Fy^b), a blood group rarely found among West Africans (Chapter 20). Red cells on which the Duffy blood group is lacking (either constitutionally or after enzymatic removal) or has been blocked by specific antibody fail to be invaded by the relevant parasite *in vitro*. Similar mechanisms are suspected in many other host-parasite combinations.

Different species of malaria parasites show preferences for different populations of erythrocytes. *P. berghei* tends to invade reticulocytes rather than older cells, thus producing higher parasitemia and mortality in young animals, where the percentage of reticulocytes is higher. A similar preference may exist in the infection of man by *P. vivax* and *P. ovale*, where parasitemia rarely exceeds 1%, compared to infection of *P. falciparum*, which invades erythrocytes of all ages and consequently causes more severe infections. The basis of this discriminatory behavior is not known, but it can probably be explained by differences in the physiologic environment inside the cells. For instance, erythrocytes with high sodium and low potassium content, such as those found in dogs and cattle, do not appear to support the growth of malaria parasites. Similarly, the association between sickle-cell hemoglobin trait and decreased severity of malaria infections may find an explanation in the reduced survival (for reasons still unclear) of parasites in sickled erythrocytes.

Certain intestinal parasites have precise requirements with respect to oxygen tension, pH, and other physiologic parameters. Conditions unfavorable for parasite establishment or survival will be created by modifications of environmental factors, such as changes in bacterial flora.

Failure of parasites to survive or grow within host tissues may be due to the unavailability of an essential nutriment. This appears to be true of the effect of a milk diet on murine malaria, which has been traced to the low content of milk in p-aminobcnzoic acid, a growth factor for the parasites.

Humoral and Cellular Defense Mechanisms

Humoral Factors.   The toxicity of fresh serum from many animal species for various parasites is well documented. For instance, *Trypanosoma brucei* is sensitive to the lytic action of fresh human serum. Sera from man and many animals agglutinate and lyse to various degrees culture promastigotes of different *Leishmania* species. The nature of the lytic factor(s) is still unclear, but in certain cases at least, antibodies and complement appear to be involved. Although these antibodies can be called "natural" in that they do not result from previous exposure to the microorganism, they cannot be called "nonspecific" since they must have arisen from contact with cross-reacting antigens. For instance, toxicity of normal guinea pig serum for *Leishmania enriettii* has been traced to the occurrence of antibodies directed against a β-D-galactosyl determinant of the parasite membrane, an antigenic configuration commonly found in nature.

Cellular Factors.   Major nonspecific defense mechanisms exist at the cellular level. If parasites gain access into phagocytic cells (Chapter 10), they may be destroyed by intracellular digestive processes. Certain microorganisms can avoid lysis, using escape mechanisms such as prevention of lysosome-phagosome fusion or resistance to lysosomal enzymes. On the other hand, the efficacy of such natural defense mechanisms may be enhanced in a nonspecific way. Various biologic substances such as endotoxin, or concomitant infections with antigenically unrelated microorganisms, can raise considerably the microbicidal potential of macrophages, a phenomenon known as macrophage activation (Chapter 11).

Immunopathology of Parasitic Infections

Although immunologic defense mechanisms appear to be relatively ineffective in parasitic diseases, immune response to the host against parasite antigens may lead to a variety of inflammatory reactions that can play an important role in the pathologic manifestations of disease. This is particularly true when the infecting parasite itself is of low pathogenicity.

Obviously, the persistence of parasite in the host results in the persistence of foreign antigens. The development of the corresponding immune response will always trigger effector mechanisms in various degrees. When these reactions are limited in time and space, the main effect can be beneficial in favoring the elimination of the parasite. Adverse effects often predominate when more extensive inflammatory reactions lead to tissue lesions or generalized allergic manifestations. The respective role of cell-mediated or humoral effector mechanisms in the immunopathology of parasitic disease is generally difficult to define since both types of reactions coexist in most situations. In addition, a relative deficiency of the immune response at the afferent or efferent level may result from the effect of immunopathologic reactions such as the formation of immune complexes.

The pathologic expression of the immune response against parasites depends partly on the type of host response and partly on the nature of the parasite. For example, antibody-dependent reactions will be influenced on one hand by the nature (class, subclass, avidity) and the concentration of the antibodies produced against parasite antigens. On the other hand, the localization of the corresponding antigens on or into parasitic cells and the distribution of parasites or parasite products in host tissues will determine the site and the effects of the immune reaction. The following examples from human or experimental pathology demonstrate the involvement of immunopathologic mechanisms in parasitic diseases.

In African trypanosomiasis, some features of the disease are due to toxic effects directly resulting from the proliferation of the parasite. This is probably true for the acute hemolytic anemia occurring in animals infected with *Trypanosoma brucei*. In the absence of an appropriate immune response, hemolytic toxic factors can be demonstrated both in plasma from infected animals and in supernatants from isolated trypanosomes. However, other features of this disease in man and animals, such as myocardial lesions and possibly "sleeping sickness" encephalitis, may result from the development of antitrypanosome immune responses. Both humoral and cell-mediated immune responses appear to be involved in the immunopathology of trypanosomiasis. A few days after the infection of mice with *Trypanosoma brucei*, high parasitemia and relatively large amounts of trypanosome antigens are released into the circulation. Simultaneously, antibodies against trypanosome antigens are produced, and circulating immune complexes can be demonstrated (Chapter 19). These *circulating immune complexes* form and persist for several weeks, and, therefore, one should expect the development of some of the classic lesions associated with the formation of soluble immune complexes in the intravascular compartment. Indeed, immunofluorescence studies have shown the deposition of antigen-antibody complexes in the renal glomeruli of mice infected for six weeks with *T. brucei*. Other features of the disease are due to the fact that a large number of these trypanosomes also migrate into the extravascular compartment and infiltrate many tissues, particularly interstitial and perivascular areas in heart muscle and peripheral striated muscles. Soluble or particulate trypanosome antigens localized in such tissues react directly with corresponding antibodies or lymphocytes diffusing into extravascular spaces. The result is local formation of immune complexes and various cellular reactions leading to an extensive myocarditis and polymyositis with severe necrotizing inflammatory lesions. The role of the immune response in the pathogenesis of these lesions can be demonstrated by infection of genetically immunodeficient (athymic, "nude") mice, of mice rendered immunodeficient by irradiation, or of mice with an immature state of immune responsiveness (newborn mice). These mice develop an extremely high parasitemia and become anemic but do not develop significant inflammatory lesions as do mice with normal immune responses. After transfer of syngeneic spleen cells from normal mice into infected athymic nude mice, immune responsiveness is restored, and a full-blown inflammatory reaction appears at the site of localization of trypanosomes in tissues. After a similar transfer of serum containing antitrypanosome antibodies, the reconstitution of the inflammatory reactions is only partial. The lesions are probably due to the additive effect of both humoral and cell-mediated immunologic effector mechanisms. In some chronic cases, the infection may be complicated by an autoimmune reaction of the host. This may occur in American trypanosomiasis (Chagas' disease) in which antibodies reacting with heart antigens have been reported. The pathogenicity of such antibodies is still undefined.

In schistosomiasis, the long-term persistence of nonreplicating adult worm in the bloodstream and the production by female schistosomes of eggs that subsequently localize in tissues lead to most of the lesions associated with the disease. Experimental studies have shown that the development of these lesions requires an immune response of the host against worms or egg antigens. The extensive liver lesions characterizing the hepatosplenic form of the infection by *S. mansoni* are mostly due to the formation of granulomata around schistosome eggs released in portal veins and migrating into the liver. *Cell-mediated reactions* are involved in the formation of the granulomata but antibodies also react with antigens diffusing from the eggs and form immune complexes localizing in the periphery of the granuloma and within the surrounding polymorphonuclear leukocytes. In addition, soluble antigens are continually excreted by adult worms and form circulating immune complexes that may be responsible for the renal glomerular lesions occasionally complicating *S. mansoni* infections.

Helminth infections stimulate the production of large amounts of IgE antibodies. *Immediate hypersensitivity reactions* (Chapter 18), which have been extensively utilized for immunodiagnosis, are probably involved in the pathogenesis of secondary features of some helminthic infections. Symptoms of spasmodic bronchitis, bronchial asthma, and massive infiltration of the pulmonary parenchyma by leukocytes, mainly eosinophils, may be caused by the passage of *Ascaris lumbricoides* through the lungs. Similarly, immediate allergic reactions seem to be associated with repeated exposure to *Schistosoma mansoni* or to chronic filarial infections.

From the previous examples, it is obvious that a variety of immuno-pathologic mechanisms may be involved in diseases caused by a given parasite. It is likely that the predominance of some of the manifestations is partially dependent on host genetic factors, possibly related to the genetic control of the immune response. The balance between protective and adverse effects of the immune response varies considerably in individual cases. This appears clearly in chronic forms of human malaria due to an infection by *Plasmodium malariae*. The majority of patients will suppress the proliferation of parasites through various immunologic mechanisms and will only occasionally exhibit clinical manifestations directly associated with the presence of the parasite. In a minority of cases, mostly in children, *P. malariae* infections will produce severe renal disease characterized by deposition in renal glomeruli of *P. malariae* antigen-antibody complexes. Similar mechanisms may be responsible for the triggering of acute cerebral complications.

In several other parasitic diseases such as onchocerciasis and filariasis, immunopathology is suspected to play a major role in the development of the main features of the disease (e.g., blindness, elephantiasis). So far, only limited studies have been carried out to define the pathogenesis of these diseases.

Immunodiagnosis

Because immunodiagnostic tests (Chapter 26) have the potential for becoming the means for rapid and accurate diagnosis of parasitic infections, they are widely used. Antigens employed to date, however, are usually complex mixtures. In falciparum malaria alone, 30 distinct antigens have been detected in association with the asexual erythrocytic forms. Present tests have at least two drawbacks. If positive, they may not be specific enough, and if specific, they do not distinguish between present and past infections. Table 16-2 lists the immunodiagnostic tests most widely used. Immediate hypersensitivity skin tests are classically associated with helminthic infections. Enzyme-labeled antibody tests (ELISA) are coming into use because they combine great sensitivity with simplicity of performance, but the purification of antigens remains a major problem (Chapter 29). Finally, little research has been carried out to determine the potential value of immunologic techniques for detection of specific antigens or antigen-antibody complexes in the circulation, or of lower-molecular-weight antigens in urine, as a test for active parasitic infections.

Immunization Against Parasitic Diseases

Malaria

Four species of protozoa in the genus *Plasmodium* are responsible for human malaria. They are *P. malariae*, *P. vivax*, *P. falciparum*, and *P. ovale*.

Table 16-2
IMMUNODIAGNOSTIC TESTS FOR PRINCIPAL HUMAN PARASITIC DISEASES*†

Disease	Principal Manifestations	Intradermal Tests	Serologic Tests	Suggested Antigen Source for Serology
Protozoa				
Amebiasis	Diarrhea, colitis, abscesses of liver, lung, brain, ulceration of skin	None	CF, IHA, SAFA, IE, GD	Trophozoites in axenic media
Malaria	Chills, fever, anemia, CNS involvement	None	IHA, IFA, SAFA, CF	Whole organisms in blood. Sephadex G-200 fractionation
Leishmaniasis	Ulcerating lesions, skin, nose, mouth, pharynx, fever, anemia, leukopenia	DH	CF, IFA	Promastigotes from cultures
Trypanosomiasis (African)	Fever, anemia, CNS involvement	None	FA, CF, GD	Epimastigotes, trypomastigote from cultures or blood
Trypanosomiasis (American)	Fever, myocarditis, megacolon, megaesophagus	DH	CF, IHA, IFA	Epimastigotes, trypomastigote from cultures or blood
Toxoplasmosis	Chorioretinitis, hydrocephalus, anemia, jaundice	DH	DT, IHA, CF, IFA	Organisms from peritoneal exudate
Helminths				
Trichinosis	Diarrhea, pain, chills, fever	IH	CF, FT, IHA, IFA, SAFA	Whole larvae, larval extract
Filariasis	Lymphadenopathy, fever, elephantiasis, blindness	IH	CF, IHA, IFA, SAFA	Adult extracts
Schistosomiasis	Diarrhea, liver disease, portal hypertension, hydroureter, hydronephrosis	IH	CF, FT, IFA, COP	Whole cercariae, cercarial adult extracts
Echinococcosis	Tumors (liver, lung, brain, bone), anaphylactic shock	IH	CF, FT, IHA, IE	Extracts from scolices

* From Cohen, S., and Sadun, E. H. (eds.): *Immunology of Parasitic Infections.* Blackwell Scientific Publications, Ltd., Oxford; J. B. Lippincott Co., Philadelphia, 1976.

† DH—delayed hypersensitivity; IH—immediate hypersensitivity; CF—complement fixation; IHA—indirect hemagglutination; IFA—indirect fluorescent antibody; SAFA—soluble antigen fluorescent antibody; GD—gel diffusion; DT—methylene blue dye test; FT—flocculation test; IE—immunoelectrophoresis, COP—circumoval precipitin.

274

The life-cycle of the human malaria parasite is completed in a primary and intermediate host—man and the *Anopheles* mosquito. A sporozoite from the salivary gland of an infected mosquito reaches the blood of an individual bitten by the infected mosquito. Within minutes, this sporozoite invades the parenchymal cells of the liver, becoming a cryptozoite. The cryptozoite lives within the liver cells for six to nine days and produces 15,000 to 40,000 microzoites. This is the exoerythrocytic stage of malaria infection. Rupture of the liver cell and release of the thousands of merozoites initiate the erythrocytic stage, although in *P. malariae*, *P. ovale*, and *P. vivax* infection, some of the merozoites reinfect liver cells, which result in subsequent erythrocytic cycles. This reinfection is responsible for relapse in these forms of malaria; the absence of reinfection explains why there are no relapses in *P. falciparum*.

Invasion of erythrocytes by merozoites results in the formation of the characteristic ring-shaped trophozoites seen within the red blood cell. The trophozoites develop into schizonts, which mature and segment into a number of merozoites. They rupture the red blood cell and release the merozoites with their metabolic products into the bloodstream. These released merozoites may then be phagocytized by the reticuloendothelial system or may reinfect other blood cells, where the erythrocytic cycle is repeated or where some of the merozoites now develop into male and female gametocytes. A mosquito that acquires the male and female gametocyte during a blood meal is the host for the sexual stage, which results in the production of sporozoites. The cycle is completed when the sporozoite is transferred from the mosquito to a human.

Malaria may be transmitted by blood transfusion, by a contaminated syringe, or, rarely, through the placenta. Transfusion-acquired infection is most common with *P. malariae* as the parasite. Transfusion infections are readily cured by chemotherapy, as only the erythrocytic cycle is involved.

The spleen plays a major role in natural immunity to infection. Splenectomy will activate latent infection and may allow infection by species of plasmodia to which an animal is naturally immune.

Acquision of resistance by populations in regions endemic for malaria is well described. In the first three months after birth, infants are relatively free of severe infection, presumably protected by maternal antibodies. Acute malaria is chiefly a disease of infancy and early childhood. From late childhood onward, parasitemia levels decline. A protective humoral response is present; immunoglobulin G prepared from West African adults had a beneficial effect in reducing parasitemia and fever when injected into children acutely ill with malaria. The role of cellular immunity is unknown, although in animal experiments, agents that stimulate macrophages protect mice against infection with *P. vinckei*.

A WHO Scientific Working Group on Immunology of Malaria, which met in July 1976, discussed the prospects for developing a vaccine for malaria. The Group examined recent evidence for different aspects of immunity to malaria, including immunity against merozoites, sporozoites, and other stages, and evidence of nonspecific immunity. They also noted recent successes in continuous *in vitro* cultivation of human malaria parasites that open up entirely new horizons for antigen production and research on vaccines. The Group believes that vaccination against malaria is feasible and that the time is now appropriate for a major international collaborative effort to be made to develop and test such vaccines.

Bibliography

Cohen, S., and Sadun, E. H. (eds.): *Immunology of Parasitic Infections.* Blackwell Scientific Publications, Ltd., Oxford; J. B. Lippincott Co., Philadelphia, 1976.

Developments in Malaria Immunology. World Health Organization Technical Report Series No. 579, 1975.

Immunology of Chagas' disease. *Bull. WHO,* **50**:459–72, 1974.

Immunology of schistosomiasis. *Bull. WHO,* **51**:553–95, 1974.

Immunopathology of nephritis in Africa. *Bull. WHO,* **46**:387–96, 1972.

Miller, L. H.; Pino, J. A.; and McKelvey, J. J., Jr. (eds.): *Immunity to Blood Parasites of Animals and Man.* Plenum Publishing Corp., New York, 1977.

17

Disorders of the Immune System

NOEL R. ROSE

Introduction

Because humans live in an environment heavily populated with micro-organisms, one of the first indications of a defect in immunologic function is repeated infection. Not only the frequency of infection, but the nature of infectious agents, is significant. The immunologic mechanisms for handling the pyogenic gram-positive cocci, such as staphylococci and streptococci, are mainly antibody mediated, whereas those immunologic mechanisms responsible for protection against certain intracellular parasites, such as tubercle bacilli and *Toxoplasma*, are mediated by mononuclear cells (Tables 17-1 and 17-2).

Immunologic Examination

The diagnosis of immunologic disorders starts with a careful history and physical examination, followed by appropriately selected laboratory tests. Contact with cytotoxic drugs or environmental toxicants that may affect one or more components of the immunologic system should receive special attention when taking an immunologic history.

Table 17-1

ANTIBODY-MEDIATED IMMUNE DEFICIENCY SYNDROME

Recurrent, severe infections
 Pneumonitis, meningitis, otitis, septicemia, pyoderma,
 eczema
Organisms
 Staphylococci, pneumococci, streptococci, meningo-
 cococci, *Pseudomonas, Haemophilus influenzae*

Table 17-2

CELL-MEDIATED IMMUNE DEFICIENCY SYNDROME

Generalized infections
 Rubeola, varicella, cytomegalovirus, candidiasis, histo-
 plasmosis, generalized tuberculosis, toxoplasmosis,
 Pneumocystis carinii
Smallpox vaccination leading to progressive vaccinia
Severe, generalized BCG infection

As part of the physical examination, attention should be given to the skin and mucous membranes, which are important portals of entry for microorganisms. Some lymphoid tissues can be estimated during the physical examination, especially the tonsils in younger individuals and the lymph nodes and spleen in adults if they are palpable.

Additional important tests that are part of a general immunologic examination include x-ray studies to attempt assessment of the thymus and adenoids in children. Occasionally, angiography of the lymph nodes also is attempted. Examinations of the blood, including quantitative and qualitative measurement of lymphocytes, monocytes, and polymorphonuclears, are essential. Histologic examination of bone marrow, tissue biopsies, or various body fluids sometimes provides evidence about an immunologic disorder.

Nonspecific Defense Mechanisms

Because they are not immediately dependent upon the ability of lymphocytes to recognize an antigen and undergo a proliferative response, the nonspecific defense mechanisms are the first line of defense against microbial invasion. Although good tests are not yet available for assessing macrophage function, there are several means by which the phagocytic capabilities of polymorphonuclear neutrophils can be determined (Chapter 10). Neutrophils from peripheral blood can be tested for responsiveness to chemotactic stimuli in special migration chambers. The engulfment of standardized particles such as starch granules, yeast cells, or latex particles can be measured quantitatively. The ability of the neutrophil to reduce an indicator dye such as nitroblue tetrazolium indicates its oxidative metabolism. Phagocytic ingestion is usually followed by a shift from normal glucose catabolism to the hexose monophosphate shunt. Glucose phosphate dehydrogenase is an essential enzyme in this sequence. Myeloperoxidase also acts with H_2O_2 generated during the shunt to generate antimicrobial activity. The mechanism of myeloperoxidase-H_2O_2 microbicidal activity is uncertain, but it requires iodine anions that link covalently with bacterial protein. Children who lack these oxidative enzymes due to an inborn error of metabolism are unable to contend with many common microorganisms.

In phagocytosis, the critical step is killing the ingested organism. A bactericidal assay of polymorphonuclear neutrophils can be performed by mixing the phagocytes with typical gram-negative bacteria, such as *Pseudomonas*, and gram-positive organisms, such as staphylococci, and determining the number of viable organisms at various times after ingestion by the phagocytes. A similar test can be carried out with microorganisms opsonized with antibody and complement.

Another important component of nonspecific immunity is the complement system. Several accurate tests for determining the intactness of this system are now available (Chapter 8). The simplest procedure is a hemolytic assay to measure total circulating levels of complement. Low levels may indicate that the patient is unable to synthesize one or more of the components essential for lysis. The missing components may be catabolized, excreted, or fixed *in vivo* by antigen-antibody combination. Thus, total hemolytic assay is sometimes useful for following patients clinically during the diseases produced by immune complexes (Chapter 19).

In addition to total hemolytic assay, each of the components of complement can be measured individually. Some clinical laboratories are able to measure complement components in a functional (hemolytic) test. These measurements are useful in distinguishing complement activation through the classic pathway of antigen-antibody interaction from alternative pathways of activation. Tests of individual complement components are also useful for detecting congenital absence of one of the components or one of the naturally occurring inhibitors of complement. Hereditary angioedema is an example of a disease due to the congenital absence of the inhibitor of an esterase generated from the first component of complement (C1). The diagnosis is dependent upon measurement of C2 and C4.

In some cases, the components of complement are present but unable to function in hemolysis. It is easier to measure individual complement components by immunochemical procedures that do not require hemolysis. Immunochemical detection of the more plentiful complement components, C3 and C4, can be performed by a simple radial diffusion precipitation test available in most clinical laboratories.

B Cell Functions

Disorders of the B lymphocytes can give rise to hypofunction or hyper-function. Hypofunction is associated with hypogammaglobulinemia or either congenital or acquired agammaglobulinemia (pages 290–97). Hyperfunction often denotes chronic antigenic stimulation and is sometimes associated with amyloid deposition. Malignancy of the B cell is recognized as plasmacytoma, multiple myeloma, or macroglobulinemia as well as B cell lymphomas and leukemias. Therefore, careful evaluation of the B lymphocyte system is an important portion of the immunologic examination (Table 17-3).

The special cell-surface properties of B lymphocytes determine their dis-tribution in the lymphatic system. They usually populate the cortex proper and the medullary areas of lymph nodes, as well as the splenic white pulp. The ability of organized lymphoid tissues such as the spleen and lymph nodes to develop germinal centers depends upon B lymphocytes. In addition, the presence of plasma cells in the bone marrow and gut lining is indicative of normal B cell function. These determinations can be made by bone marrow aspiration or appropriate biopsies, for example, of the rectal mucosa.

Table 17-3
EVALUATION OF THE B CELL FUNCTIONS

Serum electrophoresis and immunoelectrophoresis
Levels of individual immunoglobulins in serum and secretions
Biopsy of lymphoid tissues (plasma cells)
   Bone marrow
   Lymph node
   Rectal mucosa
Blood lymphocytes
   Count and morphology
   Ig-bearing cells
   EA rosettes
   EAC rosettes
   Transformation with PWM or LPS
Immunoglobulin catabolism
   Urinary and intestinal loss
Immune responses
   Schick test, Dick test
   Preexisting antibodies—isohemagglutinins, mumps, herpes, polio, streptolysin O, sheep
     erythrocytes
   Antibody response to active immunization—typhoid H and O, diphtheria and tetanus
     toxoid, *Haemophilus influenzae*, pneumococcus capsular polysaccharide
   Abnormal responses
     Autoantibodies
       Serum
       Biopsies
     Monoclonal protein

The number of B lymphocytes in the peripheral blood can be quantitated because of their unique surface markers. B lymphocytes bear antigenic determinants of immunoglobulins, which can be demonstrated by means of fluorescein-tagged antiglobulin sera raised in rabbit or goat. In addition, B lymphocytes contain special receptors for immunoglobulin Fc and for the third component (C3) of complement. These receptors can be detected by rosette formation, that is, the clustering of red blood cells coated with the appropriate reagent (Fc or C3) around the lymphocyte. Rosette formation not only permits the laboratory to enumerate B cells but may be used to separate them by differential centrifugation, if desired. B lymphocytes also have receptors for antigen, although in a blood film only a small number of lymphocytes will be able to combine with any particular antigen. Therefore, it is not feasible to quantitate B cells reactive with a particular antigenic determinant by direct counting.

For the functional evaluation of B cells, it is convenient to use nonspecific stimulators. Such reagents are available in the form of certain plant extracts. For example, a mitogen can be prepared from pokeweed (PWM) that, in the human, seems to stimulate mainly the B lymphocytes of peripheral blood. Bacterial lipopolysaccharides (LPS) also stimulate B cells, although T cells must also be present. Lymphocyte stimulation can be determined by direct observation of a lymphocyte culture after three or four days of growth or, more easily, by measuring uptake of a DNA precursor, such as tritiated thymidine. In a patient with normal numbers of B lymphocytes, their failure to undergo proliferative change indicates some sort of maturational arrest.

B lymphocytes are important because of their ability to differentiate into plasma cells and secrete immunoglobulins. The normal immunoglobulin level of serum and other fluids can be determined with great accuracy by using specific goat or rabbit antisera to individual immunoglobulin classes. The radial diffusion precipitation test is employed to measure levels of each of the three major immunoglobulin classes, IgG, IgM, and IgA (Chapter 4). Automated procedures are also available for these measurements. In addition, some specialized immunoglobulins can be measured. For example, a radioimmunoassay for IgE levels is useful in patients with allergic diseases (Chapter 18). IgA is the major immunoglobulin in secretions. Secreted IgA can be quantitated in saliva samples. IgD is usually not measured in serum but seems plentiful on the surface of many B lymphocytes where it can be measured by fluorescein-tagged specific antisera (Chapter 27).

Qualitative examination of immunoglobulins can be performed by immunochemical means as well as by ordinary zonal electrophoresis. Immunoelectrophoresis is especially useful, because it provides both electrophoretic and immunochemical criteria of immunoglobulin characterization. The test is particularly important in malignancy of the B cell system, where uncontrolled proliferation of a single clone of B cells gives rise to hypergammaglobulinemia.

In understanding an abnormally low immunoglobulin level, it is sometimes useful to know whether the defect is in protein biosynthesis, increased catabolic breakdown, or loss through the kidney, gut, or burned skin. It should not be overlooked that protein-losing syndromes, such as the nephrotic syndrome, severe burns, or exudative enteropathy, may result in lowered immunoglobulin levels, just as do acquired or congenital agammaglobulinemias. In addition, it should be recognized that synthesis of immunoglobulins is under feedback regulation, so that elevated levels of an abnormal immunoglobulin such as a myeloma protein may suppress production of other classes of normal immunoglobulins.

The "payoff" in studies of B cell function is determining the ability of the patient to synthesize antibodies. Preexisting natural antibodies should be found in the sera of all normal individuals. Blood group isoantibodies or Forssman antibodies (to sheep red blood cells) are almost always present, so that their absence indicates defective B cell function. Antibodies to common microorganisms or their toxins are also generally present. A Schick test is a convenient way of determining the presence of diphtheria antitoxins (Chapter 26). Finally, the ability of the patient to mount an antibody response following active immunization can be tested if there is preliminary laboratory evidence of failure of the B cell system. It is important to use nonliving antigens of proven safety. Both T cell–dependent and T cell–independent antigens are used in the complete assessment of B cell function. As T cell–independent antigens, pneumococcal polysaccharides and flagellin are commonly employed, whereas killed polio vaccine and tetanus toxoid are acceptable challenge antigens in the T-dependent category.

The recognition of abnormal antibodies is an important step in the diagnosis of immunologic disease. High levels of IgE antibodies accompany many allergic diseases, such as hay fever and extrinsic asthma. A radioimmunoassay for IgE antibodies (RAST) can be used in conjunction with skin tests in an effort to identify the causative antigen (Chapter 18). In the case of immune complex diseases (Chapter 19), deposits of immunoglobulin can be detected, sometimes with complement, at the site of the lesions, such as the renal glomeruli. A number of tests for autoantibodies can be performed with appropriate tissues or blood cells.

Hypergammaglobulinemias (Gammopathies)

Hypergammaglobulinemias can be classified into two groups (Table 17-4). In one group the serum pattern shows a narrow, sharp band in zonal electrophoresis due to the increase of homogeneous immunoglobulin molecules. These molecules are assumed to be secreted by a single malignant clone of B cells. Hence, diseases demonstrating this pattern have been termed

Table 17-4

CHARACTERISTICS OF MONOCLONAL AND POLYCLONAL GAMMOPATHIES

Determination	Monoclonal	Polyclonal
Serum electrophoresis	Tall, narrow peak ("spike")	Diffuse, broad-based increase
Immunoglobulin levels	Selective increase of one immunoglobulin class; other classes usually decreased	Increase in all immunoglobulin classes
Serum immunoelectrophoresis	Localized thickening or locally strongly curved immunoglobulin arcs	Smooth, symmetric arcs
	Reaction with κ or γ antisera, but not with both	Increase in both κ and λ light-chain arcs
Urine electrophoresis (concentrated sample)	Globulin "spike"	Negative or diffuse increase
Urine immunoelectrophoresis	Reaction with κ or λ antisera, not with both	Reaction with both κ and λ antisera

monoclonal gammopathies. The corresponding homogeneous immunoglobulins are called M components. The polyclonal gammopathies, on the other hand, are characterized by the increase of many molecular classes of immunoglobulins. This molecular heterogeneity produces a broad, diffuse γ globulin elevation seen in zonal electrophoresis.

Monoclonal Gammopathies

A sharp peak or "spike" is often found first by paper or cellulose acetate electrophoresis. The next step is usually to determine the total levels of IgA, IgM, and IgG. A selective increase of only one of these immunoglobulins high enough to account for the size of the peak greatly increases the suspicion of an M component. This is confirmed if only one type of light chain (either κ or λ) is demonstrated by immunoelectrophoresis. "Spikes" similar to those produced by M components can sometimes be produced by high levels of lipids, α_2 macroglobulin, haptoglobins, or hemoglobin.

Bence Jones proteins are free light chains. They appear in the urine as low-molecular-weight monomers or dimers (Chapter 3). Normal persons may excrete free light chains in small amounts in the urine (less than 100 mg/day); they are normally polyclonal, containing a mixture of both κ and λ types. Significant amounts of Bence Jones proteins can occasionally accumulate in the serum of patients with monoclonal gammopathies. They are difficult to demonstrate in serum unless antisera specific for free light chains are used.

A classification of the monoclonal gammopathies can be based on clinical and immunochemical criteria (Table 17-5). Most M components are associated with neoplasms of the plasmacytes, lymphocytes, or reticular cells.

Table 17-5
MONOCLONAL GAMMOPATHIES

A. Malignant monoclonal gammopathies
 Multiple myeloma (IgG, IgA, IgD, and IgE)
 Waldenström's macroglobulinemia (IgM)
 Solitary plasmacytoma
 Extramedullary plasmacytoma
 Nonsecretory myeloma
 Light (L) chain disease (Bence Jones myeloma)
 Heavy (H) chain diseases
  γ chain disease
  α chain disease
  μ chain disease
 Malignant lymphoma
 Chronic lymphocytic leukemia
B. Monoclonal gammopathies associated with other disorders
 Cancer
 Chronic infections
 Cold hemagglutinin syndrome
 Amyloidosis
  Primary
  Secondary
 Papular mucinosis
 Cerebroside lipidosis
 Pyoderma gangrenosum
C. Monoclonal gammopathies without coexisting disorders ("benign monoclonal gammopathy")

Myelomas and Plasmacytomas. The hallmarks of multiple myeloma are generalized skeletal lesions, plasma cell infiltration of the bone marrow, and synthesis of an M component. The same clinical picture may be seen irrespective of the immunochemical type of M component. Although multiple myeloma is a relatively common disease, solitary plasmacytoma, in which the plasma cell infiltration is restricted to only one bone, is exceptional. Soft tissue (extramedullary) plasmacytomas are rare.

An M component can be demonstrated in almost all clinically typical cases of myeloma and plasmacytoma by adequate immunochemical studies of both serum and urine. In some remaining cases, study of bone marrow specimens for cellular immunoglobulins by immunofluorescence has shown that an M component is present intracellularly but apparently is not secreted. In a few cases an M component is not seen.

The most frequent immunochemical class of myeloma is IgG (approximately 60%). IgA myelomas are less common (25%). IgD myelomas are much less frequent (1%), and, for unknown reasons, the protein almost always has λ-type light chains and rarely reaches high levels in serum. Even fewer cases of IgE myeloma have been described to date.

A Bence Jones protein can be the only M component secreted, and the disease has been called Bence Jones myeloma or light-chain disease. Hypo-gammaglobulinemia is frequent in these patients, but the clinical picture does not differ in other respects from myeloma associated with an M component in the serum. Bence Jones proteins are found in about 16% of all myelomas.

The frequency with which Bence Jones proteinuria is found depends on the method of detection. The original thermosolubility test depends upon the observation of Bence Jones that the urinary protein coagulates with moderate heating (60° C) and dissolves at higher temperatures (100° C). It has been replaced by more accurate electrophoresis and immunoelectrophoresis of concentrated urine. Routine screening methods for measuring proteinuria are not reliable in detecting Bence Jones protein. Even the sulfosalicylic acid or the concentrated nitric or hydrochloric acid ring tests give false negative results in about 5% of the cases with significant Bence Jones proteinuria.

Heavy-Chain Diseases. There are three types of heavy-chain disease, depending upon whether the abnormal protein is related to the heavy chain of IgG, IgA, or IgM. These diseases have quite different clinical pictures. Moreover, in each case the abnormal protein is not always the intact heavy chain but rather a fragment corresponding closely to the Fc portion of the molecule, frequently containing the "hinge" region.

γ CHAIN DISEASE. This malignant monoclonal gammopathy is characterized by the presence of partial heavy chains of IgG (γ chains) in serum and urine. The amino acid sequences differ in all the proteins studied but usually include most of the constant portion. The diagnosis is based on the clinical findings resembling malignant lymphoma and the demonstration of immunoglobulin fragment in the serum and urine. The abnormal proteins in serum and urine have a similar electrophoretic mobility and characteristically have a broader boundary than the usual monoclonal spike. This boundary suggests a polyclonal abnormality. However, the monoclonal nature of the protein is demonstrated by the fact that it belongs to a single subgroup of IgG. On immunoelectrophoretic analysis, these proteins react with anti-IgG antisera but not with anti-κ or anti-λ antisera.

α CHAIN DISEASE. The presence in serum and urine of a monoclonal immunoglobulin devoid of κ and λ chain activity and immunochemically related to the heavy chains of IgA (α chains) suggests α chain disease. It is the most common form of heavy-chain disease. The diagnosis is based on clinical features of progressive malabsorption. Lymph nodes adjoining the small intestine and the mesentery show a preponderantly plasmacytic infiltration. Most of the cases described are in individuals from the Mediterranean region.

Laboratory diagnosis depends on identification of the abnormal protein. The electrophoretic pattern of the serum may show a diffuse increase in the β region rather than a monoclonal spike. Only low levels of α chains are found in the urine. The abnormal protein reacts with anti-IgA (anti-α chain) antisera but not with anti-κ or anti-λ antisera.

μ Chain Disease. μ chain disease has been recognized in patients having a clinical syndrome similar to chronic lymphocytic leukemia. Some patients excrete κ Bence Jones proteins in large amounts. Osteolytic lesions are sometimes present. The laboratory diagnosis of μ chain disease is based on rapidly migrating band immunoelectrophoresis that is detected with anti-IgM antisera (anti-μ chains) but fails to react with anti-κ or anti-λ antisera.

Waldenström's Macroglobulinemia.   Macroglobulinemia is a malignant lymphoproliferative disorder associated with the secretion of a monoclonal 19 S IgM. Higher-molecular-weight polymers and sometimes 7 S monomers are present in serum in addition to the major 19 S component.

The clinical picture is similar to a lymphoma or chronic lymphocytic leukemia rather than to myeloma. Osteolytic lesions are rare. The bone marrow frequently shows large numbers of lymphocytes as well as increased numbers of plasma cells. Bence Jones proteinuria is frequently present.

The laboratory diagnosis is based on elevated IgM levels. The Sia water test (dilution in distilled water) is simple to perform but is positive in only about 50% of the cases. If available, the analytic ultracentrifuge can be used to document an increased 19 S peak and the presence of a (normally invisible) 27 S peak. A hyperviscosity syndrome is often encountered in patients with IgM levels of 2 gm or more. A significant drop in serum viscosity is produced by reduction with 0.1 M mercaptoethanol.

Monoclonal Gammopathies Associated with Other Disorders.   M components are frequent in patients with lymphoreticular cancer, such as lymphocytic leukemia, lymphosarcoma, and malignant lymphoma. M components in various nonlymphoreticular neoplasms have been reported but are not documented. An unusual monoclonal λ IgG has been found in cases of papular mucinosis. A monoclonal IgG has also been reported in cases of cerebroside lipidosis (Gaucher's disease), and a high incidence of monoclonal IgA has been described in pyoderma gangrenosum. Many other disorders have been described in association with an M component, but whether these are more than chance associations is difficult to ascertain.

Cold hemagglutinins appear after certain infections such as mycoplasmal pneumonia and infectious mononucleosis. It is a usually transient polyclonal IgM response. Occasionally, the cold hemagglutinin is a monoclonal IgM, almost invariably of the κ type, which reacts specifically with the red cell I antigen in the cold. Idiopathic chronic cold agglutinin disease has been considered a form of Waldenström's macroglubulinemia. However, most cases probably represent benign clonal proliferation.

Amyloidosis is a frequent complication of myeloma and macroglobulinemia. A major component of amyloid fibrils purified from human primary amyloid and the para-amyloid of myeloma as well as from tissues of mice with myeloma has been recently reported to be related to the variable region of light chains

(Chapter 4). However, not all types of amyloid have light-chain fragments as a major component, and the so-called secondary amyloid seen in chronic infections or rheumatoid disease may have a different chemical composition.

Monoclonal Gammopathies Without Coexisting Disorders. The term "benign monoclonal gammopathy" is used to describe the presence of M components in apparently healthy persons. This M component is being recognized with increasing frequency in about 1% of the population over 25 years and increases to 3% in those over 70 years of age.

The M proteins may be present for years without any overt disease. In some patients the abnormal protein disappears spontaneously. Occasionally, there is progression to a characteristic picture of myeloma or macroglobulinemia.

Other Serum Protein Abnormalities. *Cryoglobulins* precipitate at temperatures below 37° C. The amount and thermal properties of the cryoglobulins vary from patient to patient. Chances of producing symptoms increase when the temperature at which cryoprecipitation occurs is close to 37° C and when the cryoglobulin is present in high concentration. Symptoms due to cryoglobulinemia are extremely variable. They include cold sensitivity (e.g., Raynaud's phenomenon) and manifestations ranging from mild circulatory impairment to overt vascular occlusion.

Pyroglobulins are proteins that precipitate irreversibly when heated to 56° C. They resemble Bence Jones proteins, but the two can be distinguished by immunoelectrophoresis with antisera to light chains.

Polyclonal Gammopathies

Diffuse (polyclonal) hypergammaglobulinemia can be found in a variety of unrelated diseases, including many chronic bacterial and parasitic infections, liver disease, sarcoidosis, and connective tissue disorders. Usually all immunoglobulin classes are proportionally increased, but sometimes a single class is elevated. For instance, IgA can be markedly increased in Laennec's cirrhosis, in rheumatoid arthritis, or in chronic obstructive emphysema whereas IgG predominates in acute hepatitis, and IgM in biliary cirrhosis. In trypanosomiasis there may be a marked polyclonal increase of IgM. Although not pathognomonic, it is useful in screening tests (Chapter 16).

Intrauterine infections (syphilis, cytomegalovirus disease, toxoplasmosis, rubella) can induce fetal synthesis of antibodies of the IgM class. Quantitation of IgM levels in cord serum is, therefore, of value in detecting prenatal infections (Chapter 4). Specific tests (e.g., for rubella) can be adapted to distinguish the IgM antibodies produced by the infant from the IgG antibodies passively received from the mother.

T Cell Functions (Table 17-6)

T cells can be identified by their special localizing properties in organized lymphoid tissue. Biopsies of lymph nodes show that paracortical zones of the lymph nodes and periarteriolar sheaths of the spleen contain most of the T cells.

T cells (and B cells) can be quantitated in peripheral blood because of their special surface markers. T cells have the natural ability to form rosettes with sheep erythrocytes. These so-called E rosettes can be employed to count T cells. Unfortunately, it is somewhat difficult to demonstrate other unique antigenic determinants on human T cells. However, specific antisera have been produced in rabbits and goats which, after appropriate absorption, react only with T cells. Using fluorescent labeling (Chapter 27), these anti-T sera can be used for T cell enumeration.

Table 17-6
EVALUATION OF T CELL FUNCTIONS

Examination for thymus and adenoids by radiography
Biopsy of lymphoid tissues
   Lymph node (paracortical areas)
   Tonsils and adenoids
Blood lymphocytes
   Count and morphology
   E rosettes
   Heterologous anti-T
Delayed hypersensitivity
Skin tests (candidin, trichophytin, SK-SD, mumps)
   Induced hypersensitivity DNCB
in vitro correlates
   Lymphocyte blast transformation
      Mitogen induced (PHA, Con A)
      Antigen induced
   Macrophage migration inhibitory factor

For the functional assay of T cells, antigen-induced lymphoblast transformation is feasible, if a suitable antigen is known. For instance, the purified protein derivative of tuberculin (PPD) will raise tritiated thymidine uptake of peripheral T cell cultures if the patient is PPD sensitive. Because only a small number of T cells respond to any particular antigen, it is usually easier to measure T cell function by means of nonspecific mitogens. Several excellent T cell mitogens are available, although they differ in the subpopulation of T cells stimulated. There are two commonly used T cell stimulators; one is phytohemagglutinin (PHA) and the other is concanavalin A (Con A) (Chapter 11).

Although only a relatively small proportion of T cells respond to a particular foreign antigen, a rather large number respond to transplantation antigens of other humans (Chapter 22). This interesting observation can be used to provide another test for T cell blastogenesis. Peripheral lymphocytes of two humans (not identical twins) can be mixed in culture for five days and the amount of mutual stimulation determined by tritiated thymidine incorporation. It is possible to do this mixed lymphocyte reaction (MLR) (Chapter 22) as a one-way test by preventing proliferation of one of the partners with a mitotic inhibitor, such as mitomycin C. T cells that have been stimulated in mixed cultures are also cytotoxic for appropriate target cells. This cytotoxicity is determined by adding test cells labeled with radioactive chromium that is released into the medium if the target cells are attacked by stimulated T lymphocytes.

Following stimulation, T lymphocytes secrete pharmacologically active lymphokines (Chapter 11). Several of these lymphokines can be measured conveniently in the clinical laboratory. The best-known factor is called macrophage migration inhibitory factor (MIF) and interferes with the normal migration of macrophages. The MIF test is a valuable quantitative indicator of T cell function *in vitro*. The major difficulty in performing the assay is obtaining a suitable source of macrophages. Fortunately, the human lymphokine seems to be effective on guinea pig peritoneal macrophages so that an indirect MIF test can be performed by incubating patient lymphocytes with the test antigen, centrifuging, and mixing the supernatant with guinea pig macrophages. Sometimes laboratories prefer to use the patient's own blood leukocytes for measuring inhibition. The result of the test for leukocyte inhibitory factor (LIF) differs somewhat from the classical MIF. Tests for other lymphokines can be done in research laboratories but are not yet available on a regular basis.

Analogous to immunoglobulin synthesis in the study of B cell function is the ability of the patient to develop a delayed hypersensitivity response, which serves as an indicator of the integrity of his T cell system (Chapter 11). Like natural antibody, most patients have delayed dermal hypersensitivity to common antigens. It can best be determined by performing skin tests with a variety of microbial products, such as trichophytin, candidin, or the streptococcal products streptokinase and streptodornase (SK/SD) (Chapters 13 and 14). Mumps vaccine is useful in patients who have had mumps. Some pediatric clinics are using phytohemagglutinin as a skin test reagent when children are negative with the common microbial products.

If skin tests to common antigens are negative, deliberate sensitization can be performed to determine the integrity of the T cell system. Generally, it is done by applying a simple chemical to the skin in order to produce contact dermatitis. Dinitrochlorobenzene (DNCB) is widely used for this purpose (Chapter 14). It should be mentioned that this test has the slight possibility of producing nasty necrotic reactions and, therefore, should not be employed unless there is preliminary evidence of T cell deficiency.

Null or K Cells

At this time, quantitation of null cells is usually performed by subtraction; that is, the percentage of circulating T cells and B cells is added and subtracted from 100%. A test for killer or K cell function can be performed by using as a standard target the chicken erythrocytes labeled with chromium (Chapter 9). Antibody to the chicken erythrocytes plus human peripheral lymphocyte suspensions are mixed with the labeled red blood cells and the amount of chromium release determined.

Immunodeficiency Disorders

The common denominator of immunodeficiency disorders is heightened susceptibility to infection. Because of the integrated nature of the immunologic system, one rarely finds a lesion in one portion of the immunologic apparatus that does not have ramifications throughout the system. Nevertheless, it is often possible to identify the site of the primary defect and relate it to blocks of particular steps of immunologic maturation. Figure 17-1 depicts points in immunologic development where blocks might occur, leading to immunologic deficiency disorders. In addition to lesions in specific antibody-mediated immunity (Chapter 3) and cell-mediated immunity (Chapter 11), defects in complement (Chapter 8) or phagocytosis (Chapter 10) may be responsible for immunodeficiencies. Such deficiencies may be acquired or primary.

Acquired Immunodeficiencies

The acquired immunodeficiencies are usually secondary to another disease or to some form of treatment. Severe loss of protein through the gut, kidney, or skin results mainly in depletion of IgG. Lymphopenia may also result from prolonged gastrointestinal disease. Malignant tumors sometimes displace lymphoid tissue in bone marrow or lymph nodes and thereby impede development of cellular or humoral immunity. Hodgkin's disease and sarcoidosis are noteworthy in producing profound depressions in cellular immunity. Certain bacterial (Chapter 13), viral (Chapter 15), or fungal (Chapter 14) pathogens that affect lymphocytes also reduce cellular immunity. Measles exemplifies this phenomenon.

In everyday practice, the most common form of secondary immunodeficiency results from treatment with cytotoxic, antimetabolic, or antiinflammatory agents. Heightened susceptibility to infection is the major limitation in the use of immunosuppressant drugs in tissue transplantation (Chapter 22) or cancer chemotherapy (Chapter 24).

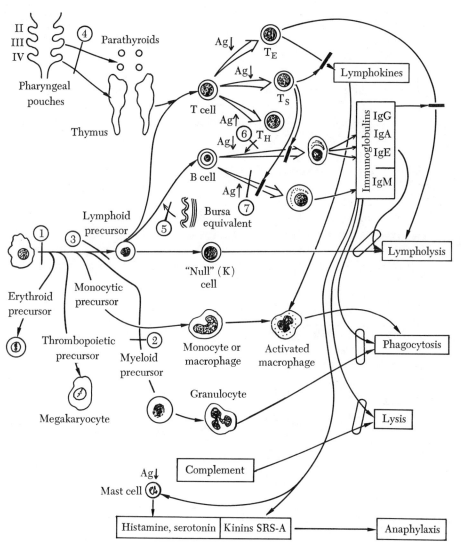

Figure 17-1. Schematic outline depicting points where interruption might occur in immunologic development (Chapter 1). *1*, Reticular dysgenesis; *2*, chronic granulomatous disease; *3*, severe combined immunodeficiency; *4*, thymic aplasia (DiGeorge); *5*, hypogammaglobulinemia (Bruton); *6*, common variable hypogammaglobulinemia; *7*, Wiskott-Aldrich syndrome; *8*, complement deficiency.

Primary Immunodeficiencies

Immunodeficiency diseases have been classified in five major categories by the World Health Organization (Table 17-7). Although few cases of primary immunodeficiency fall precisely into pigeonholes, X-linked hypogammaglobulinemia (Bruton's agammaglobulinemia), congenital thymic aplasia (DiGeorge syndrome), and severe combined immunodeficiency diseases serve as prototypes of lesions in humoral, cellular, and combined systems, respectively (Table 17-8). Although relatively rare as pure entities, they greatly aid in understanding the immunologic basis and clinical approach to this group of diseases.

X-Linked Hypogammaglobulinemia.   In 1952 Bruton described a male child with profound hypogammaglobulinemia, the first clinical description of an immunodeficiency disease. In most instances, the disease becomes evident at about five to six months of age when the maternal antibodies transferred to the infant have declined. Initial symptoms consist of repeated infections due to pyogenic bacteria, such as staphylococci, streptococci, pneumococci, and *Haemophilus influenzae*. At first, the patient may seem to

Table 17-7
Classification of Immunodeficiency Disorders

I. Antibody deficiencies
    X-linked hypogammaglobulinemia
    Selective deficiencies IgA
                IgM
                IgG subclasses
    Immunodeficiency (IgA) with ataxia-telangiectasia
    Common variable hypogammaglobulinemias
    Transient hypogammaglobulinemia of childhood
II. Cellular deficiencies
    Thymic aplasia (DiGeorge syndrome)
    Cellular immunodeficiency with normal B cells (Nézelof syndrome)
    Chronic mucocutaneous candidiasis
III. Combined deficiencies
    Immunodeficiency with hematopoietic aplasia (reticular dysgenesis)
    Severe combined immunodeficiency disease
        Autosomal recessive
        X linked
        ADA deficiency
    Immunodeficiency with thymoma
    Immunodeficiency with dysostosis
    Immunodeficiency with thrombocytopenia and eczema (Wiskcott-Aldrich syndrome)
IV. Phagocytic dysfunction
    Chronic granulomatous disease
    Glucose-6-phosphate dehydrogenase deficiency
    Myeloperoxidase deficiency
    Chediak-Higashi syndrome
V. Complement abnormalities

Table 17-8
Immunodeficiencies: Typical Disease Patterns

	Bruton's Disease (X-Linked Hypo-gammaglobulinemia)	DiGeorge Syndrome (Congenital Thymic Aplasia)	Swiss Agamma-globulinemia (Severe Combined Immunodeficiency Disease)
Onset	5-6 months	Birth	5-6 months
Agents of infection	Pyogenic bacteria	Viral, fungal, protozoan agents	Viral, fungal protozoan, bacterial agents
Immunoglobulin levels	Low	Normal or low	Low
Antibody response	Poor	Impaired to certain antigens	Impaired
B lymphocyte numbers	Low	Normal	Low
Germinal centers	Absent	Present	Absent
Plasma cells	Absent	Present	Absent
T lymphocyte numbers	Normal	Low	Low
Paracortical lymphocytes	Normal	Absent	Absent
Suggested primary	"Bursa equivalent"	Thymus	Stem cell
Proposed treatment	Repeated injections of γ globulin	Fetal thymus transplant	Transplant of histo-compatible bone marrow
Inheritance	Sex-linked recessive	Sporadic	Sex-linked recessive; autosomal recessive

respond well to antibiotic therapy; however, as the bouts of infection become more and more frequent, the child fails to thrive. The laboratory diagnosis is based on the deficiency of all five immunoglobulin classes. IgG is almost always less than 200 mg/100 ml and may be undetectable. Occasional patients have normal amounts of the other immunoglobulins. IgE is sometimes elevated. Levels of natural blood group antibodies are low, and the patients fail to respond to immunization with diphtheria or tetanus toxoid. Obviously, individuals suspected of having an immunodeficiency should not be given live vaccines. Intestinal biopsy shows few or no plasma cells in the lamina propria. Levels of circulating B lymphocytes are depressed but T lymphocytes are normal or even increased in number. Cell-mediated immunity (Chapter 11) is generally intact; delayed hypersensitivity reaction to the common allergens and induced contact responses to DNCB are demonstrable. Patients with hypogammaglobulinemia usually respond well to injections of pooled human gamma globulin given every three to four weeks.

The immunologic lesion in patients with Bruton's disease is found in the generation of B lymphocytes. Study of lymphoid tissue reveals a depletion of the thymic-independent areas, with absence of germinal center formation. A facsimile of hypogammaglobulinemia can be produced in chickens by neonatal removal of the bursa of Fabricius. Although the bursal equivalent in man has not yet been identified, many investigators equate it with gut-associated lymphoid tissue. The disease may be attributed to a failure of the bursa equivalent to function or to the absence of the B lymphocyte progenitor.

Selective Immunoglobulin Deficiencies.   In the common form of late onset IgG immunodeficiency, IgG is moderately depressed (less than 250 mg/100 ml) and IgM and IgA levels vary from depressed to elevated. Circulating B cells are usually normal in number. Isohemagglutinins are absent or present in low titers, and the patient produces little or no antibody following immunization with standard antigens. Cellular immunity is intact. The disease usually presents clinically as recurrent pyogenic infections of the respiratory tract or skin. In contrast to infantile hypogammaglobulinemia, patients may not become symptomatic until they are 15 to 35 years of age. Genetic studies have indicated several possible modes of inheritance, including X linked and autosomal recessive; usually no clear-cut genetic transmission can be demonstrated. Recent investigations by Waldmann and his colleagues have shown that abnormal suppressor T cells are present in the peripheral blood of many patients with common variable immunodeficiency. Autoimmune disease (Chapter 25) is commonly associated with the delayed-onset forms of IgG hypogammaglobulinemia, especially a rheumatoid arthritis–like disease and systemic lupus erythematosus. Patients are usually benefited by treatment with gamma globulin.

The most common immunodeficiency disease is selective IgA deficiency. Its incidence has been estimated at about 1:500 to 1:1000 in the general population. The usual presenting symptoms are recurrent bacterial or viral infections (Chapters 13 and 15) of the respiratory tract, indicating the importance of IgA in local immunity. IgA deficiencies frequently coexist with other disorders, especially ataxia-telangiectasia and malabsorption syndrome. The basis of these associations is unknown. Autoimmune diseases (Chapter 25), such as systemic lupus erythematosus and rheumatoid arthritis, are also unusually frequent in patients with IgA deficiency. Allergies (Chapter 18) are several times more common than in the general population. However, a large proportion of patients with selective IgA deficiencies are entirely asymptomatic. Sometimes this is attributed to the presence of secretory IgG or low-molecular-weight (7 S) IgM in secretions.

Patients with selective IgA deficiencies should not be treated with whole gamma globulin since they are capable of forming antibodies directed against IgA. Following infusion of whole plasma, some of these patients have developed anaphylactic reactions (Chapter 18). IgA-deficient plasma may be used, but it is usually more practical to employ aggressive treatment of the infections with antibiotics together with appropriate forms of treatment for coexisting diseases.

In addition to the gamma globulin disorders described above, selective deficiencies of IgM or individual subclasses of IgG have been described. These patients sometimes show heightened susceptibility to a broad range of infections (Chapters 13 through 16) and to autoimmune disease (Chapter 25). Not infrequently, infants and children develop transient hypogammaglobulinemia. One or more of the immunoglobulin classes may be lowered for periods up to several months. During these periods, the patients may be unresponsive to active immunization. It is important to distinguish this transient disease from congenital persistent hypogammaglobulinemia by peripheral lymphocyte counts and lymph node or intestinal biopsies. Patients with congenital hypogammaglobulinemia usually have low B cell levels and no plasma cells visible in the intestinal tract and peripheral lymph nodes.

Congenital Thymic Aplasia with Hypoparathyroidism (DiGeorge Syndrome). DiGeorge described a syndrome characterized by tetany appearing within the first 24 hours of life and abnormal facies marked by low-set ears and notched pinnae, nasal clefts, short philtrum, hypertelorism, and micrognathia. Congenital heart disease and sometimes early congestive heart failure were evident in some patients. Within a few days or weeks after birth, unusual susceptibility to infection appeared. Infections were most frequently fungal (e.g., *Candida albicans*) (Chapter 14), viral (e.g., hepatitis) (Chapter 15), or protozoan (e.g., *Pneumocystis carinii*). The initial manifestations of hypocalcemia are due to parathyroid abnormality. The thymus shadow is absent on chest roentgenogram. Evaluation of T cell immunity reveals a low lymphocyte count and, especially, a diminished number of T cells and poor response to PHA and Con A and to allogeneic cells. Lymphocytes are sparse in the paracortical areas of the lymph nodes. The majority of patients also have some impairment of humoral antibody production, especially of IgG antibody.

During the sixth to eighth weeks of intrauterine development, the thymus and parathyroid glands develop from evaginations of the third and fourth pharyngeal pouches. The glands migrate caudally during the twelfth week of gestation. At the same time, the right side of the aortic arch, the philtrum of the lip, and the outer ear differentiate. DiGeorge syndrome may result from interference with normal embryonic development at approximately 12 weeks of gestation.

Successful treatment of DiGeorge syndrome has been possible in a few cases by implantation of embryonic thymus in order to provide the microenvironment where stem cells can differentiate into T cells. Complete, long-lasting immunologic reconstitution was obtained with at least partial correction of the T cell defect. Surprisingly, most of the circulating T cells were of donor origin. These results challenge the assumption that the stem cells of patients with DiGeorge syndrome are normal, and that only the inductive effect of the thymus on maturation of T cells is deficient.

Other defects in T cell immunity from patients show partial arrest of thymic function. Spontaneous improvement of cell-mediated immunity occasionally occurs in patients with "partial" DiGeorge syndrome. The term "Nézelof's syndrome" was sometimes applied to cases with normal immunoglobulin, circulating B cell levels, and reduced cellular immunity, but without evidence of hypocalcemia, congenital heart disease, and abnormal facies.

Other Cellular Deficiencies. Chronic mucocutaneous candidiasis occurs in children of both sexes. Skin tests to *Candida albicans* may be negative, while other skin tests remain positive (Chapter 14). A similar unresponsiveness to *Candida* antigen may be observed in the *in vitro* stimulation of lymphocytes, or in the generation of migration inhibitory factor (Chapter 11). Antibody-mediated immunity is intact. In some patients, autoantibodies can be demonstrated to adrenal, parathyroid, or other endocrine glands.

Patients may present initially with multiple endocrinopathies or with chronic *Candida* infection of skin, nails, and mucous membranes (Chapter 14). Successful treatment of the infection sometimes leads to spontaneous restoration of immunologic functions, with positive skin tests or *in vitro* responses to *Candida albicans*. Some patients relapse after eradication of *Candida* infection; they may have a primary immunologic deficit. Transfer factor obtained from *Candida* skin test–positive donors has been beneficial in at least half of the patients, particularly if combined with treatment of the *Candida* infection.

Severe Combined Immunodeficiency Disease (Swiss-Type Agamma-globulinemia). The usual form of this disease is autosomal recessive, although there is an X-linked recessive form. Symptoms appear early and include slowed growth rate, chronic diarrhea, pneumonia, otitis media, and other infections. Infants with this disease are particularly susceptible to *Pneumocystis carinii*, cytomegalovirus, and *Candida* infections, as well as measles, generalized vaccinia, herpes, and overwhelming gram-negative sepsis. Use of live vaccines (such as polio) is extremely hazardous. Transfusions are also dangerous because they may result in the engraftment of incompatible donor lymphocytes to produce a graft-vs.-host reaction (Chapter 23).

The basic defect in this disease is believed to be a failure of differentiation of the stem cell into T and B cells. Hematopoietic, myelopoietic, and thrombopoietic precursors are usually normal. In rare cases, referred to as reticular dysgenesis, all of the stem-cell functions are impaired. These infants usually die within the first few weeks of life with overwhelming infection as well as a deficiency of all types of blood cells.

In the classic form of severe combined immunodeficiency disease, both T and B cell functions are severely depressed. The thymus shadow is absent, marked lymphopenia is present, and responses of peripheral lymphocytes to mitogens and allogeneic cells are greatly reduced. Maternal IgG may be present for the first five or six months of life, but active antibody production is diminished, corresponding to the lowered numbers of circulating B cells in the infant.

Several forms of this disease are associated with deficiencies of particular enzymes. The absence of adenosine deaminase (ADA) and nucleoside phosphorylase has been described; both enzymes are involved in pyrimidine metabolism.

Treatment of this disorder depends on restoration of the stem cell by means of bone marrow transplantation (Chapter 22). The bone marrow is usually matched by both HLA and mixed lymphocyte culture (MLC) tests. Unless careful MLC matching is carried out, graft-vs.-host reactions (Chapter 23) will develop. In the absence of a suitable bone marrow donor, other forms of treatment have been attempted. They include transplantation of fetal liver and fetal thymus. In addition, repeated transfusion of erythrocytes as a source of adenosine deaminase has been successful in a few cases.

Other Immunodeficiencies Involving Both T and B Cells. Wiskott-Aldrich syndrome consists of eczema, recurrent pyogenic infection, and thrombocytopenia. The infants, usually male, become symptomatic during the first year of life, often with bleeding caused by thrombocytopenia as the presenting sign. Later, they develop chronic bacterial infections such as otitis media and pneumonia, and sometimes meningitis. A recalcitrant form of eczema often appears by one year of age. Patients are particularly susceptible to infection with organisms possessing polysaccharide capsules (pneumococcus, meningococcus, and *Haemophilus influenzae*). Bronchial asthma may develop later.

The immunologic findings consist of normal IgG, low IgM, and sometimes elevated IgA and IgE levels. Patients fail to form antibodies following immunization with polysaccharide antigens. T cell immunity is generally normal initially, although it may decline with growth. The affected children rarely survive beyond ten years of age.

A form of immunodeficiency is associated with thymoma. Infections may occur in the respiratory, gastrointestinal, or urinary tracts, or on the skin. Marked hypogammaglobulinemia is often present (pages 292–94). Some patients have deficient T cell responses, as determined by delayed hypersensitivity skin tests (Chapter 11) and the response to mitogens. Thymoma is also associated with muscular weakness as seen in myasthenia gravis, or with a regenerative anemia, thrombocytopenia, or autoimmune disease.

Deficiencies of Phagocytosis. CHRONIC GRANULOMATOUS DISEASE. Chronic granulomatous disease is an X-linked disorder, although a rare autosomal recessive form has also been described. Clinical manifestations appear during the first two years of life. The patients develop repeated infections due to normally nonpathogenic bacteria, such as *Staphylococcus epidermidis, Escherichia coli, Proteus vulgaris, Klebsiella,* and *Enterobacter aerogenes,* or to fungi such as *Candida* and *Aspergillus.* Immunologic examination reveals normal immunoglobulin levels, response to toxoids, intact T and B cell functions, and normal complement levels. Tissue biopsies show granuloma formation in many organs. The phagocytic cells have normal chemotactic responses and are capable of engulfing microorganisms. However, the neutrophils fail to kill the ingested organisms. The most characteristic laboratory finding is markedly reduced nitroblue tetrazolium reduction. This finding indicates that the neutrophils of patients with chronic granulomatous disease do not shift to anaerobic metabolism following ingestion of bacteria and, therefore, fail to accumulate H_2O_2 and kill intracellular bacteria. The importance of H_2O_2 is emphasized by the fact that organisms such as *Haemophilus*, *Neisseria*, and *Streptococcus*, which produce H_2O_2 and lack catalase, do not cause problems in these patients.

The survival of patients with chronic granulomatous disease depends on prompt bacteriologic diagnosis and institution of appropriate antimicrobial treatment. Therapy using white blood cell infusions has been attempted, but experience is still limited. Even with careful attention, the risk of chronic pulmonary and gastrointestinal disease and osteomyelitis is high. Survival beyond the second decade is unusual.

GLUCOSE-6-PHOSPHATE DEHYDROGENASE DEFICIENCY. Some patients with a clinical picture similar to chronic granulomatous disease lack leukocyte glucose-6-phosphate dehydrogenase activity. It is responsible for a decreased shift to the hexose monophosphate shunt and decreased hydrogen peroxide activity, so that leukocytes are unable to kill certain microorganisms at a normal rate. The nitroblue tetrazolium test may be normal, but a specific deficiency of white blood cell glucose-6-phosphate dehydrogenase is demonstrable by cytochemical stains.

MYELOPEROXIDASE DEFICIENCY. The leukocytes of some patients with increased susceptibility to bacterial (Chapter 13) or mycotic (Chapter 14) infections are deficient in peroxidase activity, as demonstrated by benzidene staining of the neutrophils. Intracellular killing of bacteria is delayed, but the leukocytes have normal oxygen consumption, normal hexosemme-phosphate shunt activity, and normal hydrogen-peroxide production.

CHÉDIAK-HIGASHI SYNDROME. Chédiak-Higashi (C-H) syndrome is characterized by partial albinism affecting the eyes and skin; sensitivity to light; rapid, involuntary eye movements; and recurrent infections by a variety of pyogenic bacteria.

The primary immunologic defect in this disease is the inability of cells of the granulocytic series to form normal primary granules. These primary granules are specialized lysozomes containing acid-dependent hydrolases. Victims of C-H syndrome have giant cytoplasmic granules in their white blood cells and platelets. Resultant abnormalities include reduced intracellular killing by neutrophils and decreased chemotaxis. The retarded intraphagocyte killing is not the result of depressed H_2O_2 formation, but is attributable to the inability of cells to degranulate normally. Therefore, patients are susceptible to streptococcal and pneumococcal infection, as well as to infection by those organisms usually found in chronic granulomatous disease.

JOB's SYNDROME. In this variant of chronic granulomatous disease, patients have a specific phagocytic defect that permits *Staphylococcus aureus* to produce "cold" abscesses of skin, lymph nodes, or subcutaneous tissue. Phagocytes from these patients ingest bacteria normally but are unable to kill staphylococci.

Deficiencies of Complement. Several complement deficiencies have been associated with increased susceptibility to infection. A deficiency of Clq was first detected in several patients with X-linked hypogammaglobulinemia or severe combined immunodeficiency disease. The cause of the deficiency is uncertain but may be related to hypercatabolism rather than to depressed synthesis. The Clq deficiency may increase susceptibility to infection in patients with other immunodeficiency disorders.

Several patients with C2 deficiency have been described. It is transmitted as an autosomal recessive trait. Homozygotes have 0.5% to 4% of normal C2 and heterozygotes have 30% to 60% of the normal value. The depressed hemolytic activity of their sera is restored by purified C2. Activation of the alternative pathway is normal. Several of the patients had symptoms of systemic lupus erythematosus (including antibody to DNA) as well as increased susceptibility to infection.

At least two forms of C3 deficiency have been described in humans. The first form is associated with a deficiency of C3 inactivator, and the second is associated with increased destruction of C3 and decreased synthesis. The patients had approximately half the normal amount of C3 and were susceptible to a variety of bacterial infections. A similar form of C5 deficiency has also been described. The patients showed leukocytosis and hypergammaglobulinemia as well as normal levels of total hemolytic complement. In many cases, hemolytic assays for C5 are also positive, but chemotaxis is ineffective and can be corrected by adding normal C5.

Summary

The immunologic system, like other organs of the body, is complex. Its proper function depends on the integrity of each component and on a delicately balanced system of checks and balances. The organ is subject to abnormal increase or decrease in function due to congenital or acquired illness and may undergo malignant change. It is now possible to dissect these disorders with a high degree of precision. The major cell type involved can be defined and a reasonable idea of the basis of the defect made evident.

Bibliography

Alper, C. A.; Abramson, N.; Johnston, R. B., Jr.; Jandl, J. H.; and Rosen, F. S.: Increased susceptibility to infection associated with abnormalities of complement-mediated functions and of the third component of complement (C3). *N. Engl. J. Med.*, **282**:349–54, 1970.

Bellanti, J. A.: *Immunology*, 2nd ed. W. B. Saunders Co., Philadelphia, 1978.

Bergsma, D., and Good, R. A. (eds.): *Immunologic Deficiency Diseases in Man.* Birth Defects Original Article Series, Vol. 4, No. 1. National Foundation Press, New York, 1968.

Bruton, O. C.: Agammaglobulinemia. *Pediatrics*, **9**:722–28, 1952.

DiGeorge, A.: Congenital absence of the thymus and its immunological consequences; concurrence with congenital hypoparathyroidism. In Bergsma, D., and Good, R. A. (eds.): *Immunologic Deficiency Diseases in Man.* Birth Defects Original Article Series, Vol. 4, No. 1. National Foundation Press, New York, 1968.

Fudenberg, H. H.; Good, R. A.; Goodman, H. C.; Hitzig, W.; Kunkel, H. G.; Roitt, I. M.; Rosen, F. S.; Rowe, D. S.; Seligmann, M.; and Soothill, J. R.: Primary immunodeficiencies. *Pediatrics*, **47**:927–46, 1971.

Fudenberg, H. H.; Stites, D. P.; Caldwell, J. L.; and Wells, J. V. (eds.): *Basic and Clinical Immunology.* Lange Medical Publications, Los Altos, Calif., 1976.

Giblett, E. R.; Anderson, J. E.; Cohen, F.; Pollara, B.; and Meuwissen, H. J.: Adenosine-deaminase deficiency in two patients with severely impaired cellular immunity. *Lancet*, **2**:1067–69, 1972.

Hitzig, W. H.; Biro, Z.; Borsch, H.; and Huser, H. J.: Agammaglobulinemia and alymphocytosis with atrophy of lymphatic tissue. *Helv. Paediatr. Acta*, **13**:551–85, 1958.

Karnovsky, M. L.: Chronic granulomatous disease; pieces of a cellular and molecular puzzle. *Fed. Proc.*, **32**:1527–33, 1973.

Osserman, E. F.: Multiple myeloma and related plasma cell dyscrasias. In Samter, M. (ed.): *Immunological Diseases*, 2nd ed. Little, Brown & Co., Boston, 1971.

Rose, N. R.: The immune system: how it works. *Med. Opinion*, **5**:31–35, 1976. The immune system: the patient work-up. *Med. Opinion*, **6**:41–47, 1977.

Rose, N. R., and Friedman, H. (eds.): *Manual of Clinical Immunology.* American Society for Microbiology, Washington, D.C., 1976.

Ruddy, S.; Gigli, I.; and Austen, K. F.: The complement system of man. *N. Engl. J. Med.*, **287**:489–95, 545–49, 592–96, 642–46, 1972.

Waldenström, J.: *Diagnosis and Treatment of Multiple Myeloma.* Grune & Stratton, Inc., New York, 1970.

Waldmann, T. A.; Durm, M.; Broder, S.; Blackman, M.; Blaese, R. M.; and Strober, W.: Role of suppressor T cells in pathogenesis of common variable hypogammaglobulinemia. *Lancet*, **2**:609–13, 1974.

18

Diseases of Immediate Hypersensitivity

CARL E. ARBESMAN AND ROBERT E. REISMAN

Introduction

In this chapter the concept of immunologic injury mediated by undesirable or harmful properties of antibodies will be introduced.

Immediate hypersensitivity reactions are due to the reaction of humoral antibodies with a specific antigen that results in the production of cellular injury and inflammation. Two general types of these reactions have been described. In anaphylaxis of man and animal and in human atopy, the antibodies are fixed to cells where they react with the antigen; subsequently, they release chemical mediators. Clinical examples of these processes are hay fever, asthma, and anaphylactic reactions.

The second example of hypersensitivity associated with humoral antibodies is the Arthus, or serum sickness, reaction. This reaction is mediated by antigen-antibody complexes and results in vascular injury. Serum sickness, some forms of glomerulonephritis, and perhaps pulmonary hypersensitivity syndromes such as farmer's lung represent examples of this type of immunopathology. Immune complex disease is discussed in detail in Chapter 19. Selected clinical aspects of this type of reaction and its relationship to the anaphylactic reaction are presented in this chapter.

Anaphylaxis

In 1902 Portier and Richet, studying the effects of extracts of the sea anemone in dogs, found that a second injection of a nontoxic dose caused an immediate violent reaction often leading to death. They coined the term "anaphylaxis," meaning "against protection." Subsequently, similar reactions have been produced in various laboratory animals, and the underlying immunopathogenesis is now clearly elucidated.

Anaphylaxis is produced in animals by the following methods. An antigen, which is nontoxic, is injected into an animal by one of several routes (intravenous, intraperitoneal, or intradermal) (Figure 18-1). This first injection of the antigen is called the sensitizing dose. Antibodies to the antigen develop over a period of 2 to 21 days (latent period). These antibodies are present in the serum and also fixed to cells in certain tissues. This latent period varies, depending on the amount and type of antigen used, the route of sensitization, and the species of animal. After this latent period, a second injection of the same antigen (called the challenging or shocking dose) is given intravenously or by intracardiac puncture. Alternatively, antigen may be administered by aerosol. The second or challenging dose usually is five to ten times greater than the first, sensitizing dose of antigen.

Following the challenging dose, there is a reaction between the antigen and the cell-fixed antibodies. The fixed antigen-antibody complexes act on

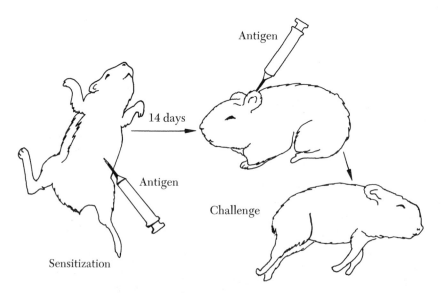

Figure 18-1. Active anaphylaxis. Two weeks after active sensitization, challenge with the same antigen results in an anaphylactic reaction and death. See text for details.

certain cells, primarily basophils and mast cells, to release mediators, causing characteristic pathophysiologic changes and clinical symptoms. These symptoms vary in different species, depending on the tissues involved and the mediators liberated.

The guinea pig has been the laboratory model for anaphylaxis for many years. Following the administration of the challenging antigen, symptoms develop immediately, consisting of restlessness, ruffling of the skin, sneezing, coughing, pruritus, incontinence, respiratory distress resembling asthma, convulsions, and death. Bronchoconstriction and hyperinflation of the lungs are important gross pathologic findings. As the major pathologic manifestations occur in the bronchial tree, it is referred to as the shock organ in guinea pig anaphylaxis. In the rabbit the pulmonary arterioles are the shock organ, and the clinical picture is one of right-sided heart failure. The hepatic venules are the shock organ of the dog, and the major clinical manifestations are emesis and bloody diarrhea. The gastrointestinal tract, particularly the small intestine, is primarily involved in rats and mice (Table 18-1).

An increasing number of chemical mediators have been detected during anaphylaxis (Chapter 1). The major mediators released initially from basophils and mast cells are histamine, eosinophilic chemotactic factor (ECF), slow-reacting substance of anaphylaxis (SRS-A), platelet-activating factor (PAF), and heparin. Subsequent secondary cellular and tissue reactions lead to release of other mediators including prostaglandins, 5-hydroxytryptamine (serotonin), and kinins. Among the many pharmacologic properties of these substances are the induction of smooth muscle contraction, increased vascular permeability, glandular hypersecretion, and blood hypocoagulability. Secondary physiologic changes result. These include hypoxia, shock, tissue necrosis, and hemorrhage. Table 18-1 lists the major

Table 18-1
COMPARISON OF ANAPHYLACTIC REACTIONS IN DIFFERENT ANIMAL SPECIES

Species	Shock Organ	Symptoms	Principal Mediators
Guinea pig	Bronchioles	Bronchoconstriction Seizures	Histamine SRS-A Serotonin Kinins
Rat	Intestine	Circulatory collapse Peristaltic activity	Histamine SRS-A Serotonin
Mouse	Intestine and lung	Respiratory distress Prostration	Histamine Serotonin
Rabbit	Pulmonary vasculature	Right-heart failure	Histamine SRS-A Serotonin
Dog	Hepatic vein	Emesis Diarrhea	Histamine

manifestations of anaphylaxis, shock organs, and mediators in various animal species. Human anaphylaxis is discussed below (page 309).

Active Anaphylaxis

This model of anaphylaxis involves sensitization and challenge by antigen, as described above. In almost all species studied, the antibodies responsible for active anaphylaxis have similar properties. These antibodies are generally heat labile, migrate as fast γ or slow β globulins in electrophoresis, and are capable of sensitizing the skin of animals of the homologous species (i.e., homocytotropic antibodies; see Chapter 4). They do not fix to the skin of other animal species. These properties are similar to those associated with the human anaphylactic or "reaginic" antibody IgE. Thus, antibodies mediating similar biologic responses in various animals and man appear to have the same physiochemical characteristics.

Passive Anaphylaxis

Passive anaphylaxis is accomplished by systemic transfer of serum-containing antibody to a normal animal, which is subsequently challenged with the same antigen, usually 24 to 48 hours later. The animals need not be of the same species, but the symptoms are characteristic of the recipient animal and do not depend on the antigen used (Figure 18-2).

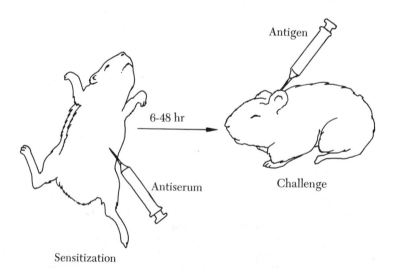

Figure 18-2. Passive anaphylaxis. Following systemic passive sensitization with antiserum, challenge with antigen results in anaphylaxis.

Passive Cutaneous Anaphylaxis (PCA)

Sensitization of the skin of a normal recipient animal by intradermal injection of antibody-containing serum is followed four to six hours later by an intravenous injection of the challenge antigen and Evans blue dye. The antigen-antibody reaction releases mediators that cause capillary permeability, and the dye leaking through the damaged vascular tissue marks the area of reaction (Figure 18-3).

The PCA technique has been useful in working out some of the immunologic conditions necessary for passive sensitization. Critical factors are the immunoglobulin type and the species of donor and recipient. Passive sensitization of animals of the same species, including man, is accomplished by the IgE antibody.

Generally IgE is unable to fix to cells of unrelated species. For example, guinea pig IgG_1 (the equivalent of IgE in that species) will fix to the skin of another guinea pig but not to the skin of a rabbit. Human reaginic antibody

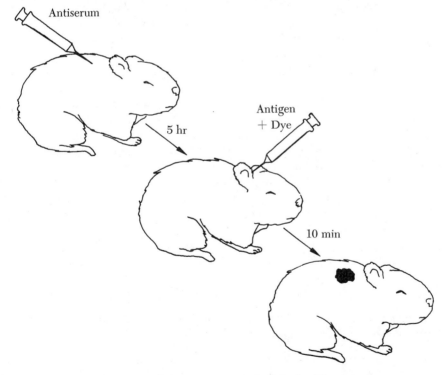

Figure 18-3. Passive cutaneous anaphylaxis. The intravenous injection of antigen results in a reaction at the site of passive skin sensitization. The reaction is clearly demonstrated by use of a marker dye.

Table 18-2
ANTIBODIES INVOLVED IN IMMEDIATE
HYPERSENSITIVITY IN VARIOUS SPECIES

Guinea pig	IgG_{1a}	IgG_{1b}	IgE
Rat	IgG_a	IgE	
Mouse	IgG_1	IgE	
Rabbit	IgE		
Dog	IgE		
Monkey	IgE		
Man	IgE	IgG(?)	

can sensitize human and primate tissues, but will not sensitize tissues of other animals.

A second major homocytotropic antibody of the IgG type has been described in several species. After immunization of guinea pigs and mice, IgG_1 antibodies are found in high concentration in their sera. In rats, the homocytotropic antibodies are in subclass IgG_a. These antibodies are heat stable and can attach to skin cells for a short period of time. Hence, challenge must be performed within a few hours. A second heat-stable homocytotropic antibody has also been described in the guinea pig (IgG_{1b}), differing primarily in the optimum latent period for the PCA reaction and persistence at passively prepared skin sites. Several recent studies have suggested that humans may also possess an IgG homocytotropic antibody with similar biologic activity.

Antibodies of the IgG type are able to sensitize skin of other species, but usually do not sensitize animals of the same species. Guinea pig γ globulin–type IgG can sensitize rabbit skin but will not sensitize tissue of other guinea pigs. Human IgG can be used successfully to sensitize guinea pig tissue, but cannot be passively transferred to human skin. Table 18-2 lists the antibodies involved in immediate hypersensitivity in various species.

Further complexities of this aspect of sensitization are related to species differences. Guinea pig tissue can be sensitized by rabbit, dog, monkey, and human IgG antibodies, but not by antibodies from the rat, chicken, goat, cow, or horse.

Reversed Passive Anaphylaxis (Figure 18-4)

Injection of antigen is followed by administration of serum-containing antibodies to the same antigen.

Desensitization

If sensitized animals are given a nonlethal challenging dose of antigen, the animals may become specifically refractory to anaphylaxis caused by

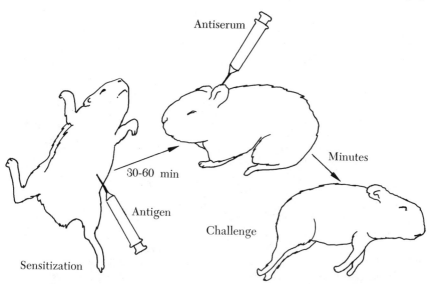

Figure 18-4. Reversed passive anaphylaxis. Antiserum is administered shortly after antigen, resulting in anaphylaxis.

further doses of antigen, even of the usually lethal dose. This refractory state is probably due to neutralization of humoral antibody. The phenomenon is referred to as desensitization. This model has a pertinent analogy to similar situations in humans.

In Vitro *Anaphylaxis*

Following systemic sensitization, either active or passive, antibody becomes fixed to cells of certain tissues of the body. The isolated tissues can then be used for *in vitro* studies. Antibody readily fixes to mast cells of the guinea pig ileum and the uterus. Either of these sensitized tissues is placed in a muscle bath containing a buffered saline solution. One end is attached to the bottom of the bath and the other end is attached by a thread to either a muscle lever or a transducer. The antigen is then added to the bath. The subsequent antigen-antibody reaction causes degranulation of the mast cells followed by the release of mediators that cause contraction of the muscle, which is recorded on a kymograph or polygraph (Figure 18-5). This technique is called the Schultz-Dale reaction. Lung tissue from the sensitized animal also contains cell-fixed antibodies. When such tissues are minced into small fragments and washed free of blood, mediators are released following the addition of specific antigen. The mediators are primarily histamine, slow-reacting substance (SRS-A), and eosinophilic chemotactic factor (ECF) and can be measured quantitatively by chemical or biologic techniques.

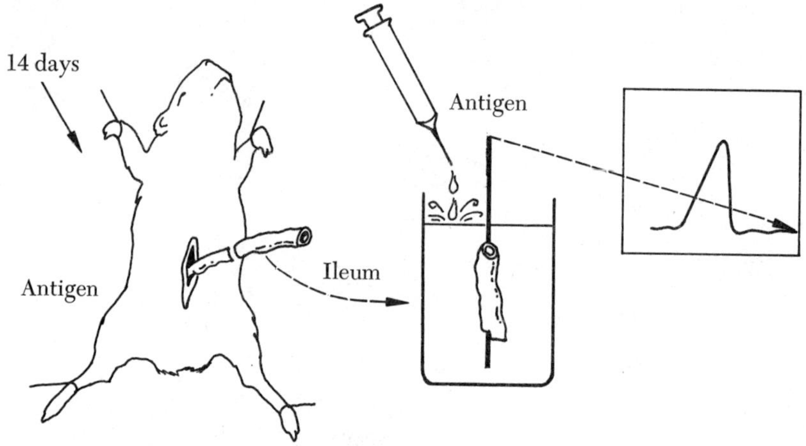

14 days

Antigen

Antigen

Ileum

Figure 18-5. Active *in vitro* anaphylaxis; Schultz-Dale reaction. Smooth muscle from an actively sensitized animal is placed in a solution. Addition of antigen results in a muscle contraction, which is recorded on a polygraph. See text for details.

A modification of these methods is referred to as "*in vitro* sensitization." A suitable tissue, such as ileum, uterus, or lung, from a nonsensitized animal, is placed in the serum of a sensitized animal, allowing the antibody to fix to the cells. After washing and the addition of antigen, the specific chemical mediators are released (Figure 18-6).

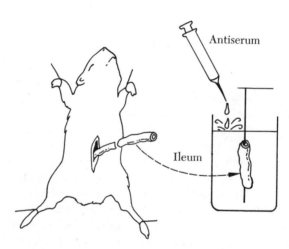

Antiserum

Ileum

Figure 18-6. Passive *in vitro* sensitization; Schultz-Dale reaction. Smooth muscle from a normal nonimmunized animal is placed in a muscle bath and passively sensitized with antiserum. Subsequent addition of antigen results in a muscle contraction, which is recorded on a polygraph.

Table 18-3

MANIFESTATIONS OF ANAPHYLAXIS IN MAN

1. Dermal: Flushing erythema, urticaria, angioedema
2. Respiratory: Laryngeal edema, bronchospasm
3. Gastrointestinal: Nausea, vomiting, diarrhea
4. Circulatory collapse: Pressuric oppression in chest, apnea, fall in blood pressure
5. Genitourinary: Uterine contractions

Anaphylaxis in Man

Anaphylactic reactions in humans may follow injection or ingestion of drugs, biologic preparations such as sera, insect stings, and food. The clinical pattern may vary. Edema of the upper airway, particularly the larynx, seems unique to humans. Other symptoms include urticaria, bronchospasm, emesis, diarrhea, hypotension, and shock. Man probably has several shock organs. Histamine is the principal mediator, although several others may also be involved. Varying symptoms can simulate those produced by various species of animals (Table 18-3).

Almost all individuals who have had anaphylactic reactions have a history of previous exposure to the antigen. For example, anaphylaxis from penicillin rarely, if ever, occurs after the first exposure. In contrast to animals, however, the latent period varies from days to years.

With a few exceptions, the antibodies mediating human generalized anaphylaxis are IgE. The biologic activity of IgE is discussed below. The rare exceptions are instances of IgG-mediated anaphylaxis. Reactions occur in patients who are usually IgA deficient and have antibodies to IgA following a transfusion that contains IgA. The reaction to γ globulins by hypogammaglobulinemic patients may be mediated by an IgG-type antibody to aggregated IgG.

Atopic Disease

Asthma, allergic rhinitis (hay fever), eczema, and urticaria are clinical examples of one type of immediate hypersensitivity. These allergies are quite common, affecting approximately 10% of the population. They are often referred to as atopic diseases. Clinically atopy is characterized by hereditary transmission and the presence of eosinophilia. Immunologically, atopic disease is analogous to experimental animal anaphylaxis.

The antibody involved in these reactions is classically termed reagin or skin-sensitizing antibody. Biologically it is extremely potent, present in small quantities, yet capable of causing severe allergic reactions. Studies in recent years have identified these antibodies as a unique class of immunoglobulins, IgE (Chapter 4). These antibodies are capable of reacting with many different types of allergens, such as pollens, airborne fungi, animal danders, household dusts, drugs, and foods. These antibodies have the unusual characteristic of being able to passively sensitize tissues of homologous species.

In contrast to that of animal, the human reaginic antibody is not usually induced by artificial immunization. It develops as a result of natural exposure by inhalation and/or ingestion in some individuals, apparently because of genetic disposition. For example, ragweed hay fever cannot be induced in normal individuals. Injection or nasal insufflation of tetanus toxoid may lead to reagin formation in atopic, but not in nonatopic, individuals. However, production of reagin is not entirely a selective phenomenon. Injections of ascaris extract will induce reagin in almost all individuals. High levels of IgE develop in response to parasitic infections, but the exact role of IgE in parasitic disease is still unclear. The possibility that IgE antibodies function as part of host defense mechanisms is a subject of current investigation.

Reagin titers increase following exposure to allergen as, for instance, during the ragweed pollen season. They also increase early in the course of specific immunotherapy with antigen extracts, but as this therapy continues, reagin levels diminish.

The physiochemical properties of IgE have been reviewed in Chapter 4. IgE is measured in serum in quantities of nanograms per milliliter in contrast to milligram amounts of other immunoglobulins. Its biologic activity stems from its unique property to fix to tissue and cells, specifically mast cells and basophils. Upon contact with antigen, chemical mediators, particularly histamine, are released from cell granules, resulting in clinical allergic manifestations.

The discovery of patients with IgE myeloma provided large amounts of this protein. Antisera to IgE were thus readily produced, and subsequently *in vitro* methods of total IgE determination have become available. Serum concentrations of IgE greater than 1500 ng/ml can be determined by the simple Mancini gel diffusion technique employing IgE antiserum in the agar (Chapter 6). However, most serum IgE concentrations are below this level, and more sensitive techniques utilizing radioimmunodiffusion are then required. One technique employs ^{125}I-labeled specific anti-IgE goat serum mixed with agar. Serum samples are placed in wells in the agar. After 48 hours the agar plates are washed and x-ray film applied. The x-ray film is developed 24 to 48 hours later, and rings showing radioactivity due to the IgE/anti-IgE reaction can be observed. By comparing the diameter of these rings with a known standard, the amount of IgE in the serum can be determined (Chapter 6). Typical results are shown in Figure 18-7. This method is simple, readily reproducible, and useful in studying large numbers of samples. Its sensitivity is limited to IgE concentrations above 20 ng/ml.

Serum IgE levels can also be measured by a solid-phase radioimmunoassay, similar to the radioallergosorbent test used to measure specific IgE antibodies, which is described below (pages 312–14). Purified anti-IgE is

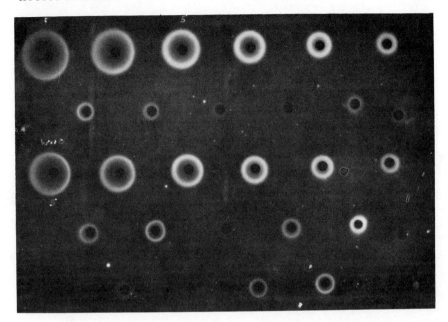

Figure 18-7. Measurement of serum IgE by radioimmuno-diffusion. Levels determined by comparison of diameters of rings with those induced by known standards.

coupled to cellulose discs. These coupled discs are then incubated with various serum samples and known concentrations of IgE. Following washing, radiolabeled purified anti-IgE is added. After further washing, the radio-activity on the disc is counted. From these data, the amount of IgE in the unknown serum samples can be determined.

Serum IgE levels are generally elevated in atopic patients with allergic rhinitis and asthma and particularly in those with atopic dermatitis. Elevations are occasionally noted in other conditions (Table 18-4).

Table 18-4
DISEASES ASSOCIATED WITH INCREASED LEVELS OF IgE IN SERUM

1. Atopic eczema
2. Allergic asthma
3. Allergic rhinitis*
4. Parasitic disease
5. Pemphigoid
6. Bronchopulmonary aspergillosis
7. Impaired cellular immunity (e.g., advanced Hodgkin's disease)

* Increased during pollen season; increased early with immunotherapy.

The usual way of detecting specific reagin is by scratch or intradermal skin testing. This technique is used regularly in clinical medicine. A small amount of allergen is placed in the skin. If reaginic antibody is present, a wheal-and-flare reaction develops within ten minutes. This reaction is due to release of histamine by tissue mast cells. In a reversed fashion an injection of anti-IgE antibody (produced in animals) results in a similar reaction in almost all individuals. The only exceptions to this latter reaction are rare individuals lacking IgE.

Demonstration of reagin in the serum of humans is done by the classic Prausnitz-Küstner (PK) reaction. Serum from an allergic individual is injected intradermally into a nonatopic recipient. Twenty-four to forty-eight hours later, the site is challenged with the appropriate allergen and a wheal-and-flare reaction quickly ensues. Control tests at a nonsensitized skin site must be negative. The sensitized site remains reactive to challenge for up to six weeks. This test demonstrates the ability of reagin to passively sensitize normal tissue mast cells for long periods of time.

The PK reaction can be blocked by prior injection of the skin site with IgE before sensitization. This IgE occupies the receptor sites of the mast cell, thus preventing the specific reaginic antibody from attaching to these tissues.

Human reaginic antibody is also able to fix to monkey skin, ileum, and lung. Appropriate experiments (PCA, Schultz-Dale, and histamine release from chopped lung) can be carried out. Monkey tissue serves as an excellent substrate for measuring human reagin. Tissues of other animals cannot be sensitized with human IgE.

Recently several investigators have shown that rat mast cells can be sensitized with human IgE and that degranulation can be noted after addition of the appropriate antigen. These findings seem to contradict the usual concepts of fixation of anaphylactic antibody only by the same species. One proposed explanation is that human and rat IgE have similar chemical structures.

IgE also fixes to basophils. Following addition of allergen to basophils from blood of allergic individuals, histamine release can be detected. Similarly, cells from nonallergic individuals can be passively sensitized with serum from patients who have reagin, and histamine is released following antigen challenge.

The measurement of histamine release from basophils has led to a better understanding of the biologic mechanism of IgE (Chapter 10). The Fc fragment of IgE is attached to the receptor site on the basophil. Histamine release from granules in the basophils occurs when two IgE molecules are bridged by antigen attached to the Fab receptor sites. This is shown diagrammatically in Figure 18-8. Bridging by antibody to IgE can also evoke histamine release.

Specific IgE antibody activity has been measured *in vitro* by the radio-allergosorbent test (RAST). An allergen, such as ragweed, is linked to

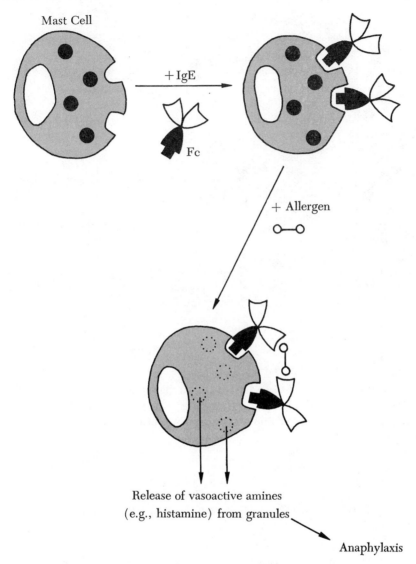

Figure 18-8.   Present concepts of the immunopathogenesis of histamine release from mast cells and basophils by allergen-IgE complexes.

cellulose by cyanogen bromide. A patient's serum is added to these antigen-coated particles. If specific antibody is present, it will attach to these particles. After washing, radioactive anti-IgE is added. It will bind to the particles, provided the IgE antibody combined with the antigen. This is an excellent method of quantitating IgE antibody or reagin. The technique is shown diagrammatically in Figure 18-9.

RAST Test

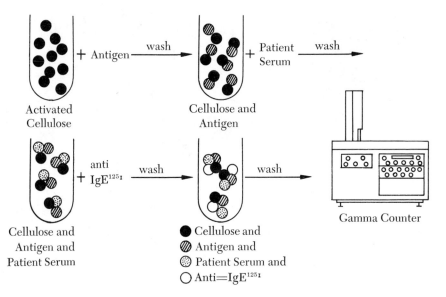

Figure 18-9. Radioallergosorbent test (RAST). See text for details.

Clinical application of the RAST includes diagnosis of specific allergy, the determination of IgE antibody activity over a period of time by analysis of sequential serum samples, and standardization of the potency of allergenic extracts.

Relationship to Immune Complex Disease*

Another type of immediate hypersensitivity reaction has been noted occasionally in humans. Rarely, following an injection of a drug, such as penicillin, a local hemorrhagic necrotic reaction develops four to six hours later at a site. It has been compared with the reaction in rabbits described by Arthus (Table 18-5). A better example of the Arthus reaction in humans is the late-onset skin test reaction, which occurs four to six hours after testing patients who have pulmonary hypersensitivity syndromes such as aspergillosis or pigeon breeder's disease with the appropriate antigen. Biopsy of such reactions has confirmed the presence of antigen, antibody, complement, and vascular injury.

* A detailed discussion of this subject is presented in Chapter 19.

Table 18-5
IMMEDIATE HYPERSENSITIVITY

	Anaphylactic	Arthus
Heredity	+	−
Eosinophilia	+	−
Antibody	IgE	IgG
Complement	−	+
Time of onset	5–15 minutes	4–6 hours
Pathology	Edema	Vasculitis
	Capillary permeability	Necrosis
	Wheal and flare	
Pulmonary reaction		
Primary tissue	Bronchioles	Alveoli
Prognosis	Reversible	With repeated exposure, irreversible

Serum Sickness

Serum sickness represents the systemic counterpart of the Arthus reaction. This problem was first described in humans and subsequently produced experimentally in animals. The pathologic and immunologic reactions in experimental serum sickness are described in Chapter 19. Human disease is quite analogous.

Primary serum sickness in humans results from administration of heterologous serum. Prior to the antibiotic era and the modern active immunization programs, biologic products prepared in the horse, such as pneumococcal antiserum and tetanus and diphtheria antitoxin, were commonly prescribed. Serum sickness was a frequent reaction. Symptoms usually occurred about seven to ten days following administration of the heterologous serum and consisted of joint pain and swelling, urticaria, fever, and lymphadenopathy. Generally the illness is self-limited with full recovery within a week. On occasion more severe manifestations, such as neuropathy, nephritis, and vasculitis, would occur. Acute glomerulonephritis due to serum sickness was the cause of death in a few patients receiving large amounts of an experimental anticancer horse serum.

Today the use of animal serum preparations is greatly reduced. Some biologic products do remain, such as antirabies serum, snake venom antisera, diphtheria antitoxin, botulinum antitoxin, and antilymphocyte globulin. Clinical serum-sickness-like symptoms occur frequently following their use as well as following the administration of drugs like penicillin. Knowledge of the immunopathogenesis of serum sickness may also apply to these drug-induced reactions.

Immunologically, human serum sickness is similar to the experimental model. Small amounts of IgG-precipitating antibody can be detected during the acute phase. Higher levels of free antibody are present following recovery.

Presumably antigen-antibody complexes are responsible for at least some of the clinical symptoms. Immunopathologic studies of patients dying of serum sickness confirm the presence of antigen and antibody in renal glomeruli.

Serum sickness in humans is also associated with the presence of reaginic antibody (IgE). This antibody is found concomitant with the clinical disease and is probably responsible for some of the symptomatology, particularly urticaria. Until recently, the presence of IgE appeared to be an important immunologic aspect differentiating human serum sickness from the animal model. However, an IgE antibody has now been described in the experimental animal model of serum sickness. Furthermore, it has been postulated that the IgE antibody plays a most important role in the pathogenesis of immune complex disease in the following manner. Reaction of antigen with IgE antibody leads to the release of vasoactive amines from basophils and platelets. These chemical mediators, in turn, cause increased permeability of blood vessels, thus allowing the complexes to invade the tissue.

Similar immune mechanisms involving antigen-antibody complexes may be operative in other human diseases, such as systemic lupus erythematosus, quartan malaria, and some forms of acute glomerulonephritis (Chapters 16 and 19).

Immune complexes may also involve the lung, causing pulmonary hypersensitivity diseases. The antigens responsible for this disorder are organic dusts and thermophilic actinomycetes (Chapter 14). Table 18-6 shows some of the common pulmonary hypersensitivity diseases and their causes. A similar pathogenesis might be the cause of pulmonary reactions from some drugs and *Bacillus subtilis* enzymes.

Clinical symptoms consist of cough, fever, and malaise, starting about four to six hours after exposure to antigen and lasting up to 18 to 24 hours.

Table 18-6
PULMONARY HYPERSENSITIVITY SYNDROMES

Disease	Etiology
Farmer's lung	*Micropolyspora faeni*
Bagassosis	*Micropolyspora vulgaris*
Mushroom worker's disease	Both thermoactinomycetes
Siberosis (oak bark or cork dust)	Thermoactinomycetes and other fungi
Malt worker's lung	*Aspergillus fumigatus* and *clavatus*
Maple bark stripper's disease	*Crystostroma corticale* (coniosporium)
Sequoisis (redwood)	Graphium
Cheese washer's lung	*Penicillium* sp. and aerobacidum
New Guinea thatched roof inhabitant's lung	Unknown
Bird fancier's lung	Pigeon's and parakeet's serum protein
Pituitary snuff-taker's lung	Pork and beef proteins
Wheat weevil disease	*Sitophilus granarius*
Laundry detergent worker's lung	Enzymes of *Bacillus subtilis*
Smallpox-handler's lung	Unknown
Coffee and sisal worker's lung	Unknown

Infiltrates can be found on chest radiographs. Chronic exposure may lead to permanent lung damage. Immunologically, patients have precipitating IgG antibodies and lymphocytes reacting with these antigens. Studies of the pulmonary lesions have revealed the presence of antigen, antibody, and complement (Chapter 27). More recent investigations, however, have suggested that cellular hypersensitivity mechanisms may be most important. Frequently, patients also have reaginic antibodies, and their role in this disease complex is not clear.

This type of hypersensitivity differs considerably from bronchial asthma. The antibody involved is primarily IgG. It is complement dependent, in contrast to the IgE of the atopic asthmatic. Symptoms on exposure to the allergen in asthma occur much more rapidly, and recovery is quicker. There is usually no elevation in temperature or pulmonary infiltrates in asthma. The differences between these two types of immediate hypersensitivity that involve humoral antibodies are listed in Table 18-5.

Summary

The immunopathophysiologic reactions of immediate hypersensitivity in man and animals have been described. The IgE-mediated anaphylactic reaction is rapid in onset, does not require complement, and can be fatal. The Arthus reactions require IgG and complement and may cause permanent cell damage and infiltrates. The mechanism of these reactions mediated by humoral antibodies differs completely from that of the delayed type of hypersensitivity (Chapter 11).

Bibliography

Arbesman, C. E., and Reisman, R. E.: Serum sickness and human anaphylaxis. In Samter, M. (ed.): *Immunological Diseases*, 2nd ed. Little, Brown & Co., Boston, 1971, p. 465.

Bloch, K. J.: Reaginic and other homocytotropic antibodies: diverse immunoglobulins with common function. In Goodfriend, L.; Sehon, A. H.; and Orange, R. P. (eds.): *Mechanisms in Allergy. Reaginic Mediated Hypersensitivity*. Marcel Dekker, New York, 1973.

Bryant, D. H.; Burns, M. W.; and Lazarus, L.: Identification of IgG antibody as a carrier of reaginic activity in asthmatic patients. *J. Allergy Clin. Immunol.*, **56**:417, 1975.

Cochrane, C. G.: Initiating events in immune complex injury. In Amos, B. (ed.): *Progress in Immunology*. Academic Press, Inc., New York, 1971, p. 143.

Dixon, F. J.: Experimental serum sickness. In Samter, M. (ed.): *Immunological Diseases*, 2nd ed. Little, Brown & Co., Boston, 1971, p. 253.

Ishizaka, K.: Experimental anaphylaxis. In Samter, M. (ed.): *Immunological Diseases*, 2nd ed. Little, Brown & Co., Boston, 1971, p. 202.

Ishizaka, T., and Ishizaka, K.: Biology of immunoglobulin E. In Kallos, P.; Waksman, B. H.; and DeWeck, P. (eds.): *Prog. Allergy*, 19:60–121, 1975.

Movat, H.: *Inflammation, Immunity and Hypersensitivity*. Harper & Row, Publishers, New York, 1971.

Pepys, J.: *Hypersensitivity Diseases of the Lungs Due to Fungi and Organic Dusts*. S. Karger, Basel/New York, 1969.

Plaut, M., and Lichtenstein, L. M.: Cellular and chemical basis of the allergic inflammatory response: component parts and control mechanisms. In Middleton, E.; Reed, C. E.; and Ellis, E. F. (eds.): *Allergy: Principles and Practice*. C. V. Mosby Co., St. Louis, 1977.

Rose, N. R., and Milgrom, F.: The immunological basis of hypersensitivity. *Postgrad. Med.*, 45:168–74, 1969.

Sherman, W. B.: The atopic diseases—introduction. In Samter, M. (ed.): *Immunological Diseases*, 2nd ed. Little, Brown & Co., Boston, 1971, p. 767.

19

Immune Complex Diseases

Giuseppe A. Andres

Introduction

The term "immune complex disease" characterizes experimental or spontaneous conditions in which the basic immunologic mechanism responsible for the lesions results from *in situ* formation of antigen-antibody complexes (Arthus reaction), or from deposition in various tissues of antigen-antibody complexes formed in the circulation (serum sickness).

Injection of antigen into the skin of a sensitized animal induces an edematous, hemorrhagic, and, eventually, necrotic lesion first described by Maurice Arthus in 1903. The Arthus reaction is produced by combination, within the wall of the vessels, of precipitating antibody with antigen. In experimental animals or in man, *in situ* formation of antigen-antibody complexes, with resulting Arthus-type reactions, may be the consequence of abnormal release of autologous antigens that normally do not enter the circulation in significant amounts, such as thyroglobulin or sperm constituents.

Serum sickness is the classic example of immune complex disease formed by circulating antigen-antibody complexes. The intravascular reaction of antigen with antibody forms macromolecular complexes, which, if soluble, circulate in the host, react with serum mediators and blood cells, and produce a variety of acute or chronic inflammatory lesions at the sites of

319

deposition. Serum sickness is important as a model for animal and human diseases for the following reasons: (1) The study of acute serum sickness produced by a single intravenous injection of antigen and the study of chronic serum sickness induced by prolonged daily injections of antigen show that rabbits develop glomerular diseases that cover the spectrum of the most frequent forms of human glomerulonephritides. (2) The use of isotopically labeled antigen and the fluorescent antibody technique makes it possible to demonstrate and to quantitate antigen, antibody, and complement, presumably as immune complexes in the lesions simultaneously with their development. (3) The deposition of circulating immune complexes may produce an initial injury that subsequently stimulates other pathogenetic mechanisms. (4) The formation of circulating immune complexes may be initiated by production of autoantibodies against autologous antigen present in the circulation. (5) Viral antigens may promote the formation of chronic immune complex diseases.

Pathogenicity of Antigen-Antibody Complexes

The mechanisms by which immune complexes exert their damage are only partially known. Immune complexes in moderate antigen excess are the most important for the production of inflammation in tissues because they are soluble and able to circulate. Some of their molecular characteristics have been established. (1) They are formed by antibodies fixing to the tissues and reacting with complement. (2) The properties of the antibody are more important than those of the antigen for the biologic activity of the immune complex. (3) The capacity to fix to tissues and to react with complement is localized in the Fc portion of the antibody molecule. (4) The biologic activity seems to be associated with a change in the property of optical rotation, thus suggesting an alteration of the tertiary configuration of the antibody molecule. This hypothesis is confirmed by the observation that γ globulin aggregated by heat or chemical bonding shows similar changes in optical rotation and comparable biologic activities.

At the cellular level, the immune complexes have the capacity to (1) produce degranulation of mast cells and liberate pharmacologically active substances; (2) react with leukocytes and liberate histamine, from platelets; (3) cause contraction of smooth muscles; (4) induce cellular proliferation; and (5) attract polymorphonuclear leukocytes by chemotaxis. These numerous cellular effects account for most of the lesions produced by immune complexes. The type of histologic damage, and in part the clinical symptoms of disease, are determined by the quantity and quality of immune complexes deposited in tissues, by their concentration and period of persistence in the circulation, and by the mediators of the inflammatory reaction. Small immune complexes, such as those formed by two antigen molecules and one antibody molecule (Ag_2Ab), remain in the circulation for long periods of time but do not have the ability to fix complement. Large, insoluble immune complexes formed by an excess of antibody are quickly removed from the circulation by the phagocytotic activity of the reticuloendothelial cells and do not circulate. Medium-size complexes remain in the circulation for a long period of time, fix complement, and are trapped in vascular structures with phlogogenic effects. Large concentrations of soluble immune complexes for short periods of time usually produce an accumulation of polymorphonuclear leukocytes, cellular proliferation, and necrosis. Low levels of soluble immune complexes for long periods of time favor their deposition in the walls of vessels without remarkable proliferation and exudation.

Experimental Lesions Produced by Antigen-Antibody Complexes

Arthus-Type Reaction

A vascular inflammatory reaction is produced when soluble antigen is injected locally into animals that have precipitating antibody in the circulation (active Arthus reaction). The same phenonemon can be produced when the antigen is in the circulation and the antibody is injected locally (passive Arthus reaction). The source of the antibody is not important since it can come from animals of the same or any other species. A necrotizing vasculitis results from the formation of antigen-antibody complexes within the wall of the vessels. The immune complexes react with complement and attract the polymorphonuclear leukocytes, which infiltrate the walls of the vessels and discharge lysosomal enzymes. Nitrogen mustard and specific antisera against polymorphonuclear leukocytes, which temporarily deprive animals of circulating neutrophils, prevent the development of lesions. The polymorphonuclear leukocytes phagocytize the antigen-antibody complexes and degrade them rapidly.

In situ formation of antigen-antibody complexes may be a pathogenetic feature of autoimmune thyroiditis developing in mice immunized with thyroglobulin or of autoimmune orchitis in vasectomized rabbits. In these conditions, antigen-antibody complexes are formed in the basement membranes of the thyroid, or of the testis, between antigens (thyroglobulin or sperm antigens) leaking out of tubules or follicles and antibodies coming from the circulation.

Acute Serum Sickness

Pathologic Features.   Acute serum sickness is usually produced in rabbits by a single intravenous injection of a large amount of foreign protein. The incidence of lesions is variable and mainly dependent on the differences in antibody response. The renal glomeruli, the heart (endocardium and myocardium), the spleen, the joints, and the arteries are the organs or the structures most frequently involved.

The glomerulitis is characterized by proliferation of mesangial and endothelial cells with partial or complete obliteration of capillary lumens. A small number of neutrophils may be present. Focal necrosis is rare. The lesions are irregularly distributed and heal rapidly without leaving traces of sclerosis. By electron microscopy focal electronopaque aggregates of foreign material are sometimes observed on the epithelial side of the basement membrane ("humps"). The immunofluorescence study shows fine granular deposits of antigen, antibody, and complement, presumably in the form of immune complexes, along glomerular capillary walls and in the mesangium. The deposits correspond to the electronopaque aggregates observed by electron microscopy.

In the heart, inflammatory changes of aortic and mitral valves are sometimes present together or without interstitial infiltration of mononuclear cells in the myocardium. Similar lesions may be seen in the synovial membranes. In the spleen perivascular granulomatous lesions result from accumulation of mononuclear cells and macrophages. The medium-sized muscular arteries of the kidney, heart, pancreas, and mesentery show infiltration of neutrophils, macrophages, and eosinophils and areas of fibrinoid necrosis.

Pathogenesis.   The immunologic events that characterize the pathogenesis of acute serum sickness can be studied in rabbits injected with radiolabeled bovine serum albumin (BSA) (Figure 19-1). The serum level of BSA declines in three phases. In the first phase, the level of BSA rapidly falls as the antigen equilibrates between intra- and extravascular spaces. Then follows a slow, nonimmune decline lasting a little more than a week, reflecting the catabolism of the protein. The third phase persists two or three days and is characterized by rapid elimination of the antigen from the circulation as a consequence of antibody production and formation of immune complexes (immune elimination). The first immune complexes to be formed are small, because they are in extreme antigen excess, and remain in the circulation for a prolonged period of time. As more antibody becomes available, the immune complexes enlarge and their proportion of antibody increases. They react with complement, as demonstrated by an abrupt drop of serum complement level, and produce acute proliferative and exudative lesions at the sites of localization. Finally, the immune complexes become so large that they are rapidly removed from the circulation by reticuloendothelial cells. Following elimination of the antigen, free antibody appears in the circulation.

The severity of glomerulitis is usually related to the rapidity of immune elimination and to the amount of antigen deposited in the glomeruli. After immune elimination, the amount of BSA detectable in glomeruli by immuno-

I°BSA Elimination-Circulating BSA Anti-BSA Complexes: Dev. of Lesions

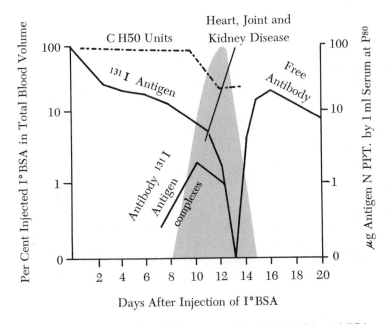

Figure 19-1. The elimination curve of circulating BSA–anti-BSA complexes in a rabbit injected with ^{131}I-labeled BSA. With the disappearance of Ag-Ab-Cx in the circulation there is a decrease of C level and development of morphologic lesions. After elimination of Ag-Ab-Cx, free Ab appears in the circulation and the inflammatory lesions rapidly heal. (From Dixon, F. J.: The role of antigen-antibody complexes in disease. *Harvey Lect.*, **58**:21–52, 1963.)

fluorescence decreases, whereas host immunoglobulins and complement increase. This is, at least in part, due to a progressive direct localization of circulating antibody on free antigenic sites of immune complexes already localized in the glomerular capillary. The phenomenon is dependent on glomerular filtration and terminates when substitution of low-affinity antibody with high-affinity antibody is complete and the latter saturates all available antigenic sites. The resulting formation of insoluble complexes in high-antibody excess corresponds to healing of glomerular lesions. Therefore, circulating complexes formed initially in antigen excess are nephritogenic, whereas subsequent accumulation of immunoglobulins and complement in extravascular sites does not continue to produce glomerular injury.

Three main factors influence the localization of complexes in vascular structures. The first, already mentioned, is the physiopathologic property of the tissues. Thus, the greatest amount of complexes is deposited in the glomeruli, and mainly in the glomerular mesangium, owing to the rich renal blood flow and the filtering function of the glomerulus and the marked phagocytic activity of mesangial cells. The focal and irregular deposits within the walls of arteries and veins are probably favored by a local increase in permeability induced by spasm. The second factor is the size of the immune complexes. Only complexes of 19 S or greater are entrapped in the vessel wall. Finally, release during immune elimination of vasoactive substances that increase vascular permeability greatly facilitates the deposition of immune complexes. Histamine and serotonin are released in large part from platelets, and platelet depletion or antagonists of histamine and serotonin interfere with the development of lesions. In acute serum sickness, the immunologic release of vasoactive amines from platelets requires the presence of sensitized leukocytes and of the antigen (leukocyte-dependent histamine release). After appearance of antigen-antibody complex in the circulation, there is formation of IgE antibody, which binds to the surface of basophils. When these sensitized cells combine with the specific antigen, they give off a soluble factor that induces platelet aggregation and release of their vasoactive amines. Immunologic mechanisms of histamine release dependent on complement do not seem equally essential.

Two host factors that may be involved in the lesions of acute serum sickness are the polymorphonuclear leukocytes (Chapter 10) and complement (Chapter 8). Immunofluorescence studies show presence of complement in the lesions. One way in which complement mediates the damage is by chemotactic attraction of polymorphonuclear leukocytes. This effect depends on formation of a C5,6,7 complex. The polymorphonuclear leukocytes, however, do not have a prominent role. The occurrence of transient glomerulitis in rabbits deprived of polymorphonuclear leukocytes suggests that the latter injury is mainly the result of the brief action of pharmacologic agents.

Finally, in the most severe forms of acute serum sickness the formation of antigen-antibody complex in the circulation may produce intravascular coagulation leading to the deposition of fibrinogen products within vascular structures. This effect could involve platelets since immune complexes promote clotting of platelet-rich plasma.

Chronic Serum Sickness

Pathologic Features.   The most reproducible model of chronic serum sickness is that induced in rabbits by repeated intravenous injections of a foreign protein over a long period of time. The rabbits develop proteinuria, hypoproteinemia, and elevated serum cholesterol and urea levels. The most common lesion is membranous glomerulonephritis characterized by thickening of glomerular capillary walls with little or no cell proliferation. As the disease progresses, proliferation of mesangial cells and sclerosis become more evident. By electron microscopy diffuse electronopaque aggregates of foreign material are seen on the epithelial side of the basement membrane, corresponding to the granular deposits of antigen, immunoglobulins, and complement visualized with the immunofluorescence technique. The subepithelial deposits may persist for a long period of time, or even increase, after cessation of antigen injection.

The majority of the immune complex deposits occur in renal glomeruli. However, in some rabbits, particularly those with active immune responses requiring correspondingly large amounts of antigen injected in multiple daily doses, extraglomerular (tubular basement membranes) and extrarenal immune deposits may occur as well. These rabbits develop a systemic immune complex disease involving lung, spleen, heart, choroid plexus, gastrointestinal tract, and serous membranes.

Pathogenesis. The most important pathogenetic factors in chronic serum sickness are the quantity and the quality of immune response. Rabbits immunized with foreign proteins may be divided into three main groups according to their antibody production. The first includes animals that are vigorous producers of precipitating antibody. They may develop a rapidly resolving acute glomerulitis in the first week. Then, as soon as the rabbits have made sufficient antibody to achieve permanent antibody excess, the antigen is quickly removed from the circulation in the form of insoluble antigen-antibody aggregates. The majority of these animals do not develop chronic lesions. Only a few may show mesangial proliferation as a consequence of glomerular deposition of insoluble immune complexes (pages 330–35). The rabbits of the second group are immunologically tolerant and do not develop disease. The fate of the antigen is no different from that of rabbit albumin. The third group includes rabbits that form an amount of antibody too small to cause precipitation of the antigen but sufficient to result in formation of circulating immune complex. In the greatest majority of these rabbits, immune complexes are present in the circulation throughout much of the time and chronic membranous glomerulonephritis does occur.

Studies performed with radiolabeled antigen (BSA) show that the amount of antigen deposited in the glomeruli and the severity of the lesions are usually proportional to the amount of antigen injected. Before the onset of proteinuria the amount of antigen deposited in the glomeruli is relatively small and mainly localized in the mesangial area. Two to three weeks after the beginning of the injections, at the onset of proteinuria, the mechanism of mesangial phagocytosis is apparently overcome and the amount of antigen deposited in the glomeruli increases. In the same period, the immune complexes accumulate in the peripheral capillary walls producing functional injury.

The size of the immune complexes and the quality of the antibody are important factors in the pathogenesis of chronic serum sickness. The immune complexes deposited in the glomerular capillary walls are 19 S or greater. Rabbits producing precipitating antibody seem to develop more consistent and severe lesions. However, other studies show that chronic serum sickness is frequent also in rabbits producing nonprecipitating antibody. Antigens with low valences fail to precipitate with antibodies. Therefore, it is possible that the rabbits that recognize only a limited number of antigenic sites present in the multivalent foreign protein may produce nonprecipitating antibody. The recognition of only a few sites would not allow the formation of a complex lattice, and the complexes would persist in the circulation and exert vascular damage.

Complement factors participate in the production of injury in chronic serum sickness. It is known from immunofluorescence study that complement is seen in both chronic and acute serum sickness (Chapter 8). But in chronic serum sickness the polymorphonuclear leukocytes may subsequently release hydrolytic enzymes from their lysosomes with phlogogenic effects.

An efficient pathogenetic mechanism of perpetuating disease, which does not depend on further glomerular localization of circulating immune complexes, is that of continuous exchange of either antigen or antibody within immune complexes already fixed in glomerular structures. Studies performed with radiolabeled antigen and antibody show that during chronic serum sickness the immune complexes deposited in glomeruli have free antigen and/or antibody valences capable of binding large amounts of circulating antigen or antibody during periods of antigen or antibody excess, respectively. In such pathologic conditions the entrapped complexes behave like immunoadsorbents, which fix antigen or antibody molecules that pass through the glomerular capillary walls during filtration. This alternate pathogenetic pathway explains why it is possible to stop the progression of chronic serum sickness glomerulitis, or to ameliorate its course, by maintaining a large and constant excess of circulating antigen.

The circulating immune complexes have no immunologic relationship to the tissues that they damage. The factors that predispose to their localization are mainly nonimmunologic. The characteristic accumulation of immune complexes on the epithelial side of the glomerular basement membrane is probably determined by the physiopathologic properties of the capillary wall. Polysaccharides, like glycosaminoglycans of basement membranes, enhance the precipitation of antigen-antibody complex *in vitro* because the latter are sterically excluded from the polysaccharides. The two main parameters that influence the solubility of immune complexes in the presence of polysaccharides are the molecular size of the proteins and the concentration of the polysaccharides. It is possible that similar mechanisms may cause precipitation of immune complexes *in vivo*. It may also be that the immune complexes, while traversing the basement membrane, may become less soluble and tend to aggregate as a result of the reduction of antigen excess in the environment. The subepithelial deposits are then sequestered from the phagocytic activity of the polymorphonuclear leukocytes and may interfere with the secretory activity of the epithelial cells, which normally provide some components to the maintenance of glomerular basement membrane.

In a minority of rabbits producing large amounts of antibody, it is possible to observe focal glomerular lesions characterized by hypercellularity, sinechiae, increase in mesangial matrix, and glomerulosclerosis. In these animals the condition of antibody excess may lead to intermittent formation of insoluble immune complexes in the circulation. Intravenous injection of antigen into hyperimmunized rabbits produces formation of large insoluble precipitates in the lumens of pulmonary and glomerular capillaries. Since fibrinogen products are demonstrable in glomerular lesions by immuno-fluorescence, it is possible that the coagulation process may also play a role in this less frequent glomerulonephritis mediated by insoluble immune complexes.

Autologous Immune Complex Disease

Rats injected intraperitoneally with homologous kidney in Freund's adjuvant develop immune complex glomerulonephritis. This disease is known as "autologous nonglomerular immune complex glomerulonephritis" in order to distinguish it from other forms of autoimmune glomerulonephri-tides. The immune complexes are formed in the circulation between auto-antibodies and an antigenic fraction contained in the brush border of the proximal convoluted tubules. Gamma globulins eluted from the diseased glomeruli react with the brush border of the proximal convoluted tubules but not with the glomeruli. When human tubular material is used as in antigen, the greatest part of the antigen present in the glomerular lesions is of rat origin. It seems, therefore, that the autoantibody, whose formation is elicited by the cross-reacting human tubular antigen, combines in the circulation with autologous antigen continuously released from the brush border. The histology (Figure 19-2) resembles that of human membranous glomerulonephritis. There is diffuse thickening of glomerular capillary walls with little or no cellular proliferation. Immunoglobulins (Chapter 4) and complement (Chapter 8) are distributed in a granular manner along glomerular capillary walls and diffuse subepithelial deposits are observed by electron microscopy. Since the disease persists indefinitely, even without continuous injection of antigen, it must be assumed that the original stimula-tion set in motion a persistent production of autoantibody.

Other antigens have been used for the production of autologous immune complex disease, and thyroglobulin appears to be the most effective. The requirements essential for the induction of autologous immune complex glomerulonephritis are (1) that the antigen is capable of eliciting formation of autoantibody, and (2) that the antigen is present in small amounts in the circulation.

Chronic Allogenic Disease

A membranous glomerulonephritis with the immunohistologic features of chronic immune complex disease develops in F_1 hybrid mice injected with parental spleen cells. It appears likely that this disease is induced by a graft-vs.-host reaction (Chapter 23) leading to glomerular deposition of immune

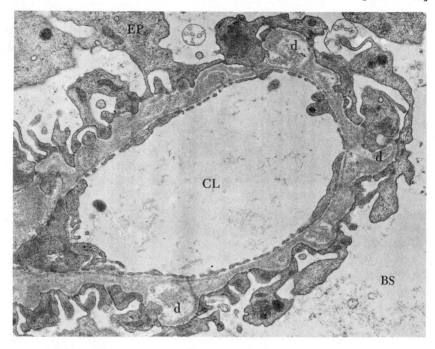

Figure 19-2. Autologous nonglomerular ICx glomerulonephritis in a rat. Deposits (*d*) of immunoglobulins are present on the epithelial (*EP*) side of the basement membrane. *CL*, capillary lumen; *BS*, Bowman's space. × 5600.

complexes containing transplantation antigens provided by the host, specific transplantation antibodies produced by the donor's cells, and complement.

Immune Complex Diseases Associated with Viral Infections in Animals

Viral immune complex diseases may be experimentally produced or may develop spontaneously in animals. Mice infected at birth with lymphocytic choriomeningitis virus develop glomerular lesions with accumulation of viral protein, specific antibody, and complement in the glomerular capillary walls (Figure 19-3). The tissues of such animals contain large amounts of infectious virus whereas circulating antibodies are not readily detectable. Therefore, it was thought that these animals were "tolerant" to viral antigens. During viral infection, circulating soluble viral antigens stimulate the production of a small amount of antibody. The resulting immune complexes tend to accumulate in glomerular structures, where they produce

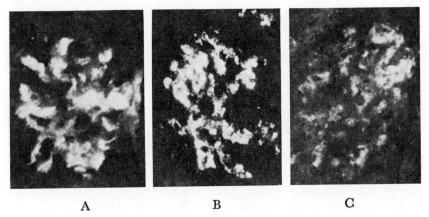

A B C

Figure 19-3. Localization of fluorescent Ab to mouse immuno-globulins (*A*), mouse C3 (*B*), and lymphocytic choriomeningitis virus (*C*) in the glomerular capillary walls and in the mesangium of a mouse neonatally infected with lymphocytic choriomeningitis virus. × 120.

injury. This experimental model shows that glomerular deposition of immune complexes may be the only detectable evidence of immune disease. In addition, a pathologic process may result from vascular deposition of immune complexes derived from an infectious agent that is not directly injurious to the tissues.

A second type of immune complex disease related to viral infection is that of New Zealand black (NZB) and white (NZW) mice and their hybrids (NZB/W) (Chapter 25). These animals have several immunologic peculiarities associated with the occurrence of immune complex glomerulonephritis and, less frequently, hemolytic anemia and lymphoma. The glomerulonephritis results from the apparent association of murine leukemia virus (Gross virus) with an autoimmune response to mouse nuclear antigens. The fatal membranous and proliferative glomerulonephritis that develops in the majority of NZB/W mice is characterized by granular deposition of immune complexes in glomerular structures. The antigens that have been identified in the lesions are native and denatured DNA, viral antigens, RNA, and antigens of the erythrocytes. Studies on eluates obtained from nephritic kidneys indicate that the antibodies reactive with nuclear antigens account for almost half of the eluted IgG, whereas antibodies reactive with Gross virus antigen are present in a significant but lesser amount (especially in the male). In NZB/W mice, a neonatal infection with either lymphocytic choriomeningitis (an RNA virus) or polyoma (a DNA virus) greatly enhances antinuclear response and the severity of nephritis. It is possible that the viral infection may accelerate cell breakdown, thus increasing the degree of exposure to the antigen and the consequent formation of immune complexes.

Other examples of viral immune complex diseases in animals are Aleutian disease of mink, lactic dehydrogenase virus infection of mice, oncornavirus, polyoma, Coxsackievirus B, cytomegalovirus infections, equine infectious anemia, and hog cholera (Chapter 15).

Immune Complexes in Human Diseases

Serum Sickness

Acute serum sickness was a frequent event when large amounts of foreign serum were used for the treatment of pneumonia, diphtheria, tetanus, and other diseases. A mild proteinuria was sometimes observed. Today, acute serum sickness is a rare, benign disease. Glomerular deposition of circulating antigen-antibody complexes has been observed in patients treated with large amounts of horse antihuman lymphocyte globulin.

Glomerulonephritis

On the basis of immunofluorescence study of renal tissues obtained from patients with glomerulonephritis, it seems that deposition of circulating nonglomerular antigen-antibody complex is the pathogenetic mechanism most frequently responsible for this disease. The antigens involved in most cases are unknown.

In *systemic lupus erythematosus glomerulonephritis* nuclear antigens are clearly implicated in a manner that mimics the disease of the New Zealand mice. DNA has been shown in the circulation of patients who, at other times, had antibody to DNA. Moreover, DNA has been found in the glomerular lesions together with specific antibody and complement. The immunopathologic findings are comparable to those of experimental chronic serum sickness (Figure 19-4). The presence of increased titers of serum antibodies to viruses and the observation of endothelial structures similar to nucleoprotein strands of myxovirus have raised the hypothesis that also in human systemic lupus erythematosus a viral infection may influence the development of the disease (Chapter 25).

In *malaria glomerulonephritis* there is evidence that exogenous antigen of *Plasmodium malariae*, specific antibodies, and complement are deposited in glomerular lesions, thereby producing membranous and proliferative changes. Although most of the patients have blood smears positive for *P. malariae*, the presence of the antigen in glomerular deposits can be demonstrated only in a minority of cases (Chapter 16).

Clinical, bacteriologic, and epidemiologic data support the view that *acute poststreptococcal glomerulonephritis* is a disease due to hypersensitivity to certain types of group A hemolytic streptococci. The immunopathologic

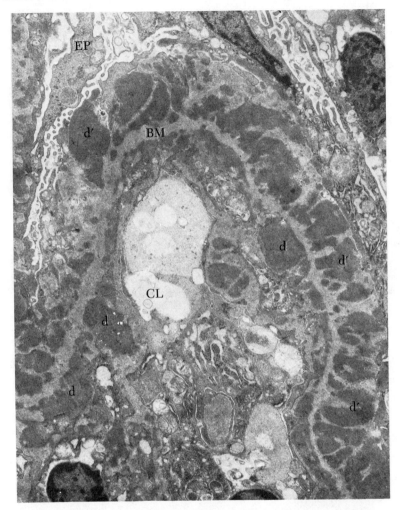

Figure 19-4. Electronopaque deposits localized on the epithelial (*d*) and endothelial (*d'*) sides of the glomerular basement membrane (*BM*) in a patient with SLE membranous glomerulonephritis. × 6400.

lesions of glomeruli resemble those of acute serum sickness. Granular deposits of immunoglobulins and complement (Figure 19-5) are present along glomerular capillary walls, corresponding to the focal subepithelial deposits seen by electron microscopy ("humps") (Figure 19-6). In rare, severe cases in which the renal tissue was obtained at the beginning of the disease, antistreptococcal sera reacted with glomerular structures. Also, γ globulins obtained from patients weeks after development of acute post-streptococcal glomerulonephritis seem to bind in the glomeruli from early biopsies. However, in the great majority of patients, streptococcal antigens

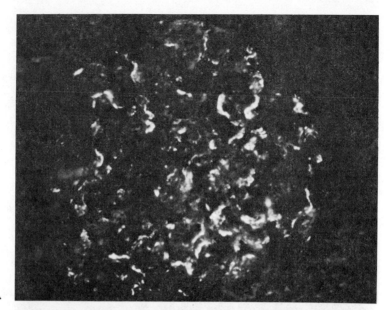

A

B

Figure 19-5. *A.* Focal, granular staining of glomerular capillary walls with fluorescent antibody to human C3 in a patient with acute poststreptococcal glomerulonephritis. × 160.

B. Immunofluorescent staining of a glomerulus from a rat with nephrotoxic nephritis. The nephrotoxic rabbit antirat kidney serum localizes in the glomerular basement membranes in a characteristic continuous linear form, different from the irregular and granular staining visible in glomerular pathology produced by circulating Ag-Ab-Cx. × 160.

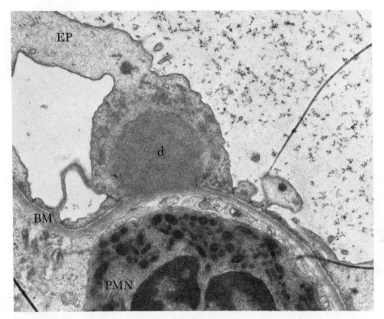

Figure 19-6. Focal deposit ("humps") (*d*) between the epithelial cytoplasm (*EP*) and the basement membrane (*BM*) in the glomerulus of a patient with acute poststreptococcal glomerulonephritis. *PMN*, polymorphonuclear leukocyte. × 5600.

are not detectable. Therefore, the precise etiology of poststreptococcal glomerulonephritis is still not clear (Chapter 13).

Membranous glomerulonephritis is a disease frequently responsible for nephrotic syndrome in adults. The glomerular capillary walls are thickened because large deposits containing immunoglobulins and complement are present between the basement membrane and the epithelial cytoplasm (Figures 19-7 and 19-8). There are scarce proliferation and exudation, at least in the initial phase. These findings are similar to those in autologous nonglomerular immune complex glomerulonephritis. Since there is no evidence of an exogenous stimulus, the most probable hypothesis is that membranous glomerulonephritis results from a prolonged exposure to circulating antigen-antibody complexes, containing unknown autologous antigens.

Hypocomplementemic membranoproliferative glomerulonephritis is a severe disease characterized by persistently low levels of serum complement and by fairly uniform proliferation of mesangial cells, which induces "splitting" of glomerular basement membranes and obliteration of capillary lumens. The membranous lesions are due to subendothelial deposits containing immunoglobulins and complement, or complement alone. In the serum of the patients a factor that can activate complement components from C3 onward (C3 nephritic factor) has been isolated (Chapter 8). This factor might be a complement inhibitor or a complex of antibody and complement. Properdin,

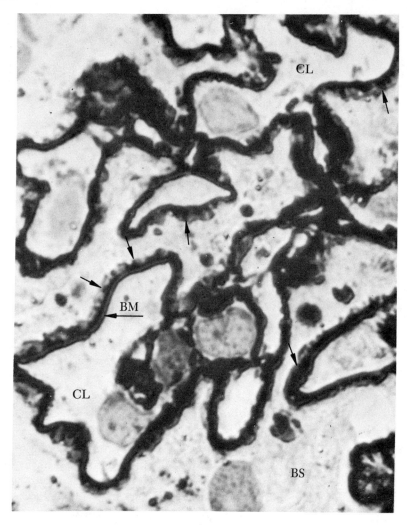

Figure 19-7. Thickening of glomerular capillary walls in a patient with membranous glomerulonephritis. Silver-positive deposits (arrows) are present on the epithelial side of glomerular basement membrane (*BM*). *CL*, capillary lumen; *BS*, Bowman's space. Silver-methenamine staining. × 1600.

which is frequently localized in glomerular lesions together with C3, could also participate in the activation of complement. Therefore, the nephritic factor or properdin may initiate an inflammatory reaction at C3, providing an alternative pathway that circumvents the need of immune complexes in the genesis of membranoproliferative glomerulonephritis.

In patients with *cancer* of the bronchi or in patients with persistent *Australia antigenemia* following posttransfusion hepatitis, the underlying glomerulo-

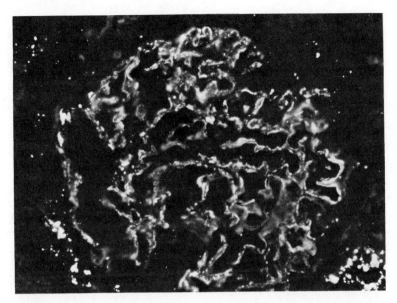

Figure 19-8. Granular localization of fluorescent antibody to human IgG in the glomerular capillary wall of a patient with membranous glomerulonephritis. × 160.

nephritides seem to be produced by antigen-antibody complexes. Australia antigen, or tumor-associated (specific) antigens, have been demonstrated in the glomerular lesions together with immunoglobulins and complement.

Another condition in which circulating antigen-antibody complexes may be associated with glomerular lesions is *idiopathic mixed cryoglobulinemia*. The immune complexes are presumably composed of IgM antibodies combined with altered IgG. Such patients may develop a glomerulonephritis with granular deposits of IgM and IgG in glomeruli (Chapter 17).

Periarteritis Nodosa

Periarteritis nodosa appears to be induced by a hypersensitivity reaction similar to acute serum sickness. The main evidence is represented by the histologic similarity. The clinical picture of periarteritis nodosa, however, is quite different because it follows a severe and progressive course. In some instances, allergic reactions to drugs have been of etiologic importance. More recently in patients with periarteritis nodosa, immune complexes containing Australia antigen have been demonstrated in the circulation and in the arterial lesions.

Rheumatoid Arthritis

Immune complexes, or factors with immunologic properties of immune complexes, have been detected in rheumatoid synovial fluids with the aid of several techniques. The present available data suggest that in the rheumatoid joints immune complexes activate the complement sequence, generating a variety of biologically active materials, some of which are chemotactic for the polymorphonuclear leukocytes. The leukocytes ingest the immune complexes and release hydrolytic enzymes from their lysosomal granules. These inflammatory enzymes appear to be the direct cause of proliferative and degenerative changes in synovial membranes.

Renal Allografts

After grafting, there is a release of histocompatibility antigens into the circulation and formation of cytotoxic antibody. Immune complexes containing histocompatibility antigens, specific antibody, and complement could be implicated in chronic rejection of renal allografts in patients treated with immunosuppressive agents. However, immunohistologic changes compatible with chronic serum sickness are rarely observed in glomerular structures of patients whose original disease was not glomerulonephritis. Definite demonstration of histocompatibility antigens and specific antibodies in glomerular lesions has not yet been reported. Therefore, this problem must be considered unresolved.

Bibliography

Andres, G. A.; Seegal, B. C.; Hsu, K. C.; Rothenberg, M. S.; and Chapeau, M. L.: Electron microscopic studies of experimental nephritis with ferritin-conjugated antibody: localization of antigen-antibody complexes in rabbit glomeruli following repeated injections of bovine serum albumin. *J. Exp. Med.*, **117**:691–704, 1963.

Bigazzi, P. E.; Kosuda, L. L.; Hsu, K. C.; and Andres, G. A.: Immune complex orchitis in vasectomized rabbits. *J. Exp. Med.*, **143**:382, 1976.

Clagett, J. A.; Wilson, C. B.; and Weigle, W. O.: Interstitial immune complex thyroiditis in mice. *J. Exp. Med.*, **140**:1439, 1974.

Cochrane, C. G.: Mechanisms involved in the deposition of immune complexes in tissues. *J. Exp. Med.*, **134**:75x–89x, 1971.

Dixon, F. J.: The role of antigen-antibody complexes in disease. *Harvey Lect.*, **58**:21–52, 1963.

Dixon, F. J.; Feldman, J. D.; and Vazquez, J. J.: Experimental glomerulonephritis: the pathogenesis of a laboratory model resembling the spectrum of human glomerulonephritis. *J. Exp. Med.*, **113**:899–920, 1961.

Koffler, D.; Schur, P. H.; and Kunkel, H. G.: Immunological studies concerning the nephritis of systemic lupus erythematosus. *J. Exp. Med.*, **126**:607–24, 1967.

Lewis, R. M.; Armstrong, M. Y. K.; André-Schwartz, J.; Muftuoglu, A.; Beldotti, L.; and Schwartz, R. S.: Chronic allogenic disease. I. Development of glomerulonephritis. *J. Exp. Med.*, **128**:653–79, 1968.

McCluskey, R. T., and Vassalli, P.: Serum sickness (immune complex disease). In Movat, H. Z. (ed.): *Inflammation, Immunity and Hypersensitivity.* Harper & Row, Publishers, New York, 1971, pp. 426–57.

McCluskey, R. T.; Vassalli, P.; Gallo, G.; and Baldwin, D. S.: An immunofluorescent study of pathogenetic mechanisms in glomerular diseases. *N. Engl. J. Med.,* **274**:695–701, 1966.

Wilson, C. B., and Dixon, F. J.: Quantitation of acute and chronic serum sickness in the rabbit. *J. Exp. Med.,* **134**:7s–18s, 1971.

20

Blood Groups

JAMES F. MOHN

Introduction

For blood transfusion to have become the practical, therapeutic reality it is today, two major obstacles had to be surmounted. The resolution of these problems led to the development of our modern system of blood banking with the ready availability of well-preserved, stored blood that has made possible new remedial measures such as hemodialysis and exchange transfusion and, in conjunction with advances in anesthesiology, great surgical progress permitting radical extirpative treatment of malignant tumors, open cardiac surgery, and renal and other organ transplants, to list but a few examples. These hindrances could be generically categorized as (1) immunologic—unfavorable reactions caused by any incompatibility between the blood of a recipient and that of a donor had to be recognized and understood, and (2) biochemical—difficulties caused by coagulation of donor blood had to be prevented by perfection of techniques and equipment and especially by the development of nontoxic anticoagulants. Only the immunologic question will be dealt with here, limited to the two blood group systems of major clinical importance.

All the early attempts at intravenous transfusion in man toward the end of the seventeenth century consisted exclusively in the use of animal blood such as that of lambs and dogs, frequently resulting in distressing and even fatal consequences to the unfortunate recipients. This undesirable reaction was apprehended two centuries later in 1875 when Landois observed that agglutination of the erythrocytes of one animal species usually occurred when they were mixed *in vitro* with the serum of another species. The fundamental concept embodied in this discovery was the inference that this hemagglutination was due to the presence of antigens on the red cell surface interacting with serum antibodies. Of almost equal importance, this finding established the species specificity of the erythrocytic elements of blood.

Twenty-five years later Karl Landsteiner first noted similar agglutination of human red blood cells by human sera, a totally intraspecies reaction. Based on the hemagglutination patterns he obtained when blood specimens from five of his colleagues and himself were examined in a cross-hatch experiment where each serum was mixed separately with each saline cell suspension, he divided these test samples, and subsequently the blood of all humans, into three distinct serologic groups. He was fully cognizant of the important role blood group antigenic differences played in blood transfusion and used this information in laying the foundation for safe transfusion practice.

Perhaps of even greater importance than the practical application of this knowledge in reducing sharply the immunologic hazard, thus establishing firmly the prospect of blood transfusion as a potential, invaluable addition to the physician's armamentarium, this discovery of the human blood groups represents the origin of a new immunologic principle or antigenic system, called isospecificity (*isos*, Greek—equal). It is based on the existence of different antigens occurring within a single animal species, isoantigens, and their corresponding, specific antibodies, isoagglutinins, with their interaction resulting in the phenomenon of isoagglutination. In the case of the blood groups, since erythrocytes are involved, it is often referred to as isohemagglutination.*

The fourth and rarest group in this ABO blood group system was discovered in 1902 by von Decastello and Sturli, Landsteiner's pupils and associates.

Almost 40 years followed with little enlargement of our knowledge of erythrocytic antigens, except for the initial descriptions of the basic antigens in the MN and P blood group systems by Landsteiner and Levine in 1927. These two systems had no impact on the practice of blood transfusion. It appeared that the ABO blood groups were the only ones of any clinical importance. Then in 1939, Levine and Stetson reported their serologic findings in the case of a secundiparous woman who experienced an almost fatal hemolytic reaction following the transfusion of blood donated by her husband to compensate for her postpartum hemorrhaging when she delivered prematurely a stillborn fetus. Their careful examination revealed

---

* The prefix *iso-* used in this chapter has been replaced in most fields of immunology by *allo-*.

that the husband's red cells actually were not compatible with his wife's serum prior to the transfusion and that her serum in addition to reacting with his erythrocytes agglutinated those of approximately 77% (80/104) of ABO compatible donors. Since this mother had never been transfused previously and did possess antibodies capable of reacting with her husband's cells prior to receiving his blood, they postulated that as she lacked this new antigen, which they failed to name, she had been immunized by the red cells of her fetus, which contained this antigen because it was inherited from the father. Thus, these antibodies in the mother's serum reacted with this same antigen on the father's cells when she was transfused with his blood.

The following year, Landsteiner and Wiener published the results of their experimental studies on the immunization of rabbits with the red cells of *Macacus rhesus* monkeys. The antisera produced not only agglutinated the erythrocytes of the monkeys tested, as might have been anticipated, but also remarkably the red cells of about 85% of the human samples of Caucasian origin, which they subsequently called Rh positive, the 15% that failed to react, Rh negative. The direct implication of this observation in clinical medicine followed in the same year when Wiener and Peters showed unequivocally that the reactions in three cases of homospecific ABO group transfusions were caused by anti-Rh antibodies probably produced in these Rh negative recipients by previous transfusions of presumably Rh positive donor blood.

Shortly thereafter, in comparative examinations employing the same set of randomly selected human blood specimens, the antibodies in the serum of Levine and Stetson's original case seemed to be indistinguishable from the anti-Rh antibodies produced in rabbits injected with rhesus monkey red blood cells. With this apparent identity of the fetal antigen (hypothesized to have produced antibodies by active immunization of the mother) to the Rh antigen, Levine, Burnham, Katzin, and Vogel, based on their determinations of the Rh groups and detection of anti-Rh antibodies in an extensive examination of 350 cases, demonstrated that erythroblastosis fetalis, now more properly referred to as hemolytic disease of the newborn, was directly related to fetomaternal Rh incompatibility. It was statistically significant that in this series 90% of mothers with children so afflicted were Rh negative whereas 100% of the fathers and living children so afflicted were Rh positive in contrast to the random, normal Caucasian population distribution of 85% Rh positive and 15% Rh negative.

The discovery of the Rh blood group system had an enormous influence not only on the field of human blood groups but on immunology in general because (1) isoimmunization within a blood group system was established as the cause of some hemolytic transfusion reactions and (2) isoimmunization of pregnancy was demonstrated to be the cause of hemolytic disease of the newborn, which very often involves the Rh blood group system.

Since 1940 our knowledge of the human blood groups has increased at a great rate and several other systems are of clinical importance. The presently

Table 20-1
HUMAN BLOOD GROUP SYSTEMS

Year Discovered	System	Common Antigens or Groups
1900	ABO	A_1, A_2, B, O
1927	MNSs	M, N, S, s
1927	P	P_1, P^k
1939	Rh	D, C, c, E, e
1945	Lutheran	Lu^a, Lu^b
1946	Kell	K, k
1946	Lewis	Le^a, Le^b
1950	Duffy	Fy^a, Fy^b
1951	Kidd	Jk^a, Jk^b
1954	Diego	Di^a, Di^b
1956	Cartwright	Yt^a, Yt^b
1956	I	I, i
1962	Xg	Xg^a
1965	Dombrock	Do^a, Do^b
1965	Colton	Co^a, Co^b

accepted, distinctly separate systems, together with some of their common antigens or groups, are shown in Table 20-1.

The discovery of "new" antigens on human erythrocytes can be achieved only when the equivalent, specific antibodies become available. The three main reasons for the rapid strides in our acquisition of information on the human blood groups are as follows: (1) The etiologic linking of the Rh antigen with hemolytic disease of the newborn led to the establishment of prenatal testing with the resultant examination of many thousands of blood specimens that previously never would have reached a laboratory. (2) The increasing use of whole blood or packed red cell transfusions, routinely given in multiple units of two or more and often repeatedly to the same patient, coupled with more intense study of the occasional reactions resulting therefrom has provided new antisera. (3) Advances in blood group serologic techniques, especially in the development of methods for detecting antigen-antibody reactions not necessarily or regularly resulting directly in agglutination, because the antibodies are primarily of the sensitizing or coating variety, so-called incomplete antibodies, particularly the introduction of the antiglobulin test, have permitted many antibodies resulting from isoimmunization, produced either by transfusion or pregnancy, to be more readily detectable or even detectable at all.

Landsteiner had hoped that one day blood groups would distinguish one person from another just as fingerprints now do. At his death in 1943 four blood group systems existed whereas today at least 15 are recognized. In the diagnostic laboratory of a large hospital blood bank, approximately 13,000 different phenotypic combinations could be recognized using the common, commercially available blood group antisera. Employing all the specific blood group antisera currently known, a collection including some great rarities generally available only in a few, specialized, blood group research centers, at least 300,000 different phenotypic combinations could be demonstrated. There is no doubt that the ability to identify individuals by their blood group or hemagglutinogen patterns exists and is becoming increasingly practicable.

ABO Blood Groups

Basic Properties or Characteristics

The four groups are based on the presence of two different antigens on the red blood cell membranes and two corresponding antibodies in the sera. The erythrocytic agglutinogens are named A and B. They are fully potent antigens capable of both iso- and heteroimmunization. The agglutinins (or lysins) in the serum (plasma) are referred to as anti-A, those specific for the A antigen, and anti-B, those specific for the B antigen. These antibodies belong to both the IgM and IgG immunoglobulin classes, predominantly to the former but the so-called immune variety particularly to the latter. Either variety is capable of binding complement both *in vitro* and *in vivo* and consequently can produce intravascular hemolysis under the appropriate incompatibility conditions within this system. The composition of these groups with respect to both the red blood cell and the serum properties is shown in Table 20-2.

According to Landsteiner's quite inflexible law, mutually exclusive opposites (antigens and antibodies) *must* always be present. It should be stressed that this refers only to adults and infants over three to six months of age but never to newborn infants. Examples of adults lacking the expected anti-A or/and anti-B agglutinins are extremely rare and usually represent some fascinating phenomenon when properly investigated and identified. They may be instances of agammaglobulinemia or hypogammaglobulinemia, of chimerism, of dispermy or the first indication of one of the rare variants of blood group A such as the A_x, A_{bantu}, A_{end}, A_{finn}, A_{el}, or A_m phenotypes. Whenever the expected agglutinins are not present, blood and saliva speciment from the propositus and his family should be examined.

Table 20-2
SEROLOGIC PROPERTIES OF THE ABO GROUPS

Group	Erythrocytic Antigens	Serum Antibodies
O	—	Anti-A and anti-B
A	A	Anti-B
B	B	Anti-A
AB	A and B	—

Determinations

In testing for a person's ABO group, it is imperative that both the cell and the serum properties be determined. It is customary, first, to examine for the antigenic characteristics of the erythrocytes and then to confirm them independently by testing the serum for its agglutinin content.

The reagents used in testing the red cell suspensions are monospecific antisera of human origin, anti-A from a group B donor and anti-B from a group A donor. Such antisera of sufficient titer and potency to pass the government licensing standards are obtained exclusively from volunteers stimulated by injections of small amounts of A or B specific substances of porcine and equine origins, respectively.

The test cells employed in detecting the agglutinins in the serum confirmation or serum check phase consist of saline suspensions of known group A and group B erythrocytes. Separate suspensions of subgroup A_1 and A_2 red cells are superior to a single suspension of pooled group A cells. The former may provide the first clue to the existence of one of the uncommon group A variant bloods.

Incidence and Racial Distribution

The frequencies of these four ABO groups in North America among persons of Caucasian and Negro ancestry are as follows:

	Whites	Blacks
O	43 to 47%	48 to 53%
A	38 to 41%	24 to 28%
B	9 to 13%	17 to 23%
AB	3 to 5%	3 to 4%

The frequencies found among populations native to widely separated geographic areas provided another application of these blood groups to an entirely different science, physical anthropology. The impetus for this came in 1919 from the pioneering investigations of the Hirszfelds, who first established that the distribution of the ABO blood groups varied from one population to another. They found that the frequencies were related to a certain extent to geographic locations; the frequency of the A antigen decreased from west to east as that of the B antigen increased. To classify the various populations studied, they proposed a "biochemical index" as an expression of the ratio of A to B antigen. This consisted of the sum of the frequencies of groups A and AB divided by the corresponding sum of groups B and AB in the formula $I = (A + AB)/(B + AB)$. Employing this formula, they distinguished three groups:

European	$I = \geqslant 2.5$
Intermediate	$I = 1.3$ to 1.8
Asio-African	$I = \leqslant 1.0$

Table 20-3

EXAMPLES OF ABO BLOOD GROUP FREQUENCIES

Group	Distribution (%)					
	U.S. WHITES	POLISH	TADZHIKS	SIAMESE	JAPANESE	BANTU
O	43–47	33.1	29.7	35.0	47.3	47.9
A	38–41	39.3	29.3	18.8	12.7	24.3
B	9–13	19.1	31.5	40.2	38.7	24.7
AB	3–5	8.5	9.5	6.0	1.3	3.1
Index		1.73	0.95	0.58	0.35	0.98

All the data accumulated from innumerable surveys since the original concept was espoused by the Hirszfelds confirmed that the frequencies of the ABO groups do remain constant over long periods of time, representing an excellent example of balanced polymorphism. Thus, the relative frequencies of the A and B antigens are a stable characteristic of a particular race.

A few examples illustrative of the different percentage distributions of the ABO groups are given in Table 20-3. The Polish figures represent the population of Wrocław. The Tadzhiks, a people of Iranian descent, are from Afghanistan. The Japanese data were acquired from the population of Tsushima, an island of the Korea Strait in the Kyushu district. The Bantu, members of numerous Negro tribes of central and southern Africa, reported here were from South Africa.

Blood group determinations of North American Indians have revealed a high frequency of group O, especially among those with little or no admixture with peoples of other ethnic origins (Table 20-4). For the figures shown, the Cherokee are from Kansas, the Chippewa from Minnesota, the Navaho from New Mexico, and the Nootka from Puget Sound. From these data, the earliest aboriginal population of North America must have belonged exclusively to blood group O. This would indicate that these original inhabitants migrated, as most anthropologists now believe, from Asia prior to the introduction of the A and B antigens into the parent population of these immigrants.

As was implied earlier, if negligible race-crossing exists, the relative frequencies of the ABO groups in any given population will remain constant for years or even centuries. A striking example in confirmation of this can be

Table 20-4

ABO BLOOD GROUP FREQUENCIES OF SOME NORTH
AMERICAN INDIANS (PURE)

Group	Distribution (%)			
	CHEROKEE	CHIPPEWA	NAVAHO	NOOTKA
O	95.6	87.6	99.1	96.7
A	3.7	12.4	0.9	3.3
B	0.7	0.0	0.0	0.0
AB	0.0	0.0	0.0	0.0

Table 20-5

ABO BLOOD GROUPS AMONG THREE DISTINCT POPULATIONS
LIVING IN HUNGARY

Population	Distribution (%)				Index
	O	A	B	AB	
Gypsies	33.6	20.5	37.9	8.0	0.62
Germans	40.8	43.5	12.6	3.1	2.97
Hungarians	31.0	38.0	18.8	12.2	1.62

found in Hungary where three distinct populations have lived and worked together but remained intact with respect to marriage customs and affiliations (Table 20–5).

The gypsies, of Hindu origin, migrated from India where they originated. During the several hundred years they have lived in Hungary, there has been little intermarriage between them and the other racial populations. They demonstrate the modern Hindustani distribution of the ABO groups with an Asio-African index of 0.62. German settlers migrated into Hungary at the beginning of the eighteenth century. They established colonies in which they retained their original language and customs and did not intermarry with the native Hungarians. Their ABO group frequencies are the same as the present-day German distribution with a European index of 2.97. The native Hungarian population possesses a modern distribution quite unlike either of the previous two groups with an intermediate index of 1.62.

Ontogenesis

Antigens. The A antigen has been demonstrated on the erythrocytes of a fetus as young as 37 days. Absorption studies have shown that fetal red blood cells contain much less A and B antigenic activity than corresponding adult cells. This was confirmed directly by radioactivity measurements using ^{125}I-labeled IgG fractions of rabbit antihuman group A_1 erythrocyte heteroantisera. The number of A antigen sites per red blood cell was estimated to be 810,000 to 1,170,000 on adult group A_1 cells whereas it was 250,000 to 370,000 per group A_1 cord cell, at least a threefold difference. In examinations of erythrocytes from fetuses of different ages using the anti-serum-absorption technique, no quantitative alteration could be detected throughout fetal life. The change to the adult level of antigen sites is not one that gradually evolves during fetal life but occurs some weeks after birth through a mechanism that might be related or similar to the transformation of hemoglobin F (fetal) to hemoglobin A (adult).

The agglutinogens, however, are sufficiently developed to be readily demonstrable at birth, and reliable determinations of a newborn infant's ABO group can be carried out by an examination of cord blood.

Antibodies. In contrast to the readily detectable presence of these isoantigens at birth, only about 35 to 40% of newborn infants possess demonstrable isoagglutinins. Whether or not these antibodies are found in the serum of a particular child depends to a considerable extent on the ABO blood group of the mother and the child. For example, in a homospecific pregnancy where the mother and infant both belong to blood group O, these isoagglutinins may be found in the sera of 80% of the children or more. In contrast, the antibodies may be found in only 20% of group A children born to group O mothers, an example of a heterospecific pregnancy.

In 1928, Hirszfeld first postulated that the anti-A and/or anti-B agglutinins present in the sera at birth were all passively derived from the mother by transplacental filtration. This was based on two observations. First, isoagglutinins were demonstrable only in newborn infants when they were present in the mother, and even then in small amounts. Thus, he did not find any anti-B antibodies in the sera of group A newborn infants when their mothers belonged to group AB. Second, he showed that no newborn infant possessed antibodies capable of reacting with any A or B receptors on the mother's erythrocytes. He proposed that most of the maternal isoagglutinins incompatible with the red blood cells of the fetus were neutralized or absorbed by the A or B blood group specific substances in the fetal body fluids and tissues.

Those isoagglutinins present at birth regularly disappear from the infant's circulation, usually within the first seven to ten days of life, but occasionally may persist with gradual diminution in titer up to two weeks. There then exists a hiatus of two to three months, occasionally as long as six months, when no antibodies at all may be found in the infant's serum. Thereafter, the child's own isoagglutinins, of the proper specificity in accord with Landsteiner's law, are produced and appear in the serum, rapidly rising in titer to the age of five to ten years. Then they gradually diminish in amount.

It is because of this situation that in the pretransfusion major compatibility procedure in preparation for any transfusion of an infant in the first seven to ten days of life, the maternal serum rather than the infant's own serum is routinely used in the *in vitro* cross-match test with the donor's erythrocytes.

Inheritance

Conclusive proof that the A and B agglutinogens are inherited as simple mendelian dominants, thus instituting the hereditary nature of the ABO blood groups, was produced by von Dungern and Hirszfeld in 1910. However, the genetic theory of two independent pairs of allelic genes at different chromosomal loci that they proposed to explain the mechanism of inheritance did not withstand the test of time. It failed to satisfy the ABO group frequencies in certain populations where statistical data that became available could not account for the kinds of children resulting from marriages in which at least one parent belonged to group AB.

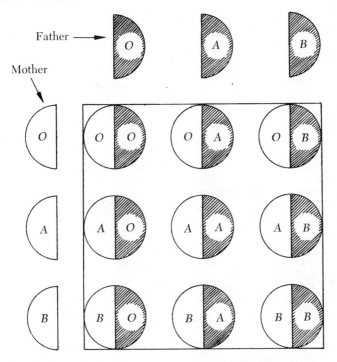

Figure 20-1. Scheme of the possible ABO group genotypes according to Bernstein's three allelic gene theory of inheritance.

The accepted manner of inheritance was expounded by Bernstein in 1924. He showed that the antigens comprising the four ABO groups were inherited as mendelian characters by means of three allelic genes at only one locus on a single pair of chromosomes, where any one of the three genes may be situated, a type of heredity known as multiple allelism. These genes, *A*, *B*, and *O* (originally designated *R*), operate in the fashion that *A* and *B* are dominant at *O* and codominant if combined in the genotype *AB*. This infers that an anti-A serum will detect all individuals carrying the *A* gene and an anti-B serum will do likewise for all those carrying the *B* gene (Figure 20–1).

This system provides for the existence of six different genotypes, based on three possible varieties each of sperm and ova (Table 20–6).

There are two important inheritance laws that derive from this scheme and now have been firmly established by the accumulated statistical data. They are: (1) The agglutinogens A and B cannot appear in the blood of a child unless they are present in the blood of one or both parents. (2) Combinations of a group AB parent with a group O child and a group O parent with a group AB child are impossible.

The possible groups of children from the various mating combinations with respect to the ABO groups of the parents are listed in Table 20–7.

Table 20-6

ABO GENOTYPES ACCORDING
TO BERNSTEIN'S THEORY OF
INHERITANCE

Phenotypes	Genotypes
O	*00*
A	*AA, AO*
B	*BB, BO*
AB	*AB*

The scientifically indisputable facts of the manner of inheritance in this blood group system are used in a practical way by the application of blood group determinations in cases of disputed paternity.

Subgroups of A

The existence of two subgroups of A was discovered by von Dungern and Hirzfeld in 1911 when they observed that the erythrocytes from a small number of group A specimens were weakly agglutinated by two and not at all by one of the group B sera they were using. That this was regular and not a chance finding was confirmed by appropriate absorption studies. Pursuing this approach, Landsteiner and Witt, by absorption and antibody elution experiments, showed that two distinct varieties of anti-A agglutinins, anti-A and anti-A_1, could be separated from group B sera that were reactive with two qualitatively different A agglutinogens, A and A_1, one of these being present on the red cells of both subgroups and the other limited to one of the subgroups. In a follow-up study, Landsteiner and Levine (1926) confirmed the existence of these two qualitatively different subgroups and

Table 20-7

POSSIBLE ABO GROUPS OF CHILDREN
WITH VARIOUS PARENTAL ABO GROUP
COMBINATIONS (BERNSTEIN'S THEORY)

Groups of Parents	Groups of Children
O × O	O
O × A	O, A
O × B	O, B
A × A	O, A
A × B	O, A, B, AB
B × B	O, B
O × AB	A, B
A × AB	A, B, AB
B × AB	A, B, AB
AB × AB	A, B, AB

introduced the notations now commonly employed, group A_1 and group A_2. The properties of these two subgroups are:

Subgroup	Erythrocytic Antigens	React with anti-A	anti-A_1
A_1	AA_1	+	+
A_2	A	+	−

This division also holds true for group AB where the subgroups A_1B and A_2B are recognized. The estimated frequencies of these subgroups among Caucasians of group A are A_1, 78 to 80%, and A_2, 20 to 22%; and of group AB are A_1B, 75 to 80%, and A_2B, 20 to 25%.

Specific, naturally occurring anti-A_1 agglutinins of low thermal amplitude are detectable at room temperature in the sera of 2 to 8% of group A_2 and in 25 to 39% of group A_2B persons.

The three different types of reagents presently available for determining these subgroups are (1) absorbed anti-A serum (group B), prepared by progressive removal of the anti-A agglutinins with consecutive absorptions using small amounts of group A_2 red blood cells leaving behind the specific anti-A_1 agglutinins; (2) naturally occurring anti-A_1 sera of sufficient potency from individuals of group A_2B, used in tests usually performed at incubation temperatures from 4° to 15° C; and (3) anti-A_1 lectin, a specific phytohemagglutinin, made as a saline extract of the seeds of *Dolichos biflorus*, probably the most useful of all these reagents that agglutinate group A_1 and A_1B erythrocytes very strongly in high dilutions.

The potency of the agglutination produced by anti-A serum with erythrocytes of these subgroups can be rated as $A_2 < A_1$ and $A_2B < A_1B$ and A_2. That there is also a quantitative difference between these subgroups has been demonstrated by the same radioactivity measurements mentioned above in the section "Ontogenesis." The number of A antigen sites per group A_1 red blood cell has been estimated at 810,000 to 1,170,000 compared to 240,000 to 290,000 per group A_2.

Acquisition of the complete group A_1 characteristics of erythrocytes is a developmental process that occurs several weeks after birth. It is impossible to obtain reliable subgrouping determinations on the red cells of newborn infants. Although the A property is clearly distinguishable, as mentioned above (page 345), the red cells of the majority of babies at birth react as if they belong to subgroup A_2, for they fail to be agglutinated by most anti-A_1 reagents. *Dolichos biflorus* lectin is usually the best in attempting to make this distinction, but in most instances genetically group A_1 newborn infants are still not determinable from group A_2 since they so often lack the adult spectrum of antigenic groupings.

The occurrence of these subgroups is not a random phenomenon. Soon after their discovery extensive family studies clearly indicated that these were inheritable characteristics. Consequently, the three allelic gene theory of

Bernstein has been expanded to include four allelic genes, A_1, A_2, B, and O. With the three commonly available antisera, anti-A, anti-A_1, and anti-B, six phenotypes can be distinguished of the ten possible genotypes. The number of genotypes now includes homozygous A_1A_1 and A_2A_2 and heterozygous A_1A_2, A_1O, and A_1A_2, which can only be distinguished exactly by blood grouping entire families. The genotypes A_1B and A_2B can be determined directly.

There are two important clinical applications of the existence of these two subgroups of A. First, it is vitally important in all laboratory determinations of the ABO groups of patients or blood donors that the anti-A serum be of sufficient potency to detect all weak subgroup A_2 cells or they could erroneously be classified, before an examination of the serum for its antibody characteristics, as group O or, in the case of actual group A_2B cells, as group B. The second point of importance relates to ABO hemolytic disease of the newborn, predominantly involving group A_1 infants with group O mothers. Genetically group A_2 infants escape this disease; only genetically group A_1 babies are affected, even if the erythrocytes of such genetically group A_1 infants with severe disease are not reactive at birth with anti-A_1 reagents. This is presumably also the reason that premature infants are protected from this serologic form of the disease, as their erythrocytes react even more weakly than those of full-term babies.

A and B Antigens in Tissues and Secretions

The A and B antigens have now been demonstrated on many cells other than erythrocytes; in fact, the cells of almost the entire body are stigmatized by the same blood-group-specific characteristics as the erythrocytes of the individual. As a consequence, Witebsky proposed many years ago that the term "blood groups" should be replaced by "cell" or "tissue groups."

With the possible exception of blood platelets, they cannot be demonstrated on cells other than red blood cells by direct agglutination tests. Generally, their presence is detected by any of three methods: (1) specific absorption of agglutinins from standard anti-A or anti-B sera; (2) complement-fixation tests with alcoholic extracts of organs and rabbit antihuman erythrocyte heteroantisera; or (3) specific inhibition of agglutination by aqueous extracts of organs tested with human, nonimmune sera.

The concentrations in different organs vary widely with the largest amounts found in the submaxillary gland, esophagus, stomach, pancreas, and gallbladder; moderate amounts in the parotid gland, lung, liver, adrenal, and kidney; and trace amounts in the testis and spleen. None has been detected in the brain, ocular lens, hair, compact bone, or cartilage. Other practical applications include the knowledge that these antigens are on blood platelets, which has considerable significance in the transfusion of platelet concentrates where the greatest useful survival time in the circulation of the platelet-deficient recipient occurs when they are the same ABO blood group as the patient. There is also reason to believe that ABO incompatibility may influence the success of corneal grafts.

Water-soluble A and B specific substances have been found in normal secretions such as saliva, gastric juice, bile, urine, amniotic fluid, and sweat as well as in pathologic secretions such as pleural, pericardial, ascitic, and hydrocele fluids, and pseudomucinous ovarian cyst fluid, an especially rich source with his concentrations. However, they are never present in cerebrospinal fluid. They may be demonstrated in these body fluids by two techniques: (1) direct precipitation, a method not suitable for general usage since it requires potent antisera such as rabbit antihuman erythrocyte heteroantisera or immune human isoantisera; and (2) specific inhibition of agglutination, a sensitive method that can be designed to detect microgram quantities, especially if naturally occurring or nonimmune human anti-A or anti-B sera are used. The relative concentrations in various secretions, compared to the antibody absorbing potency of a 50% suspension of human group A_1 erythrocytes, expressed as the dilution ranges of a series of specimens within which complete inhibition of agglutination was achieved, are as follows:

Gastric juice	256–524,288
Saliva	256-131,072
Semen	128–8192
Amniotic fluid	64–256
Erythrocytes (50% susp.)	8–32
Urine	2–16
Cerebrospinal fluid	0

From these results it is obvious that certain secretions of a group A person may contain enormous amounts of A antigen in comparison with the A activity demonstrable on erythrocytes as measured by their absorption capacity.

This secretion was found to be an inherited characteristic under the control of a pair of mendelian genes, Se and se. Without exception, the Se gene is dominant to the se gene and, when present in either the homozygous or heterozygous state, conveys the ability to secrete either A or B water-soluble substance, depending on the ABO group of the individual. Nonsecretors represent the homozygous state sese genotype. With the known exception of North American Indians and Australian aborigines, all other peoples examined in Europe and American have revealed the following frequencies: secretors, 77 to 78%; and nonsecretors, 22 to 23%. This represents an independent gene system with no linkage to the ABO genes, a situation of genetic independence yet with intimate association.

There are two distinct forms of the A and B antigens, differences among individuals only in regard to the water-soluble substances being responsible for the existence of secretor and nonsecretor types. These are: (1) Alcohol-soluble; glycolipid. This is the variety of the membrane antigens that is present in all tissues and on red blood cells except the brain and in all persons whether they are secretors or nonsecretors. This type is not present in secretions and is not influenced by the *Se* gene. (2) Water-soluble: poly-saccharide. This is easily extracted from the tissues of secretors but does not occur in aqueous extracts of the organs of nonsecretors. It is not on the erythrocytes, and its presence in most fluids of secretors except the spinal fluid is determined by the *Se* gene. The largest quantities are found in glandular organs, with the concentrations in different glands closely paralleling the concentrations in the corresponding secretions.

Rh Blood Groups

Basic Properties or Characteristics

Antigens. The major antigen of clinical importance and the first one discovered in this system, the D antigen, also referred to as Rh_0 antigen by some, is present on the erythrocytes of about 85% of Caucasians, referred to as $Rh_0(D)$ positive, and absent in about 15%, named $Rh_0(D)$ negative. For transfusion purposes it is only necessary to know whether patients and blood donors are $Rh_0(D)$ positive or $Rh_0(D)$ negative. These awkward appearing and sounding designations are intended to emphasize specifically that this is the result of testing for precisely this significant antigen of several now known to comprise the Rh system. The use of the Rh symbol, instead of replacing it completely with the more sensible notation D, has been maintained out of the common usage that arose in medical practice from earlier days when it was believed that Rh was a single antigen, and people were either positive or negative with respect to its presence. Many clinical services still refer simply to a person being Rh positive or Rh negative; this is scientifically imprecise.

Rapidly within a two to three-year span after the initial findings concerning this antigen, other examples of antibodies produced by isoimmunization in transfusion or in pregnancy resulting in hemolytic disease of the newborn were encountered. These antibodies produced agglutination patterns suspicious for or indicative of the detection of antigens somehow related to the original D antigen but with completely different reaction rates with blood specimens of white persons. Analyzing the statistical data available at the time on families studied by English investigators using four of these different antisera, Sir Ronald Fisher brilliantly observed that the agglutination patterns produced by two of them were antithetical and postulated that they identified antigens controlled by allelic genes. Although the remaining two clearly did not yield such antithetical reaction patterns, he predicted that under proper immunologic circumstances permitting isoimmunization,

Table 20-8

FREQUENCIES OF REACTION RATES OF THE FIVE BASIC ANTI-Rh SERA IN CAUCASIAN POPULATIONS

Antisera		General	English		Swedish	
FISHER-RACE	WIENER	POSITIVE %	POSITIVE %	NEGATIVE %	POSITIVE %	NEGATIVE %
Anti-D	Anti-Rh_0	85	83.2	16.8	84.5	15.5
Anti-C	Anti-rh'	70	67.8	32.2	67.8	32.2
Anti-E	Anti-rh"	30	28.7	71.3	31.0	69.0
Anti-c	Anti-hr'	80	81.3	18.7	81.9	18.1
Anti-e	Anti-hr"	98	97.6	2.4	96.9	3.1

antibodies identifying antigens antithetical to these two latter varieties of antisera would be produced. Two years after his hypothesis was proposed, one of the antisera was found and all of the reactions expected of it within the Rh system were observed, confirming this perspicaciously conceived scheme.

To describe his interpretations and to name these specific antigens and their corresponding antibodies for future reference, Fisher proposed the symbols C and c, D and d, and E and e for the corresponding members of each pair of antigens. Unfortunately, a different notational system was advocated at about the same time by Wiener with the net result of introducing a degree of confusion for the beginning reader of this body of scientific literature. The observed frequencies of the reaction rates in Caucasian populations with the existing five basic antisera identified by the two notational systems are given in Table 20–8.

From these findings and the accumulated data of many investigators in this field, it became obvious that an individual's complete Rh antigenic (gene) complex (or genotype) contained six components, three inherited from each parent. Without taking into account any of the known variants of the D, C, or E antigens, the following eight different combinations are possible: cde, cDe, CDe, cDE, Cde, cdE, CDE, and CdE. These can be paired in 36 different ways to constitute a person's complete Rh antigenic pattern (genotype). For example, an individual's Rh complex may be cde/cde, CDe/cde, CDe/CDe, or cDE/cDE.

The frequencies of the occurrence of seven of these eight basic Rh complexes (or chromosomes) in Caucasians and Negroes are listed in Table 20-9. The CdE combination is so very rare that it does not appear at all in most surveys.

Although the existing antigens D, C, E, c, and e are usually expressed coequally when inherited, that is to say detectable on the erythrocytic membrane by the corresponding antisera, these antigens vary widely in their immunogenicity or capability of inducing antibody formation. The D antigen is by far the most antigenic in reference to eliciting antibody

Table 20-9
FREQUENCIES OF THE RH GENE COMPLEXES OR CHROMOSOMES

CDE Fisher	Short Symbol	% Distribution				
		U.S.		ENGLISH	NEGROES	
		WHITES	BLACKS		BANTU	LUO
cde	r	41.09	25.00	39.03	11.84	4.15
CDe	R_1	40.71	15.79	40.15	2.56	0.00
cDE	R_2	13.69	9.13	14.50	4.27	0.00
cDe	R_0	2.60	46.75	2.62	64.91	81.74
Cde	r'	0.45	1.48	1.19	7.07	4.69
cdE	r''	0.36	0.62	0.97	0.00	4.69
CDE	R_z	0.15	1.04	0.27	0.00	0.00

production and the most important one medically with respect to blood transfusion and hemolytic disease of the newborn. Relatively speaking, the others are biologically poor antigens that do not evoke an antibody response anywhere near the frequency of the D antigen. Under the proper immunologic circumstances, however, anyone homozygous for any of the Rh antigens theoretically has the potential of producing antibodies to the antithetical antigen. For example, a mother of the Rh antigenic pattern CDe/CDe could produce anti-c antibodies to the red cells of a fetus of the Rh group CDe/cde. Actually it is just such an occurrence that does provide the anti-c sera used in determining the probable Rh genotype of an individual. Fortunately, because of the low potency of the antigens other than the D antigen, this occurs infrequently. If these antigens were of equal immunogenicity, it would be necessary to pair Rh antigenic complex with Rh antigenic complex in matching a donor for a recipient of a blood transfusion. With respect to the Rh antigens other than D, a rating of their immunogenicity in decreasing sequence would be in the order of c, E, C, and e.

Concerning the ontogenesis of the Rh antigens, a newborn infant can readily and accurately be determined as $Rh_0(D)$ positive or $Rh_0(D)$ negative by tests on the cord blood. That these antigens are well developed long before birth has been proved by the detection of D antigen on the erythrocytes of fetuses estimated to be from 11 to 17 weeks of age. The earliest detectability of the D antigen, in fact a complete probable Rh genotyping of cDE/cde, was on erythrocytes from the cord blood of an embryo estimated to be about six weeks of age from the crown-to-rump measurement of 32 mm.

There are far fewer D antigenic receptor sites per adult erythrocyte than A or B. In fact, the magnitude of this difference is immense. For instance, the red cells of the most common Rh genotype among North American whites, CDe/cde, of a group A_1 person contain anywhere from 50 to 115 times more A sites than D sites per cell. The number of D antigen sites per erythrocyte has been estimated for various probable Rh genotypes using ^{125}I-labeled antigammaglobulin anti-D reagent (Table 20-10).

For this reason, hemagglutination produced by anti-D antibodies is much weaker than that by anti-A or anti-B. As a consequence, greater care must be taken in reading the reactions when determining whether someone is $Rh_0(D)$ positive or $Rh_0(D)$ negative, especially in test tube techniques when shaking the centrifuged cells to resuspend them for macroscopic reading.

Table 20-10

Rh Genotype	D Antigen Sites
CDe/cde	9,900–14,600
cDe/cde	12,000–20,000
cDE/cde	14,000–16,600
CDe/CDe	14,500–19,300
CDe/CDe	23,000–31,000
cDE/cDE	15,800–33,300

Antibodies. In sharp contrast to the fundamental characteristic of the ABO blood group system, anti-Rh antibodies are never present normally. They always result from isoimmunization produced by (1) pregnancy with a fetus carrying an Rh antigen foreign to the mother, most frequently D; (2) transfusion, currently very frequently due to the D antigen since all transfusions are now routinely matched for this major antigen by restricting $Rh_0(D)$ positive blood to $Rh_0(D)$ positive recipients and $Rh_0(D)$ negative donor bloods to $Rh_0(D)$ negative patients; and (3) intentional stimulation of volunteers for reagent antiserum production.

These antibodies may belong either to the IgM or the IgG immunoglobulin class. With respect to their pathogenetic role in hemolytic disease of the newborn, only IgG antibodies are significant since they alone can traverse the placental barrier and enter the circulation of the fetus. It is frequently observed in isoimmunization to fetal erythrocytic D antigens that saline-active or IgM agglutinins that appear in the maternal serum early in the pregnancy disappear and are replaced by albumin-active or IgG antibodies as the pregnancy proceeds to term.

An important contrast to the isoagglutinins of the ABO blood group system exists in the fact that anti-Rh agglutinins irrespective of their specificity have never been demonstrated to produce hemolysis either *in vitro* or *in vivo*. Consequently, they cannot effect any intravascular hemolytic phenomena if D positive erythrocytes are inadvertently transfused into a recipient whose serum contains anti-D antibodies. In the latter circumstance, the hemolytic process that results, broadly defined as a premature shortening of the life-span of the donated red blood cells, is by definition extravascular and is manifested by a rapid, selective sequestration of the antibody-coated erythrocytes in the sinusoids of the spleen.

It was fortuitous that Levine and Stetson were able to demonstrate antibodies *in vitro* in their original case by using the classic, serologic milieu of saline solution. Subsequent investigators studying typical cases of hemolytic disease of the newborn, where 100% showed the perfect, theoretic setup with respect to clinical, hematologic, biochemical, and pathologic signs in the newborn and the expected Rh groups of the mother and father, were not able to detect agglutinins in the maternal sera by this customary technique in more than 50% of the cases. In our experience, this was true in only 30 to 40% with potent antibodies detectable in only 3 to 5% of these.

This seeming discrepancy with respect to Levine's theory of the pathogenesis of hemolytic disease of the newborn was dismissed by the almost simultaneous, independent finding of a new serologic variety of anti-Rh antibodies by Race and by Wiener in 1944 named, respectively, the incomplete or blocking antibodies. This was a fundamental discovery of cardinal consequence in immunology with respect to our understanding of the nature of antibodies, serving as an impetus to the investigations that ultimately led to the definition of the immunoglobulin classes. The indirect procedure they reported for detecting these antibodies that fail to agglutinate D positive erythrocytes in saline solution was cumbersome to perform and not too sensitive in that it revealed antibodies in, at most, only 60% of those maternal sera that were nonreactive in saline solution. This was soon replaced by a more efficient and reliable technique when it was discovered that incomplete anti-D antibodies would effect agglutination directly by substituting human group AB serum for saline solution as a diluent for titrating the maternal serum under investigation and for suspending the D positive test cells.

Following many additional investigations on this variety of anti-Rh antibodies, three general procedures useful for demonstrating the presence of these incomplete antibodies have emerged.

1. Use of high-protein or macromolecular diluents. Human group AB serum (or other ABO compatible serum) was replaced by 20% bovine serum albumin solution, which proved to be more effective and could be made readily available in large volumes. The best all-protein diluent for this purpose has been shown to be a mixture of equal parts of undiluted, human group AB serum (or other ABO compatible serum) and 30% bovine serum albumin solution. Synthetic preparations such as dextran and polyvinylpyrrolidone (PVP) have been used to a much lesser extent (Chapter 6).

2. Indirect antiglobulin technique. In this test advantage is taken of the fact that the incomplete antibodies do effect the first phase of agglutination. Specifically, they unite with the D antigenic receptor sites on the erythrocytes, commonly expressed as coating or sensitizing the cells, and this antigen-antibody union will withstand several washes with saline solution to remove the other serum proteins. The presence of these antibody molecules on the red cell surface is then determined by the addition of rabbit, goat, or sheep antihuman globulin serum, which bridges the gap between the incomplete Rh antibody-sensitized cells and permits a lattice formation with subsequent agglutination (Chapter 6).

3. Enzyme pretreatment of test cells. Mild treatment of D positive red cells with trypsin, papain, ficin, or bromelin is extremely effective in allowing the incomplete antibodies to produce direct agglutination of such treated test cells in saline solution (Chapter 6).

The saline-active, complete anti-Rh agglutinins were shown by ultracentrifugal analysis to have a sedimentation constant of 19 S and by electrophoretic migration to be IgM globulins. The albumin-active, incomplete antibodies similarly were shown to have a sedimentation constant of 7 S and to be IgG globulins.

An example of the effects of these different procedures in demonstrating the presence of incomplete anti-D antibodies in a maternal serum is depicted in Table 20–11.

Racial Distribution

The frequency data obtained on some selected populations of different ethnic origins examined with anti-D sera are listed in Table 20–12.

Table 20-11

Titration of Incomplete Anti-D Serum (Seb) vs. CDe/cE(R_1R_2) Cells by Several Serologic Techniques

Anti-D Serum (Seb)	0.9% Saline	Undiluted Human Serum	20% Bovine Albumin	Human Serum + Bovine Albumin	Indirect Antiglobulin	Ficin-Treated Cells in Saline
Undiluted	−	++++	++++	++++	++++	++++
1:2	−	++++	++++	++++	++++	++++
1:4	−	+++	++++	++++	++++	++++
1:8	−	+++	++++	++++	++++	++++
1:16	−	++	++++	++++	+++	++++
1:32	−	+	+++	++++	+++	++++
1:64	−	(+)	+++	++++	++	+++
1:128	−	±	+++	++++	+	+++
1:256	−	−	++	+++	(+)	+++
1:512	−	−	++	+++	−	+++
1:1024	−	−	+	++	−	+++
1:2048	−	−	(+)	++	−	++
1:4096	−	−	±	+	−	++
1:8192	−	−	−	+	−	++
1:16,384	−	−	−	(+)	−	+
Diluent	−	−	−	±	−	−

Table 20-12
FREQUENCIES OF THE D ANTIGEN IN
VARIOUS POPULATIONS

| Population | Phenotypes % | |
	D+	D−
English	85.16	14.84
Ethiopians	95.79	4.21
Bantu	94.85	5.15
Eskimos	99.96	0.04
Chinese	99.40	0.60
Japanese	99.56	0.44
Indonesians	99.32	0.68
Papuans	100.00	0.00
Basques	71.46	28.54
Berbers	71.26	28.74

The Bantu are from South Africa and the Eskimos represent those living in western Alaska. The Indonesians studied were from Djakarta, the Chinese from Peking, and the Japanese from Tokyo. The Basques are from an ancient and long-isolated population of a peculiar ethnic type inhabiting the Pyrenees mountain region and a sector of the Bay of Biscay in Spain. The Berbers, Caucasians belonging to a group of Moslem tribes who are Hamites, the chief native race of North Africa west of Tripoli, are from Aït Moghrad.

According to Mourant, the present distribution of the uniform frequency of D and d genes in most countries of northern and central Europe could only have emerged from a mixing in the last few thousand years of two populations, one entirely or almost entirely $Rh_0(D)$ positive and one all or nearly all $Rh_0(D)$ negative. As can be seen from this table, many populations of Asia and Africa have very high D antigen frequencies. In Europe, only the Basques have a significantly lower frequency of D antigen today, which is shared by the Berbers of North Africa, to whom they may be related. Most population geneticists agree that they represent the remnants of the original population in which the D antigen was either absent or present in a very small percentage.

Inheritance

Shortly after the discovery of the first and clinically still the most important Rh antigen, the D antigen, family studies revealed clearly that it was inherited as a mendelian character. A person who is $Rh_0(D)$ positive may be either homozygous, D/D, or heterozygous, D/d, whereas someone who is $Rh_0(D)$ negative is always homozygous, d/d. Similarly, family studies have indicated unequivocally that the D antigen cannot appear in the blood of a child unless present in the blood of one or both parents.

The same facts prevail when families are analyzed for the C and c pair of antigens and the E and e pair of antigens. The same three basic patterns exist as is true for the D antigen. An individual whose red cells are agglutinated by anti-C serum may be either homozygous, C/C, or heterozygous C/c, and, if not, must be homozygous, c/c. An analogous situation exists if the E and e antigens are considered. In tests for the latter two pairs of antigens, however, homozygosity or heterozygosity can be determined directly since anti-c and anti-e sera are available in addition to the anti-C and anti-E. Unfortunately, no example of anti-d serum has been found, which is surprising in view of the hundreds of thousands of sera that have been screened for antibodies. Either the d antigen is extremely impotent or, more likely, it appears to be a nonentity, a situation that would imply that the *d* gene is probably an amorph like the *O* gene. Thus, the exact complete Rh genotype of a person cannot be determined directly.

However, since direct examinations for the presence of C and c antigens and E and e antigens are possible, the results they yield with respect to homozygosity or heterozygosity for these antigens allow an estimate of the most probable Rh genotype based on statistical analyses of existing family data. For example, the likelihood of a white person who tests to be homozygous for the C antigen, C/C, also being homozygous for the D antigen, D/D, with a probable Rh genotype of *CDe/CDe* is 95.4%. Similarly, among whites if a person were found to be heterozygous for the C antigen, C/c, the chance of his being also heterozygous for the D antigen, D/d, with the probable Rh genotype of *CDe/cde* is about 93.8%.

Combining the three pairs of antigens, it is definite that a child cannot possess the D antigen, the C or c antigens, or the E or e antigens if any one of these is absent from both parents.

The passage of time and the accumulation of knowledge especially based on studies of bacterial genes have gently nudged aside the emotional need to marshal arguments for or against either of the two theories proposed in the early days of Rh studies concerning the exact mechanics of inheritance. The Fisher-Race theory called for the existence of three separate but topographically extremely close gene loci on a single pair of chromosomes, one locus for the *D* and *d* genes, another for the *C* and *c* genes, and a third for the *E* and *e* genes. It implied that three pairs of allelomorphic antigens were controlled by three closely linked, if not absolutely linked, genes. This linkage theory is based on each gene determining the presence of a particular antigen on the red cells in an uncomplicated fashion. In contrast, Wiener's theory specified a single Rh gene locus on a single pair of chromosomes with a series of multiple alleles at one locus, analogous to the ABO inheritance, requiring that the single gene determined the presence of three "factors."

The D^u Antigens

Individuals whose red cells were agglutinated by only a few anti-D sera, being completely negative with the majority of antisera used, were reported by Stratton in 1946. That this was not a chance finding dependent simply on technique or the potency of the anti-D sera was confirmed when studies on the families of the propositi clearly indicated this to be an inheritable property.

There are many varieties of the D^u antigen based on the different grades of reactivity observed when erythrocytes from many such individuals are tested with a battery of anti-D sera of both the complete, saline-active and incomplete, albumin-active types. Examples of high-grade D^u erythrocytes are agglutinated by some complete anti-D sera in saline, like the original cases, and by only a few incomplete (albumin) anti-D sera in a medium of 20% albumin or suspended in the individual's own serum. Low-grade D^u positive cells are not agglutinated directly by either serologic variety of anti-D serum in its own respective medium. Agglutination of erythrocytes of this category is accomplished only by using an indirect antiglobulin technique after sensitizing the cells with incomplete (albumin) anti-D sera. The lowest grade of D^u antigen, and the most difficult to detect, is found in certain persons whose red cells give positive reactions only with selected incomplete (albumin) anti-D sera by the indirect antiglobulin technique. In such latter instances it is important, if this condition is suspected, since it may be according to the probable Rh genotype as it has been determined up to this stage, that several albumin-active anti-D sera previously selected for their known reactivity with weak D^u variant cells must be used in these tests rather than depending on a single example of anti-D serum. The particular grade of reactivity of the D^u antigen variant (high, low, lowest) observed in the propositus is very likely to be found as the same level occurring in other family members who possess the D^u antigen, indicating this is probably an inherited trait.

Carefully conducted examinations of many blood specimens of the apparent Rh genotypes *Cde/cde*, *cdE/cde*, or *cde/cde* from both whites and blacks have proved that a certain percentage of these actually are D^u positive. Such results are shown in Table 20–13.

Whether or not an individual is D^u positive is of some importance since the D^u antigen is very common in Negroes who could erroneously be grouped as $Rh_0(D)$ negative were they not examined specifically for the D^u antigen. Although there are reported instances of $Rh_0(D)$ negative persons of the Rh

Table 20-13

FREQUENCIES OF THE D^u ANTIGEN (D^u GENOTYPES)
IN Rh GROUPS NEGATIVE FOR THE D ANTIGEN

	% D^u Positive		
APPARENT	WHITES	BLACKS	ACTUAL
Cde/cde	44.7	83.7	*CD^{u}e/cde*
cdE/cde	20.6	100.0	*cD^{u}E/cde*
cde/cde	0.5	26.6	*cD^{u}e/cde*
All genotypes	1.6	5.5	

genotype *cde/cde* on contact with the D^u antigen having produced anti-D antibodies exhibiting a fairly normal and expected reaction rate on randomly selected blood specimens, these have almost all been in cases of deliberate immunization of volunteers to produce antisera or of isoimmunization of pregnancy with a D^u positive fetus. Apparently, this is not a major problem in blood transfusion, as had originally been suspected. Most blood banks routinely examine all blood donors appearing to be $Rh_0(D)$ negative for the presence of the D^u antigen. Those found to be D^u positive are labeled as $Rh_0(D)$ positive and not used for $Rh_0(D)$ negative recipients. This may be an unnecessary precaution since recently some investigators have deliberately transfused $Rh_0(D)$ negative volunteers with full transfusion units of D^u positive blood without the appearance of anti-D antibodies in the sera of the volunteers.

Isoimmunization of pregnancy in D^u positive women carrying $Rh_0(D)$ positive fetuses has resulted in the production of anti-D antibodies with severe and even fatal hemolytic disease of the newborn as a result. In this situation, with this kind of an antigenic stimulus, the D^u antigen does not block the production of anti-D antibodies.

Bibliography

Hartmann, G.: *Group Antigens in Human Organs.* Ejnar Munksgaard Forlag, Copenhagen, 1941. Reprinted in Camp, F. R., and Ellis, F. R. (eds.): *Selected Contributions to the Literature of Blood Groups and Immunology.* Blood Transfusion Division, U.S. Army Medical Research Laboratory, Fort Knox, Ky., 1970.

Hirszfeld, L.: *Konstitutionsserologie und Blutgruppenforschung.* Springer-Verlag, Berlin, 1928. Translated and reprinted in Camp, F. R., and Ellis, F. R. (eds.): *Selected Contributions to the Literature of Blood Groups and Immunology*, Vol. III, Part 1. Blood Transfusion Division, U.S. Army Medical Research Laboratory, Fort Knox, Ky., 1969.

Kabat, E. A.: *Blood Group Substances.* Academic Press, Inc., New York, 1956.

Mohn, J. F., and Lambert, R. M.: Immunohematologic procedures. In Rose, N. R., and Bigazzi, P. E. (eds.): *Methods in Immunodiagnosis.* John Wiley & Sons, Inc., New York, 1973.

Mohn, J. F., and Plunkett, R. W.: Preliminary studies on anti-A agglutinins formed in human volunteers in response to stimulation with A substance. In Rose, N. R., and Milgrom, F. (eds.): *International Convocation on Immunology.* S. Karger, Basel/New York, 1969.

Mohn, J. F.; Plunkett, R. W.; Cunningham, R. K.; and Lambert, R. M. (eds.): *Human Blood Groups.* Proceedings of 5th International Convocation on Immunology. S. Karger, Basel, 1977.

Mollison, P. L.: *Blood Transfusion in Clinical Medicine*, 5th ed. Blackwell Scientific Publications, Ltd., Oxford, 1972.

Mourant, A. E.; Kopeć, A. C.; and Domaniewska-Sobczak, K.: *The Distribution of the Human Blood Groups and Other Polymorphisms,* 2nd ed. Oxford University Press, London, 1976.

Prokop, O., and Uhlenbruck, G.: *Human Blood and Serum Groups.* John Wiley & Sons, Inc., New York, 1969.

Race, R. R., and Sanger, R.: *Blood Groups in Man,* 6th ed. Blackwell Scientific Publications, Ltd., Oxford, 1975.

Stratton, F., and Renton, P. H.: *Practical Blood Grouping,* Blackwell Scientific Publications, Ltd., Oxford, 1958.

Strumia, M. M.; Crosby, W. H.; Gibson, J. G., 2nd; Greenwalt, T. J.; and Krevans, J. R. (eds.): *General Principles of Blood Transfusion.* J. B. Lippincott Co., Philadelphia, 1963. Published originally in *Transfusion,* **3**:303–46, 1963.

Wiener, A. S.: *Blood Groups and Transfusion,* 3rd ed. Charles C Thomas, Publisher, Springfield, Ill., 1943.

Witebsky, E.: Interrelationship between the Rh system and the AB system. *Blood,* **3**:66–79, 1948.

Witebsky, E.; Klendshoj, N. C.; and McNeil, C.: Potent typing sera produced by treatment of donors with isolated blood group specific substances. *Proc. Soc. Exp. Biol.,* **55**:167–70, 1944.

Zmijewski, C. M., and Fletcher, J. L.: *Immunohematology,* 2nd ed. Appleton-Century-Crofts, New York, 1972.

21

Tissue-Specific, Organ-Specific, and Heterophile Antigens

Felix Milgrom

Species Specificity of Whole Serum

At the beginning of the twentieth century, Fisch in the United States and Wassermann and Schüze in Germany noted that milk or serum originating from various species differ in antigenic structure. The term "species specificity" was created. A species-specific antigen may be defined as an antigen that is present in all members of a given species and differs from an analogous antigen in other species. In most of the early experiments on species specificity, antisera were prepared in rabbits by injections with whole sera of various species origin. Nuttall collected 30 such antisera and tested them against sera from animals of various species by means of test tube precipitation. Strongest reactions were always noted with the corresponding antigen. Strong cross-reactions occurred with sera of closely related species and weaker cross-reactions or negative results were observed with sera from distant species. This may be exemplified by results of an experiment that was selected by Landsteiner for illustration of the pattern of interspecies cross-reactions (Table 21-1). It may be seen that rabbit antisera to human serum produced the strongest reactions with human serum. The reactions were weaker with sera of anthropoid apes, still weaker with sera of Old World monkeys, and weakest with sera of American monkeys. Absorption of such an antiserum with sera of subhuman primates would result in a reagent combining with human serum only.

Antisera to a serum from an animal of one vertebrate class would usually give a greater or lesser degree of cross-reactions with sera of other animals of the same class, but, by and large, no cross-reactions would be observed with sera from animals belonging to another vertebrate class.

Besides being of considerable theoretic interest, studies on species specificity also found medicolegal application. The species origin of blood stains or tissue debris may be identified by means of proper species-specific antisera in criminal trials. In addition, the species origin of food products has been studied in order to detect possible adulteration or mislabeling.

The species of animal used for production of antisera to species-specific antigens is of considerable importance. For example, rabbit antisera can clearly distinguish the differences in the serologic structure of sera from animals of various families and even species belonging to the same mammalian class. On the other hand, rabbit antisera are poor reagents for distinguishing the species differences among avian sera, e.g., the difference between chicken and pigeon serum. These observations brought Landsteiner to coin the term "faulty perspective." In our example, the rabbit is a species far removed from the birds; consequently, upon immunization it is overwhelmed with strong antigens common to sera of all birds and cannot distinguish relatively subtle differences between chicken and pigeon serum. The best procedure for distinguishing the differences between two taxonomically close species is "cross-immunization" in which members of two such species are selected for reciprocal immunization. To adhere to our example, a chicken antiserum to pigeon serum would clearly distinguish the sera of these two species since it would produce strong reaction with pigeon serum but no reaction with chicken serum. Conversely, pigeon antichicken serum would combine with chicken but not with pigeon serum.

Table 21-1
REACTIONS OF RABBIT IMMUNE SERA TO
HUMAN SERUM WITH SERA OF PRIMATES*

The Strength of Reactions Was Established on the Basis of the Volume of the Precipitates and Expressed in Relative Terms

	Immune	Serum
	1	2
Man	100	100
Orangutan	47	80
Cynocephalus mormon	30	50
Ceropithecus petaurista	30	50
Ateles vellerosus	22	25

* From Landsteiner, K.: *The Specificity of Serological Reactions.* Harvard University Press, Cambridge, 1946, p. 14.

Specificity of Individual Serum Proteins

Whereas in early studies on species specificity whole serum was used as an antigenic entity, more recently individual serum proteins have been investigated. The results were similar. For example, γ globulin has definite species specificity, but still, cross-reactions among γ globulins of various mammals may be readily demonstrated. In Figure 21–1 the results of an experiment are presented in which human and bovine γ globulins were tested against rabbit antisera to human or rabbit γ globulins. Both antisera formed precipitation lines with human as well as with bovine γ globulins, and these lines merged into reactions of partial identity. As could have been expected, in each instance the line of homologous reaction extended in the form of a spur over the line of heterologous reaction (Chapter 6). A similar pattern of reactions would be observed in a study of any other serum protein, e.g., albumin. Such experiments show that analogous serum proteins carry definite species specificity but in addition they show antigenic similarity even if they originate from different species. On the contrary, there is no antigenic similarity among different kinds of serum proteins even if they originate from the same species. This is exemplified in Figure 21–2, which shows that precipitation lines formed by bovine γ globulin and bovine albumin cross each other in a reaction of nonidentity. It may be concluded that in the

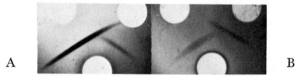

A   B

Figure 21-1.   Partial identity reactions between human and bovine γ globulins. Lower wells: Plate *A*, rabbit antiserum to bovine γ globulin; plate *B*, rabbit antiserum to human γ globulin. Upper wells in both plates: Left, γ globulin fraction of bovine serum; right, γ globulin fraction of human serum.

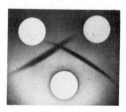

Figure 21-2.   Nonidentity reaction between bovine γ globulin and albumin. Upper left well: Gamma globulin fraction of bovine serum. Upper right well: Albumin fraction of bovine serum. Lower well: Rabbit antiserum to bovine serum.

process of evolution there is a gradual development of antigenic structures leading to species specificity whereas the ontogenic differentiation of substances serving various purposes results in the emergence of completely different antigenic structures. This brings our discussion to the problem of "tissue specificity."

Tissue Specificity

A tissue-specific antigen may be defined as an antigen characteristic for only one particular tissue. To some extent, γ globulin may be considered a tissue-specific antigen for plasma cells and albumin an antigen characteristic for liver cells. Both these proteins, however, are shed off to the circulation and reach most of the animal's tissues. For this reason, before recognition of individual serum components as separate antigens, serum was considered an exclusively species-specific antigen, which also implied that it is present in the entire body of an animal of a given species.

The ubiquity of serum proteins interfered with detection of tissue-specific antigens. This was especially the case in the first four decades of the twentieth century when precipitation in a fluid medium and complement-fixation tests were used for most studies on tissue specificity. By means of these procedures it was extremely difficult, if at all possible, to recognize a minor tissue-specific antigen in the presence of strong serum antigens in tissue extracts. Therefore, it is not surprising that the first tissue-specific antigens were demonstrated in eye lens, an organ free of serum. In 1903, Uhlenhuth injected rabbits with homogenates of bovine lens; the antisera obtained in this way combined not only with antigenic preparations of bovine lens but also with those from other animal species, including nonvertebrate classes. From these results it has been concluded that lens antigens are devoid of species specificity. Subsequent investigations showed, however, that there exist several lens-specific antigens, which have been developed in the course of the evolution of this organ. Those lens antigens that are phylogenetically oldest have indeed little species specificity in that they are present in all vertebrates. Other antigens, however, which evolved later, show quite well-pronounced species specificity.

In studies on brain specificity conducted in the 1920s, Witebsky and his associates identified a lipid antigen that had similar or identical structure in brains from animals of all the vertebrate classes. This property would indicate that this antigen had emerged early in evolution. Over 30 years after its original discovery the chemical nature of this antigen was defined as galactocerebroside. Besides this antigen, several other brain-specific antigens have been described subsequently. Of these, the basic protein is of particular interest. This chemically well-defined substance plays a predominant role in eliciting allergic encephalomyelitis (Chapter 25). The basic protein shows

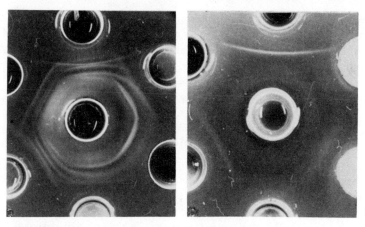

A   B

Figure 21-3. Reactions produced by rabbit antiserum to bovine aorta. Peripheral wells in both plates: Bovine tissue antigens (clockwise from the uppermost well)—aorta extract, spleen extract, liver extract, kidney extract, adrenal extract, and serum. Central well in *A*: Antiserum to bovine aorta. Central well in *B*: The same antiserum adsorbed with bovine serum. It may be seen that absorption of the antiserum with bovine serum resulted in the disappearance of most lines that were not characteristic for aorta. Some residual non-aorta-specific lines may still be recognized. They would disappear after additional absorption of the antiserum with tissues other than aorta. (From Milgrom, F.; Intorp, H. W.; and Witebsky, E.: Studies on antigenic structure of bovine aortic intima. *J. Immunol.*, **99**:164–70, 1967. © 1967 The Williams & Wilkins Co., Baltimore.)

very little species specificity as evidenced by the fact that antigenic preparations derived from the brains of various species origin readily elicit allergic encephalomyelitis in guinea pigs. Other brain components have various degrees of species specificity.

Thyroglobulin, the antigen characteristic of the thyroid gland, has also been studied since the 1920s. Thyroglobulin carries definite species specificity in addition to tissue specificity. Rabbit antisera to human and to bovine thyroglobulins would react with these antigens to give patterns of reactions very similar to those presented for γ globulins in Figure 21-1. The role of sensitization with thyroglobulin in production of autoimmune thyroiditis has been discussed in Chapter 25. It would be beyond the scope of this chapter to discuss all known tissue-specific antigens.

Methods for Detection and Characterization of Tissue-Specific Antigens

Rabbit has been the species most frequently used for raising the antisera. The species selected as donor of tissues used for immunization is usually one of readily available slaughter animals such as ox, sheep, or pig. Human tissues obtained at autopsy or surgery are also frequently used for immunization. Immunization is performed with tissue suspensions or tissue extracts, which are frequently incorporated into Freund's adjuvant in order to strengthen the immune response.

The most useful *in vitro* procedure for studies on tissue specificity is double-diffusion gel precipitation. Rabbit antiserum to a particular mammalian tissue (referred to as tissue A) is tested against extract of this tissue and extracts of other tissues from the same species (Figure 21–3). In most instances, the antiserum produces many precipitation lines with extracts of A and non-A. The lines formed with A, which have their counterparts in non-A, are readily sorted out as being due to reactions with antigens that are not characteristic for A. Several of these lines frequently represent reactions with serum proteins that contaminate antigenic preparations used for immunization and for *in vitro* tests. Some lines may be formed with cytoplasmic antigens that are nontissue specific. In several instances a line with A may be recognized that has no counterpart lines in reactions with non-A. Such a line is likely to be A specific.

Absorption of the antiserum is usually helpful for detection of tissue-specific reactions. Removal of antibodies to serum proteins is readily achieved by dissolving lyophilized serum in the antiserum. Frequently, absorption with serum does not suffice to abolish all nontissue-specific reactions. In such a case, lyophilized extracts of tissues other than A may be used for additional absorption. The objective of obtaining a tissue-specific reagent is usually achieved by such absorption procedures. Extracts of many tissues other than A must be tested before one can definitely identify tissue specificity. Sometimes an antigen may be shared only by two tissues, e.g., brain and testicle or pituitary and adrenal.

Interspecies cross-reactions are usually studied. If positive results are obtained with extracts of A from all or most mammalian species, the study is extended to other vertebrate classes. Studies for interspecies cross-reactions usually include the antibody-producing species (in our example, the rabbit). Positive reactions with extract of A from this species indicate that at least some tissue-specific antibodies may be autoantibodies in that they would combine with the extract from the tissue A of the antibody-producing animal itself.

Besides gel precipitation, passive agglutination is a procedure frequently used in studies on tissue specificity. This procedure is especially valuable if the tissue-specific antibodies are too weak to be detected by precipitation tests. For this test, convenient carrier particles, usually erythrocytes, are coated with extracts of A and non-A as well as with serum and tested against various dilutions of antiserum. Assessing tissue-specific reactions by means of passive agglutination is more difficult than by means of precipitation. Two approaches are usually taken: (1) Antiserum extensively absorbed with non-A is tested against particles coated by A and non-A. If a residual reaction occurs with A only, this is a strong indication for tissue specificity of this

Table 21-2
TANNED CELL HEMAGGLUTINATION TEST

Influence of Absorptions on the Reaction of Rabbit Anti-bovine-adrenal Serum with Red Blood Cells Coated by Saline Extracts of Bovine Organs and by Bovine Serum

| | Highest Dilution of Antiserum Giving Definite Agglutination of Cells Coated by | | | |
| | EXTRACT OF BOVINE | | | BOVINE |
	ADRENAL	SPLEEN	KIDNEY	SERUM
Unabsorbed antiserum	7290	2430	2430	> 7290
Antiserum absorbed by bovine				
Adrenal extract	< 10	< 10	< 10	< 10
Spleen extract	2430	< 10	< 10	< 10
Kidney extract	2430	< 10	< 10	10
Serum	2430	270	810	< 10

reaction (Table 21–2). (2) The reaction between anti-A and particles coated by A is inhibited by extracts of various tissues. If the inhibition is accomplished to a much higher extent by A than by non-A, this again is an indication for tissue specificity.

Several other serologic procedures including complement fixation, immunofluorescence, and tests with radiolabeled antigens and antibodies have been also successfully employed for studies on tissue specificity.

Once a tissue-specific antigen is identified, studies on its physicochemical properties are usually performed. If the tissue-specific reaction can be detected by means of gel precipitation, then information concerning the nature of antigen is obtained by means of immunoelectrophoresis and staining of the precipitation lines with histochemical reagents. Thereafter, isolation and purification of the antigen are attempted by a variety of procedures, including column chromatography, gel filtration, curtain electrophoresis, and gradient ultracentrifugation. Frequently, the information about the chemical nature of the antigen is derived from studies on degradation by such reagents as nucleases, proteases, and periodate.

Physiologic Role and Localization of Tissue-Specific Antigens

The physiologic role of most tissue-specific antigens is unknown, thyroglobulin being an outstanding exception in this respect. In recent years, extensive studies on the antigenic properties of hormones with well-defined physiologic activities have been performed. A hormone may be justifiably called a tissue-specific antigen of the particular endocrine gland even though it is excreted into the circulation. Hormonal immunoassays based on detection and quantitation of a hormone by means of an immune serum are of considerable practical importance. Detection of chorionic gonadotropin in urine by means of an antiserum to this hormone serves as a useful test for pregnancy (Chapter 29).

Whereas some tissue-specific antigens are shed off to the circulation, as is the case with serum proteins and hormones, others are sequestered, intracellular components. The above-discussed antigens of lens, brain, and thyroid gland may be classified as such antigens even though some minute amounts of thyroglobulin "leak" into the circulation. The confinement of tissue antigens may account for their autoantigenic potentialities. One could conceive that these antigens have no access to the immunologic apparatus under physiologic conditions and, therefore, do not elicit self-recognition. If proper immunizing procedures are employed, formation of tissue-specific autoantibodies may be quite readily achieved. Autoimmune responses and pathologic lesions induced by them are discussed at length in Chapter 25. It should be stated here, however, that antisera with tissue-specific autoantibodies may serve as excellent reagents for detection of some tissue antigens such as those of brain, thyroid gland, adrenal, heart, testicle, and others.

Heterophile Specificity

Heterophile antibodies are defined as antibodies combining with an antigen that apparently is completely unrelated to the antigen that stimulated their formation. Heterophile antigen may be defined as an antigen stimulating formation of heterophile antibodies or an antigen combining with them.

The Forssman System

The discovery of Forssman in 1911, even if not the first, was the most important discovery of a heterophile antigen-antibody system. Forssman demonstrated that rabbits immunized with suspensions of guinea pig tissues formed antibodies combining with sheep erythrocytes. The antigen shared by guinea pig tissues and sheep erythrocytes has been called Forssman antigen. The first studies on the physicochemical nature of Forssman antigen showed that it is a thermostable, ethanol-soluble substance of apparently lipid nature. More recent studies demonstrated that the Forssman antigen is a glycolipid.

Forssman antigen appears in tissues of many animal species that are referred to as Forssman positive, and it is absent from tissues of other animal species called Forssman negative. Inspection of Table 21–3 shows clearly that the distribution of the Forssman antigen among various species is quite haphazard, e.g., mouse is Forssman positive, but closely related rat is Forssman negative. Among Bovidae, sheep and goat are positive but ox and

Table 21-3
DISTRIBUTION OF THE FORSSMAN ANTIGEN IN THE ANIMAL
KINGDOM

Forssman-Positive Species	Forssman-Negative Species
Guinea pig	Rabbit
Sheep, goat	Ox, deer
Horse	Pig
Dog, fox	Man, chimpanzee
Cat, lion, tiger	
Camel	
Hamster	
Mouse	Rat
Chicken, turkey	Goose, duck
Ostrich	
Carp	Herring
Eel	
	Shellfish

deer are negative. Obviously, only Forssman-negative animals are capable of forming Forssman antibodies. Rabbit is the prototype of such animals. Man is a Forssman-negative species; however, the human blood group A antigen is closely related to the Forssman antigen. Forssman antigen is also present in some but not all plants and bacteria. According to Landsteiner, such random, haphazard distribution of an antigen is characteristic for carbohydrates. As we discussed above (pages 364–65), structure of protein antigens reflected in species specificity follows closely the evolutionary pathway.

Injection of rabbit antiserum containing Forssman antibodies into the circulation of a guinea pig kills the animal with symptoms closely resembling anaphylactic shock. Some investigators have called this phenomenon inverse anaphylaxsis in view of the fact that, opposite to the usual experimental design for anaphylactic shock (Chapter 18), in inverse anaphylaxis the antigen is bound to the tissues and antibody administered to the circulation.

The Hanganutziu-Deicher System

Another type of heterophile antibodies was described by Hanganutziu in 1924 and Deicher in 1926. These antibodies were noted in patients who received therapeutic injections of foreign species sera such as diphtheria antitoxin of horse origin. These antibodies combined with sheep erythrocytes, but they obviously were not of Forssman nature since they reacted with erythrocytes of many Forssman-negative animals including ox. They have frequently been called serum sickness antibodies, which is a misnomer since their appearance is not related to symptoms of serum sickness. A preferable term is Hanganutziu-Deicher or HD antibodies. The corresponding antigen (HD antigen) is a glycolipid. Recent observations showed that HD antibodies appear in a small proportion of human patients suffering from various diseases even though they never received an injection of a foreign species serum.

The Paul-Bunnell System

Medically, the most important heterophile system was described by Paul and Bunnell, who in 1932 reported that sera of patients suffering from infectious mononucleosis agglutinate sheep erythrocytes. It was subsequently shown that these antibodies (to be referred to as Paul-Bunnell or PB antibodies) react also with bovine erythrocytes. Because bovine erythrocytes are poorly agglutinable, the reaction with them is usually studied by means of a complement-mediated lysis. The fact that they react with Forssman-negative bovine erythrocytes and that they are not removed by absorption with Forssman-positive guinea pig tissues clearly proved that PB antibodies differ from Forssman antibodies. Table 21–4 shows the most important features distinguishing Forssman, HD, and PB antigens. Davidson's differential test for infectious mononucleosis is based on the demonstration that agglutination of sheep erythrocytes by patient serum is abolished by absorption with bovine erythrocytes but not with guinea pig kidney suspension.

The reaction of infectious mononucleosis sera with bovine erythrocytes involves more antigenic sites than the reaction with sheep or horse erythrocytes. The PB antigen of bovine erythrocytes is a glycoprotein. PB antibodies belong, as a rule, to the IgM class and only in rare instances are they found in the IgG fraction of serum. They are independent of antibodies to the Epstein-Barr virus broadly recognized as the causative agent of infectious mononucleosis. They are also independent of a variety of other antibodies found in infectious mononucleosis sera such as antibodies against Newcastle disease virus, antibodies to blood group i antigen, or antibodies eliciting lysis of human lymphocytes at low temperatures.

The antigenic stimulus responsible for formation of PB antibodies is a mystery. The present author advocated for many years the thesis that the stimulus is exerted by a "novel" antigen that appears on the patient's cells as a result of infection with the virus of infectious mononucleosis. Convincing evidence supporting this hypothesis was obtained in recent studies which demonstrated PB antigen in the tissues, particularly in the kidneys, from a patient who died of heart failure when suffering from infectious mononucleosis.

Table 21-4
DISTRIBUTION OF HETEROPHILE ANTIGENS

	Sheep Erythrocytes	Bovine Erythrocytes	Guinea Pig Kidney
Forssman	+	−	+
Hanganutziu-Deicher	+	+	+
Paul-Bunnell	+	+	−

Cell Surface Antigens

Most of the antigens present on cell membranes are water insoluble and are nonextractable by the usual techniques. Therefore, these antigens cannot be readily studied by such procedures as gel precipitation or passive agglutination, which are capable of detecting soluble antigens only. Detection of cell-surface antigens can be achieved in the simplest way by means of a plain agglutination procedure. However, this procedure requires a stable cell suspension and, therefore, can be employed only for studies of some cells, primarily erythrocytes. In contrast, nucleated cells of most tissues cannot be obtained in suspensions stable enough to permit application of agglutination. For studies of surface antigens of nucleated cells, membrane immuno-fluorescence, cytolysis, cytotoxicity, and mixed agglutination procedures proved to be convenient tools.

By means of mixed agglutination tests it was shown that predominant antigens of the surface of living mammalian nucleated cells are characterized by pronounced species specificity. In studies of cell-surface antigens, inter-species cross-reactions are obviously also encountered but they are considerably weaker than homologous reactions. Evidence has also been presented that some of the cell-surface antigens may be characteristic for the given cells, e.g., thymus cells.

Interesting observations were made on interspecies cell hybrids, which were obtained by fusion of murine and human cell cultures. The resulting man-mouse hybrid cells had surface antigens characteristic of both species. When upon propagation of hybrid cells the human chromosomes were deleted, the cells lost the antigens characteristic for man but retained those characteristic for mouse.

Of the antigens discussed in previous parts of this chapter, tissue- and species-specific antigens appear mostly as water-soluble components of cell cytoplasm and body fluids. Heterophile antigens discussed above are found intracellularly but they also appear on the cell surface. The latter location accounts for the toxicity of Forssman antibodies.

Summary

Saline extracts of vertebrate tissues usually contain antigen(s) characteristic for the given tissue. Besides their tissue specificity, such antigens usually carry also species specificity. Antigens excreted to the circulation such as serum proteins and hormones are characteristic for the species but they reflect also the specificity of their function and origin. Therefore, they also can be considered tissue-specific antigens. The major antigens of mammalian cell surface are saline nonextractable antigens, which are characteristic for the species. In contrast to the protein antigens, heterophile antigens, which are carbohydrates, do not follow the evolutionary pathway and appear in a haphazard way in various species.

Studies on species and tissue specificity, as well as hererophile specificity, have constituted a fruitful field of immunologic research, which has had important implications for studies on normal and pathologic tissues, for studies on autoimmune disorders, and for developing important sero-diagnostic procedures.

Bibliography

Coombs, R. R. A., and Franks, D.: Immunological reactions involving two cell types. *Prog. Allergy*, 13:174–212, 1969.

Dumonde, D. C.: Tissue-specific antigens. *Adv. Immunol.*, 5:245–412, 1966.

Forssman, J.: Die heterogenetischen Antigen, besonders die sog. Forssman-Antigene und ihre Antikörper. In Kolle, W.; Kraus, R.; and Uhlenhuth, P. (eds.): *Handbuch der pathogenen Mikroorganismen, III*. Urban & Schwarzenberg, Berlin/Wien, 1930, pp. 469–526.

Glade, P. R.: *Infectious Mononucleosis*. J. B. Lippincott, Philadelphia, 1973.

Halbert, S. P., and Manski, W.: Organ specificity with special reference to the lens. *Prog. Allergy*, 7:107–86, 1963.

Kabat, E. A., and Mayer, M. M.: *Experimental Immunochemistry*. Charles C Thomas, Publisher, Springfield, Ill., 1961.

Kano, K., and Milgrom, F.: Heterophile antigens and antibodies in medicine. *Curr. Top. Microbiol. Immunol.*, 77:43–69, 1977.

Landsteiner, K.: *The Specificity of Serological Reactions*. Harvard University Press, Cambridge, Mass., 1946.

Milgrom, F.: Tissue specificity. In Rose, N. R., and Milgrom, F. (eds.): *International Convocation on Immunology*. S. Karger, Basel/New York, 1969, pp. 270–78.

Nuttal, G. H. F.: *Blood Immunity and Blood Relationship*. Cambridge University Press, Cambridge, 1904.

Springer, G. F.: Blood-group and Forssman antigenic determinants shared between microbes and mammalian cells. *Prog. Allergy*, 15:9–77, 1971.

Uhlenhuth, P., and Seiffert, W.: Die biologische Eiweissdifferenzierung mittels der Präcipitation mit besonderer Berücksichtung der Technik. In *Handbuch der pathogenen Mikroorganismen, III*. Urban & Schwartzenberg, Berlin/Wein, 1930, pp. 365–468.

Witebsky, E.: Die serologische Analyse von Zellen und Geweben. *Naturwissenschaften*, 17:771–76, 1929.

22

Transplantation Immunology

FELIX MILGROM, KYOICHI KANO, AND
MAREK B. ZALESKI

Introduction and Definitions

The interest in transplantation was undoubtedly generated by its possible medical application. The idea of the replacement of diseased tissues with normal tissues as a therapeutic measure has appealed to physicians and laymen for centuries. This interest has been expressed in ancient myths and medieval pictures before progress in surgery made it possible to graft tissues and organs in animals and man. At the beginning of the twentieth century, however, it was realized that the recipient's own tissues would be accepted, whereas tissues from other donors would be rejected. Definite evidence for the immunologic nature of the rejection of foreign grafts was presented by Medawar in 1944. It is now broadly recognized that rejection of foreign grafts is one of the expressions of immunologic surveillance that is responsible for elimination of foreign antigens including pathogenic microorganisms that invade an animal.

For our further discussion we will define the terms that are used in this chapter.

1. *Autograft:* a transplant taken from the recipient. Provided that the surgical procedures are proper, the autograft is permanently accepted, since it does not contain any foreign antigens. Autotransplantation has been successfully employed in plastic surgery for decades.

2. *Homograft:* a transplant from another individual of the same species. In some instances the donor may be genetically identical with the recipient; such a graft is called syngeneic. In humans, only a graft from a monozygotic twin is syngeneic. In animals, a syngeneic graft is usually taken from a donor of the same inbred strain as the recipient. Inbred strains of animals have been raised by brother-to-sister mating for many generations. This eventually resulted in animals that are homozygous for all inherited traits and, at least for practical reasons, are genetically identical. Many inbred strains of mice and rats are readily available. There are also a few inbred strains of guinea pigs, rabbits, hamsters, and chickens. A syngeneic graft, like an autograft is almost always permanently accepted. Here, except for weak sex-linked antigens, this graft has no antigens foreign to the recipient and, therefore, no stimulus that would engender an immune response of the recipient. *Allogeneic homograft or allograft* is a graft originating from a donor that belongs to the same species as the recipient but is genetically different. In the transplantation nomenclature the term "homograft" is quite frequently used without an adjective. In such instances, this term denotes allogeneic homograft. An allograft is usually rejected within a few days or weeks. Here the graft contains antigens absent from the recipient and, therefore, the recipient mounts an immune response that leads to the rejection.

3. *Xenograft or heterograft:* a transplant from a donor belonging to a species other than recipient. In view of pronounced antigenic disparity, a xenograft is usually rejected more quickly than an allograft.

Allograft Rejection

Mechanisms underlying allograft rejection have been extensively studied since the 1940s, and from these studies a field of transplantation immunology has emerged. Most experiments were performed using skin allografts because of the simple surgical procedures involved and an easy clinical follow-up of these grafts.

With a few exceptions, a recipient who had no previous contact with the donor's antigens produces no immediate response to a skin allograft. Vascular connections are established, and for a few days the allograft is indistinguishable from an autograft. Usually, the first signs of rejection are noted five or six days after transplantation, and in 10 to 12 days the graft is completely sloughed off and replaced by eschar. The rejection of skin allografts is a necrotizing reaction with accumulation of predominantly mononuclear cells such as lymphocytes and macrophages.

The process of rejection leaves the recipient hypersensitive to the allograft. This hypersensitivity may be readily demonstrated by challenging the recipient with a second skin graft. The rejection process is now more rapid than with the first graft. The rejection would be accomplished within, for example, five days rather than ten days. In many instances, no vascular connections are established between the recipient and the second graft. Sometimes, the second graft appears like a parchment and then it is called a white graft. The terms "accelerated rejection" and "second-set rejection" have been used to distinguish the rejection of an allograft by a sensitized animal from the "first-set rejection" produced by a normal, nonsensitized animal.

Hypersensitivity to allograft is systemic in that accelerated rejection can be observed not only in the area in which the first graft was placed but also in practically any other part of the recipient's body. This hypersensitivity is not organ specific since skin, for example, presented as a first graft may condition the recipient to reject, in an accelerated way, a second graft consisting of another organ, such as the kidney. On the other hand, this hypersensitivity is donor specific in that the accelerated rejection is observed only if the second graft originates from the same donor as the first or from a donor that is antigenically related to the donor of the first graft.

Transplantation Antigens in Vertebrates

The cytoplasmic membranes of all cells contain a wide variety of molecules which, if the cells are grafted, come into contact with the immunologically competent cells of the allogeneic recipient. The latter recognizes some of the surface molecules as foreign and mounts an immune response directed against these molecules, which ultimately leads to allograft rejection. The cell-surface molecules triggering the response resulting in allograft rejection are called transplantation or histocompatibility antigens. In the mouse, a multitude of distinct histocompatibility antigens have been identified; each is genetically determined by an allele at a specific locus. Thus far, over 60 histocompatibility loci have been recognized in the murine genome. The exact or tentative positions are known for some loci but others still await genetic assignment. Figure 22–1 presents the chromosomal location of loci with reasonably well-established positions.

It may be noted that several different symbols are used to designate different loci. The symbol *H* (histocompatibility) designates loci with genes that determine antigens primarily involved in allograft rejection (classic histocompatibility antigens). The role played in allograft rejection by the products of genes at other loci shown in Figure 22–1 is still controversial. The symbols generally reflect the cell type on which products of a particular gene are commonly demonstrated: *Ea* on erythrocytes, *Ly* on lymphocytes, *Thy* on thymocytes, *Pca* on plasma cells, and *Tla* on leukemic cells. The products of these genes always trigger the production of serum antibodies, but only in some instances do they become responsible for the rejection of certain types of allografts.

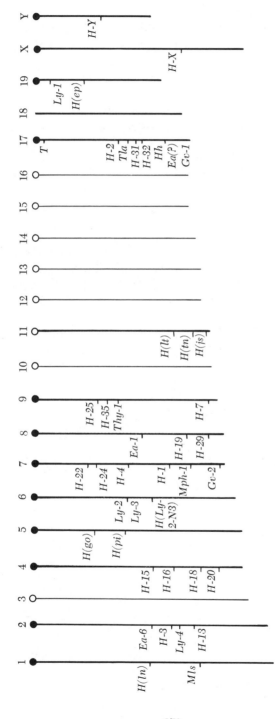

Figure 22-1. Localization of histocompatibility loci within the murine genome. Each heavy line represents a chromosome to which at least one histocompatibility locus has been assigned, whereas thin lines represent chromosomes without histocompatibility loci. Terminal dot symbolizes centromere.

Each of the indicated loci has at least two alleles but frequently more than two. Virtually all the information presently available comes from studies on inbred mice that were derived from a small original stock; hence, the true polymorphism of the species, including the wild population, is under-represented. It should be stressed that as many as 20 identified histocompatibility loci for minor transplantation antigens have not as yet been assigned a position in any particular chromosome.

Earlier studies employing grafts of malignant tumors and normal skin in mice have demonstrated that one of many histocompatibility antigens invariably produces particularly vigorous rejection of all incompatible allografts, usually within 10 to 14 days. The other antigens are significantly less potent in their capability to induce allograft rejection. Incompatibility, especially if restricted to one, or even a few, of these antigens, results in slow graft rejection, and occasionally some but not all first-set grafts are rejected. Therefore, two classes of transplantation antigens can be distinguished: major and minor histocompatibility antigens. Table 22-1 summarizes the most pronounced differences between these two classes of antigens.

Most of the differences between major and minor histocompatibility antigens are quantitative (Table 22-1). However, at least one difference appears to be qualitative: in all animal species studied thus far, relationship was established between some immune responses and major histocompatibility antigens. No relationship with the minor histocompatibility antigens was demonstrated. The *Ir* genes, which determine the magnitude of immune responses to a wide variety of antigens, have been mapped inside or close to

Table 22-1
COMPARISON OF MAJOR AND MINOR HISTOCOMPATIBILITY ANTIGENS

Characteristic	Histocompatibility Antigens	
	MAJOR	MINOR
Genetic determination	Complex of loci	Single locus
Recognized polymorphism	Up to a hundred alleles	Two to four alleles
Association with *Ir* loci	Always found	Not found
Usual time of first-set rejection of incompatible skin graft	< 3 weeks	> 3 weeks
Frequency of rejection of first-set skin graft	100%	10 to 100%
Effect of immunosuppression on allograft rejection	Relatively weak	Relatively strong
Effect of preimmunization on allograft rejection	Usually not impressive	Significant
Induction of humoral antibodies	Common	Rare and irregular
Induction of tolerance	Difficult	Relatively easy
Involvement in mixed lymphocyte and graft-vs.-host reactions	Invariably strong	Variable
Involvement in physiologic T and B cell collaboration	Essential	None

the major histocompatibility system. The nature of the products of the *Ir* genes and their relationship to transplantation antigens are still the subject of dispute. However, it is well established that a particular *Ir* gene determines the magnitude of the immune response to a given antigen without affecting the responsiveness to other antigens.

Mixed Lymphocyte Reaction (MLR)

In 1964, Bain and Löwenstein mixed two allogeneic white cell populations and placed the mixture in a tissue culture. Several days later, they found that approximately 30% of lymphocytes in the culture were transformed to lymphoblasts. This phenomenon was initially called mixed leukocyte culture (MLC) phenomenon and now is usually referred to as mixed lymphocyte reaction (MLR). Initially, MLR has been quantitated by differential counting of the smears of cultured cells and determining the percent of lymphoblasts. Presently, quantitation is achieved by pulse labeling of cultures with ^{3}H thymidine and then measuring the amount of the radio-activity associated with the DNA of lymphoblasts.

The immunologic character of the MLR seems to be firmly established on the basis of its specificity and the role played by immunologic memory in this reaction. It is commonly believed that the MLR consists of stimulation of a small fraction of T cells by products of major and, in some instances, minor histocompatibility loci. However, the possibility that B cells may also be stimulated to some extent cannot be excluded. According to presently available data, the stimulating structures are expressed primarily on B cells but also to some extent on T cells, and the stimulating potency of these cells depends on the genetic disparity between the responding and stimulating cells under investigation. Although there is no doubt that stimulating structures are determined by loci mapped inside or close to the major histocompatibility loci, the relationship between stimulating structures and antigens responsible for allograft rejection remains to be resolved. Until the precise determination of such a relationship is possible, the term "lymphocyte activating determinants" (Lad) is used for sites responsible for the MLR. The Lad are determined by a presently undefined number of *Lad* loci (page 387).

When the normal lymphocytes from two unrelated individuals are mixed the positive MLR represents a result of simultaneous transformation and proliferation of cells from both individuals. In MLR employed as a part of the donor-recipient matching procedures for clinical transplantation, it is essential to determine the presence or absence of transformation of prospective recipient cells. Transformation of prospective donor cells is relatively unimportant. To distinguish between the two components of MLR, a technique called one-way MLR has been developed. Unlike two-way MLR, in which cells of both individuals act as stimulator and responder for each other, in one-way MLR the cells of the prospective donor are prevented from responding; hence, they are acting only as stimulator for the cells of the prospective recipient. The cells are rendered unresponsive by pretreatment with cytostatic substances such as dactinomycin or mitomycin, or by exposing them to ionizing irradiation. Identification of stimulator and responder cells is also important for many investigative purposes.

The MLR is not an exclusive property of structures determined by major histocompatibility loci. In several cases, incompatibility restricted to minor loci resulted in a pronounced MLR. The stimulating capability of structures determined by minor loci varies from virtually undetectable (e.g., incompatibility at a single *H* locus in mice) through moderate (e.g., *Thy-1* incompatibility or multiple minor *H* loci incompatibilities) to stimulation as strong as that produced by incompatibility at a major locus (e.g., *M*-locus incompatibility). In addition, the magnitude of the MLR elicited by incompatibility at minor loci was found to be influenced by alleles at the *MLR-capacitating* locus (*MLRC*), and a similar influence has been suggested in the case of MLR elicited by incompatibility at the major locus. In both instances, the control could be analogous to that determined by *Ir* genes involved in the humoral responses to a variety of antigens.

Major Histocompatibility Complex in Mice

For obvious reasons, the main effort of researchers has been devoted to defining the genetic determination, immunochemical nature, cellular localization, and mode of action of major histocompatibility antigens. These efforts were originally clouded by unexpected complexity, which, at certain times, made any comprehensive interpretation virtually impossible. Ultimately, however, significant progress has been made, to a great extent promoted by the concept that major histocompatibility antigens are the products of several closely linked loci forming the major histocompatibility complex (MHC). Indeed, the adoption of this concept permitted the interpretation of data and the explanation of phenomena that otherwise appeared highly controversial. In virtually all vertebrate species thus far studied, man, mice, rats, dogs, pigs, monkeys, guinea pigs, and chickens, the MHC was found to have a similar structure. The murine MHC was studied most extensively.

Figure 22–2 represents a simplified structure of the MHC of mice, also called the *H-2* complex.* It consists of five distinct regions, *K*, *I*, *S*, *G*, and *D*, separable from each other by crossing over and characterized by the presence of at least one locus with several alleles. Except for those determined

---

* Since the H-2 complex was the first murine histocompatibility system to be discovered, this complex might have been named *H-1*. However, the name *H-2*, originally assigned to the locus coding for antigen II discovered by Gorer, has been retained as the name of murine MHC.

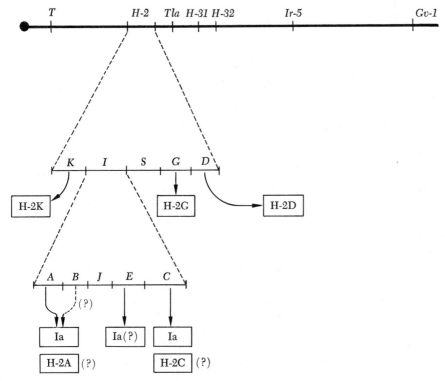

Figure 22-2. Simplified map of the murine chromosome 17 and genetic structure of the *H-2* complex. Symbols in boxes represent the products (transplantation antigens) determined by alleles at appropriate region or subregion.

by the *S* region, the molecules determined by loci in the *H-2* complex are found in the cell membranes of various cells and can be detected and characterized by two major features; they trigger the production of specific antibodies and are implicated in the immune responses resulting in allograft rejection.

The *I* region is further subdivided into five subregions, *A*, *B*, *J*, *E*, and *C*, characterized by appropriate loci with genes that code for specific cell-surface molecules.

Essentially, two types of molecules are determined by the loci of the *H-2* complex, the *H-2* and Ia.* These two types of molecules are, in many respects, quite similar but, at the same time, they function in sufficiently different ways that they should be described separately.

It should be mentioned that some authors tend to include the closely linked loci *Tla*, *H-31*, *H-32*, and even *T* into the murine MHC.

---

* For the sake of simplicity, products of any other loci of the *H-2* complex are disregarded in this discussion. For relevant data, see Klein, 1975.

H-2 Antigens

Antigens determined by murine MHC, which are distributed in essentially all tissues and are apparently involved in allograft rejection, are generally classified as H-2 antigens. There are five discrete *H-2* loci within the *H-2* complex, but a significant body of information has been collected with regard to the products of two of these loci, *H-2K* and *H-2D*. Because of their general similarities, the products of these two loci will be discussed jointly.

From a chemical point of view, the products of the *H-2K* and *H-2D* genes, i.e., H-2K and H-2D molecules, are glycoproteins (about 45,000 daltons). *In vivo*, the molecules are associated noncovalently at a 1:1 ratio with β_2 microglobulin (β_2m) (11,600 daltons; Chapter 3). Two H-2 molecules can form a dimer of 90,000 daltons with a disulfide bond between the polypeptide chains, but some believe that this may represent an artifact caused by isolation procedures. The protein moiety of the H-2 molecule constitutes approximately 90% of the molecular weight, which corresponds to a poly-peptide chain composed of 300 to 350 amino acids. The polypeptide is particularly rich in glutamic (13%) and aspartic (9.5%) acids but, otherwise, is neither rich nor poor in any particular amino acid.

The carbohydrate moiety of about 3300 daltons constitutes close to 10% of the molecular weight of the H-2 molecule. It consists of a short core chain of mannose and glucosamine from which three short side chains of sialic acid-galactose-glucosamine extend outward. The core chain is linked with asparagine of the protein moiety by fucosyl-N-glucosamine.

H-2 molecules are determined by codominant genes at the *H-2K* and *H-2D* loci. The alleles present at the *H-2K* and *H-2D* loci of an individual strain together with alleles at other loci of MHC form the *H-2* haplotype. At each of the *H-2* loci, there are at least eight unrelated alleles designated by small letters. If all minor variants are considered, the number of alleles becomes significantly greater. A particular allele determines the glyco-protein molecule, which is distinguishable from the products of other alleles by its antigenic properties. Antigenic properties reside in the protein moiety and the carbohydrate portion is identical for all H-2 molecules. An average H-2 molecule has three to ten antigenic determinants called specificities and designated by Arabic figures. Table 22–2 summarizes the specificities found in the eight most common allelic products of the *H-2K* and *H-2D* genes and shows some specificities that can be assigned to either H-2K or H-2D molecules. In fact, there are over 56 specificities already recognized by monospecific antisera.

It is quite evident that either H-2K or H-2D molecules contain two types of specificities. On the one hand, there are two series of mutually exclusive (allelic) specificities: 16, 17, 18, 19, 23, 26, 31, and 33 for H-2K molecules; and 2, 4, 9, 12, 16, 18, 30, and 32 for H-2D molecules. These specificities are

Table 22-2
ANTIGENIC SPECIFICITIES OF H-2K AND H-2D MOLECULES DETERMINED BY SOME
H-2 ALLELES

H-2K Molecule	Allele	H-2D Molecule
5, 27, 28, 29, **33**, 25, 36, 39, 46	*b*	2, 6, 27, 28, 29
3, 8, 27, 28, 29, **31**, 34, 46, 47	*d*	3, **4**, 6, 13, 27, 28, 29, 35, 36, 41, 42, 43, 44, 49
7, 8, **26**, 27, 28, 29, 37, 39, 46	*f*	6, **9**, 27
1, 3, 5, 8, 11, **23**, 25, 45, 47	*k*	1, 3, 5, **32**, 49
1, 5, 7, 8, **16**,* 34, 37, 38, 46	*p*	1, 3, 5, 6, **16**,* 35, 41, 49
1, 3, 5, 11, **17**, 34, 45	*q*	3, 6, 13, 27, 28, 29, **30**, 49
1, 3, 5, 8, 11, **18**,* 25, 45, 47	*r*	1, 5, 6, **18**,* 49
1, 5, 7, **19**, 42, 45	*s*	3, 6, **12**, 28, 36, 42, 49

* Specificities that could not be definitely assigned to one of two molecules because of the absence of appropriate recombinants.

restricted to a single allele; hence, they are called private. Typically, they give rise to relatively strong antibodies. On the other hand, there are specificities that are present in two (e.g., 25) or even seven (e.g., 5) different molecules. The specificities that are shared by many allelic molecules are called public.

Of the entire H-2 molecule, about 65% of the protein moiety displays an apparent chemical dissimilarity between allelic products, and the remaining 35% displays remarkable similarity within the H-2K variety as well as between H-2K and H-2D varieties. Antigenic specificities are probably associated with the variable part of the molecule.

Incompatibility, restricted to the *H-2*K and *H-2D* loci, causes an apparent though weak MLR in most if not all cases. This finding has several possible explanations. The *K* as well as the *D* regions may consist of two closely linked loci, one coding for appropriate H-2 molecules and the other for the appropriate Lad molecule. Alternatively, the H-2K and H-2D themselves act as stimulating structures in MLR. In the latter case, one could postulate that within the H-2 molecule, one portion is predominantly responsible for allograft rejection and another portion is triggering MLR. One should not overlook still another alternative—that the MLR evoked by H-2 molecules is qualitatively different from that elicited by the products of the *I* region.

Figure 22–3 represents schematically the relationship between H-2 molecules and the cytoplasmic membrane. The integration of the molecules into the membrane is accomplished by a small segment of the protein moiety that can be detached by papain without appreciable effect on the antigenic properties of the molecule. Detailed analysis showed that H-2 molecules are distributed independently of each other and other cell membrane molecules within the cytoplasmic membrane. There is a definite relationship between the H-2D and Tla molecules in the membrane; usually increased H-2D molecules are accompanied by decreased Tla molecules.

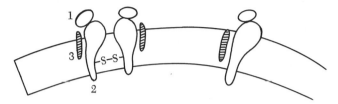

Figure 22-3.   Schematic representation of H-2 molecules in the cell membrane. *1*, Carbohydrate portion; *2*, protein portion; *3*, β_2 microglobulin. The extracellular space is in upper part of figure.

The H-2K and H-2D molecules are found in the cell membranes of virtually all cells of the body, but their concentration is variable. Thus lymphocytes and bone marrow cells contain significantly more H-2 antigen than, for example, thymus or muscle cells.

The products of recently identified *H-2G* locus are poorly defined. Thus far, only one serologic specificity, 7, has been described. Only two allelic products of this locus can be distinguished, one associated with the *H-2* haplotypes, *f*, *k*, *p*, and *s* and possessing specificity 7, and the other associated with the remaining haplotypes and lacking specificity 7. Specificity 7 is detectable in a particularly high density on erythrocytes as compared with lymphocytes. Little is known about the structure of H-2G molecules.

Products of the *H-2A* and *H-2C* loci, previously called jointly the *H-2I* locus, are unknown, and they may, in fact, be identical to Ia molecules.

Ia Antigens

The molecules determined by genes at the *I* region of the murine MHC are classified as Ia (*I* region–associated) antigens. Characteristically, they have a more restricted distribution than H-2 molecules, and they trigger the production of antibodies that are cytotoxic for certain populations of lymphocytes but do not agglutinate erythrocytes. There are at least three loci with several alleles coding for Ia antigens since, thus far, three discrete molecules have been identified and associated with the *IA*, *IE*, and *IC* subregions.

Chemically, all Ia molecules are glycoproteins of 26,000 or 35,000 daltons, sometimes forming dimers through disulfide bonds. Contrary to the H-2K and H-2D molecules, no association was found between Ia molecules and β_2m.

Serologic analysis of the Ia molecules revealed two series of specificities, similar to H-2 molecules, which tentatively can be classified as private (2, 4, 10, and 14) and public. Table 22–3 shows the distribution of 22 known specificities of the Ia molecules in the eight most common *H-2* haplotypes.

The *IB* subregion does not have any specificity positively assigned to it, and there are some doubts concerning its existence. The *IJ* subregion has

Table 22-3

SPECIFICITIES OF TWO IA MOLECULES DETERMINED BY ALLELES AT UNRELATED
H-2 COMPLEXES

Ia Molecule Determined by Alleles at *IA/IB* Subregions	*H-2* Allele	Ia Molecule Determined by Alleles at *IC* Subregion	Ia Molecule Determined by Alleles at *IE* Subregion
3, 8, 9, 15, W20	*b*	—	—
8, 11, 15, 16	*d*	6,7	—
1, 5, **14**,* 17, 18	*f*	—	—
1, **2**,* 3, 15, 17, 18, 19	*k*	7	22
5, 13	*p*	6, 7, W21*	—
3, 5, 9, **10**,* 13, 16	*q*	—	—
1, 3, 5, 12, 17, 19	*r*	7	—
4, 5, 9, 12, 17, 18	*s*	—	—

* Specificities found exclusively in a given allele (private).

been identified on the basis of determining surface marker of suppressor T cells, which seems to be different from "classic" Ia molecules. Finally, the recently described *IE* subregion seems to determine Ia.22 specificity, thus far found only in the *H-2*^{k} haplotype and those derived from it.

The exact relationship between H-2A and H-2C molecules and Ia molecules is impossible to ascertain at present. Therefore, one cannot determine whether Ia molecules can act as classic transplantation antigens. Rejection of allografts incompatible at the *I* region is usually accompanied by the production of antibodies to Ia just as antibodies to H-2 appear after rejection of *H-2* incompatible grafts. On the other hand, it is quite likely that *Ia* loci and Ia molecules are identical to some *Lad* loci and Lad molecules, respectively, because *H-2*–identical but *I*-incompatible cells give strong MLR, which can be blocked by antibodies to Ia antigens of stimulating cells. Further support of this suggestion is given by the association of cellular distribution of Ia molecules and MLR-stimulating properties of various cells. To explain the differences in stimulating capability of Ia and H-2 molecules, one could postulate that there is higher polymorphism of the MLR-stimulating segment of Ia molecules than of the analogous segment of H-2 molecules.

Because of space limitations, we cannot dwell on other functions ascribed to Ia molecules or, more generally, to gene products of the *I* region. An interesting suggestion appears to be that Ia molecules have the function of products of the *Ir* genes.

Human Transplantation Antigens

Unlike the previously described experiments in laboratory animals, studies on human transplantation antigens faced obvious difficulties, since man is an outbred species. Early experiences in clinical renal transplantation clearly showed that incompatibility in the ABO blood group system often resulted in acute rejection of the grafts.

The survival rate of ABO-compatible renal allografts was the lowest in unrelated donor-recipient combinations, intermediate in parent-child combinations, and best in sibling-sibling combinations. Furthermore, survival time of ABO-compatible skin grafts exchanged between siblings showed a clear-cut bimodal distribution with two distinct survival times of 22 days and 13 days. These results indicated the possible presence of a major histocompatibility complex determining strong transplantation antigens independent from ABO antigens. Following the discovery of the HLA antigens and establishment of HLA serology, it was found that all skin grafts with a mean survival of 22 days came from HLA-identical siblings and the remaining grafts from HLA-nonidentical siblings. Thus, the HLA system proved to be the major histocompatibility complex in man.

From our present knowledge of histocompatibility loci in laboratory animals, it is generally assumed that minor histocompatibility loci must exist in man. In fact, several reports indicate that some ABO-compatible renal grafts from siblings identical for HLA antigens were rejected in spite of adequate immunosuppressive treatment. This situation appears similar to the rejection of experimental allografts incompatible at multiple minor histocompatibility loci. Sera of patients who rejected ABO-compatible HLA-identical renal grafts often contained alloantibodies different from HLA antibodies.

ABO System

As mentioned previously, the early experience of surgeons with ABO-incompatible renal grafts prompted them to avoid ABO incompatibility in renal transplantation.* Experimental evidence later confirmed these observations. Preimmunization of group O individuals with group A_1 erythrocytes or even with soluble A substance resulted, in most instances, in white graft rejection of A_1 skin grafts. On the other hand, O grafts and A_2 grafts survived in such recipients for 9 to 13 days. Interestingly enough, most of B skin grafts transplanted to O recipients immunized with A substance went through white graft rejection, and the remaining B grafts were rejected in an acute fashion. Apparently, the immunized O recipients could not discriminate B grafts from A grafts, suggesting that "cross-reacting" antibodies combining with A and B play a role in the rejection of this homograft. Furthermore, A individuals immunized with B substance rejected B skin grafts in an accelerated fashion, and B individuals immunized with A

---

* A graft that does not have ABO antigens combining with the recipient's antibodies is considered ABO compatible. Accordingly, similar to classic experience with blood transfusion, O grafts may be placed into any recipient, A grafts into A or AB recipient, B grafts into B or AB recipient, and AB grafts into AB recipient only.

substance produced accelerated rejection of A skin grafts, which indicated that A and B determinants are fully immunogenic in regard to transplantation immunity. The serology and genetics of ABO system are discussed in Chapter 20.

Major Histocompatibility Complex in Man

In 1958, Dausset discovered a leukocyte alloantigen called "Mac" using leukoagglutination technique with immune sera obtained from volunteers who were injected with allogeneic leukocytes. This finding was followed by discoveries of several other leukocyte alloantigens apparently belonging to the same system. However, further information about this highly complex system had to wait for the development of a reliable serologic procedure, the microdroplet lymphocytotoxicity test of Terasaki and his coworkers, and for a genetic hypothesis of two segregant series proposed by Dausset and Ivanyi. Since 1964, international collaborative efforts in the form of periodic workshops have been devoted to the serologic as well as genetic investigations on this highly polymorphic system.

The *HLA* is a small segment on the autosome no. 6, which is similar to the murine *H-2* complex and consists of several discrete but closely linked loci (Figure 22–4). Genes at loci *A*, *B*, and *C* determine serologically detectable antigens, and gene products of locus *D* are usually demonstrated by MLR. As seen in Table 22–4, there are multiple alleles at each of these loci, 20 alleles at the *A* locus, 31 at the *B* locus, at least 6 at the *C* locus, and at least 11 at the *D* locus. The sum of gene frequencies for alleles at the *A* locus is close to 100% and so in the sum of allelic gene frequencies at the *B* locus.

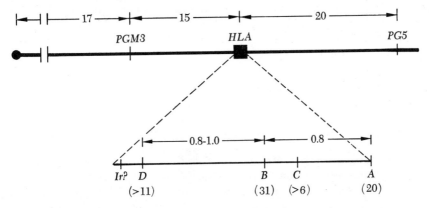

Figure 22-4. Schematic illustration of the human chromosome number 6 with enlargement of the HLA complex. Numbers between two loci indicate recombinant units. PGM3 and PG5 denote phosphoglucomatase 3 and urinary pepsinogen 5, respectively.

Table 22-4

NOMENCLATURE OF *HLA* ALLELES ADOPTED BY THE WHO COMMITTEE IN 1975*

Locus D	Locus B	Locus C	Locus A
DW1 (10)	*B5* (10)	*CW1* (5)	*A1* (11)
DW2 (8)	*B7* (11)	*CW2* (8)	*A2* (24)
DW3 (9)	*B8* (7)	*CW3* (15)	*A3* (12)
DW4 (8)	*B12* (11)	*CW4* (11)	*A9* (13)
DW5 (8)	*B13* (2)	*CW5* (7)	*A10* (5)
DW6 (5)	*B14* (3)		*A11* (9)
	B18 (7)		*A28* (5)
	B27 (4)		*A29* (2)
	BW15 (7)		*AW23* (3)
	BW16 (3)		*AW24* (10)
	BW17 (6)		*AW25* (1)
	BW21 (3)		*AW26* (5)
	BW22 (2)		*AW30* (4)
	BW35 (10)		*AW31* (1)
	BW37 (1)		*AW32* (4)
	BW38 ⎤ (3)		*AW33*
	BW39 ⎦		*AW34*
	BW40 (5)		*AW36*
	BW41 (2)		*AW43*
	BW42		

* Numbers in parenthesis are gene frequencies (%) in Caucasians. (Summary report on "Transplantation and Immunology Research," NIAID, Nov., 1974.)

On the other hand, the sum of gene frequencies for alleles at the *C* or *D* locus did not reach 50%. This means that new alleles at *C* or *D* loci will probably be found in the future, but there is little or no "space" for new alleles at *A* and *B* loci. The validity of this genetic model was finally ascertained by the demonstration of crossovers between all four loci constituting the *HLA* complex. The crossover between the *A* and *B* locus was found to occur at the ratio of 0.8% and the rate of crossovers between the *B* and *D* locus was determined to be 0.8 to 1.0%.

Antigens determined by the *C* locus have been studied recently. They appear, at present, much less important than the antigens determined by *A* and *B* loci and will not be discussed further.

HLA Loci A and B

HLA antigens determined by the *A* and *B* loci were most extensively studied in the past ten years. As mentioned above, the microdroplet lymphocytotoxicity test has been most widely employed for the detection of these antigens. However, there are many other serologic tests available such as leukoagglutination, platelet complement fixation, indirect immunofluorescence, and mixed agglutination. Anti-HLA sera used in these serologic tests are posttransplantation sera, sera of volunteers immunized with allogeneic cells, posttransfusion sera, and sera of multiparous women. For clinical HLA serotyping, selected sera from multiparous women are mainly employed. Attempts were made to obtain HLA-typing reagents in foreign species, and some limited success in this endeavor was reported.

Frequencies of alleles at A and B loci are listed in Table 22–4. The most frequent allele in the Caucasian population is $A2$. It should be stressed, however, that marked racial differences occur in frequencies of some *HLA* alleles. For example, $A1$ and $A3$ are rarely found in Oriental populations, and the frequency of $A9$ is significantly higher in Orientals than in Caucasians.

Somatic cells of an individual usually possess four HLA antigens, two determined by alleles at locus A and two by alleles at locus B. An individual who is homozygous either at the A or the B locus possesses only three HLA antigens, and in an individual homozygous at both loci, only two HLA antigens can be detected. Regardless of the homozygosity, a single germ cell of an individual possesses one A locus allele and one B locus allele. The antigens thus far discussed are analogous to the private specificities of the murine H-2 antigens. In addition, several cross-reacting specificities were discovered in this system, which are analogous to public specificities of the murine H-2 antigens, and they are shared by individuals possessing different "private" HLA specificities.

The mode of inheritance of antigens determined by A and B loci was extensively studied at the Fourth International Histocompatibility Workshop in 1970, in which each participant tested families of his choice with the same set of coded sera. The results of these blind tests clearly showed that the HLA antigens determined by the alleles at the A and B loci are inherited as simple codominant mendelian traits. Unless a crossover between A and B loci takes place, alleles at A and B loci of a given haplotype are inherited together.

By examining HLA phenotypes of members belonging to two generations of a family, one usually can deduce two paternal and two maternal *HLA* haplotypes. Haplotype determination in a given family is extremely important whenever a family member is to be selected as a donor for organ transplantation. Table 22-5 exemplifies such haplotype determination. By

Table 22-5
SEGREGATION OF *HLA* A AND B LOCUS ALLELES IN A FAMILY

	Locus A				Locus B			
	$A1$	$A2$	$A3$	$A9$	$B5$	$B7$	$B8$	$B12$
Father	+	−	+	−	−	+	+	−
Mother	−	+	−	+	+	−	−	+
Children: I	+	+	−	−	+	−	+	−
II	+	+	−	−	+	−	+	−
III	+	−	−	+	−	−	+	+
IV	−	+	+	−	+	+	−	−
V	−	−	+	+	−	+	−	+

inspecting segregation of paternal antigens in this family, it can be noted that *A1* and *B8* are inherited together by children I, II, and III, and *A3* and *B7* by children IV and V. Therefore, the paternal haplotypes are *A1–B8* and *A3–B7*. In a similar way, maternal haplotypes are *A2–B5* and *A9–B12*. If, in a given family, one assigns letters *a* and *b* to paternal haplotypes and *c* and *d* to maternal haplotypes, the possible genotypes of the children would be *ac*, *ad*, *bc*, and *bd*. Accordingly, the likelihood that two siblings have an identical genotype is 25%.

Some *HLA* haplotypes appear more frequently than others in a given population. An excess of a particular haplotype over the expected frequency calculated from the gene frequencies is called linkage disequilibrium (Δ). For example, *A1–B8*, *A3–B7*, and *A2–B12* haplotypes are frequent among Caucasians, showing Δ values of 654, 523, and $243/10^4$, respectively. There are marked differences in frequencies of some *HLA* haplotypes among different races; e.g., *A1–B8* and *A3–B7* haplotypes are rarely found among Oriental populations. These facts are important when one performs clinical HLA typings or studies the association between HLA antigens and various diseases.

Physicochemical structure of HLA antigens determined by *A* or *B* locus has been elucidated. Similar to H-2 antigens shown in Figure 22–3, HLA antigens consist of a glycoprotein of 43,000 daltons and a β_2-m molecule of 11,000 daltons, which is attached to the glycoprotein noncovalently. The antigenic determinant is present on the polypeptide of the glycoprotein close to its N terminal, and the C terminal of the polypeptide is buried in cell membrane. Papain cleavage site of the glycoprotein appears to be located near the C terminal. Such treatment of cell membrane releases the glycoprotein molecule together with β_2-m without altering the antigenic specificity. Biologic functions of carbohydrate in the glycoprotein and of β_2m remain to be determined. Structural similarity of the HLA molecule to IgG molecule (Chapter 4) has been suggested. Glycoprotein with its variable portion containing HLA determinant has been considered analogous to the heavy chain and the β_2-m to the light chain of IgG (Chapter 3). HLA and IgG molecules are also similar in some serologic properties. Upon immunization with these molecules, animals of heterologous species invariably respond to species-specific antigens of both molecules. On the other hand, alloantigens of these molecules, HLA determinants, and IgG allotypes, which are physically linked to the species antigens, are recognized by alloimmune sera.

Similar to H-2 antigens, HLA antigens determined by *A* or *B* loci are distributed in practically all cells and tissues. They are particularly abundant in lymphoid organs such as spleen, lymph nodes, and peripheral lymphocytes. Their concentration in lung, liver, and kidney is lower than in lymphoid organs, and the concentrations in aorta, muscle, and brain are the lowest. Some of the antigens were also found in plasma or milk in a form of soluble substances.

HLA Locus D

The importance of MLR in man as donor-recipient matching test was recognized shortly after its discovery, since mixed cultures of cells originating from identical twins gave consistently negative results. Following the development of one-way stimulation techniques, extensive studies have been carried out to obtain immunogenetic and cytologic information on human MLR.

MLR was interpreted as *in vitro* response of a T lymphocyte to allogeneic structures (Lad) of a stimulating lymphocyte upon physical contact of these two cells. Some investigators called Lad lymphocyte-defined (LD) antigens, since these structures are quite difficult to identify serologically. For understanding of further discussion, one should keep in mind that in negative MLR, two allogeneic cells and, therefore, the donors of these cells share the same Lad, while any disparity between the two individuals with regard to the Lad results in positive MLR. The human Lad appear to be predominant on B lymphocytes, although there is evidence for the presence of Lad on some T lymphocytes and other cells. Whatever the exact chemical structure of the human Lad, the MLR seems to correspond to the recognition phase of alloimmune responses in transplantation. Recent studies revealed that MLR results not only in blast transformation of responding T lymphocytes and their subsequent proliferation, but it also generates cytotoxic lymphocytes capable of destroying proper target cells *in vitro*.

The *D* locus determining the Lad responsible for the MLR was mapped to the left of the *B* locus of the *HLA* complex (Figure 22-4). These conclusions were based on the results of extensive family studies in which MLR was employed to study histocompatibility between any two children of a given family. As stated previously, about 25% of such children are identical for the *A* and *B* alleles. The vast majority (99%) of such children pairs when tested by MLR against each other would give a negative result. However, about 1% of such pairs would give strongly positive MLR. This finding, reported for the first time by Bach and Amos, indicated that products of a locus different from but closely linked to either *A* or *B* are responsible for triggering MLR. Subsequently, the locus called *D* has been mapped 0.8 to 1.0 cM to the left of the *B* locus. In fact, incompatibility limited to the *A* and *B* loci leads to negligible MLR as compared with the MLR elicited by incompatibility limited to the *D* locus.

Cells from unrelated individuals in the vast majority of instances give a positive MLR regardless of differences or identity at the *A* and *B* loci between reacting cells. However, in the case of haplotypes displaying strong linkage disequilibrium, *A1–B8* and *A3–B7*, as many as 10% of pairs identical at the *A* and *B* loci give negative rather than positive MLR. This indicates the existence of the linkage disequilibrium between the alleles at the *D* locus on one hand and alleles at *B* or at both *A* and *B* loci on the other hand, in addition to the already discussed disequilibrium between some alleles at the *A* and *B*.

Establishing the existence of the *D* locus with alleles determining MLR required HLA-matching procedures for products of this locus in addition to the products of *A* and *B* loci. Thus, MLR became an important adjunct to serotyping, particularly when either one or both parents of an individual were homozygous at the *A* and *B* loci, hence producing single haplotype and "spuriously" identical siblings. The latter, in spite of being identical for the *A* and *B* alleles, can still differ in the *D* allele. Furthermore, it is advisable to test for the *D* locus compatibility between serologically identical siblings in order to avoid mismatch at the *D* locus due to crossover.

For the past several years, it has been recognized that matching of the recipient with the prospective donor for the *D* allele is quite important for the clinical outcome of renal grafts, even those from unrelated donors. However, application of the MLR test for the *D* locus matching of unrelated individuals is not practical because the ordinary test requires at least four to five days of incubation and the test itself, while detecting incompatibility, cannot identify the specificities determined by a given *D* allele. To resolve the latter problem, two promising procedures have recently been explored to type for the products of the *D* locus. One procedure utilizes as stimulator cells a panel of selected cells that are homozygous at the *A*, *B*, and *D* loci and carry a distinct allele at the *D* locus. If some cells of the panel fail to stimulate cells of a given individual, it can be interpreted as evidence that this individual shares at least one *D* allele with the donor stimulator cells. Another method called primed lymphocyte typing uses as responder cells a panel of lymphocytes primed with haploidentical cells, i.e., parent cells primed by cells of one of their children. If the cells of a tested individual stimulate primed cells into a rapid MLR ("secondary response"), the tested individual shares the *D* allele of the stimulator cells used for priming.

Several attempts are currently being made in order to detect the structures controlled by *D* locus using serologic techniques, first of all immunofluorescence. No definite statement can be made about these attempts at present.

Cellular and Humoral Immunity in Graft Rejection

As stated above (pages 377–78), allograft rejection is an immunologic phenomenon that can be related to the immune response to transplantation antigens present in the graft but absent from the recipient. A great deal of experimentation was devoted to identifying more precisely the immunologic mechanisms responsible for this rejection. Since humoral antibodies may frequently be detected in the recipient's serum after allograft rejection, several investigators suggested that the graft rejection may be mediated by humoral antibodies themselves. Experimental evidence supporting this contention was produced for allografts composed of dispersed cells, e.g., lymphoid or epithelial cells. Such grafts are quite readily destroyed by cytotoxic action of humoral antibodies to transplantation antigens and complement.

Similar evidence has been sought for the role of humoral antibodies in the rejection of skin grafts. Most studies were performed as passive transfer experiments. Antiserum from an animal sensitized by an allograft or by immunization with allogeneic tissues was injected into a normal animal, which was then challenged with a skin allograft that originated from an animal syngeneic with the donor of tissues used to procure the antiserum. In most of these experiments the animals treated with antibody-containing sera rejected the challenging grafts by a first-set rejection, pointing to the fact that hypersensitivity was not transferred by serum. In view of the generally unsuccessful transfer experiments with humoral antibodies, cell-mediated immunity has been implicated in the rejection of skin allografts (Chapter 11). A considerable body of evidence supporting this hypothesis was obtained in experiments on passive transfer of allograft hypersensitivity with lymphoid cells. An animal was sensitized with a graft or immunized with cells from an allogeneic donor. The lymphoid cells of the sensitized animal were transferred into another animal belonging to the same inbred strain. This procedure was selected in order to avoid destruction of the transferred cells in the recipient animal. The state of immunity established by means of transfer of syngeneic immune lymphocyte is called adoptive immunity. When the animal that received sensitized cells was challenged with a skin graft from the original donor (or a genetically identical donor), accelerated rejection was observed. From these experiments it was concluded that cell-mediated rather than humoral immunity is primarily responsible for the rejection of solid tissue allografts. This conclusion seems to be valid as far as rejection of skin allografts is concerned; on the other hand, this conclusion is not always correct with respect to some other solid tissue grafts.

With the incompatibility at MHC, the rejection of an allograft by cellular immunity is usually accomplished within ten days by an unprimed recipient and within four to six days by a primed recipient. The hallmark of this rejection is infiltration by mononuclear cells, lymphocytes, and macrophages. Figure 22–5 shows an early phase (a) and a late phase (b) of rejection of renal allograft in a rabbit.

The way in which previously described products of MHC participate in allograft rejection has not yet been finally elucidated. Some investigators have proposed that a mechanism similar to MLR triggers proliferation of the recipient's T lymphocytes in the case of incompatibility with the donor's cells, first of all in murine I loci or human D locus. The rejection itself occurs after proliferation and is due to the killer effect exerted by T lymphocytes. This effect may be simulated *in vitro* by cell-mediated lympholytotoxicity (CML) (Chapter 9). In this test, cultures of target lymphocytes preexposed to a mitogen and labeled by ^{51}Cr are mixed with stimulated "killer" lymphocytes. The killer effect is measured by the release of radioactivity. CML has been used in experiments that were performed to identify the

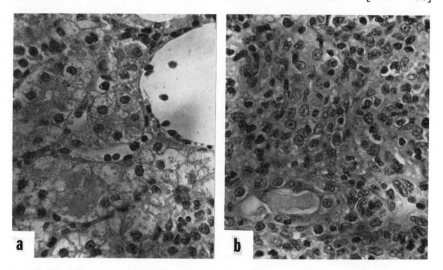

Figure 22-5. Rabbit kidney allograft in the process of cell-mediated rejection. *a*. Early accumulation of lymphocytes in peritubular capillaries. *b*. Almost total obliteration of kidney parenchyma by lymphocytes and macrophages. (From Milgrom F.; Klassen, J.; and Fuji, H.: Immunologic injury of renal homografts. *J. Exp. Med.,* **134**:193s–207s, 1971.)

nature of antigens on target lymphocytes. Studies in mice showed that incompatibility for antigens determined by K and D loci is primarily responsible for the killer effect. However, more recent investigations indicated that antigens determined by genes at the *IA* and *IC* regions may also serve as targets for CML. In man, antigens determined by the B locus play a predominant role as targets for CML. In addition to these antigens, those determined by A and C loci, and possibly even by D locus, may serve as targets.

From the available data on human renal transplantation, it is reasonable to assume at present that in the induction phase of alloimmune responses of nonimmunized recipients, D locus products may play a decisive role and, therefore, influence significantly the prognosis of the grafts. On the other hand, in immunized recipients, matching for the A and B locus antigens may be of greater importance than matching for the D locus.

The final answer about the identity of transplantation antigens (in the strict sense of this term) determined by MHC may not come until experiments become feasible in which immunization of recipients with highly purified antigens determined by each locus of the complex is followed by grafting of tissues with or without the particular antigen.

In the last decade, transplantation surgeons noted that a renal graft occasionaly undergoes "hyperacute" rejection in that the blood flow through the graft ceases within a few minutes or a few hours. This type of rejection was observed primarily in recipients of second or third grafts, and

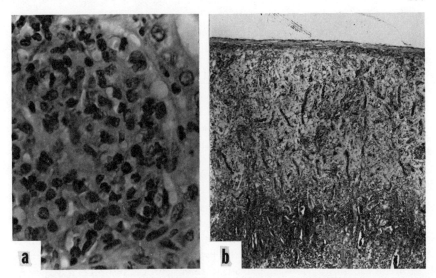

Figure 22-6. Rabbit kidney allograft in hyperacute rejection. *a.* Polymorphonuclear leukocytes in glomerular and peritubular capillaries. *b.* Renal cortical necrosis in a kidney left *in situ* for 48 hours after rejection. (From Milgrom, F., *et al.*; *J. Exp. Med.*, **134**:193–207, 1971.)

it was also noted in ABO-incompatible combinations in which the recipient had antibodies to A or B antigen present in the graft. The hallmarks of this rejection are the accumulation of polymorphonuclear leukocytes in glomerular and peritubular capillaries (Figure 22–6 *A*) and, if the graft is left long enough *in situ*, renal cortical necrosis (Figure 22–6 *B*). The hyperacute rejection of renal allografts could be clearly related to the recipient's humoral antibodies directed against the donor's transplantation antigens. This was also confirmed by extensive animal experiments that suggested that occlusion of interlobular arteries may play the decisive role in this antibody-mediated rejection. The accelerated rejection of skin allograft taking the form of a white graft may also be due to humoral antibodies, according to the available evidence.

As stated previously, xenografts undergo violent rejection in most instances. There is reason to believe that humoral antibodies play the most important role in rejection of these grafts.

Organ Transplantation in Man

Renal grafts are by far the most important in human clinical transplantation. This procedure has been conducted for about 20 years and has been developed to the point where it may be considered today as a therapeutic measure. According to the world registry, the number of renal grafts performed to date is over 46,000. The longest survival time for a kidney graft has been over 20 years for a syngeneic kidney and over ten years for allogeneic kidneys. The one-year graft survival has exceeded 70% for kidneys originating from living, related donors and 50% for kidneys from cadaveric donors. The rejection of the renal grafts is by no means synonymous with the recipient's death, as reflected by higher one-year survival figures of the recipients than of the grafts: over 80% for recipients of grafts from related donors and over 60% for recipients of grafts from cadaveric donors. Patients who rejected one graft frequently enjoyed good function of the second graft, and some patients had the third or even the fourth renal grafts functioning well. As mentioned, the best function and longest survival are observed in renal allografts originating from HLA-identical siblings. All renal allograft recipients are maintained on immunosuppressive regimes. The drugs routinely used are azathioprine and steroids. Many clinicians supplement this therapy by administration of gamma globulin fraction of heteroimmune sera, usually horse sera, to human lymphocytes or thymocytes.

One of the most serious side effects of renal transplantation is the appearance of malignant tumors in the recipients. In some rather rare instances, growth of an allogeneic tumor transplanted with the organ was observed, and this included cases with metastases of such tumors. The growth of the allogeneic tumor was made possible by the immunosuppressive therapy, and in most instances the tumors disappeared after cessation of immunosuppression (and removal of the graft). A much more serious consequence of the renal homograft is *de novo* formation of a malignant tumor by the recipient. According to material assembled by Penn, the incidence of malignant tumors in renal graft recipients is about 100 times greater than in the general populations. The observed tumors, in decreasing order of frequency, have been: cancers of the skin and lips, solid lymphomas, carcinoma of the cervix of the uterus, and lung carcinoma. Interestingly, the lymphomas showed more frequent involvement of the central nervous system than similar tumors in nongrafted patients. Whether this high incidence of tumors in human allograft recipients is exclusively due to immunosuppressive therapy is debatable. According to the data assembled by some investigators, in addition to immunosuppression, stimulation of the patient by foreign transplantation antigens plays a role in tumor formation.

In recent years, hyperacute rejection of renal grafts mediated by humoral antibodies has been avoided by cross-matching performed before transplantation, and the cell-mediated rejection is to a great extent prevented by immunosuppressive therapy. The success of renal graft survival for periods exceeding one year is impressive and undeniable. Recently, several investigators noted that renal grafts that had enjoyed good function for several months or even years eventually undergo slow deterioration. This includes grafts from HLA-identical siblings. Morphologic studies of such late rejection showed deposition of IgM and, in most cases, of IgG and complement along the glomerular basement membranes in a linear or finely granular pattern. Electron microscopy showed deposition of electron-opaque deposits along the glomerular basement membrane. In the vast majority of cases, these were subendothelial and only in a few cases sub-epithelial deposits.

These findings were consistent with the hypothesis that the glomerular lesions under study were induced by humoral antibodies either directly combining with glomerular basement membrane or deposited from the circulation in the form of immune complexes (Chapter 19). The simplest mechanism explaining this lesion is the recurrence of the original disease in the recipient. Whereas this explanation is undoubtedly correct in some cases, it certainly cannot account for all of them. Significantly, late deterioration of renal grafts with a similar glomerular lesion was observed in grafts placed into recipients whose original renal disease was not of immunologic origin.

Another hypothesis that attracted some investigators was that transplantation antigens of the renal graft combine in the circulation with the corresponding antibodies produced by the recipient, and then the complexes are deposited on the glomerular basement membrane of the graft. Significantly, in many recipients of renal grafts, circulating immune complexes were shown several weeks or months after transplantation even though they could not be demonstrated in pretransplantation serum samples.

Still another explanation for late deterioration of renal grafts postulates that antigens are released from the graft that are not transplantation antigens but are shared by the recipient and that these antigens stimulate formation of antibodies in the recipient. Obviously, such antibodies may be considered autoantibodies. There is experimental evidence that autoantibodies may have pathogenic effects on the renal graft, either directly or through immune complex formation.

Interestingly, the majority of renal graft recipients form IgM antibodies against IgG (Chapter 26), which resemble rheumatoid factor. A hypothesis was proposed that these antibodies are formed in response to IgG transplantation antibodies, which underwent molecular transformation in their reaction with the corresponding antigens. The possible role of the rheumatoid-like factor in the outcome of the graft remains a matter of conjecture.

Cardiac grafts elicited well-understood general interest since their broadly publicized initiation in 1968. Cardiac grafts are more difficult to manage than renal grafts. Thus far, close to 400 such grafts were performed, and the longest survival of a functioning graft has been 9 years. Liver grafts proved to be more difficult than originally anticipated. A total of about 300 hepatic grafts have been conducted; the longest survival time has been over seven years. Both heart and liver grafts are still experimental, but they may become therapeutic procedures similar to kidney grafts. On the other hand, the results obtained with transplantation of other organs in man including lung, pancreas, and intestine do not, thus far, hold much promise.

Bone marrow grafting had been attempted for the first time in the 1960s, and since then, several hundred grafts have been performed worldwide. Bone marrow grafting has been contemplated as a possible therapeutic measure in (1) severe congenital immunodeficiencies, (2) aplastic anemias, (3) certain hemoglobulinopathies, and (4) terminal leukemias. Although bone marrow grafting produced some degree of success in the first three groups of diseases, it has been unsuccessful in the leukemias.

The failure of bone marrow grafts can be attributed to three major causes. (1) Grafted cells fail to lodge in the recipient and are slowly eliminated without an overt immunologic reaction. (2) Immunologic rejection is due either to preexisting immunity, most commonly seen in patients receiving massive transfusions, or to allograft reaction developing *de novo*. To minimize the incidence of rejection, proper matching for HLA and MLR of donor and recipient is essential. (3) The most common cause of bone marrow graft failures is the development of graft-vs.-host reaction (Chapter 23).

Summary

The field of transplantation is one of the youngest but most exciting fields of immunology. The body of knowledge accumulated in this field is great, and the speed with which this field has progressed in the last two decades is unprecedented. On the one hand, clinical transplantation of tissues moved from science fiction to reality. The miracle of a man living for many years with another man's kidney or heart has to be placed among the most spectacular achievements in the history of science. On the other hand, the definition of the major histocompatibility complex is certainly the leading discovery of immunogenetics.

With the hope created by the science of transplantation, disappointments have also been experienced. The "nonspecific" immunosuppression used for the maintenance of allograft is a necessary evil. At the end of the rainbow of our efforts, we see specific immunosuppression that we have to learn to institute. With increasing demand, the number of available allografts will be far from sufficient. Eventually the field of transplantation will face the enormous task of application of xenografts, but at the moment, this is still science fiction.

Bibliography

Amos, D. B.: Genetic and antigenic aspects of human histocompatibility systems. *Adv. Immunol.*, **10**:251, 1969.

Benaceraff, B. (ed.): *Immunogenetics and Immunodeficiency*. University Park Press, Baltimore, 1975.

———: Biochemistry and biology of Ia antigens. *Transpl. Rev.*, **30**, Munksgaard, Copenhagen, 1976.

Ceppellini, R.: Facts about transplantation antigens in man. In Amos, B. D. (ed.): *Progress in Immunology*. Academic Press, New York, London, 1971, p. 973.

Ceppellini, R., and van Rood, J. J.: The HLA system. I. Genetics and molecular biology. *Sem. Hematol.*, **11**:233, 1974.

Götze, D. (ed.): *The Major Histocompatibility System in Man and Animals*. Springer-Verlag, Berlin, Heidelberg, New York, 1977.

Joint Report of the Fourth International Histocompatibility Workshop: In Terasaki, P. I. (ed.): *Histocompatibility Testing 1970*. Munksgaard, Copenhagen, 1970, p. 17.

Klein, J.: *Biology of the Mouse Histocompatibility-2 Complex*. Springer-Verlag, New York, Heidelberg, Berlin, 1975.

Milgrom, F.; Klassen, J.; Kano, K.; and Fuji, H.: Renal graft rejection by humoral antibodies. In Miescher, P. A. (ed.): *Immunopathology*, Proceedings of the Sixth International Symposium. Schwabe & Company, Basel, 1971, p. 236.

Mitchison, N. A.; Greep, J. M.; and Hattinga Verschure, J. C. M. (eds.): *Organ Transplantation Today*. Williams & Wilkins, Baltimore, 1969.

Najarian, J. S., and Simmons, R. L.: *Transplantation*. Lea & Febiger, Philadelphia, 1972.

Rapaport, F. T., and Dausset, J.: *Human Transplantation*. Grune & Stratton, New York, 1968.

Snell, G. D.; Dausset, J.; and Nathenson, S.: *Histocompatibility*. Academic Press, New York, San Francisco, London, 1976.

van Rood, J. J.: The HLA system. II. Clinical relevance. *Sem. Hematol.*, **11**:253, 1974.

23

Graft-Versus-Host Reactions

MAREK B. ZALESKI

Introduction

A normal recipient of an allogeneic graft rejects such a graft due to the action of immunologically competent cells directed to the transplantation antigens of the graft. If, however, an immunologically unresponsive recipient receives the allogeneic graft containing immunologically competent cells, these cells react against the transplantation antigens of the host. Such a graft-vs.-host reaction (GVHR) was theoretically predicted by Simonsen and Dempster in the early 1950s, and the experimental evidence was supplied by Simonsen and by Billingham and Brent in the late 1950s.

Prerequisites of GVHR

There are three basic prerequisites for the development of the GVHR.

1. The host must be at least partially unable to react against transplantation antigens of the graft. Such impairment is most commonly encountered in the following situations.

a. Since essentially all histocompatibility genes are fully codominant, an

F_1 hybrid expresses phenotypically the antigens of both parents and is unable to respond to these antigens. The experimental model, which consists of grafting the parental cells into the F_1 host, is one of the most often employed in studies of GVHR and serves as the basis of further discussion in this chapter.

b. Due to immunologic immaturity, embryos and, in some species, newborn individuals are unresponsive to a variety of antigens, including transplantation antigens.

c. Under natural as well as experimental conditions, various factors can diminish or abolish the immunologic responsiveness of an animal. The list of such factors consists of genetically determined immune deficiencies, unresponsiveness induced by sublethal irradiation, cytostatic drugs, and acquired tolerance (Chapter 12).

2. Histoincompatibility must exist between the host and graft with the host having transplantation antigens that are absent in the grafted cells. Similar to allograft rejection (Chapter 22), the GVHR is most pronounced when incompatibility involves major histocompatibility antigens. Detailed studies have demonstrated that in mice, two classes of antigens are involved in the GVHR elicited by major histoincompatibility. On the one hand, antigens determined by the *I* region and also the *G* region of the host's *H-2* complex appear to be the most potent in stimulating competent cells of the graft into proliferative reaction. These antigens seem to be identical to the Lad involved in MLR. On the other hand, antigens determined by the *K* and *D* regions of the *H-2* complex appear to be the most potent in generating the effector cells that ultimately interact and damage the cells of the host. Until recently, the two classes of antigens were believed to be quite distinct and recognized by two different cell populations present in the graft. One cell would recognize H-2K and/or H-2D antigens and generate effector cells directed against these antigens. The generation of effector cells would be significantly helped by the cells that recognize Lad structures without generating effector cells against them. This concept has been based on the observation that cells generated by an incompatibility limited to the *I* region were incapable of damaging *I*-incompatible target cells. However, these observations may reflect merely the insensitivity of the cell-mediated lymphotoxicity (CML) assay. Recently published reports have demonstrated effector cells directed against Ia antigens of the target cells. These data, together with observations that incompatibility limited to the *K* region can elicit a proliferative response, seem to indicate that the original distinction of two classes of antigens is largely artificial, and it may reflect quantitative, rather than qualitative, differences between the antigens. The effector response in GVHR appears to be directed to the carrier portion of the H-2K and H-2D molecules and not to the portion containing serologically detectable specificities (Chapter 22). It has been repeatedly demonstrated that the intensity of the GVHR is not related to serologically detectable differences between graft and host, and one can see pronounced GVHR with little

serologic differences and vice versa. Apart from incompatibility for major antigens, incompatibility for minor antigens can elicit GVHR, although special conditions must often be fulfilled to visualize GVHR. Most typically, the GVHR against minor antigens requires either increased numbers of grafted cells or preimmunization of the donor of these cells.

3. The graft must contain a sufficient number of immunologically competent cells capable of recognizing the transplantation antigens of the host. It has been shown that T cells are the major, if not the sole, culprit in eliciting GVHR. Involvement of the T cells was directly demonstrated by abolishing GVHR after experimental removal of T cells from the graft by treating it with antibodies selectively killing or blocking T cells. Further analysis of the cells responsible for GVHR showed the involvement of two discrete subpopulations of T cells. Cantor showed a synergistic effect of the cells obtained from lymph node and thymus. As an interpretation of these observations, it has been postulated that there are two types of T cells— nonrecirculating, precursor cells (T_1) and recirculating amplifier cells (T_2). The potency of any given graft to evoke GHVR reflects not so much the absolute content of T cells as it does the proportion between the two types of T cells (Chapter 3).

Cellular Pathogenesis of GVHR

There is striking parallelism between the magnitude of the early phase of GVHR and the magnitude of MLR. It is believed that the one-way mixed lymphocyte reaction (MLR) (Chapter 22) represents an *in vitro* model of the GVHR observed *in vitro*. This conclusion is based on observations indicating that in both instances (1) T cells are predominantly responsible for recognition of antigen and subsequent cell proliferation; (2) major histocompatibility antigens appear to determine the magnitude of both reactions; and (3) incompatibility at the *I* region appears to determine both the most pronounced mixed lymphocyte reaction (MLR) and the early phase of GVHR. Table 23–1 shows the remarkable parallelism between the magnitude of MLR and early phase of GVHR, the latter being measured by spleen index assays (see below). However, when GVHR is measured in terms of mortality, including both the early phase and its later consequences mediated by effector cells, one can see that incompatibilities at the *K*, *D*, and *I* regions result in a similar intensity of GVHR.

Thus, MLR is an apparent oversimplification of the phenomena contributing to the overall picture of GVHR *in vivo*. Nevertheless, it seems plausible that in both instances, a strictly defined clone of T cells recognizes the appropriate transplantation antigen and thus initiates the reaction. Data indicate that such a clone is surprisingly large and consists of anywhere from 1 to 5% of all T cells. In the first stage of MLR and GVHR, the T cells

Table 23-1
MAGNITUDE OF MLR MEASURED BY THE RATIO OF ^{3}H-THYMIDINE INCORPORATION INTO STIMULATED AND NONSTIMULATED LYMPHOCYTES, AND MAGNITUDE OF GVHR MEASURED BY THE SPLEEN INDEX (SI) AND THE MORTALITY ELICITED BY INCOMPATIBILITIES AT DIFFERENT REGIONS OF THE *H-2* COMPLEX*

Incompatibility at							GVHR		
K	IA	IB	IC	S	G	D	*MLR*	*SI*	*Mortality*
├————————————————————————┤ (K–D)							+++	+++	+++
├———————————————┤ (K–IC)							+++	n.t.	+++
├——┤ (K)							+	+	++
					├———┤ (G–D)		+	+	++
├——┤ (K)					├———┤ (G–D)		++	++	n.t.
├————————————————————————┤ (K–D)							+++	+++	++

* Based on data kindly supplied by J. Klein.

undergo blast transformation leading to a transient but pronounced proliferative activity, which is followed by generation of the specific effector cells. Although the presence of effector cells generated in MLR can be demonstrated by means of CML (Chapter 9), their presence in GVHR can only be inferred from the clinical symptoms.

In the classic experiment, parental lymphoid cells are injected intravenously or intraperitoneally into F_1 recipients. Within 24 hours, the injected cells reach all organs of the recipient. Some investigators believe that grafted cells become selectively entrapped in spleen and lymph nodes where the grafted T cells recognize transplantation antigens of the F_1 hybrid. The host's leukocytes, lymphocytes, and possibly neutrophils are the major source of antigenic stimulus for grafted cells, whereas other cells are of little importance in this respect. As a result of the recognition, the process of blast transformation and proliferation ensues. This proliferation is responsible for the fact that in early stages of the GVHR, as many as 90% of the mitotic figures are of graft origin. The degree of proliferation of the grafted cells varies within broad ranges and depends on the graft-host combination. Proliferation of grafted cells may not be an absolute prerequisite of GVHR, but rather an amplifying phenomenon. In some instances, only a few cells seem to proliferate while most of the subsequent effector cells become recruited into reaction without prior transformation and proliferation.

In the early stage of GVHR, the transformed and proliferating grafted cells remain fixed in the lymphoid organs of the host and do not enter the recirculating pool. There are insufficient data concerning the fate of progeny of proliferating grafted cells. It is assumed that grafted cells become effector cells which, upon contact with host cells, inflict damage on the host. At least three not mutually exclusive mechanisms causing this damage should be considered: (1) contact cytotoxicity analogous or identical to the CML phenomenon observed *in vitro*; (2) antibody-mediated cytotoxicity in which antibodies produced by grafted cells react with target cells of the host and complement causing lysis of these cells; (3) nonspecific cytotoxicity caused either by the grafted cells themselves or by the products of their stimulation. This nonspecific cytotoxicity affects not only host cells but injures grafted cells as well.

Whichever the mechanism of injury during GVHR, the reaction itself has a finite duration, which is easily comprehensible if one considers that the reaction is triggered in a limited population of normal cells. The estimates of duration of GVHR in different experimental models range from one day to several months, but it seems that an average grafted cell displays an effective "hostility" toward the recipient for about 14 days. The cessation of activity of grafted cells against host antigens does not imply saving the host. In some instances, the host may survive the acute phase of GVHR and then almost fully recover; in other instances, the consequences of acute GVHR result in the death of the host in spite of a lack of an overt graft activity.

The following mechanisms attributed to either grafted cell or host activity are most often responsible for limiting the duration of GVHR:

1. Induction of specific tolerance of grafted cells to a host antigen. Such tolerance can affect immunologically competent cells of the graft or, more likely, its hematopoietic precursors of lymphocytes.

2. Senescence of reactive cells, which, after becoming highly differentiated into cytotoxic effector cells, have a limited capability of self-renewal and ultimately become extinct.

3. Allergic death of activated grafted cells due to their exposure to gigantic excess of the host antigens.

4. Production by the grafted cells of blocking antibodies analogous to enhancing antibodies (Chapter 24) that bind to the host cells, rendering them resistant to attack by the grafted cells. Autoantibodies produced by host B cells that become activated by T cells of the graft can be included in this category.

5. A complete repopulation of the host hematopoietic tissues by grafted cells may ultimately render the host nonimmunogenic, since the host's leukocytes appear to provide major antigenic stimulus for GVHR.

6. An immune reaction mounted by the host and directed against the grafted cells results in their rejection. Although in some instances this mechanism seems to be plausible, e.g., in grafting male parent cells into female F_1 host, or grafting allogeneic cells into a temporarily unresponsive host, in other instances this concept requires introduction of the unorthodox hypothesis of noncodominant histocompatibility genes. Indeed, it has been reported that an allele at Hh locus* may be recessive, therefore being expressed in parental cells but not in F_1 hybrids. As a result, F_1 hybrids

---

* Hh locus (or loci) determining antigen present on hematopoietic cells has been mapped in the vicinity of H–2 complex of mice.

may mount the allograft reaction against grafted parental cells and reject them. This phenomenon is known as hybrid resistance.

7. Allogeneic inhibition phenomenon could in some instances be blamed for curtailing of the survival, at least from a functional point of view, of the grafted cells.

8. Some data indicate that the host may produce inhibitory factors with activity directed against graft cells.

In different models, different mechanisms may be involved, and more than one mechanism may contribute to the termination of the GVHR.

To conclude the remarks concerning the cellular pathogenesis of GVHR, one is compelled to discuss the involvement of the host's cells. Hematopoietically derived host cells appear to be essential for initiating GVHR by supplying the antigenic stimulus for grafted cells. The same cells seem to be the primary target for the effector cells generated during GVHR. The ensuing cytotoxic reaction results in various degrees of cell and tissue damage, which is accompanied by inflammatory reactions within and in the vicinity of the foci of injury and, sometimes, this is followed by the repair processes mediated by the connective tissue cells of the host. These repair processes are held responsible for the host cell proliferation seen in lymphatic organs, particularly in the latter stages of the GVHR. Interestingly, in MLR with parental cells, a similar proliferation of F_1 cells can be observed. It is speculated that the host's cell proliferation concerns predominantly B cells, which become unspecifically activated by T cells of the graft. In fact, it seems that T cells of the host not only do not proliferate, but they may even exert an inhibitory effect on the host's cell proliferation.

Signs and Symptoms of GVHR

Local GVHR

In this type of reaction, the cells are grafted locally, subcutaneously, or under the renal capsule, and the changes occurring at the site of the injection and in its vicinity are evaluated.

In the first case, injection of cells results in a cutaneous lesion that closely resembles a delayed hypersensitivity reaction. Macroscopically, there are induration, erythema, and necrosis, and microscopically, one can see aggregation of mononuclear cells, many of them undergoing blast transformation and proliferation. One should, however, keep in mind that the local changes reflect the combined reaction of the grafted cells and the inflammatory reaction of the host. The local injection of parental cells may produce prominent changes in the regional lymph node draining the site of injection. The histologic changes in the lymph node, which may increase up to 30 times in size, are essentially the same as those described below for the systemic GVHR.

Injection of parental cells under the renal capsule of the F_1 hybrid produces massive mononuclear infiltration of the renal cortex accompanied by extensive destruction of the renal tubules. Due to the proliferation of grafted cells and coexisting inflammation, the weight of the affected kidney increases significantly. Local changes are accompanied by an enlarged spleen, but there is no detectable activity of grafted cells in the spleen, suggesting that splenomegaly, as seen in systemic GVHR, may at least partially represent an unspecific host response to humoral factors produced in the course of the GVHR.

Systemic GVHR

The systemic GVHR ensues when parental cells are injected intravenously or intraperitoneally into appropriate F_1 hybrid. Depending on the number of grafted cells, age of the host at the time of injection, and histoincompatibility involved, systemic GVHR can take either an acute or a chronic course.

When a large number of parental cells are grafted into newborn or relatively young F_1 hybrids, the macroscopic signs of GVHR become obvious within seven to ten days after injection. There is sudden inhibition of the animal's growth (runting), and affected animals become hypoactive, assume a hunched position, often suffer from diarrhea, the fur becomes ruffled, and many animals succumb within three to four weeks. Autopsy performed at the peak of the symptoms reveals several typical signs. The hallmark of the fully developed GVHR is significant splenomegaly. In some combinations, the spleen increases three to four times its normal size. Early splenomegaly can be attributed to the proliferation of grafted cells, but in later periods, it is due to proliferation of the host's cells in response to injury and/or mitogenic factors produced in the course of GVHR. Histologically, the follicular structure of the spleen becomes obliterated, and most of the organ is occupied by blastlike cells. As the reaction progresses, foci of necrosis appear and become filled with reticular cells accompanied by a few scattered blast cells. The phenomenon analogous to splenomegaly can be induced *in vitro* when small fragments of F_1 spleens are cultured in the presence of the parental cells. In later stages, the spleen becomes hypoplastic, and so spleens of animals that died of GVHR may be normal or even smaller than normal. Splenectomy reduces the severity of GVHR; this effect has been attributed to the removal of lodging and reaction sites for grafted cells.

Parallel to splenomegaly, enlargement of lymph nodes is observed. The degree of lymphadenopathy is quite variable, depending on the location of the node. Histologically, the follicular structure is obscured, and there is massive aggregation of blastlike cells, particularly in the sinuses and paracortical areas. Similar to spleen, lymph node hyperplasia is followed by prominent hypoplasia.

In addition to the enlargement of spleen and lymph nodes, the liver also becomes enlarged. Upon histologic examination, one can almost invariably find numerous perivascular infiltrates along the branches of the portal system. The infiltrates are composed of mononuclear cells, some of which are blastlike. The origin of these infiltrates remains the subject of controversy, as they may represent the proliferation of grafted cells that have lodged in the liver or the host inflammatory reaction similar to that responsible for late splenomegaly. Some authors also observed reticuloendothelial hyperplasia, fatty degeneration, and focal necrosis of liver parenchyma.

A characteristic sign of acute GVHR is pronounced hypoplasia and hypotrophy of the thymus. This is predominantly the result of the excessive production and release of corticosteroids, since the direct attack of grafted cells appears rather unlikely.

Other changes that seem to be of importance are inflammatory and necrotic lesions of skin and intestines. The first contribute to "garden variety" symptoms, such as dyskeratosis, exfoliation, alopecia, and so on. The intestinal changes seem to be the main, but not the only, cause of diarrhea and wasting of animals. Whether the injury to epithelial tissue is due to unspecific inflammation or specific immune attack directed against epithelial cells remains to be elucidated. In this respect, it is interesting to note that in some cases of GVHR antiepithelial antibodies have been demonstrated.

Several functional abnormalities can be related directly to anatomic changes. The most important physiologic changes are immunologic, hematologic, and hepatic dysfunctions.

One can easily envision that immunologic attack against lymphoid cells of the host will make the host immunologically deficient. Indeed, a long list of reports demonstrates that GVHR results in severe immunosuppression to a variety of antigens. In addition to the purely physical damage inflicted upon competent cells of the host, alternative mechanisms such as excessive release of corticosteroids, release of immunosuppressive factor produced by and/or influencing T suppressor cells, and antigenic competition may be operational. While the first two would act on both graft and host cells, the latter would cause unresponsiveness of the grafted rather than host cells. Decreased immune responsiveness results in increased susceptibility to infections, which almost invariably complicate the clinical course of GVHR. Interestingly, GVHR in germ-free animals has a much less severe course than in conventional animals.

Concomitant with immunosuppression, some authors observed significant enhancement of responsiveness to some antigens during GVHR. This paradoxic phenomenon is explained by nonspecific activation of the macrophages or T cells of both graft and host. Under proper conditions, T cells of the graft may provide a nonspecific signal to both T and B cells of the host triggering their polyclonal proliferation accompanied by increased production of antibodies to some antigens. A similar mechanism could be involved in triggering latent autoimmune clones with resulting appearance of autoantibodies.

The hematologic findings during GVHR consist of several symptoms such as anemia, leukopenia, and blood-clotting disturbances. An attack of graft cells against stem cells of the bone marrow of the host appears to be the most likely mechanism responsible for anemia. The nature of this attack remains unknown, and it may consist of either specific immunologic destruction or unspecific inhibition by factors produced during GVHR. In addition, Coombs' positive anemia is sometimes observed during GVHR. The source of the antibodies has not been established. The lymphopenia, which can develop independently of anemia, is a common finding in GVHR. The cause of lymphopenia is not as obvious as it would appear. Besides specific antilymphocytic antibodies produced by grafted cells, one should also consider the possible lymphopenic effect of concomitant infections and, even more significantly, the lympholytic effect of corticosteroids secreted in excess.

Numerous foci of necrosis accompanying GVHR constitute a rich source of tissue thromboplastin responsible for serious disturbances in homeostasis of blood clotting. Increased blood coagulability may contribute to mortality in GVHR.

Previously described morphologic changes in the liver sufficiently account for hepatic dysfunctions during GVHR as expressed by jaundice and alteration in the level of serum enzymes.

There is no exact definition of a chronic form of systemic GVHR, but for the purpose of this discussion, GVHR that does not lead to high mortality within four weeks may be considered chronic. With some exceptions, the symptoms described in the acute form are demonstrable in chronic GVHR. In particular, lymphoid hypoplasia, skin lesions, immunosuppression, and anemia are often more readily noted in chronic GVHR. In addition to these changes, two characteristic phenomena have been described in chronic GVHR.

1. In many murine strain combinations tested, hosts suffering from GVHR developed remarkably frequent, malignant reticuloendothelial tumors. There are at least three nonexclusive mechanisms proposed as the explanation for tumorigenesis in GVHR.

Some authors have shown that the tumors are caused by the transfer of viruses from parental donor into susceptible host. Other investigators argue that the viruses are present in the latent form in host tissues and become activated to produce neoplastic transformation by the extremely intensive cell proliferation accompanying GVHR. Finally, an effect of the GVHR-associated immunosuppression must be seriously considered as a factor facilitating development and growth of tumors.

2. In some combinations, animals suffering from GVHR for long periods developed severe glomerulonephritis closely resembling immune complex nephritis with glomerular deposits containing transplantation antibodies of the donor origin (Chapter 19).

Quantitation of the GVHR

Studies of GVHR were significantly facilitated by the development of methods allowing quantitative measurement of the intensity of GVHR. Out of many proposed methods, three have won general acceptance.

Spleen Index Assay of Simonsen

This assay is based on the observation that the degree of splenomegaly during the acute phase of GVHR is directly proportional to the strength of the histoincompatibility and the number of grafted cells. The splenomegaly is expressed as spleen index (SI) representing the ratio of relative spleen weight of animals grafted with a given number of parental cells to the relative spleen weight of their littermates grafted with the same number of syngeneic cells. Figure 23–1 shows an example of spleen index assay in which SI values are plotted against the logarithms of the number of grafted cells obtained from different compartments of lymphoid tissue. The lymph node cells are the most, and thymus cells the least, potent in evoking GVHR. It

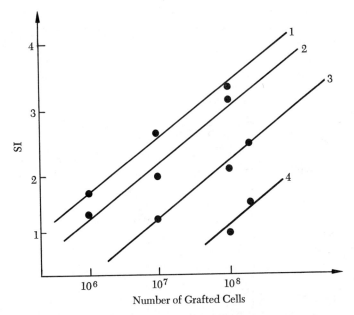

Figure 23-1. Spleen index assay of Simonsen. Each point represents a mean value of spleen index (*SI*) (ordinate) of a group of animals grafted with a certain number (abscissa) of allogeneic cells from lymph node (*1*), spleen (*2*), bone marrow (*3*), or thymus (*4*).

should be reemphasized here that splenomegaly is a result of proliferation of graft and host cells; thus it is only a partially specific indicator of immunologic phenomenon underlying GVHR. The assays measuring weight increase of regional lymph node after subcutaneous injection or weight increase of kidney after subcapsular injection of parental cells are identical in principle with the spleen assay.

Phagocytic Activity Assay of Howard

This assay is based on the phenomenon of increased phagocytic activity observed between days 7 and 40 of GVHR. The phagocytic activity is measured by means of colloidal carbon clearance from the bloodstream of tested animals. The assay permits GVHR to be quantitated without sacrificing animals. However, it does not distinguish between alteration of phagocytic activity caused by GVHR itself and alteration caused by complications such as infection or inflammation.

Liver Perivascular Infiltrates Assay of Miller and Bain

In this assay, logarithms of numbers of perivascular infiltrates detectable histologically in liver are plotted against logarithms of numbers of grafted cells. Bain, in careful studies, demonstrated that until day 6 the number of infiltrates is exponentially related to the number of grafted cells. Although some authors claim that each focus consists of descendants of a single cellular unit capable of producing GVHR, this claim was never experimentally substantiated.

GVHR in Man

GVHR is an exciting phenomenon and fruitful tool of research in the field of cellular immunology and has also been implicated in human pathology. If one remembers three basic prerequisites for the development of GVHR, it is easy to envision the occurrence of GVHR in human beings. Although apparent GVHR after massive transfusion of peripheral blood (exchange transfusion *in utero*, transfusions in patients with severe immunologic deficiencies) was observed only sporadically, the GVHR as a consequence of bone marrow grafting poses a major clinical problem. Recent data indicate that as many as 70% of the patients receiving allogeneic bone marrow graft develop GVHR, which is lethal in about 20% of the cases. At this point, it seems proper to introduce the concept of graft-vs.-host disease (GVHD), which encompasses a "proper" GVHR, as encountered in animal models, and symptoms superimposed on it and influencing the clinical picture. The distinction seems to be warranted when one remembers that in animal experiments, the host is usually in good health before GVHR is elicited, whereas in man the host is gravely ill. Thus, symptoms of GVHR blend with preexisting symptoms caused by immune deficiency (congenital or induced by disease or treatment) and concomitant infections. The earliest signs of GVHD appear from 10 to 30 days after grafting of the bone marrow. The earlier they appear, the more serious the prognosis. The clinical picture of GVHR and GVHD in man consists of dermatitis with erythematous maculopapular eruptions spreading all over the body, hepatitis with jaundice, elevated serum transaminase, and diarrhea. These symptoms, if not promptly controlled, will lead to generalized immunodeficiency and severe infections, resulting ultimately in the death of the patient.

Bibliography

Elkins, W. L.: Cellular immunology and the pathogenesis of graft versus host reactions. *Progr. Allergy*, **15**:78–187, 1971.

Klein, J.: *Biology of the Mouse Histocompatibility-2 Complex*. Springer-Verlag, New York, Heidelberg, Berlin, 1975, pp. 454–82.

McBride, R. A.: Graft-versus-host reaction in lymphoid proliferation. *Cancer Res.*, **26**:1135–51, 1966.

Simonsen, M.: Graft-versus-host reactions. Their natural history and applicability as tool of research. *Progr. Allergy*, **6**:349–467, 1962.

Snell, G. D.; Dausset, J.; and Nathenson, S.: *Histocompatibility*. Academic Press, Inc., New York, San Francisco, London, 1976, pp. 147–51, 261–62.

24

Tumor Immunology

C. John Abeyounis and Felix Milgrom

Introduction

Cancer may arise in any vertebrate tissue; it may strike man or animal at all ages. Its cause has mystified medical science for centuries. At one time, cancer was thought to be a single disease, but it is now known to encompass more than 100 distinct clinical entities. Malignancies develop in two stages: (1) one or more normal cells become transformed, whereby their growth becomes uncontrolled and disorderly, and (2) the transformed or malignant cells proliferate into a detectable mass. Many theories of carcinogenesis have been advanced; some are particularly pertinent in the light of knowledge gained in recent years.

The irritation theory, proposed in 1863 by Virchow, held that the physical or chemical action of environmental irritants was the principal culprit. It had been noted that a particular malignancy would show high incidence in persons working in certain occupations, e.g., scrotal carcinoma in chimney sweeps, bronchogenic carcinoma in coal miners, osteogenic sarcoma in radium painters, and skin cancer in farmers chronically exposed to sunlight. Furthermore, Virchow's theory has been strongly supported by a number of studies in experimental animals that showed that a variety of malignant growths can be induced by the action of physical or chemical agents.

Virchow's theory is of particular importance today since environmental factors such as chemical by-products, pesticides, food additives, and even natural substances have been implicated as carcinogenic substances. For example, aflatoxin, a product of the mold *Aspergillus flavus*, commonly found on improperly processed peanuts, and cycasin, a substance found in seeds of a palmlike plant used as food in the South Pacific, are both potent carcinogens.

The theory of embryonal rests, proposed by Cohnheim in 1877, held that cancer originates from a clone or clones of dormant embryonic cells that are activated and proliferate later in life. This view is supported by studies that show that many tumors possess antigens found in fetal tissue but not in adult tissue.

The germ theory of disease, which came to fruition at the end of the nineteenth century, stimulated the search for cancer-causing microorganisms. This culminated in the first demonstration of a viral etiology for cancer by Peyton Rous in 1911. He succeeded in inducing tumors in healthy chickens by injection of a cell-free extract prepared from tumor tissue. The viral etiology of cancer in mammals was first shown by Richard Shope in 1933. Subsequently, in the 1940s and 1950s, a number of viruses of both the DNA and RNA types were shown to induce malignancy in laboratory animals. More recently, viruses have been implicated in human cancer, e.g., Epstein-Barr virus (EBV) in Burkitt's lymphoma and herpes simplex virus type II in carcinoma of the uterine cervix (Chapter 15).

Investigations on the viral etiology of cancer led to the widely held virogene-oncogene theory, which declares that (1) viral genes are part of the genetic apparatus of normal mammalian cells and are under the control of the host cell; (2) malignant transformation results from expression in the host cell of a particular viral gene called the oncogene; and (3) a particular viral gene (or genes) may be expressed in the absence of malignant transformation, e.g., appearance of G_{IX} cell-surface antigen on normal murine cells (page 422). This work led to the further speculation that animal viruses evolved from cells.

Thus, cancer can be induced in experimental animals and most likely in man by chemicals, radiation, repeated trauma, and viruses. Many believe that such environmental factors trigger carcinogenesis by damaging the DNA and RNA of normal cells so that they are transformed and become malignant. In addition, genetic factors also appear to be involved in some malignancies. Retinoblastoma, pheochromocytoma, and xeroderma pigmentosum are among the cancers that appear to have a genetic basis. Furthermore, familial tendencies have been observed for others, such as cancer of the breast, uterus, and stomach.

Normal cells contain a variety of antigenic substances that are found both externally on the cell surface as part of the plasma membrane and internally in the cytoplasm or nucleus. These antigens may be categorized as (1) species specific, which are found in all members of the same species; (2)

tissue specific, which are found only in a certain tissue and which show various degrees of species specificity; and (3) allospecific, which are present in some, but not all, members of a species (ABO, HLA in man). Malignant cells, as a consequence of transformation, are usually antigenically altered. A particular "normal" antigen may become deleted and disappear, or its concentration may decrease. Conversely, the concentration of a normal antigen may increase in tumors; such antigens are termed "tumor-associated antigens" (TAA). The antigenic alteration may be more drastic in that a qualitative change occurs, manifested by the appearance of a new antigen foreign to the host. Such neoantigens are termed "tumor-specific antigens" (TSA), and they may be present as intracellular structures in the cytoplasm or nucleus, or more important, they may represent new cell-surface structures. TSA on the cell surface that are detected by transplantation rejection tests are termed "tumor-specific transplantation antigens" (TSTA). The term "tumor-specific cell-surface antigens" (TSCSA) is used in this chapter for TSA detected on the cell surface by serologic tests, the role of which is unknown in tumor immunity.

Immunology of Animal Tumors

Innumerable studies conducted since the beginning of this century have shown that resistance to tumors could be induced in experimental animals. Transplantable tumors available at that time grew in some animals and regressed in others. This regression was taken mistakenly as evidence for tumor immunity. With the emergence of the field of transplantation immunology, it was realized that the tumor regression seen in these early studies was due, not to the antigenic uniqueness of the tumor tissue, but to the genetic heterogeneity of the experimental animals. The tumors used in these studies were allogeneic for the recipient. They grew whenever their "virulence" overwhelmed transplantation immunity, but otherwise, especially in pre-sensitized recipients, they were rejected by an immune response to transplantation antigens.

The first evidence for the existence of TSA was provided by Gross, in 1943, who showed that a fibrosarcoma induced by the chemical carcinogen methylcholanthrene would not grow in syngeneic mice that had been immunized with a small amount of the tumor before challenge. Some investigators claimed that the tumor resistance observed by Gross was due to residual heterozygosity in the inbred mouse population, whereas others suggested that mutation in normal histocompatibility antigens could have occurred during long-term passage of the tumor.

Ten years later, more convincing evidence for tumor immunity was provided by Foley, who demonstrated tumor resistance in inbred mice immunized with a "young" methylcholanthrene-induced tumor. He showed further that this resistance was specific for the methylcholanthrene tumor, since the mice were not resistant to a syngeneic mammary carcinoma that had arisen spontaneously in the same inbred population. If resistance to the methylcholanthrene-induced tumor were due to residual heterozygosity, then resistance to the mammary carcinoma should also have been observed. Later, Prehn and Main showed that inbred mice that had been immunized with, and were subsequently resistant to, a syngeneic methylcholanthrene-induced tumor would readily accept a syngeneic skin graft. This experiment provided stronger evidence for the existence of an antigen in the tumor tissue that is absent from normal tissue. Still stronger evidence was obtained by Klein and his group who showed that an animal could be made resistant to its own (autochthonous) tumor. In an elegantly designed experiment, a tumor was induced in the leg of an inbred mouse with methylcholanthrene. The leg was amputated and the tumor was passaged in other mice of the same strain. The mouse in which the tumor was originally induced was subsequently immunized with this passaged tumor and was later resistant when challenged with a lethal dose of this tumor.

These experiments not only provided strong evidence for the existence of TSA, but also indicated that tumors induced by the same carcinogen in individual syngeneic mice may possess individual specificity. This concept of the individual specificity of chemically induced tumors was strongly supported by the studies of Globerson and Feldman. They employed two tumors, to be called A and B, which were induced in the same mouse by the same carcinogen. The syngeneic mice immunized with A were resistant to a subsequent challenge with A but were sensitive to B, whereas the opposite was true for mice immunized with the B tumor. Subsequently, TSTA with individual specificity have been demonstrated on sarcomas and hepatomas induced by chemical or physical agents such as polycyclic hydrocarbons, plastic films, ultraviolet irradiation in mice, rats, and guinea pigs (Figure 24–1).

Resistance to virus-induced tumors was demonstrated in 1961 by Sjögren and his coworkers and by Habel. Using a tumor induced with a polyoma virus (a DNA virus), they demonstrated resistance in animals that had been immunized with this tumor. Soon after, resistance was also demonstrated to tumors induced with other DNA viruses, such as SV40, Shope papilloma, and Rous sarcoma, as well as by a large group of oncogenic RNA viruses, which included the mammary tumor virus (MTV) and the murine leukemia viruses (MuLV). In contrast to what has been observed with carcinogen-induced tumors, resistance to virus-induced tumors showed virus specificity rather than individual specificity. For example, immunization with a tumor induced by polyoma virus in one mouse would evoke resistance to a tumor induced by polyoma virus in another mouse of the same or even another strain. Furthermore, resistance could be established by immunization with tumor induced by polyoma virus in another species.

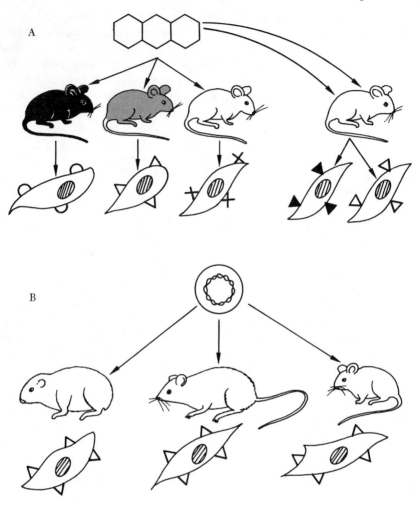

Figure 24-1. TSTA induced by (*A*) chemical carcinogens and (*B*) viruses. Each tumor induced by a chemical carcinogen has individual specificity not shared with other tumors, even when they are induced with the same chemical in the same animal. Each tumor induced by a given virus has the same specificity, regardless of the tissue or species in which it arises. Some specificities may be shared by tumors induced by closely related viruses.

Experimental tumors from both avian and mammalian species have been the object of extensive serologic characterization. Many TSCSA, as well as intracellular TSA or TAA, have been described. Much of our discussion will be devoted to murine antigens, since these have been studied most extensively and are well characterized. Of particular importance are TSTA since they are involved in control or immune rejection of malignant cells.

The important antigens found on the surface of murine cells include species-specific antigens. Generally, species antigens have wide tissue distribution; however, some murine species antigens have restricted tissue distribution. For example, murine-specific lymphocyte antigen (MSLA) is found in all mice but only on thymocytes and lymphocytes.

Other important surface antigens, referred to as alloantigens, reflect polymorphism within the species. For the most part, murine alloantigens, such as H-2, show wide tissue distribution, but some alloantigens are restricted to certain tissue. Tla are found only on thymocytes, Thy-1 and Ly on thymocytes and lymphocytes, and Pca on plasma cells. These antigens have been termed collectively as differentiation antigens. Some of these alloantigens, notably Tla and G_{IX}, may appear as normal or as tumor antigens (see below). Some antigens, such as virus envelope antigens (VEA), are closely related to infection with MuLV, whereas the viral relationship of other antigens such as the cell-surface antigens of DNA-virus–induced tumors is not so clear.

The existence of TSA was first established in experiments on chemically induced tumors using the *in vivo* technique of immune rejection of tumors transplanted into syngeneic recipients. Attempts to characterize the surface antigens of these tumors serologically have proven difficult, since sarcoma and even carcinoma cells are not readily studied *in vitro* by routine tests such as cytotoxicity (Chapter 9). On the other hand, experiments employing membrane immunofluorescence, the colony inhibition test, or the indirect ^{125}I-labeled antibody technique have demonstrated the individual specificity of these tumors. This agrees with similar specificity observed in the *in vivo* transplantation rejection experiments. However, *in vitro* tests with some chemically induced tumors have shown that there may be considerable sharing or cross-reactivity of TSCSA. These shared TSCSA appear to be embryonic antigens that have wide distribution in chemically induced tumors. It is not clear whether they can function as transplantation antigens. However, at least some TSTA are distinct from TSCSA shared with embryonal cells. In rat experiments, Baldwin showed that lymphocytes from multiparous females are cytotoxic for both tumor cells and embryonic cells. This cytotoxic activity could be blocked by sera from multiparous females. However, cytotoxic activity against tumor cells of lymphocytes from tumor-bearing rats could be blocked only by sera from tumor-bearing rats.

Serologic characterization of tumor antigens has been most fruitful in studies on virus-induced tumors. Tumors induced by DNA viruses such as polyoma or SV40 contain TSTA and TSCSA, as well as a soluble intracellular protein antigen termed "T antigen." T antigen is detectable by immunofluorescence or complement-fixation tests, is found in the cytoplasm or nucleus of the tumor cell, and is virus specific but is not part of the virion. Antibody to T antigen induced by polyoma virus reacts with polyoma-infected cells but not with SV40-infected cells, and vice versa. Anti-T antibody does not react with uninfected cells or with isolated virus. Similarly, the TSTA is virus specific and also is not part of the virion. Antiviral antibodies do not protect against the tumor, and the tumor cells do not contain infectious virus or virion antigens.

The question has been raised whether the TSTA, as well as the internal T antigens described above, are of the host cell origin resulting from derepression or whether the virus genome codes for them. There is some evidence that both antigens arise from a viral code, since both T antigen and TSTA are the same regardless of the cell type or species in which they appear. Inhibition by interferon of T antigen synthesis also supports the thesis that a viral gene codes for this antigen. However, some investigators argue that a DNA virus such as SV40 contains only sufficient DNA to code for its own structural proteins.

TSCSA on DNA-virus–induced tumors have been described using cytotoxicity, indirect immunofluorescence, colony inhibition, and isotopic antiglobulin tests. Similar to TSTA and T antigens, TSCSA are also specific for the transforming virus; they are absent from normal cells and from cells transformed by unrelated viruses.

Much of the work on the relationship of TSTA and TSCSA of DNA-virus–induced tumors supports the view that they are distinct antigens. Tumors have been described in which cells serologically positive for TSCSA lack TSTA detectable by transplantation tests (Chapter 22). Other studies support the possibility that TSCSA are normal cell structures unmasked by viral transformation. After treatment with trypsin, polyoma virus-transformed cells reacted with antibody to SV40-transformed cells.

Embryonic antigens have also been described on DNA-virus–induced tumors. Antisera produced in mice to syngeneic fetal tissue reacted with tumor cells regardless of the transforming virus. Antibody activity could be absorbed by both tumor and embryonic tissue. However, antibody prepared against tumors in syngeneic hosts reacted with tumor but not embryonic tissue. These same studies also showed that immunization with embryonic tissue failed to produce tumor resistance. On the other hand, immunization with embryonic tissue can induce some measure of resistance to DNA-virus–induced tumors. However, most investigators agree that embryonic antigens on DNA-virus–induced tumors are distinct from the TSTA.

Antigens of tumors induced by RNA viruses, notably MuLV (Gross, Friend, Moloney, and Rauscher viruses), were among the first to be described. Not only was rejection of transplanted leukemias observed, but production of antibodies cytotoxic for the leukemia cells was readily demonstrated.

Malignant transformation by MuLV gives rise to four types of tumor antigens: (1) cell-surface antigens (TSCSA), which are virus related, but not part of the virion; (2) viral envelope antigens (VEA); (3) internal virion antigens termed group-specific (gs) antigens; and (4) soluble antigens. Virus-specific TSCSA have been identified in cells infected by all MuLV. Serologic studies of these MuLV-related antigens have revealed several interesting features. The Gross antigen is found on all MuLV-induced leukemias. This is not surprising since the Gross virus is transmitted both horizontally and vertically and is widespread among mice and rats. In addition to TSCSA characteristic for each of MuLV, there are also TSCSA shared by MuLV-induced leukemia cells. For example, there are Friend-specific TSCSA, a TSCSA shared by Friend and Moloney leukemia cells, and a TSCSA shared by Friend and Rauscher leukemia cells.

MuLV-induced leukemia cells also possess TSCSA that are found on fetal tissue. Present evidence suggests that this fetal antigen is shared by Friend, Moloney, and Rauscher virus-induced leukemia cells.

A number of VEA have been described in RNA-virus–induced tumors using mouse antisera and antisera raised in other species. Some of these VEA are common to most, if not all, oncogenic RNA viruses. Some are common to certain groups of viruses, and others are specific for a given virus.

The distinction between VEA and virus-related TSCSA has been clearly shown by immunoelectron microscopic studies of leukemia cells, using rat and mouse antisera to Gross antigens. The rat antiserum, which contained antibodies to both VEA and TSCSA, reacted with the envelope of the budding virus, as well as with the leukemia cell surface. On the other hand, the mouse antiserum contained antibodies only to TSCSA. This antiserum reacted only with the leukemia cell surface, and it did not react with the viral envelope.

Group-specific antigens in RNA-virus–induced tumors are detectable by immunofluorescence (Chapter 27) and gel precipitation tests (Chapter 6). They were first demonstrated in avian leukemia-sarcoma viruses and subsequently in MuLV (gs1–5); they are not strictly tumor specific since they are part of the internal component of the virus particle. Group-specific antigens may be species and virus restricted; e.g., gs1 is found in MuLV, but not murine MTV, and it is shared by all MuLV. Another antigen termed gs3 or "interspec" is more widespread, being found in leukemia viruses of several mammalian species including the mouse, cat, hamster, and rat.

Several soluble antigens have been detected in the circulation of animals bearing RNA-virus–induced tumors. They are related to TSCSA, as well as to VEA and gs antigens. Detection of these soluble components can serve to diagnose infection by these viruses. These soluble antigens have also been detected in immune complexes, which suggests their potential pathogenic role in immune complex disease (Chapter 19) and in abrogation of immune surveillance of the given tumor.

One of the earliest TSA to be described and perhaps the best documented is the thymus-leukemia antigen (Tla) of mice. Tla was initially detected by a C57BL/6 antiserum to a spontaneous leukemia of strain A mice. This antiserum was cytotoxic for the leukemia cells used for immunization and for several leukemias of C57BL/6 origin, but not for normal C57BL/6 tissue.

Cytotoxic activity could be removed by cells of the C57BL/6 leukemia and of the spontaneous leukemia of the A strain. Activity could also be removed by normal thymocytes from A mice, but could not be removed by thymocytes of C57BL/6 or several other mouse strains. Tla is a tumor-specific antigen in C57BL/6 mice, but is a normal antigenic constituent of other murine strains such as A and C58. It was subsequently shown that mice can be divided into those in which Tla is present on normal thymocytes, designated Tla+, and those in which it is absent, designated Tla−. Tla is an antigen restricted to thymocytes in normal Tla+ mice, but may appear on leukemia cells arising in Tla− as well as in Tla+ mice. Tla can also function as a histocompatibility antigen in that skin grafts and leukemia grafts exchanged between *TL* congenic lines are rejected. Further studies have shown that Tla is not a single antigen, but a complex consisting of at least four antigens: Tla.1, Tla.2, Tla.3, and Tla.4.

Cytotoxic antibodies in high titer can be produced in Tla− mice immunized with either normal or malignant Tla+ cells. If such mice are subsequently challenged with a Tla+ leukemia, death rather than protection ensues. Furthermore, tumor cells recovered from these mice give no evidence of Tla antigens by *in vitro* tests. This loss of Tla on tumor cells is, however, only temporary, since passage of these tumor cells in untreated syngeneic hosts results in reacquisition of Tla antigen. Such loss of antigenic structure after exposure to specific antibody is called antigenic modulation. Antigens undergoing modulation may be removed from the cell surface by degradation or by pinocytosis.

Antigenic modulation in the form of phenotypic deletion has also been described in other lymphoid malignancies, such as Burkitt's lymphoma in man and murine leukemias induced by Gross leukemia virus. This phenomenon may provide a means by which tumor cells escape destruction by the host's immune response.

The study of another murine surface antigen, G_{IX}, has contributed greatly to our understanding of virus-tumor relationship. G_{IX} antibodies are produced in $(W/Fu \times Bn)F_1$ rats immunized with leukemia cells elicited by the Gross virus in W/Fu rats. G_{IX} is a murine alloantigen that is present in normal G_{IX}^+ mice only on lymphoid cells and, interestingly, sperm. Distribution of G_{IX} antigen depends on infection with MuLV. In G_{IX}^+ strains that produce MuLV, the G_{IX} antigen is present in all lymphoid tissue, whereas in the absence of MuLV, the antigen is present only on thymocytes. Similar to Tla, G_{IX} may appear on leukemia cells of both G_{IX}^+ and G_{IX}^- mice. It has been suggested that production of G_{IX} antigen represents partial expression of the MuLV genome, since cells producing MuLV may express G_{IX} regardless of the tissue type of G_{IX} genotype. It appears that G_{IX} antigen is similar or identical to the major structural component of the envelope of MuLV, gp69/71. This suggests that G_{IX} is determined by a viral gene contained in the host cell genome.

Genetic Correlates of Tumorigenesis

In the study of cancer in man and animals, several observations point to the importance of the host's genetic makeup in tumorigenesis. These include instances of familial tendencies in certain human cancers and wide strain variation in incidence of spontaneous tumors in inbred mice. Information in this regard has been obtained in studies on one of the murine leukemia-associated antigen, X.1, in which susceptibility to virus infection was determined by the host's genome.

Cells of an x-irradiation–induced leukemia of BALB/c mice bear a strong surface antigen, X.1. Despite the fact that X.1 is absent from the tissue of normal BALB/c mice, they do not respond immunologically to this antigen. However, BALB/c × C57BL/6 F_1 hybrids not only reject leukemias bearing X.1 antigen; they also produce cytotoxic antibodies to X.1. Tumor resistance and production of X.1 antibody is presumably conferred to the hybrids by a C57BL/6 gene, Rgv-1. This gene is part of the allelic genes Rgv-1, rgv-1, Rgv-2, rgv-2, which control the response of mice to Gross virus. Only those mice that are homozygous for the dominant genes Rgv-1, Rgv-2, i.e., Rgv-1/Rgv-1, Rgv-2/Rgv-2, are resistant to infection by Gross virus.

Interestingly, X.1 is associated with MuLV and is an alloantigen present on the normal lymphoid cells of some strains of mice (X.1+) but absent on cells of other strains (X.1−). Similar to Tla, X.1 may be present on MuLV-induced leukemia cells arising in X.1− mice. The term X.1 is used for this antigenic system because of its similarity to the X antigen described by Gorer and Amos over 20 years ago. These authors demonstrated protection in C57BL mice against the syngeneic EL-4 leukemia after injecting the mice with a BALB/c anti-EL-4 serum. They designated the responsible antigen X. The tumor-specific nature of X rested on the fact that anti-X serum afforded protection even after extensive absorption with normal C57BL tissue. The authors also observed that passive transfer of antiserum produced better protection against leukemia cells in hemisyngeneic hybrids than in the syngeneic strain of origin of the leukemia. This X antigen was never demonstrated by serologic tests.

Several other examples of the genetic control of virus susceptibility have been described. The expression of G_{IX} is controlled by the dominant genes Gv-1 and Gv-2; Friend virus infection is controlled by an Fv locus; the H-2 complex is involved in susceptibility to MTV, as well as to vaccinia virus and lymphocytic choriomeningitis virus.

Immunology of Human Tumors

Early studies in immunology utilized immune sera as reagents to study microorganisms and their products. This principle was applied to the analysis of cells, tissues, and body fluids and enabled detection and definition of species-specific and tissue-specific antigens. From these studies stemmed attempts to define antigens that would characterize a given pathologic process, such as rheumatic fever, amyloidosis, and above all tumors. Pioneering these studies in the late 1920s and early 1930s were Hirszfeld and his group in Poland and Witebsky and coworkers in Germany. Rabbit immune sera were used as reagents and ethanol extracts of human tumors as *in vitro* antigens. Both groups reported that they could distinguish extracts of tumor tissues from extracts of normal tissues. The possibility of misleading results due to blood group antigens was clearly recognized and avoided. Hirszfeld also noted the similarity of ethanol-soluble antigens from tumors to such antigens from caseous tissues in tuberculosis, pus, and myocardial infarction tissue. He used the term "necrotic antigens" to denote antigens appearing in various processes involving tissue necrosis.

Rapport and his group in the 1950s and 1960s described several glycolipids, termed cytolipins (H, G, etc.), characteristic for various human tumors. Through chromatographic fractionation, a component called cytolipin H, a glycosphingolipid that is unrelated to cardiolipin or Forssman antigen, was isolated. It was present in human adenocarcinomas and myelomas but absent from other tumors. Normal tissue extracts contained this antigen but in much smaller quantities.

None of the lipid components tested by Hirszfeld, Witebsky, and Rapport were really TSA in the strict sense. They represent TAA in that they are normal tissue components that are increased in quantity in tumors.

In recent years considerable interest has been focused on a group of TAA known as oncofetal antigens. The relationship between embryonic and cancerous tissue stems from the work of Schöne at the beginning of this century. This investigator, a student of Ehrlich, showed that mice immunized with fetal tissue could reject transplants of tumor tissue that would otherwise grow. This immune state could not be elicited by normal adult tissue. Hirszfeld and associates also noted the antigenic similarity between neoplastic and embryonal tissues. They demonstrated that rabbit antisera to human cancer would combine with extracts of human fetal tissues, but not extracts of normal adult tissues.

Of studies on oncofetal antigens, the most important are those first reported by Gold and colleagues in 1965. Using rabbit antisera extensively absorbed with extracts of normal tissue, they demonstrated an antigen in perchloric acid extracts of human adenocarcinomas of the gastrointestinal tract. This antigen was not detectable in the extracts of tumors growing outside the gastrointestinal tract or in extracts of normal tissues. Further experiments revealed that extracts of fetal tissues contained an identical antigen, and the term "carcinoembryonic antigen" (CEA) was coined. A theory was proposed that CEA is a normal cellular constituent of the fetal tissue that becomes repressed in the process of differentiation of the normal epithelium of the digestive tract but is derepressed in the course of malignant transformation. Several studies have demonstrated an antigen serologically identical to CEA in nonmalignant pathologic tissue, as well as in normal human colon, albeit in much lower concentration than in tumor tissue. Therefore, CEA should be considered a TAA. CEA is characterized as a glycoprotein component of the glycocalyx of the cell with an electrophoretic mobility in the β globulin region, a sedimentation coefficient of 7–8 S, and a molecular weight of 200,000.

A radioimmunoassay procedure (Chapter 29) has been developed in which CEA can be detected in serum in a concentration as low as 0.5 ng/ml. Initial work using this procedure showed that CEA was present in the vast majority of patients with colonic or rectal cancer. Disappearance of the antigen from the circulation following successful surgery was also noted.

These early investigations gave promise for a diagnostic test for malignant gastrointestinal tumors; however, subsequent studies showed that increased serum levels of CEA could also be found in patients with malignant tumors outside the gastrointestinal tract, as well as in various nonmalignant diseases. Furthermore, increased levels were found in some apparently healthy individuals. Clearly, this procedure is not a reliable diagnostic aid for gastrointestinal tract tumors, but it is useful in the management of cancer patients in terms of prognosis and in monitoring the recurrence or progression of disease.

More recent evidence suggests that CEA is a heterogeneous substance with a number of closely related specificities. It is hoped that one of these may be more useful for diagnostic purposes.

Alpha fetoprotein (AFP) is another TAA of biologic as well as clinical interest. This substance was first described in the 1960s in chemically induced mouse and rat hepatomas by Abelev. Subsequent work showed a similar antigen in fetal sera from many species, including man.

High levels of AFP are present in man between 14 and 22 weeks of fetal life, from which time it decreases to barely detectable levels at birth and disappears completely a few weeks later. Significant levels of AFP are associated with primary hepatoma, being present in sera from 50 to 80% of patients with this tumor. Detection of AFP is now used routinely for the diagnosis of this disease. This substance is also present in other disease states such as acute or viral hepatitis and testicular teratoblastoma, though with lower frequency. AFP production accompanies proliferation of liver cells either in fetuses, or in the regenerating adult liver damaged by various noxious factors and diseases including hepatoma.

A closely related substance, alpha$_2$-H ferroprotein, is also of hepatic origin. It is normally present in human fetal organs and sera, being either absent or present only in trace amounts after two months of age. Beyond that period, its presence is associated with a number of malignant diseases, including hepatoma, neuroblastoma, nephroblastoma, and lymphosarcoma.

Other oncofetal TAA that may have potential value in the diagnosis of malignant tumors include: (1) Regan isoenzyme, a placental alkaline phosphatase isoenzyme normally absent from adult human tissue except for placenta and sera of pregnant women, but present in sera of 4 to 5% of patients with various malignant tumors; (2) fetal sulfoglycoprotein antigen, a substance found in the fetal gut and in a high percentage of patients with gastric carcinoma; and (3) heterophile fetal antigen, which is detectable in precipitation tests with some sera from patients with various malignant tumors. This antigen is present in the extracts of a number of different malignant tumors, but is also found in benign tumors and in nontumorous tissue in small amounts. Heterophile fetal antigen is not species specific and is found in sera of human, bovine, porcine, canine, and feline fetuses.

Identification of TSCSA in human tumors has proven to be elusive if not illusory. There have been claims that cells from various types of tumors, including carcinomas, sarcomas, and leukemias, bear cell-surface antigens that are unique for those tumors. In addition, several TAA have been described in a number of human cancers, including melanoma, osteogenic sarcoma, bladder carcinoma, Burkitt's lymphoma, and Hodgkin's disease, as well as other lymphomas and leukemias. Although most of these studies are not well documented, one theme seems to prevail. There appears to be considerable cross-reactivity in both cellular and humoral reactions among tumors of the same type. This has been demonstrated in sarcoma, malignant melanoma, Wilms' tumor, malignant glioma, and carcinoma of the uterine cervix, endometrium, ovary, breast, bladder, kidney, and colon.

One of the best described tumors is Burkitt's lymphoma, a disease associated with EBV infection (Chapter 15). These lymphomas bear surface antigens related to EBV and a cytoplasmic virus-related nonvirion antigen termed "early antigen" (EA). Antibodies in patients' sera to the surface antigen and to EA are important in the diagnosis and prognosis of this disease.

Another antigen of interest is the Paul-Bunnell antigen associated with infectious mononucleosis. This antigen has recently been described on lymphoid cells of spleen tissue taken from patients with Hodgkin's disease and other lymphomas, as well as from patients with various leukemias.

Immune Response of Tumor-Bearing Hosts

Several observations in animals and man suggest that some measure of tumor immunity resides in the tumor-bearing host. Instances of spontaneous recovery from malignancy in man are well documented. Tumor-bearing animals are capable of rejecting a small inoculum of the same tumor when it is administered in an anatomic site different from the primary location, in which it apparently shows unhindered growth. This phenomenon is known as concomitant immunity.

Numerous studies also describe both cellular and humoral antitumor immunity in tumor-bearing humans. Many of these reports claimed that lymphocytes from cancer patients can specifically kill target cells prepared from the patient's own tumor or cells from tumors of the same histologic type obtained from other patients. Cells from histologically different tumors were not killed nor were the target cells killed by lymphocytes from normal individuals or from patients with a different disease. Specific cytotoxicity has been reported in a number of malignant conditions, including breast and bladder carcinomas, melanomas, and sarcomas. These results have been questioned by some investigators who believe that there is no specificity with regard to the target cell killed and that lymphocytes from normal individuals may exhibit similar or even higher cytotoxic activity against tumor cells. These apparently contradictory findings do not necessarily invalidate the view that specific cellular antitumor immunity is present in cancer patients. Indeed, one could conclude that such immunity is present in normal individuals as well as in cancer patients, but that the tumor did not gain a foothold in the former group.

Similar to the studies on cell-mediated immunity are the countless reports in the literature describing tumor-specific antibodies in sera from patients with a variety of malignancies. Interpretation of these findings has also proven to be hazardous. Tumor specificity has been extremely difficult to verify. Much of the work has been performed on cultured tumor cells, and it is well known that cultured cells can "acquire" antigens from the culture medium, e.g., Mycoplasma antigens, which react with human sera. Mycoplasmas are widespread in nature and are particularly troublesome because they frequently infect cultured cells. The sera of patients may also contain antibodies resulting from blood transfusions that are directed against blood group or HLA antigens. Unless the studies are well controlled, detection of such antibodies may lead to a false conclusion regarding their tumor-specific nature.

Identification of tumor-specific antibodies has shown the most promise in studies on malignant melanoma. Although this is a relatively rare disease (2 to 3% of malignancies in the United States), it is of particular immunologic interest because of the disproportionately high incidence of spontaneous regression seen in this disease when compared with other malignant conditions. Antibodies in patient sera are reactive with both intracellular and surface antigens of melanoma cells. There are conflicting claims as to whether these antigens are individual specific or whether they are shared among melanomas.

Cellular and Humoral Effectors of the Immune Response to Tumors

In the early 1960s, Klein and his group showed that lymphoid cells from immunized mice could confer tumor resistance when passively transferred to syngeneic mice. Subsequent studies by a number of investigators showed that tumor resistance could be passively transferred using spleen cells, lymph node cells, thoracic duct lymphocytes, and peritoneal exudate cells. In the late 1960s, antitumor activity of lymphoid cells was demonstrated *in vitro* by Hellström using the colony inhibition test that he devised.

Subsequent studies have shown that cytotoxic T lymphocytes are a major force in tumor destruction (Chapter 9). Tumor cells may also be destroyed by the combined action of antitumor antibody and nonsensitized lymphocytes in the antibody-dependent, lymphocyte-mediated cytotoxicity reaction (ADCC). This nonsensitized lymphocyte that bears an Fc receptor has not been fully identified; it is frequently referred to as a K cell. Neutrophils, monocytes, B cells, and K cells all have Fc receptors. Whether all of these cells are involved in this reaction is not yet clear.

Recently, it has been shown that macrophages are also involved in the killing or rejection of tumors. A number of experiments have shown that resistance to tumors could be more efficiently demonstrated with peritoneal exudate cells that are rich in macrophages than with spleen cells or lymph node cells. Some studies suggest that peritoneal exudate cells alone are effective in conferring antitumor immunity.

Tumor destruction by macrophages is believed to be accomplished by two mechanisms. Macrophages bearing cytophilic antibodies or antigen-specific receptors (from T cells) are known as armed macrophages. Such armed macrophages may bind specifically to tumor cells and become activated, after which they function nonspecifically in that they can kill not only the tumor cells but also "innocent" bystander cells. Destruction of tumor cells can also be accomplished by activated but unarmed macrophages. Activated macrophages may result from stimulation of the immune system by a variety of antigens such as BCG.

Lymphoid cells play a major role in tumor resistance. The role of humoral antibody in this regard is not so clear. Protection by humoral alloantibody against dispersed-cell or ascitic tumors such as leukemias or lymphomas can be readily demonstrated. As yet, no convincing studies have shown the efficacy of protection by humoral antibodies against solid tumors. On the other hand, it can readily be shown that sera from mice immunized with an allogeneic or even syngeneic tumor will, in the presence of complement, lyse the tumor cells used for immunization. Humoral antibodies contained in an alloantiserum can also protect against growth of ascitic tumors *in vivo*. As mentioned before, humoral antibodies play a crucial role in antitumor immunity in the ADCC reaction and in the arming of macrophages.

Immunologic Surveillance

Most immunologists accept the idea that the immune system functions as a surveillance mechanism to prevent establishment of neoplasia. This concept was first formulated many years ago by Ehrlich and more recently espoused by Thomas and Burnet. According to this view, a malignant cell that emerges from a normal population carries on its surface TSTA that are recognized as foreign. As a consequence of this recognition, the malignant cell is destroyed by the immune system of the host.

Support for the concept of immunologic surveillance stems from several clinical observations. (1) An increased incidence of cancer is seen in older people. This is presumably due to (a) a cumulative mutagenic effect of carcinogens and (b) a decline in the efficiency of the immune system. (2) There is histologic evidence of *in situ* malignant tumors in autopsies of individuals who show no other clinical signs of malignant disease. (3) There is increased frequency of malignant tumors in individuals whose cell-mediated immunity (Chapter 11) has been abrogated by immunosuppressive therapy or who have congenital defects of the immune system, such as ataxia-telangiectasia, Wiskott-Aldrich syndrome, or thymic aplasia.

There is also much experimental evidence that supports the surveillance role of the immune system. For example, a significantly higher incidence of tumors has been reported in thymectomized mice that were subsequently treated with carcinogens or injected with oncogenic viruses, as compared to similarly treated nonthymectomized controls.

On the other hand, several observations cast doubt on the surveillance concept, at least in its most simplistic form. No increased incidence of tumors has been observed in several diseases in which definite immunosuppression occurs, such as leprosy and sarcoidosis. Nude mice, which lack T cell function, do not have a high incidence of spontaneous tumors, which might have been expected according to the surveillance theory. Also, chemically induced tumors arise just as frequently in normal mice as they do in athymic or nude mice. Presence of a normally functioning T cell system apparently does not lead to a decreased incidence of tumor induction. Likewise, no increase in spontaneous tumors has been observed in immunosuppressed mice. According to the theory, immunologically privileged sites such as the anterior chamber of the eye and the brain are the sites in which tumors should develop frequently. This is not the case.

Prehn, one of the leading antagonists of the surveillance theory, believes that the response of the immune system to tumors is for the most part "too little and too late." He argues, for example, that the "sneak-through" phenomenon is evidence against surveillance. According to this phenomenon, the immunizing stimulus may be too weak in the initial stages of tumor growth to engender a sufficiently strong response. By the time an adequate response is elicited, the tumor is too large and too fast growing to be rejected. This would explain the observation that an extremely small inoculum of tumor could grow in a syngeneic host, whereas a slightly larger dose would elicit an immune response and be destroyed.

Another argument against surveillance is the concept of immunostimulation proposed by Prehn. He has shown in both *in vivo* and *in vitro* experiments that growth of a tumor may be enhanced in the presence of syngeneic lymphoid cells sensitized against the tumor. He has suggested that in the early stage of development, tumor growth is stimulated by the immune system. Later, as the tumor increases in size, the immune system may acquire inhibitory potential that may or may not succeed in preventing further growth of the tumor.

There are other lines of evidence that show that the immune system may enhance rather than inhibit tumor growth (Figure 24–2). Studies reported in the early 1900s showed that tumor growth in rats could be facilitated by prior injection of killed tissue from the same tumor. Casey obtained similar results in mice and rabbits in the 1930s and described the phenomenon as an enhancing effect. In the early 1950s, Kaliss and his group showed that this phenomenon of immunologic enhancement was due to alloantibodies directed against transplantation antigens on the tumor cells. Subsequently, it was proposed that these alloantibodies, after combining with transplantation antigens, could either prevent recognition of these antigens by the recipient animal or could block the lethal action of lymphocytes sensitized against these antigens (Chapter 12).

Subsequently, Hellström and his group performed experiments with both human and experimental tumors showing that enhancement of tumor growth could be demonstrated in a syngeneic situation. Their experiments were performed with a tumor that regresses spontaneously in some animals and persists in others. Using the colony inhibition assay, they showed that lymphocytes from both persistor and regressor animals could kill tumor cells and inhibit tumor growth. Thus, the lymphoid cells from both groups of animals possessed antitumor potential. The lethal effects of both persistor and regressor lymphocytes could be abolished by adding serum from persistor animals to the mixture. Normal serum or serum from regressor animals did not block the action of the sensitized lymphocytes. They postulated that serum from persistor animals contained a substance termed "blocking factor," which could nullify the killing effect of T lymphocytes. Blocking factor is thought to be a complex composed of "soluble" tumor antigen and its corresponding antibody. Evidence also has been presented that tumor antigen alone can block cytotoxicity; however, maximum blocking requires complexing of tumor antigen and antibody. Recently, a deblocking factor has been described, which can abrogate the activity of blocking factor and thereby allow cytotoxic lymphocytes to destroy target tumor cells.

Destruction of tumor cells may be abrogated by tumor antigen which has been shed into the circulation or by tumor antibody. Shed tumor antigens may bind specific receptors on lymphocytes and inhibit their cytotoxic activity against the tumor cells. Tumor antibody may bind to antigen on tumor cells and shield the cells from attacking lymphocytes.

It has recently been proposed that tumors may escape surveillance by another mechanism. Several years ago, evidence was presented that tumor tissue could adsorb erythrocytes sensitized by antierythrocyte antibody.

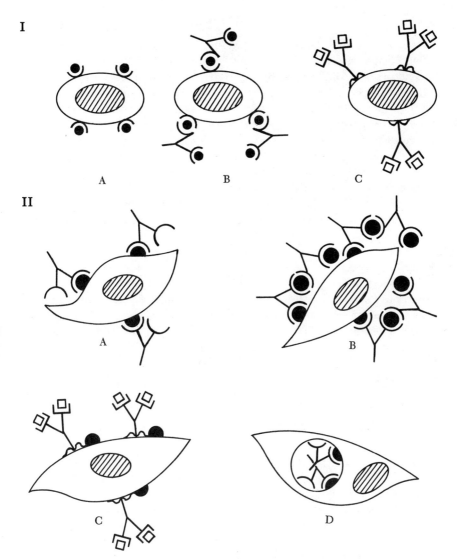

Figure 24-2. Possible mechanisms of escape from tumor immunity.
I. Cytotoxic action of lymphoid cells may be inhibited by (*A*) binding of soluble tumor antigens to corresponding receptors on sensitized T lymphocytes; (*B*) binding of immune complexes composed of tumor antigens and their antibodies to receptors on sensitized T lymphocytes; or (*C*) binding of any immune complexes to Fc receptors on K lymphocytes or macrophages participating in "nonspecific" tumor destruction.
II. Destruction of tumor cells by lymphoid cells may be blocked by (*A*) binding of specific antibody to antigenic sites on tumor cells; (*B*) binding of specific immune complexes to antigenic sites on tumor cells; (*C*) binding of any immune complexes to Fc receptors of tumor cells; or (*D*) antigenic modulation, exemplified here by pinocytotic uptake of tumor antigen following its reaction with antibody.

Subsequent studies showed that binding of sensitized erythrocytes to the tumor tissue was dependent on the Fc portion of the IgG molecule since hemadsorption could not be demonstrated by erythrocytes sensitized by the $F(ab')_2$ fragment of antierythrocyte antibody. Concurrently, normal lymphoid tissue including macrophages was shown to possess receptors that bind the Fc portion of the IgG molecule. Today it is still not clear whether hemadsorption by tumor tissue is due to infiltration of the tumor by Fc receptor–bearing cells (such as macrophages) or whether tumor cells themselves possess Fc receptors. If it is true that tumor cells may possess Fc receptors, another mechanism would be provided for the escape of tumors from surveillance in that nonspecific immune complexes could shield newly emerging tumor cells possessing Fc receptors from immune cell-mediated destruction.

There is yet another means by which tumors may escape the lethal action of immune surveillance. Recent work has shown that tumors can inhibit the migration of macrophages to sites of inflammation. Snyderman and his group have shown that this inhibition of macrophages can be produced by a soluble factor extracted from tumor tissue. This factor is a low-molecular-weight substance (10,000) produced by neoplastic cells and is capable of inhibiting the chemotactic response of macrophages. The chemotactic signal is muted to the point that macrophages are unable to "seek and destroy" tumor cells.

Immunotherapy of Malignant Diseases

The control and perhaps even the eradication of cancer from the list of major human afflictions comprise one of the principal commitments of modern medicine. Following the experience gained in taming many infectious diseases by immunologic methods, many attempts were made to utilize this knowledge for tumor therapy. These attempts were justified more by enthusiasm than by experimental evidence. Some studies were conducted in which cancer patients were administered massive amounts of heteroantisera that were believed to be cancer-specific reagents. Unfortunately, these sera were not cancer specific; on the contrary, they proved to be quite toxic for the patients. In other studies, patients were immunized with vaccines prepared from their own tumor tissue. These early attempts were, for the most part, fruitless.

Successful treatment of malignant diseases is now achieved through surgery, radiation therapy, or chemotherapy used singly or in combination. The most success has been obtained in the treatment of localized tumors. These modes of therapy too often fail in combating metastases. For many years, only chemotherapy was useful in controlling disseminated malignant cancer, but immunotherapy is believed to show some promise in this regard. Several approaches are being explored for tumor immunotherapy. These include (1) immunization with (a) nonspecific agents such as BCG or dinitrochlorobenzene (DNCB) and (b) specific agents such as tumor vaccines, and (2) replacement or supplementation of the patient's immune system by (a) adoptive transfer with lymphocytes and (b) administration of transfer factor.

Nonspecific stimulation of the immune system by immunization with BCG or other bacteria that produce an adjuvant effect, such as *Bordetella pertussis* and *Proprionibacterium acnes* (previously named *Corynebacterium parvum*), appears to be a potentially useful therapeutic procedure. Some measure of protection against leukemias and even solid tumors has been reported in experimental animals. In man, treatment of several types of malignancies, particularly leukemias, lymphomas, and melanomas, has been attempted. Some success has been claimed. This "bacterial" therapy appears to act by stimulation of lymphocytes and activation of macrophages. Treatment with a methanol-soluble extract of tubercle bacilli, which is reportedly a more active immunostimulant, is also being tried.

Nonspecific agents used with some success are those chemicals, such as DNCB, that induce delayed hypersensitivity (Chapter 11) when applied topically. They have been employed with some success in treatment of basal-cell and squamous-cell carcinomas, melanomas, and, in particular, cutaneous lymphomas. Promising results have been obtained only with cutaneous lesions. These agents induce inflammation; apparently, the inflammatory cells act in conjunction with the tumor-specific lymphocytes already in the area to destroy the tumor.

Active immunization with tumor vaccines, though one of the earliest modes of cancer immunotherapy, has shown the least promise. Most protocols called for immunization of the patient with a vaccine prepared from the surgically removed primary tumor. In many studies, the vaccine was administered with an immunopotentiating agent such as Freund's complete adjuvant (a suspension of killed tubercle bacilli in mineral oil). Clinical trials showed no significant increase in survival rates of immunized patients as compared to nonimmunized controls. It is conceivable that lack of success is due to the induction of blocking antibodies by this procedure.

Some success has been claimed in leukemia patients immunized with neuraminidase-treated leukemia cells. This treatment strips away cellular glycocalyx and presumably uncovers tumor antigens.

In the light of recent knowledge concerning the immune state of the tumor-bearing individual, cancer immunotherapy must be used with caution. Since it has been shown that the cell-mediated immune response in the tumor-bearing host can be abrogated by the blocking factor, it is crucial that the treatment does not induce the production of blocking factor or increase its concentration.

Renewed efforts in the use of tumor vaccine will most certainly center on attempts to elicit T cell but not B cell immunity with suitable preparations of tumor antigen. Promising results in immunoprophylaxis against tumors have been obtained in animal experiments. A recent report described the induction of cell-mediated immunity in mice injected with syngeneic tumor cells treated with mitomycin. This procedure elicited protection against a lethal dose of the tumor without the production of detectable levels of anti-tumor antibodies. It is hoped that this principle can be applied to tumor immunotherapy as well.

Adoptive immunization procedures in which a recipient is injected with lymphocytes from a sensitized or unsensitized donor have been successfully employed in conferring antitumor immunity in tumor-bearing animals. Several studies in animals have shown that a tumor-killing effect can be produced in tumor-bearing recipients that have been injected with lymphocytes obtained from a syngeneic donor immunized with the same tumor. Sensitized allogeneic lymphocytes cannot be used since they would be rejected by the recipient.

Since syngeneic lymphocytes are not available in man, clinical studies along these lines have centered on the grafting of allogeneic bone marrow in leukemia patients, whose own lymphoid systems have been eradicated by irradiation. Claims of remission in some leukemia patients have been reported with this method of treatment. However, since these irradiated individuals are incapable of mounting an immune response, the passively transferred allogeneic lymphoid cells can often elicit a fatal graft-vs.-host response (Chapter 23).

A recent approach to cancer immunotherapy involves the use of transfer factor (Chapter 11). This substance is described as a relatively low-molecular-weight ($\sim 10,000$) factor that is extracted from sensitized human lymphocytes. Existence of this substance in nonhuman lymphocytes has not been established. Transfer factor induces a state of delayed hypersensitivity in normal recipients, and it has been used successfully to treat certain diseases such as mucocutaneous candidiasis (Chapter 14).

Studies on patients with a variety of malignant tumors including melanoma, osteogenic sarcoma, nasopharyngeal carcinoma, and breast carcinoma, have shown that cell-mediated immunity could be elicited by the administration of "tumor-specific" transfer factor. In a few instances, some degree of tumor regression had been noted.

Bibliography

Aoki, T., and Sibal, L. R.: RNA oncogenic virus-associated antigens and host immune response to them. In Becker, F. F. (ed.): Cancer. A Comprehensive Treatise. Vol. 4: Biology of Tumors: Surfaces, Immunology, and Comparative Pathology. Plenum Press, New York, 1975.

Baldwin, R. W.: Role of immunosurveillance against chemically induced rat tumors. Transplant. Rev., 28:62–74, 1976.

Boyse, E. A.; Old, L. J.; and Stockert, E.: The TL (thymus leukemia) antigen: a review. In Grabar, P., and Miescher, P. A. (eds.): Immunopathology. Fourth International Symposium. Schwabe, Basel, 1966.

Golub, S. H.: Host immune response to human tumor antigens. In Becker, F. F. (ed.): *Cancer. A Comprehensive Treatise.* Vol. 4: Biology of Tumors: Surfaces, Immunology, and Comparative Pathology. Plenum Press, New York, 1975.

Hellström, K. E., and Hellström, I.: Lymphocyte-mediated cytotoxicity and blocking serum activity to tumor antigens. *Adv. Immunol.,* **18**:209–77, 1974.

Hersh, E. M.; Gutterman, J. U.; and Mavligit, G.: *Immunotherapy of Cancer in Man. Scientific Basis and Current Status.* Charles C Thomas, Publisher, Springfield, Ill., 1973.

Milgrom, F.: A short review of immunological investigations on cancer. *Cancer Res.,* **21**:862–68, 1961.

Morton, D. L.; Eilber, F. R.; and Malmgren, R. A.: Immune factors in human cancer: malignant melanomas, skeletal and soft tissue sarcomas. *Prog. Exp. Tumor Res.,* **14**:25–42, 1971.

Obata, Y.; Ikeda, H.; Stockert, E.; and Boyse, E. A.: Relation of G_{IX} antigen of thymocytes to envelope glycoprotein of murine leukemia virus. *J. Exp. Med.,* **141**:188–97, 1975.

Old, L. J., and Boyse, E. A.: Current enigmas in cancer research. *Harvey Lect.,* **67**:273–315, 1973.

Prehn, R. T.: Do tumors grow because of the immune response of the host? *Transplant. Rev.,* **28**:34–42, 1976.

Price, M. R., and Baldwin, R. W.: Immunobiology of chemically induced tumors. In Becker, F. F. (ed.): *Cancer. A Comprehensive Treatise.* Vol. 4: Biology of Tumors: Surfaces, Immunology, and Comparative Pathology. Plenum Press, New York, 1975.

Sato, H.; Boyse, E. A.; Aoki, T.; Irritani, C.; and Old, L. J.: Leukemia associated transplantation antigens related to murine leukemia virus. The x.1 system: immune response controlled by a locus linked to *H-2. J. Exp. Med.,* **138**:593–606, 1973.

Stockert, E.; Old, L. J.; and Boyse, E. A.: The G_{IX} system. A cell surface alloantigen associated with murine leukemia virus: implications regarding chromosomal integration of the viral genome. *J. Exp. Med.,* **133**:1334–55, 1971.

Terry, W. D.; Henkart, P. A.; Coligan, J. E.; and Todd, C. W.: Carcinoembryonic antigen: characterization and clinical applications. *Transplant Rev.,* **20**:100–129, 1974.

Tevethia, S. S., and Tevethia, M. J.: DNA virus (SV40) induced antigens. In Becker, F. F. (ed.): *Cancer. A Comprehensive Treatise.* Vol. 4: Biology of Tumors: Surfaces, Immunology, and Comparative Pathology. Plenum Press, New York, 1975.

25

Autoimmune Diseases

NOEL R. ROSE

Self-Recognition

In 1900 Ehrlich and Morgenroth became interested in the fate of extravasated blood. If goats were injected intraperitoneally with blood of a foreign species, such as the dog, they developed antibodies to the red blood cells of the dog. The blood of other goats, injected in the same manner, also caused the goats to produce antibodies. These antibodies dissolved the red blood cells of the donor goat and of most, but not all, other goats tested. Consistently, however, these antibodies failed to dissolve the red blood cells of the recipient goat itself. They acted, in effect, like typical blood-group-specific isoantibodies (Chapter 20). The fact that goats refused to form antibodies to their own red blood cells fascinated Ehrlich. His curiosity was heightened when he found that goats injected intraperitoneally with their own blood cells failed to produce any antibodies at all. He coined the term *horror autotoxicus* to describe the finding that animals usually fail to produce antibodies to antigens of their own bodies. Ehrlich speculated that, were this biologic rule to be violated, animals would produce autoantibodies that would injure their own tissues and might result in disease or death.

Many later investigators were impressed by the general validity of Ehrlich's principle. In 1949 Sir MacFarlane Burnet pointed out that the phenomenon of self-recognition (as he named it) could not be readily accounted for by the instructive theories of antibody formation then prevalent (Chapter 3). At first he suggested that all of the potentially antigenic molecules of the body possess self-markers that prevent autoantibody formation. The concept of self-markers was discarded because of the difficulty in demonstrating a single grouping or antigenic determinant present on all molecules of the body. When Burnet developed the clonal selection hypothesis, he proposed that the contract of immunologically reactive precursor cells with their respective antigens during fetal life leads to destruction of the cells and therefore elimination of the particular clone. For this reason, self-reactive lymphocytes are not present in the body except if they arise later in life due to a somatic mutation within the lymphocyte population. Burnet suggested that the progeny of such hypothetic mutants, referred to as forbidden clones, give rise to autoantibodies.

Recently several modifications of the clonal elimination hypothesis have been introduced. On the basis of experimental findings of Taylor and of Weigle that tolerance can be induced more easily in T cells than B cells, Allison suggested that certain antigens circulating in only small amounts eliminate the T cell clones, leaving self-reactive B cells in the body (Chapter 12). This hypothesis explains why it is extraordinarily difficult to evoke autoimmunity to plentiful antigens, such as serum albumin, which induce tolerance in both T and B cells, whereas it is much easier to induce autoimmunity to tissue antigens like thyroglobulin that are present in the bloodstream in small amounts and induce tolerance only in T cells.

In recent years several new explanations for tolerance—including self-tolerance—have been advanced (Chapter 12). They are based on the increasing realization that there are built-in mechanisms for regulating the immunologic response. T cells have been identified that suppress rather than promote antibody production by B cells. Suppressor T cells can also reduce the function of other T cells in producing cell-mediated immunity. Another mechanism recently proposed for controlling the immunologic response is production of antireceptor or anti-idiotype antibodies (Chapter 12).

Several lines of investigation support the concept that these regulating mechanisms are important in controlling self-recognition. Cohen and Wekerle have found that lymphocytes removed from the body can be immunized to fibroblasts of the same animals, provided they are cultured in the absence of the animal's own serum. Progenitors of self-reactive lymphocytes may be normally present in the body but held in check by regulatory controls.

Autoimmunization (Table 25-1)

Despite the array of mechanisms for preventing immune responses to self-antigens, there are now numerous examples of the experimental induction

Table 25-1

INDUCTION OF AUTOIMMUNITY

Experimental Method	Possible Natural Equivalent
Release of isolated antigen	Vasectomy
Freund's adjuvant	Chronic infectious diseases, e.g., tuberculosis, viral infections
Foreign, cross-reactive antigen	Rheumatic fever
Hapten-substituted antigen	α methyldopa–induced hemolytic anemia
Proteolyzed antigen	Collagen disease
Defect in immunologic regulation	New Zealand mice; lupus

of an autoimmune reaction. The immunologic system seems to be capable of responding readily to self-antigens that are not in contact with the circulation during embryonic growth. In order to initiate autoantibody formation, it is necessary to remove such antigens from their cloistered site and inject them into the bloodstream. Examples of isolated antigens are found in the lens of the eye and in the sperm of the testes. An anatomic barrier prevents free exchange with the blood and lymphatic circulation. When antigens of the lens and sperm are injected into the same animal, they elicit autoantibodies. It is interesting that humans undergoing surgical occlusion of the spermatic ducts (vasectomy) generally develop antibodies to their own sperm.

When one deals with antigens that are not well isolated, it is more difficult to initiate the production of autoantibodies. Injection of simple saline extracts of such tissues as thyroid or adrenal glands into the same animal rarely evoke antibody production. However, if injected with proper adjuvant, extracts of these organs are antigenic. Most commonly used is complete Freund's adjuvant. When injected with an organ extract, Freund's adjuvant diminishes self-tolerance. In addition to promoting anti-body formation, Freund's adjuvant induces cell-mediated immunity (Chapter 11). Autoimmunization using complete Freund's adjuvant often leads to damage in the equivalent organ of the immunized animal. One frequently sees a correlation between the degree of cell-mediated immunity as measured by a skin test and development of lesions in the target organ following autoimmunization. This correlation has led many investigators to propose that the lesions of autoimmune diseases in these organs are due to cell-mediated immunity.

Obviously the use of Freund's adjuvant is highly artificial. It is difficult to identify the natural equivalent of this adjuvant. Infection by some micro-organisms, such as those with acid-fast properties, may serve this function. There has been a good deal of interest in the hypothesis that pulmonary tuberculosis is associated with simultaneous production of autoantibodies to lung tissue. Bacterial lipopolysaccharides may serve as adjuvants and induce autoantibody formation and autoimmune tissue damage. Viruses may incorporate host proteins and thereby act as an adjuvant, or viral infections may alter cell membranes and make them antigenic.

Another way of inducing the formation of autoantibodies is injection of foreign, cross-reacting antigens. During the vigorous response to the foreign antigenic determinants, antibodies to the autologous determinants are also produced. Moreover, once the process has begun, further exposure to the self-antigen by itself can boost autoantibody production.

A likely natural equivalent of this experimental phenomenon is repeated streptococcal infections. Membranes of these common bacteria share antigens with the membranes of mammalian cells. Immunization with streptococci can induce antibodies reactive with the membranes of human heart muscle fibers. This mechanism may be involved in the production of rheumatic fever.

It is possible to add foreign determinants to autologous proteins by chemical coupling. For example, addition of arsenilic and sulfanilic groups to thyroglobulin renders it antigenic in the same animal. Extensive immunization with these altered antigens leads to the development of lesions in the equivalent organ of the immunized animals. This mechanism may explain the hemolytic anemia associated with certain drugs like α methyldopa that are known to couple spontaneously with surface constituents of the red blood cell.

Another means by which novel antigenic determinants can be exposed on autologous antigens is partial degradation. Macromolecules of the tissues are always in the dynamic state of breakdown and resynthesis. Enzymes present in the body are occupied with degrading these molecules to smaller units, which are normally too small to be antigenic. If, however, the process of degradation is interrupted for some reason, large fragments may be released. Partially degraded collagen has been shown to be antigenic by experimental immunization. This mechanism may be important in human connective tissue diseases such as rheumatoid arthritis, systemic sclerosis, or dermatomyositis.

All of the mechanisms described thus far depend upon changes in the antigen. An alternative possibility to explain the development of autoimmunity is that abnormalities arise in immunologic recognition. Sometimes viruses with a predilection for immunologically competent lymphocytes may disturb self-recognition. It is also possible that genetic aberrations occur in the cells responsible for immunologic recognition. Some inbred strains of mice develop autoimmune diseases with great regularity. These New Zealand (NZ) mice demonstrate that genetic and perhaps viral factors can play a role in the induction of autoimmunity (pages 441–42).

Experimental Autoimmune Diseases (Table 25-2)

The best-studied example of an experimentally induced autoimmune disease is produced by myelin, the protein that serves as insulation for the

Table 25-2
SOME EXPERIMENTAL AUTOIMMUNE DISEASES

Experimental Disease	Organ Affected	Antigen
Encephalomyelitis	Central nervous system	Basic protein
Peripheral neuropathy	Peripheral nervous system	*
Thyroiditis	Thyroid	Thyroglobulin
Parathyroiditis	Parathyroid	*
Adrenalitis	Adrenal	Heat-stable protein
Orchitis-aspermatogenesis	Testis	Acrosomal S & P proteins
Endophthalmitis	Lens	Crystallin
Uveitis	Uvea	Uveal pigment metabolite
Gastritis	Gastric mucosa	*
Insulinitis	Pancreatic islets	*
Myocarditis	Heart	*
Glomerulonephritis	Kidney	Glomerular basement membrane
Thymitis	Thymus	*
Myasthenia	Neuromuscular junction	Acetylcholine receptor

* Crude extracts of particular organ used; antigen not yet defined.

nerve fibers of the central nervous system. Injection of a well-defined basic protein isolated from myelin, with complete Freund's adjuvant, results in a demyelinating disease, autoimmune encephalomyelitis. Most investigators attribute the encephalomyelitis to the effects of cell-mediated immunity (Chapter 11). Their argument is strengthened by the observation that induction of a humoral antibody response to myelin by use of incomplete Freund's adjuvant does not induce encephalomyelitis. In fact, it interferes with production of the disease by the standard immunization procedure. Clinically, autoimmune encephalomyelitis resembles human demyelinating diseases such as multiple sclerosis. Autoimmune peripheral neuropathy can be induced in rabbits by injection of myelin isolated from peripheral nerves; it seems to mimic human idiopathic peripheral neuritis (Guillain-Barré syndrome).

There is one rather exceptional example of a human demyelinating disease clearly produced by autoimmunization. In former years the original Pasteur rabies vaccine sometimes resulted in paralytic accidents. They were probably due to antigens of rabbit brain that cross-react with the patient's own brain antigens.

Experimental thyroiditis provides a close facsimile of the human disease, chronic thyroiditis. Inflammation of the thyroid gland can be induced by injections of rabbits, guinea pigs, rats, mice, or other animals with thyroglobulin. Foreign, cross-reactive thyroglobulin or sulfanilated-arsenilited thyroglobulin of the same species can induce autoantibody production, as can partially degraded thyroglobulin. However, the most effective means of inducing autoantibody production and disease is to combine thyroglobulin of the same species with complete Freund's adjuvant or with bacterial lipopolysaccharide.

The interplay of humoral and cell-mediated immunity in producing experimental thyroiditis has still not been resolved. In some species it is possible to transfer the disease from immunized to normal animals with serum. In other species this has not been accomplished but transfer has been carried out only with lymphocytes of actively immunized animals.

OS chickens represent a selected flock that develop thyroiditis spontaneously in high incidence. By demonstrating autoantibodies to thyroglobulin, Witebsky was able to show that this process is autoimmune. The disease is much diminished by bursectomy, a procedure associated with the reduction of antibody production. Conversely, neonatal thymectomy, which diminished cell-mediated immunity, does not reduce the severity of thyroiditis in OS chickens. In fact, it leads to intensification of the disease. These findings, together with similar observations in NZ mice, suggest that the thymus normally may control the emergence of autoantibody-producing clones of B lymphocytes in animals that are genetically predisposed to autoimmune disease.

Experiments described previously have shown that immunologically competent cell populations capable of reacting with self-antigens are present throughout life. All lymphocytes responding to self-antigens are not eliminated during embryonic growth. The suppression of self-reactive clones of lymphocytes requires active monitoring.

Genetics, Aging, and Sex

Colonies of animals with a high incidence of spontaneous autoimmune disease, such as NZ mice or OS chickens, support the belief that there is a genetic tendency toward the development of autoimmunity. It was noticed many years ago that certain human autoimmune diseases occur in unexpected frequency among members of the same family. For instance, the incidence of autoantibodies to thyroglobulin is much higher in individuals who have close relatives with chronic thyroiditis or some related disorder of the thyroid gland. Such persons may also have more than the expected frequency of autoantibodies to other organs, such as the adrenal glands or the gastric lining. Recently, a statistical association of the insulin-dependent form of diabetes mellitus with the organ-specific autoimmune diseases has been reported. These observations suggest that there is an inherited tendency toward the development of autoimmunity, although the particular organ involved varies from individual to individual. The additional observation that a disproportionately large number of patients with one or another of the autoimmune diseases have the HLA-B8 haplotype further points to an association of disease susceptibility and the major histocompatibility complex (Chapter 22).

Immunologic regulation diminishes with age, and autoimmunity is generally more common in older individuals. Most autoimmune diseases are also more frequent in women than men, suggesting that the balance of sex hormones plays a role in immunologic regulation. In NZ mice, castration of males and treatment with estrogen aggravate autoimmune disease.

Autoimmune Diseases in the Human

The production of autoantibodies in man is not uncommon, although it is often difficult to show that they are the cause of disease. Some of the most important diagnostic laboratory tests in medicine are based on the production of autoantibodies. A good example of a diagnostic application of autoantibody is the Wassermann test for syphilis, which depends on the demonstration of autoantibody to a ubiquitously distributed diphosatidylglycerol, cardiolipin. It is not certain how this autoantibody arises. Perhaps the spirochete of syphilis induces its production, or possibly tissue breakdown liberates autologous cardiolipin. In any case the autoantibody is empirically associated with syphilis and provides a useful diagnostic test, even though the antibodies themselves have nothing to do with causing the disease (Chapter 13).

Table 25-3
SOME HUMAN DISEASES WITH AUTOIMMUNE MANIFESTATIONS

Disease	Antigen
A. Endocrinopathies	
Chronic thyroiditis (Hashimoto's disease) and primary myxedema	Thyroglobulin Thyroid microsomes CA_2 Thyroid cell surface
Hyperthyroidism (Graves' disease)	Thyroid cell surface—TSH receptor (stimulatory antibody)
Adrenal insufficiency (Addison's disease)	Adrenal cortex
Primary ovarian failure	Steroid-producing cells of adrenal, ovary, testis, and placenta
Diabetes mellitus (early-onset)	Islet cells
B. Gastrointestinal diseases	
Pernicious anemia and atrophic gastritis	Intrinsic factor Parietal cells
Ulcerative colitis	Colonic mucosal cells
Primary biliary cirrhosis	Mitochondria
Chronic active hepatitis	Smooth muscle
C. Diseases of the reproductive tissues	
Masculine sterility	Spermatozoa
D. Diseases of the eye	
Phacoanaphylactic endophthalmitis	Lens
Sympathetic ophthalmia	Uvea

Table 25-3—*continued*

SOME HUMAN DISEASES WITH AUTOIMMUNE MANIFESTATIONS

Disease	Antigen
E. Neurologic diseases	
Postvaccinal encephalitis and post-infectious encephalitis	Myelin or basic protein of brain or spinal cord
Polyneuritis and neuropathy (Guillain-Barré syndrome)	Peripheral nervous tissue
F. Diseases of the heart and kidney	
Postcardiotomy—postinfarction syndrome	Cardiac muscle
Rheumatic fever	Subsarcolemmal membrane of cardiac muscle
Autoimmune glomerulonephritis (Goodpasture's syndrome)	Glomerular basement membrane of the kidney (linear deposition)
Immune complex glomerulonephritis	Streptococcal of malarial antigens (granular deposition)
G. Connective tissue diseases	
Lupus erythematosus	Nuclear components (DNA, DNA-protein, RNA)
	Mitochondria, microsomes
Rheumatoid arthritis	Fc of IgG
	Collagen
Progressive systemic sclerosis	Nuclear components (extractable nuclear antigen, nucleoli)
	Collagen
Dermatomyositis	Nuclear components
	Collagen
H. Neuromuscular diseases	
Myasthenia gravis	Acetylcholine receptors
	Striations of skeletal (and cardiac) muscle; "myoid" cells of thymus
I Disease of exocrine glands	
Keratoconjunctivitis sicca (Sjögren's syndrome)	Salivary gland ducts; nuclei; IgG; thyroglobulin
J. Skin diseases	
Pemphigus vulgaris	Intercellular substance of stratified squamous epithelia
Bullous pemphigoid	Basal membrane between epidermis and dermis
K. Diseases of the blood	
Acquired hemolytic anemia	Red blood cell surface
Idiopathic thrombocytic purpura	Platelet surface
Leukopenia	Leukocyte surface

The first demonstration of the human disease resulting from autoantibody formation occurred in 1904. In a relatively rare disease called paroxysmal cold hemoglobulinuria, Donath and Landsteiner discovered an autoantibody that combines with human erythrocytes only at lowered temperatures. When restored to normal body temperature, this bound antibody is capable of activating complement to produce lysis of the red blood cell (Chapter 8).

The reaction is best shown in the body by first lowering the temperature (for example, by dipping a finger in a glass of ice water) and then restoring it to normal temperature. Only recently has the red cell antigen responsible for this phenomenon been identified as Tj^a ($P + P_1$), one of the blood group antigens (Chapter 20).

Several other forms of human hemolytic anemia are associated with autoantibody formation. These antibodies combine with the patients' erythrocytes at body temperature and promote destruction of the erythrocytes by the spleen. The demonstration of immunoglobulin to the patient's red blood cells by means of Coombs' antiglobulin test is the cornerstone in the diagnosis of human autoimmune hemolytic anemia (Chapter 20).

Table 25-3 gives a partial list of human diseases for which there is some evidence of an autoimmune reaction. The identification of autoantibodies is not necessarily an indication that a disease is autoimmune in origin. Even before the autoimmune pathogenesis of a human disease is fully documented, however, the antibodies may be reliably used for laboratory diagnosis.

Endocrinopathies

Most patients with chronic lymphocytic thyroiditis have autoantibodies to thyroid tissue. The serologic findings in human chronic thyroiditis differ from those in experimental thyroiditis in one significant respect. In addition to autoantibodies to thyroglobulin, autoantibodies to other organ-specific antigens of the thyroid are commonly found. A second antigen associated with the membranous portion of the thyroid microsome produces complement fixation with human thyroiditis sera. The antibodies localize in the cytoplasm of the thyroid cell, as shown by autoimmune diseases. This finding is taken as a strong suggestion that an accumulation of abnormalities—hormonal, infectious, metabolic, or somatogenetic—is important for the initiation of these diseases in man.

In many cases of hyperthyroidism due to Graves' disease, autoantibody to the receptor to thyroid-stimulating hormone (TSH) on the surface of thyroid epithelial cells has exerted a stimulating effect. Because of the slow but prolonged action of this antibody compared with TSH, it was termed "long-acting thyroid stimulator" (LATS) or thyroid-stimulating antibody (TsAb).

A striking feature of autoimmune thyroid disease is its overlap with certain other diseases. Patients with pernicious anemia, for instance, or with idiopathic adrenal insufficiency frequently develop thyroiditis, and vice versa. Moreover, the incidence of thyroid autoantibodies is unusually high in these patients. Therefore, if there is a genetic diathesis toward the development of autoimmunity, it must predispose to the whole group of organ-specific disorders.

Patients with idiopathic adrenal insufficiency (Addison's disease) frequently have antibodies to one or more antigens of the adrenal gland itself.

The most important antigen is found in the microsomes of the adrenal cortex; a second antigen rests in the steroid-producing cells of the adrenal, ovary, testis, and placenta. The antibodies are most easily demonstrated by means of indirect immunofluorescence (Chapter 27). In addition to its clinical and serologic overlap with thyroiditis, adrenal insufficiency, especially in children, seems to be associated with hypoparathyroidism and with the development of recalcitrant *Candida* infections (Chapter 14). The reason for the link with this particular infectious disease is still uncertain.

Patients with the early-onset, insulin-dependent form of diabetes mellitus often have antibodies to islet cells. A disproportionately great number of individuals with this form of diabetes have the haplotype HLA-B8. The same haplotype is unusually common in other forms of organ-specific autoimmunity, suggesting that it predisposes to this group of diseases.

Gastrointestinal Diseases

Patients with atrophic gastritis show lymphocytic and monocytic infiltration of the gastric mucosa. In their serum, one frequently finds autoantibodies to microsomes of the gastric parietal cells. Autoantibodies may also be demonstrated in gastric secretions. Patients with pernicious anemia show an additional antibody directed to intrinsic factor. Some of these antibodies combine with intrinsic factor but do not interfere with its ability to promote the uptake of vitamin B_{12}. Other antibodies to intrinsic factor block B_{12} binding.

In patients with inflammatory disease of the small and large bowel (ulcerative colitis or regional ileitis), antibodies to the intestinal mucosa can be demonstrated by means of indirect immunofluorescence and complement fixation. In cases of ulcerative colitis, lymphocytes from the peripheral blood have a cytotoxic action upon living mucosal cells, damaging them so that they release radioisotope-tagged internal constituents. This reaction can be performed even with fetal tissue, indicating that it is not due to the presence of adsorbed bacterial antigen upon the mucosal cells. Frequently, patients with chronic inflammatory disease of the intestinal tract develop high levels of antibody to various microorganisms inhabiting the colon. In this respect, it is difficult to differentiate cause from effect. It is quite possible that colonic disease allows microbial products to enter the bloodstream and stimulates antibody formation. On the other hand, the lipopolysaccharide antigens of certain organisms, especially *Escherichia coli*, cross-react with human fetal colonic mucosa. It might well be supposed, therefore, that an immunologic response to this or other intestinal bacteria could trigger an autoimmune process.

Chronic active hepatitis is a progressive liver disease characterized by infiltration of the parenchyma with lymphocytes and plasma cells. In the sera of many patients, antibodies are reactive with smooth muscle actomyosin and liver cell membranes.

Primary biliary cirrhosis is a chronic liver disease affecting the intra-hepatic bile ducts. Lymphocytes, sometimes accompanied by plasma cells, surround the bile ducts and invade the hepatic parenchymal tissue. Antibodies reactive with mitochondrial membranes are frequently present and of diagnostic value.

Diseases of Reproductive Tissues

Some men suffering from unexplained infertility show agglutinins for spermatozoa in their spermatic fluid or blood serum. These autoantibodies may produce head-to-head or tail-to-tail agglutination. They may well interfere with the viability or motility of the spermatozoon. Frequently, the formation of the spermagglutinins is associated with a history of occlusion of the efferent ducts. Orchitis sometimes occurs following cases of mumps, especially in older individuals. Many virologists believe that this post-infectious orchitis is attributable to autoimmunization to testicular tissue precipitated by the virus infection.

Diseases of the Eye

Sympathetic ophthalmia is a disease with chronic inflammatory changes that follow surgery or injury to the eye. It characteristically affects both the injured and the uninjured eye. Initial changes of focal lymphocytic infiltration are followed by development of granulomas with giant cells and epithelioid cells, resembling somewhat experimental uveitis. According to one investigator, antibody to uveal pigment is more readily demonstrated in patients with trauma to the eye in which uveitis failed to develop, whereas antibodies are absent from patients who do develop the disease. On the other hand, delayed skin tests to pigment are present in many patients who develop granulomatous uveitis. These apparently paradoxic results seem to indicate that circulating autoantibodies may protect uveal tissue from damage inflicted by cellular immunologic factors.

Phacoanaphyaxis or lens-induced uveitis is sometimes recognized following cataract extraction or trauma. Autoantibodies to lens have occasionally been demonstrated. The inflammatory changes may be due to an auto-immune reaction to lens antigen released during surgery or injury.

Neurologic Diseases

There are close similarities of several demyelinating diseases of the human to experimental allergic encephalomyelitis and experimental peripheral neuritis. However, up to now, in multiple sclerosis, it has not been possible to identify a circulating autoantibody to brain antigen or specific cellular sensitization to brain antigen. Just as measles virus has been associated with subacute sclerosing panencephalitis, a persistent, slowly involving infection could initiate multiple sclerosis.

Diseases of the Heart and Kidney

In rheumatic fever, laboratory studies suggest that autoimmunity to heart tissue may be induced in response to a constituent of group A streptococci that cross-reacts with heart antigen. Immunofluorescence staining reveals that sera of rheumatic fever patients react with cardiac myofibrils. Myofibrillar staining is observed best in sarcolemmal or subsarcolemmal sites of cardiac skeletal muscle. The streptococcal antigen is located mainly in the cell wall or membrane.

Following cardiac surgery or myocardial infarction, some patients develop fever and unexplained evidence of delayed cardiac inflammation. Sometimes autoantibodies to heart muscle have been demonstrated for a short period of time suggesting that a transient autoimmune reaction may become superimposed upon the original tissue injury.

Glomerulonephritis of man is most commonly associated with the deposition of antigen-antibody-complement complexes in the renal glomerular basement membrane. The detection of these immune complexes in renal biopsies is discussed in detail in Chapter 19. The antibody in this disease may be directed to an extrinsic antigen such as a streptococcal type-specific protein or to an intrinsic antigen. Among the intrinsic antigens incriminated are nuclear constituents, as seen in patients with systemic lupus erythematosus, or components of the tubular epithelium and brush border of the kidney in idiopathic glomerulonephritis. Less commonly, cases of glomerulonephritis may be associated with the production of autoantibodies to the glomerular basement membrane itself. The autoantibodies are recognized by the linear pattern they produce in immunofluorescence studies of renal biopsies. A reaction may sometimes be observed with the basement membrane of the lung. Clinically this form of autoimmune glomerulonephritis is recognized in Goodpasture's syndrome.

Connective Tissue Diseases

Systemic lupus erythematosus is often regarded as the best example of a disseminated disease related to autosensitization. Like the other connective tissue diseases, it shares certain features with the artificially induced disease, serum sickness (Chapter 19). The recognition by Hargraves in 1948 of the lupus erythematosus (LE) cell in the bone marrow of patients with the disease represented the first step in unraveling its pathogenesis. Later studies showed that the phenomenon was due to an antibody in the serum of lupus patients that combines with nuclei of human or other cells. Immunochemically this antibody can be shown to react with deoxyribonucleic acid (DNA). Other antibodies have been detected to single-stranded (denatured) DNA, ribonucleic acid (RNA), or extractable nuclear proteins. Collectively the antibodies are termed "antinuclear factors." Their demonstration by the immunofluorescent technique is an initial step in the diagnosis of lupus. In addition to antibodies to nuclear constituents, lupus patients develop auto-antibodies with some regularity to red blood cells, platelets, and clotting factors. They also show nonorgan-specific reactions with ribosomal or other cytoplasmic antigens. Recently, efforts have been made to correlate the presence of particular autoantibodies with the clinical manifestations of disease. For instance, some antinuclear antibodies react with an extractable acidic nuclear protein devoid of DNA or RNA, referred to as Sm protein. Antibody to this nuclear macromolecule is characteristic of lupus and is less common in other connective tissue diseases. Interestingly, these patients are less likely than other lupus patients to develop nephritis, and they respond better to steroid therapy. There is a second extractable nuclear protein that is degraded by ribonuclease. These antibodies are commonly found in the sera of patients with mixed connective tissue disease.

Rheumatoid arthritis is another connective tissue disease with evidence of an abnormal immunologic response. Rheumatoid factor is an antibody to γ globulin present in the serum of almost all patients. It seems to represent an autoantibody to the Fc portion of altered or aggregated IgG (Chapter 6). It may be found in any of the principal immunoglobulin classes but is most commonly an IgM. In some rheumatoid patients, complexes with the sedimentation constant of 22 S can be found, apparently representing an association of IgM rheumatoid factor with IgG. A few patients, especially those with severe symptoms of hyperviscosity, have heterogenous components sedimenting between 7 S and 19 S. These intermediate complexes seem to be composed of IgG rheumatoid factor and nonantibody IgG. The pathogenic significance of rheumatoid factor has not been clearly established. However, the presence of low complement levels in the synovial fluids of some rheumatoid patients indicates that local antigen-antibody interactions may be taking place. Rheumatoid factor is not an exclusive feature of rheumatoid arthritis. It is found in other connective tissue diseases and in certain chronic infections, especially leprosy and subacute bacterial endocarditis. In these cases, the interaction of circulating antibody with its antigen produces an unfolding of the antibody molecule that results in stimulation of the individual by otherwise secluded portions of his own IgG molecules.

Myasthenia Gravis

The first suggestion that autoantibody production may be a component of myasthenia gravis came from the observation that babies born to myasthenic mothers develop transient signs of the disease. Later, it was demonstrated by immunofluorescence that most patients with myasthenia gravis have autoantibodies to the striations of skeletal and cardiac muscle and lowered levels of complement. Since the disease itself is attributable mainly to a lesion at the myoneural junction, recently described antibodies to the acetylcholine receptors are of greater clinical importance. Of particular interest from the immunologic point of view is the common association of myasthenia gravis with germinal center formation or tumors of the thymus. Certain patients with myasthenia gravis are greatly benefited by thymectomy. These clinical observations made many years ago have given origin to many speculations about the role of the thymus in generating autoantibody-producing clones of cells or in controlling their production.

Keratoconjunctivitis Sicca

Among autoimmune diseases, keratoconjunctivitis sicca or Sjögren's syndrome assumes a position of special significance. In addition to an antibody to salivary gland demonstrable by immunofluorescence, half of the patients have high titers of antibodies to thyroglobulin. Many patients also have clinical and immunologic evidence of rheumatoid arthritis or lupus erythematosus. The disease, therefore, constitutes a bridge between the organ-specific autoimmune disorders and the systemic autoimmune diseases.

Skin Diseases

Pemphigus vulgaris is a bullous skin disease which, before the introduction of corticosteroids, was generally fatal. Patients suffering from this disease usually have antibodies in their sera or bullous fluids to the intracellular substance of stratified squamous epithelium. These are conveniently demonstrated in immunofluorescent tests using sections of primate skin or esophagus. Unusual among the autoimmune diseases is the demonstration that immunoglobulins showing the same pattern of localization can be found in biopsies taken from unaffected parts of the skin of pemphigus patients. Complement can also be demonstrated at these locations. These findings indicate that the antibody is capable of localizing in the skin *in vivo*. Perhaps they play a direct role in pathogenesis. Bullous pemphigoid can be differentiated from pemphigus vulgaris by its more benign clinical manifestations. It is immunologically different, since the autoantibody reaction is localized in the basement layers of skin or esophageal epithelium.

Diseases of the Blood

The demonstration of erythrocyte autoantibodies by means of the Coombs' antiglobulin test has become the basis for standard laboratory tests used in the diagnosis of acquired hemolytic anemia. The globulins coating human erythrocytes can be eluted and studied for their specificity. Many have been found specific for one of the Rh antigens, such as e (Chapter 20). Commonly, a mixture of antibodies to different Rh determinants is encountered. Most cases of hemolytic anemia are primary or idiopathic; that is, they are not associated with any detectable underlying disease. Sometimes, however, they are secondary to malignancies, infections, or connective tissue diseases. Drugs may also induce hemolytic anemias. Penicillin, for example, can attach spontaneously to the normal erythrocyte. Antibodies produced to penicillin can cause splenic sequestration or hemolysis of the red blood cells, which suffer the fate of an "innocent bystander" in the reaction of the drug with its specific antibody. Another form of hemolytic anemia is associated with the ingestion of certain drugs such as α methyldopa. Antibodies eluted from the patient's erythrocytes in this disease are directed to Rh antigens. Apparently, the drug confers autoantigenicity on the Rh determinant.

Some types of anemia are associated with production of cold hemagglutinins. These autoantibodies are active only at temperatures below that of the body. The antigen-antibody union can be dissolved by warming the agglutinated cells to 37° C. The antibody, which is frequently present in high titers, can react with the patient's own erythrocytes in the test tube. It is usually an IgM and is sometimes oligoclonal. The cold hemagglutinins have been reported to have only κ light chains, suggesting their biased origin from abnormal clones of antibody-producing cells. They have anti-I or anti-i specificities. Cold hemagglutinins are frequently associated in a secondary manner with parasitic, mycoplasmal, or viral infection (Table 25–4).

Leukocytes and platelets may become coated with globulins in cases of unexplained leukopenia or thrombocytopenia, respectively. Eluates from the sensitized cells contain immunoglobulins that act as autoantibodies. Unfortunately, white cells and platelets tend to clump spontaneously and to absorb serum proteins readily, making the diagnostic application of serologic tests rather difficult.

Table 25-4
SEROLOGIC FINDINGS IN AUTOIMMUNE HEMOLYTIC ANEMIAS

Clinical Nomenclature	Direct Antiglobulin Test Positive with Anti-	Hemagglutinins	Specificity of Eluate
Cold antibody type	Complement (C3)	Increased	Anti-I Anti-i Anti-Pr
Warm antibody type	IgG IgA (rarely) Complement	Normal levels	Anti-Rh Anti-En$_a$
Paroxysmal cold hemoglobulinemia	IgG (rarely) complement	Normal levels	Anti-P + P$_1$ (Donath-Landsteiner antibody)

Summary

Immunologists differ greatly in their requirements for accepting a human disease as autoimmune in origin. Some apply the term to any disease of unknown etiology with evidence of an autoimmune response, especially if the patient benefits from immunosuppressive treatment. Other investigators insist that only diseases that can be reproduced by passive transfer should be regarded as autoimmune. Although this kind of evidence is highly desirable, especially to gain some insight into pathogenic mechanisms, it can rarely be obtained in the case of human disease. In an effort to place the study of human autoimmune disease on a rational basis, several criteria were proposed by Witebsky and his coworkers in 1957. They still seem valid today. These steps are:

1. That one should demonstrate circulating autoantibodies active at body temperature or evidence of cell-mediated immunity in patients suffering from the disease;
2. That the antigen to which the antibody or cell-mediated activities are directed should be characterized and, if possible, isolated;
3. That antibodies or cell-mediated phenomena should be produced against the equivalent antigen in experimental animals;
4. That pathologic changes that are similar to those seen in the human disease should appear in the corresponding tissue of an actively sensitized animal.

The crucial concept in the application of these criteria, as in Koch's postulates for establishing the microbial etiology of human disease, is to allow the discovery of an analogous experimental model that will give an opportunity to the investigator to delineate the antigen and to demonstrate its autoantigenic capability. At the moment, only models for organ-specific autoimmunity can be produced by deliberate stimulation. However, other autoimmune diseases that occur on a genetic basis or in conjunction with a chronic viral infection have been described in experimental animals. These models help to reveal the mechanisms underlying human autoimmune diseases.

Bibliography

Autoimmunity and self-nonself discrimination. *Transplant. Rev.*, **31**:1–285, 1976.

Burnet, F. M.: *Autoimmunity and Autoimmune Disease.* F. A. Davis Company, Philadelphia, 1972.

Dameshek, W.; Milgrom, F.; and Witebsky, E. (eds.): *Autoimmunity–experimental and clinical aspects. Ann. N.Y. Acad. Sci.*, **122**, Parts I and II, 1965.

East, J.: Immunopathology and neoplasms in New Zealand black (NZB) and SJL/J mice. In Homburger, F. (ed.): *Progress in Experimental Tumor Research.* S. Karger, New York, 1970, pp. 86–134.

Ehrlich, P., and Morgenroth, J.: Ueber Haemolysine. *Berl. Klin. Wochenschr.,* **37**:453–58, 1900.

Eylar, E. H., and Hashim, G. A.: Allergic encephalomyelitis: the structure of the encephalitogenic determinant. *Proc. Natl. Acad. Sci. USA,* **61**:644–50, 1968.

Freund, J.; Lipton, M. M.; and Thompson, G. F.: Aspermatogenesis in the guinea pig induced by testicular tissue and adjuvants. *J. Exp. Med.,* **97**:711–26, 1953.

Fudenberg, H. H.; Stites, D. P.; Caldwell, J. L.; and Wells, J. V.: *Basic and Clinical Immunology.* Lange Medical Publications, Los Altos, Calif., 1976.

Halbert, S. P., and Manski, W.: Organ specificity with special reference to the lens. *Progr. Allergy,* **7**:107–86, 1963.

Helyer, B. J., and Howie, J. B.: The thymus and autoimmune disease. *Lancet,* **2**:1026–29, 1963.

Mellors, R. C.: Autoimmune disease and neoplasia of NZB mice: experimental model and its implications. In Rose, N. R., and Milgrom, F. (eds.): *International Convocation on Immunology.* S. Karger, Basel/New York, 1969, pp. 222–32.

Milgrom, F., and Witebsky, E.: Studies on the rheumatoid and related serum factors. I. Autoimmunization of rabbits with gamma globulin. *J.A.M.A.,* **174**:56–63, 1960.

Roitt, I. M.; Doniach, D.; Campbell, P.; and Hudson, R. V.: Auto-antibodies in Hashimoto's disease (lymphodenoid goiter). *Lancet,* **2**:820–21, 1956.

Rose, N. R.: Autoimmune diseases. In Grant, L.; McCluskey, R. T.; and Zweifach, B. W. (eds.): *The Inflammatory Process.* Academic Press, Inc., New York, 1973.

————: Experimental autoimmune disease. In McCluskey, R. T., and Cohen, S. (eds.): *Mechanisms of Immunopathology.* John Wiley & Sons, New York, in press.

Rose, N. R.; Kite, J. H., Jr.; Flanagan, T. D.; and Witebsky, E.: Humoral and cellular immune factors in spontaneous autoimmune disease. In Cohen, S.; Cudkowicz, G.; and McCluskey, R. T. (eds.): *Cellular Interactions in the Immune Response.* S. Karger, Basel/New York, 1971, pp. 264–81.

Rose, N. R., and Witebsky, E.: V. Changes in the thyroid glands of rabbits following active immunization with rabbit thyroid extracts. *J. Immunol.,* **76**:417–27, 1956.

Talal, N. (ed.): *Autoimmunity.* Academic Press, Inc., New York, 1977.

Waksman, B. H.: Experimental allergic encephalomyelitis and the "autoallergic" diseases. *Int. Arch. Allergy Appl. Immunol.,* **14**:1–87, Suppl. I, 1959.

UNIT III

Applied Immunology

26

Diagnostic and Therapeutic Applications of Immunology

Felix Milgrom, Noel R. Rose, and Herald R. Cox

Serologic Procedures

Since the remarkable specificity of antigen-antibody reactions was discovered at the end of the nineteenth century, serologic tests have been used for diagnostic purposes. Two major principles of this application of serologic procedures should be distinguished: (1) An antiserum with known antibody specificity serves as a reagent for the identification of the corresponding antigen. (2) A known antigen serves as a reagent for the detection of the corresponding antibody.

Antiserum as Reagent

The first principle has been widely employed in medical microbiology for the identification of pathogenic microorganisms. Appropriate antisera usually raised in rabbits have served for demonstration of numerous serotypes within many bacterial species. In all these instances the antisera are employed as additional reagents for more precise identification of isolated organisms after the initial identification has been made by establishing cultural characteristics and biochemical properties of the bacteria (Chapter 13). In many instances, however, antisera to microbial antigens have been used to detect these antigens directly in the pathologic material. By means of proper immune sera, specific soluble substances of pneumococci can be detected in serum, pleural effusion, cerebrospinal fluid, or urine of patients suffering from pneumococcal infections, and the serotype of the invading pneumococci may be ascertained. In the Ascoli test, a defined antiserum has been used to detect a thermostable antigen of the anthrax bacilli in the extracts from tissues of an animal suspected of having anthrax infection. Identification of pathogenic organisms in direct films from the pathologic material may be greatly facilitated by staining the organisms with fluorescein-conjugated antibodies. In this procedure, the serologic test adds the information on the antigenic structure of the organisms to the information on their morphologic and tinctorial properties.

Antibody-containing sera have been also used as important and useful reagents for the detection and quantitation of noninfectious antigens. Demonstration of C-reactive protein in patient serum is a valuable test indicating an acute inflammatory process. Serum level of several hormones can be conveniently established by means of proper antisera, and the demonstration of chorionic gonadotropin in urine serves as a diagnostic test for pregnancy (Chapter 29). Quantitation of immunoglobulins in human sera is a valuable test for the diagnosis of immune deficiency diseases, myelomas, and macroglobulinemia (Chapter 17). Finally, diagnosis of hepatomas and adenocarcinomas of the gastrointestinal tract based on detection of tumor-associated antigens in the patient's sera has been attempted (Chapter 24).

Antigen as Reagent

The term "serodiagnosis" is usually employed to denote the procedures that follow the second of the two above-mentioned principles, i.e., the detection of antibodies in patient serum by means of a known antigen. This principle was first employed by Widal, who described agglutination of typhoid bacilli by sera of patients suffering or recovering from typhoid fever. Serodiagnostic procedures have been used in everyday clinical practice as the most valuable tools for the diagnosis of many infectious and, in recent years, also noninfectious diseases.

Considerable knowledge and experience are needed for proper interpretation of serodiagnostic tests. This may be exemplified by a short discussion of the Widal test, which is based on titration of patient serum for agglutinins to typhoid bacilli and other salmonellae. (1) A positive test permits the diagnosis of salmonellosis, but it gives only vague information concerning the *Salmonella* species responsible for the infection. This is obvious if one bears in mind that salmonellae share many somatic and flagellar antigens. (2) The test becomes positive in the second week of disease in only a small proportion of patients; after three weeks it is positive in roughly 80% and after four to six weeks it is positive in practically all patients. Therefore, a negative result early in the disease is meaningless, but a negative result late in the disease is strong evidence against salmonellosis. (3) The titer of the reaction has to be interpreted on the basis of the knowledge of the titers encountered in the normal population of the given geographic area. In areas with prevalent salmonelloses, the large part of the population would have antibodies resulting from previous clinical or subclinical infections. Therefore, in such populations antibody titers of 50 or even 100 may be meaningless. On the other hand, in populations with a low incidence of salmonelloses, titers of 50 usually have diagnostic value. (4) The history of previous infection or vaccination is of considerable importance since, once elicited, antibodies may persist for several years.

It becomes obvious that in an individual case the most valuable information for interpretation of the results of a serodiagnostic test may be gained by comparing the antibody titers early and late in the disease. A rise of the titer during the course of the disease provides strong evidence that the patient has really suffered from the disease for which the test was performed. This generalization holds for many serodiagnostic tests, especially those performed in viral infections (Chapter 15). Since in many viral diseases antibodies in the patient's serum may remain from a previous infection, comparison of titers of the "acute" and "convalescent" serum specimens is the most important criterion for establishing the diagnosis. Because of the short duration of many viral diseases, the diagnosis based on the result of the test is frequently made after the patient's recovery. Such retrospective diagnosis is still of considerable importance for community medical practice and for epidemiologic reasons.

In some instances, tracing the titer of antibodies in the course of an infectious disease may serve to evaluate treatment and to predict the course of the disease. Quantitative complement-fixation (Wassermann) and flocculation tests for syphilis may serve to exemplify this. If, following the penicillin treatment of early syphilis, the titer of Wassermann antibodies steadily decreases until eventually the test becomes negative, this finding can be taken as evidence for effective treatment and a good prognosis. On the other hand, if the titer remains uninfluenced by treatment, levels off after initial decline, or increases (without or after decline), it is an alarming indication that the treatment was not effective. Increase of titer may be interpreted as a "serologic relapse," which usually precedes clinical relapse.

Serodiagnostic tests do not necessarily measure immunity to infectious disease. Some antibodies to microbial agents may play a definite role in recovery and specific protection as, for example, antibodies to specific soluble substances of pneumococci or antibodies to bacterial exotoxins. Other antibodies directed against harmless bacterial components such as flagellar antigens are of no importance for either recovery or protection. Still, since these antibodies are being formed as a result of infection, their demonstration is of diagnostic value. In this connection, it may be remembered that several infectious diseases are accompanied by the appearance of antibodies that can be demonstrated by means of antigens not derived from the particular microorganism. Outstanding examples of such antibodies are the Wassermann antibody in syphilis, which is directed against a cardiolipin (Chapter 13), and heterophile antibody in infectious mononucleosis, which reacts with a thermostable antigen on erythrocytes of ox, sheep, and horse (Chapter 21). The node of formation of these antibodies is poorly understood even though their detection serves useful diagnostic purposes.

As mentioned previously, detection of some antibodies may measure specific protection to the given disease. This is especially true for antibodies to bacterial toxins such as diphtheria toxin and scarlatinal (erythrogenic) toxin. The Schick test and the Dick test are the procedures that demonstrate antitoxic immunity to diphtheria and scarlet fever, respectively. Even though these tests undergo conversion in the course of the disease, they have hardly been used as diagnostic tests in clinical cases of diphtheria or scarlet fever. On the other hand, they have been used extensively for studying immunity in the population and also for selecting sensitive individuals for vaccination.

Serologic Tests in Noninfectious Diseases

Serodiagnostic tests have also been used in noninfectious diseases, including immunologic disorders of various organs and tissues (Chapter 25). In many instances, these tests are based on the detection of tissue-specific antibodies such as antibodies to the constituents of thyroid gland, which appear in the course of chronic thyroiditis, antibodies to striated muscles, which may be found in myasthenia gravis, or antibodies to glomerular basement membrane, which are characteristic of Goodpasture's disease. Detection of antibodies to nuclear components has been used regularly in diagnosis of disseminated lupus erythematosus, and detection of antibodies to denatured IgG has served as a valuable diagnostic procedure for rheumatoid arthritis.

Sensitivity and Specificity of Serologic Tests

In order to assess the clinical value of a serodiagnostic procedure, both sensitivity and specificity are usually analyzed.

Sensitivity is measured by the proportion of positive results that the test gives in patients suffering from a given disease. Most serodiagnostic tests reach a sensitivity close to 100%, but only in some stages of the disease. The Widal test attains such a high sensitivity level four to six weeks after onset of symptoms and the Wassermann test at the stage of secondary eruption, about two months after infection. Obviously one cannot expect any high sensitivity of serodiagnostic tests early in the disease, since several days or even a few weeks have to pass before antibodies reach detectable levels. In acute infections, especially in viral diseases, the high sensitivity of tests is usually not observed before recovery. In chronic infections, some tests remain positive as long as the infection persists, whereas other tests become negative as least in some patients.

In considering the specificity of a serodiagnostic test, one has to stress that this term is used in the clinical sense. From an immunologic point of view, any reaction of an antigen with its corresponding antibody is a specific reaction, and only those reactions would be considered "nonspecific" which mimic serologic reactions without being antigen-antibody reactions. For a clinician, a specific serodiagnostic reaction is the one that is positive in the disease for which the particular test has been developed and a nonspecific reaction is positive in any other disease or in normal human beings. No serodiagnostic test can be ideally specific. Cross-reactions between various microorganisms account for the fact that a serodiagnostic test designed for one infectious disease may quite frequently be positive in another disease. Antibodies detected by a serodiagnostic test might have been elicited by some previous clinical or subclinical disease or by vaccination. In newborn infants, antibodies are frequently of maternal origin and therefore their detection does not necessarily reflect the actual disease in the baby. In order to interpret properly the results of a serodiagnostic test, a clinician has to have considerable knowledge concerning the conditions in which this test gives positive results in the absence of the particular disease ("false positive results," "nonspecific results"). It is, for example, important to know that the Wassermann test is frequently positive in other treponemal diseases, leprosy, disseminated lupus erythematosus, and some parasitic diseases. It is also positive in a few (about 1 in 5000) apparently normal human beings. The latter information is important for the evaluation of results in serologic mass examinations of syphilis, which include millions of people.

The specificity of serodiagnostic tests is usually measured in negative terms by the proportion of positive results that are encountered in a given population free of the disease for which the test is designed.

The sensitivity of all serodiagnostic tests may be increased quite easily by various technical modifications. Increased sensitivity is usually accompanied by decreased specificity. Therefore, in well-established serodiagnostic tests a middle road has been taken that resulted in tests that are sufficiently, though not ideally, sensitive and specific. Occasionally, oversensitive tests are employed that are designed to exclude a particular disease most reliably. Obviously, in developing such tests, specificity is sacrificed for extreme sensitivity.

Active Immunization

Bacterial Vaccines

Antibodies, whether antibacterial or antitoxic, play a major role in immunity to most bacterial infections; in one the bacterium is rendered

Table 26-1

ESSENTIAL DATA CONCERNING PRODUCTS FOR ACTIVE IMMUNIZATION

Bacterial Vaccines	Basic Preparation	Storage °C	Expiration Date, Month	Usual Dose
BCG vaccine, NF XIV (*The National Formulary*, Fourteenth Edition)	Dried, living culture, bacillus Calmette-Guérin strain, *Mycobacterium tuberculosis*, variety *bovis*. Contains no antimicrobial agent	2–5	6	Intradermal, 0.1 ml reconstituted vaccine. Percutaneous, 1 drop reconstituted vaccine on skin surface, administered by multiple-puncture method
Cholera vaccine, USP XIX (*The United States Pharmacopeia*, Nineteenth Revision)	Sterile suspension of killed cholera vibrios (*Vibrio cholerae*). Equal portions of the Inaba and Ogawa strains. Contains suitable antimicrobial agent	2–8	18	Intramuscular or subcutaneous, 0.5 ml, then 1.0 ml 4 weeks. A 0.5 ml booster dose repeated every 6 months if necessary
Pertussis vaccine, NF XIV	Sterile bacterial fraction or suspension of killed pertussis bacilli (*Bordetella pertussis*). Contains suitable preservative	2–8, avoid freezing	18	Subcutaneous, 3 injections of 0.5 or 1.0 ml each, spaced at least 4 weeks apart
Adsorbed pertussis vaccine, NF XIV	Sterile bacterial fraction or suspension of killed pertussis bacilli (*Bordetella pertussis*). Precipitated or adsorbed by addition of aluminium hydroxide or aluminium phosphate, and resuspended	2–8, avoid freezing	18	Intramuscular, 3 injections of 0.5 or 1.0 ml, as specified in labeling, spaced at least 4 weeks apart
Plague vaccine, USP XIX	Sterile suspension of killed plague bacilli (*Pasteurella pestis*). Contains suitable preservative	2–8, avoid freezing	18	Intramuscular, 2 injections of 0.5 ml each, spaced at least 4 weeks apart, and a third booster dose of 0.2 ml 4 to 12 weeks later
Typhoid vaccine, USP XIX	Sterile suspension or frozen and dried solid, containing killed typhoid bacilli (*Salmonella typhosa*)	2–8	18	Subcutaneous, 2 or 3 injections of 0.5 ml each, spaced at least 4 weeks apart; 0.5 ml every 3 years thereafter

more susceptible to phagocytosis, whereas in the other the bacterial toxin is neutralized (Chapter 13). However, in the case of certain bacteria, such as mycobacteria (tubercle and leprosy bacilli), the defense of the body against these organisms appears to be primarily due to specific cellular mediated immunity (Chapter 11).

The word "vaccine" was originally given to the material used for immunization against smallpox, a glycerinated suspension of vesicles obtained from calves that had vaccinia (cowpox). This material was first used by Jenner in 1796 when he used cowpox to protect a child against smallpox (variola) (Chapters 1, 15). Later the term was extended to include all antigenic materials prepared from viruses, and still later to those made from bacteria and rickettsiae as well.

Bacterial vaccines are suspensions of killed or attenuated bacteria in physiologic salt solution. They may contain a preservative such as thimerosal or phenol. Bacterial vaccines are divided into two main classes: (1) stock vaccines and (2) autogenous vaccines. Stock vaccines are those prepared from stock cultures maintained in the laboratory and consist of strains expressly selected for their capacity to stimulate production of immunity. Autogenous vaccines are those prepared from the patient's own infectious agent. The offending organisms obtained from the blood or lesion of the individual are used to prepare the vaccine.

A simple or monovalent vaccine is one made from a single strain or species of microorganism, and a mixed or polyvalent vaccine is one that contains two or more different species. Table 26–1 presents the essential data concerning a number of bacterial vaccines that are commonly used.

Exotoxins

Exotoxins are the strongest poisons known in pharmacology. Purified diphtheria toxin would kill susceptible animals in a dose of 1 μg/kg, and a purified botulinum toxin is about 50 times more lethal.

Bacterial exotoxins are produced by several gram-positive organisms, including *Corynebacterium diphtheriae*, *Clostridium tetani*, *Clostridium botulinum*, *Clostridium oedematiens*, *Clostridium septicum*, *Clostridium welchii*, *Staphylococcus aureus*, *Streptococcus pyogenes*, and *Bacillus anthracis*. They are also produced by a few gram-negative organisms, including *Shigella dysenteriae*, *Vibrio cholerae*, and *Pasteurella pestis*. Whereas some organisms produce only one toxin (e.g., *Corynebacterium diphtheriae*), other organisms produce many toxins with different pharmacologic and antigenic properties (e.g., *Clostridium welchii* and *Streptococcus pyogenes*).

Characteristically all bacterial exotoxins are proteins. Diphtheria toxin is a heat-labile protein with a molecular weight of 72,000. It is produced under aerobic conditions in media with iron concentrations suboptimal for the bacterial growth. Recent experiments showed that this toxin may be an enzyme. Through a rather complex chain of biochemical processes, diphtheria toxin interferes with protein synthesis and brings about the death of the cell. Significantly, all cells are sensitive to the action of diphtheria toxin. On the other hand, some species (man, horse, and guinea pig) are much more susceptible to this toxin than others (rat and mouse). Upon injection into an animal, diphtheria toxin produces local hemorrhage; congestion and necrosis in the regional lymph nodes are also noted. Systemic manifestations of toxemia include adrenal hemorrhage, as well as pleural and pericardial effusions. Death results from circulatory failure. Upon injection of diphtheria toxin even in a high dose into a susceptible animal, there is always a latent period of 6 to 15 hours before the first symptoms are noted, and death seldom occurs before 24 hours.

The power of diphtheria toxin preparations is measured in minimal lethal doses (MLD). According to Ehrlich's definition, one MLD is the minimal dose of diphtheria toxin capable of killing a guinea pig weighing 250 gm within four days. Bacterial filtrates of strongly toxogenic strains of diphtheria bacilli would contain 1000 to 2000 MLD/ml.

Toxoids

Under a variety of conditions, bacterial exotoxins lose their toxicity without losing antigenicity. Ehrlich introduced the term "toxoid" to name such a pharmacologically inactive toxin preparation. For practical purposes, e.g., production of preparations used for immunization, toxoid is obtained by incubation of toxin with formaldehyde at 37° C for three to four weeks. To explain the properties of toxin and toxoid, Ehrlich postulated that a toxin molecule contains two separate chemical groups, the toxophore group responsible for pharmacologic activity and the haptophore group determining the antigenic properties. In these terms, toxoid is a toxin deprived of its toxophore group. Neutralization of toxin by antitoxin has to result from the reaction of the antibody with the haptophore group. The toxophore group is not destroyed in a neutral toxin-antitoxin mixture. As a matter of fact, if an excess of toxoid is added to such neutral mixtures, free toxin molecules are released and the preparation becomes toxic. This would indicate that the neutralization effect is due to the steric hindrance by antibodies, which results in functional inactivity of the toxophore group. The interpretation of Ehrlich seems to fit well the data accumulated in several decades of subsequent experimentation. However, the toxophore group by itself may be weakly antigenic, and some antitoxic antibodies may act through the blocking of this group. The toxoids are available both in unprecipitated form, usually designated as fluid, and in precipitated or adsorbed form. Precipitation is accomplished by the addition of alum, aluminium hydroxide, or aluminium phosphate. The precipitated and adsorbed forms claim to yield higher levels of immunity. Such precipitated or adsorbed products are relatively insoluble, and upon injection the insoluble mass persists for quite some time in the tissues before being completely absorbed. A fairly high incidence of so-called sterile abscesses follow the use of precipitated and adsorbed toxoids, but as a rule these are of no important consequence.

The clinical protection afforded against diphtheria by active immunization is quite impressive. The protection is not absolute, as is the case with all active immunization procedures, but the incidence of clinical diphtheria among those immunized is certainly no more than about 10% of that among the nonimmunized. It is believed that communities that maintain rates of active immunization of 35% or more of the children under five years of age, and 50% of the children of school age, are free from danger of significant outbreaks of diphtheria.

Active immunization against tetanus is strongly advised for allergic individuals and for those who are hypersensitive to horse serum, as well as children, farmers, horsemen, hunters, those in military service, public utility workers in field duty, veterinarians, and others whose duties and occupations frequently expose them to injuries favoring the development of tetanus infection.

Table 26–2 presents essential data concerning a number of toxoids and multiple antigens that are commonly used.

Viral Vaccines

The immunity to viruses (Chapter 15) differs from the immunity to bacterial infections in that it is almost always long lasting. After infection and recovery, virus is not entirely eliminated from the body, but residual virons are believed to remain protected within certain infected cells. Thereafter, small quantities of virus may be periodically released to the lymphoid tissues where the immune status can be maintained.

The greatest success in immunizing against viral infection has been achieved by the use of living, attenuated viruses, lacking the invasiveness and pathogenicity of the parent strain, but retaining the same antigenic structure. In most cases, the immunity induced by living, viral vaccines is of higher degree and longer duration than that produced by inactivated or killed vaccines.

Yellow fever vaccine represents a most successful, attenuated, living, viral immunizing agent. The vaccine is based on the original findings of Theiler that white mice, when inoculated intracerebrally, are susceptible to yellow fever, and that a fixed virus with a shortened incubation period and heightened virulence for mice can be produced by repeated passage through these animals. Consequently, Theiler and his associates carried out a long series of investigations that resulted in the chicken-embryo-adapted 17D yellow fever vaccine. Inoculation of monkeys by neural routes showed that the 17D strain, between the eighty-ninth and one hundred-fourteenth chicken embryo tissue culture passages, had lost to a great extent its power to produce fatal encephalitis. The reason for this relatively rapid change in virulence of the 17D strain was and still is completely unknown. After further

Table 26-2

Essential Data Concerning Products for Active Immunization

Toxoids	Basic Preparation	Storage, °C	Expiration Date, Months	Usual Dose
Diphtheria toxoid, USP XIX	A sterile solution of formaldehyde-treated growth products of diphtheria bacillus (*Corynebacterium diphtheriae*)	2–8	24	Intramuscular or subcutaneous, 3 injections of 0.5 to 1.0 ml each, spaced at least 4 weeks apart, and a 4th booster dose 6 to 12 months later
Adsorbed diphtheria toxoid, USP XIX	A sterile suspension of diphtheria toxoid precipitated or adsorbed by addition of alum, aluminum hydroxide, or aluminum phosphate to formaldehyde-treated solution of growth products of diphtheria bacillus	2–8	24	Intramuscular, 2 injections of 0.5 to 1.0 ml each as specified in the labeling, spaced at least 4 weeks apart, and a third booster dose 6 to 12 months later
Tetanus toxoid, USP XIX	A sterile solution of formaldehyde-treated growth products of tetanus bacillus (*Clostridium tetani*)	2–8	24	Subcutaneous, 3 injections of 0.5 or 1.0 ml each, as specified in the labeling, spaced at least 4 weeks apart, followed by 0.5 ml one year later and every ten years thereafter
Adsorbed tetanus toxoid, USP XIX	A sterile suspension of tetanus toxoid precipitated or adsorbed by addition of alum, aluminum hydroxide, or aluminum phosphate to formaldehyde-treated solution of growth products of tetanus bacillus	2–8	24	Intramuscular, 2 injections of 0.5 each, as specified in the labeling, spaced at least 4 weeks apart, followed by 0.5 ml one year later and every 10 years thereafter

Diphtheria and tetanus toxoids, NF XIV	A sterile solution of a suitable mixture of fluid diphtheria toxoid and fluid tetanus toxoid	2–8	24	Intramuscular or subcutaneous, 2 injections of 0.5 or 1.0 ml each, as specified in the labeling, spaced at least 4 weeks apart. A third booster dose 12 months later
Adsorbed diphtheria and tetanus toxoids, USP XIX	A sterile solution prepared by mixing suitable quantities of adsorbed diphtheria toxoid and adsorbed tetanus toxoid, each having been precipitated or adsorbed by some agent, such as alum, aluminum hydroxide, or aluminum phosphate	2–8	24	Intramuscular, 2 injections of 0.5 or 1.0 ml each, as specified in the labeling, spaced at least 4 weeks apart. A third booster dose 12 months later
Diphtheria and tetanus toxoids and pertussis vaccine, NF XIV	A sterile suspension of killed pertussis bacilli (*Bordetella pertussis*) in a suitable mixture of diphtheria toxoid and tetanus toxoid	2–8	18	Intramuscular or subcutaneous, 3 injections of 0.5 or 1.0 ml each, as specified in the labeling, spaced at least 4 weeks apart. A fourth booster dose 12 months later
Adsorbed diphtheria and tetanus toxoids, USP XIX	A sterile suspension of the precipitate obtained by treating a mixture of diphtheria toxoid and tetanus toxoid with alum, aluminum hydroxide, or aluminum phosphate	2–8	18	Intramuscular, 2 injections of 0.5 each, as specified in the labeling, spaced at least 4 weeks apart. A fourth booster dose of 0.5 ml 12 months later and further boosters every 10 years thereafter

465

Table 26-3

ESSENTIAL DATA CONCERNING PRODUCTS FOR ACTIVE IMMUNIZATION

Viral Vaccines	Basic Preparation	Storage °C	Expiration Date, Months	Usual Dose
Influenza virus vaccine, USP XIX	A sterile, aqueous suspension of suitably inactivated influenza virus prepared from the extraembryonic fluids of influenza virus-infected chicken embryos. May contain an adsorbent such as aluminum phosphate or protamine	2–8	18	Intramuscular or subcutaneous, 2 injections of 0.5 ml each, as specified in the labeling, spaced 6 to 8 weeks apart
Live attenuated measles virus vaccine, USP XIX	A preparation derived from a strain of measles virus found suitable for human immunization; grown on cultures either of chicken embryo tissue or of canine renal tissue	2–8	12	Subcutaneous, 0.5 ml, single injection
Live attenuated mumps virus vaccine	A preparation derived from a strain of mumps virus found suitable for human immunization; grown in cultures of chicken embryo tissue	2–8	12	Subcutaneous, one injection of 0.5 ml
Poliomyelitis vaccine, USP XIX	A sterile suspension of inactivated poliomyelitis virus types 1, 2, and 3. Virus strains are grown separately in primary cultures of monkey kidney tissue; after inactivation are combined in suitable proportions	2–8	12	Intramuscular or subcutaneous, 2 injections of 1.0 ml each, 4-to 6 weeks apart; a third booster dose of 1.0 ml at least 6 months later, then a 1.0 ml booster every 2 to 3 years

Name	Description	Storage temperature	Expiration (months)	Dosage
Live oral poliovirus vaccine, USP XIX	A preparation of one or a combination of the three types of live, attenuated polioviruses that have been grown separately in primary cultures of monkey kidney tissue. Vaccine is free from any known microbial agent other than the attenuated poliovirus or polioviruses declared in the labeling	Preserve at temperature recommended by manufacturer	12 when stored at −10° or less	Oral, one dose of each monovalent type in the volume indicated in the labeling as representing one dose, 6 to 8 weeks apart, and a fourth, reinforcing dose of the trivalent vaccine 8 to 12 months later; or trivalent vaccine in the volume representing 2 doses, 6 to 8 weeks apart, and a third, reinforcing dose 8 to 12 months later
Rabies vaccine, USP XIX	A sterile preparation, in liquid or dried form, of killed, fixed rabies virus. Virus is obtained from the brain tissue of rabbits, or from duck embryos that have been infected with fixed rabies virus	2–8	Liquid vaccine, 6; dried vaccine, 18	Subcutaneous, the labeled dose once a day for 14 to 21 days, depending on the severity of exposure
Smallpox vaccine, USP XIX	Contains the living virus of vaccinia that has been grown in the skin of a calf, or in the membranes of the chicken embryo. It is available in liquid and in dried form	Keep liquid vaccine below 0° Keep dried vaccine 2–8°	Liquid vaccine, 3; dried vaccine, 18	Percutaneous, the contents of one capillary tube, or one drop of reconstituted vaccine, by the multiple-puncture method
Yellow fever vaccine, USP XIX	An attenuated strain (17D) of living, yellow fever virus propagated in the living chicken embryo. The processed vaccine, free from any microbial agents, is dried from the frozen state and stored under dry nitrogen	Preferably below 0° Never above 5° C	12	Subcutaneous, 0.5 ml reconstituted vaccine, repeated every 10 years

Table 26-3—*continued*

ESSENTIAL DATA CONCERNING PRODUCTS FOR ACTIVE IMMUNIZATION

Viral Vaccines	Basic Preparation	Storage °C	Expiration Date, Month	Usual Dose
Live measles and rubella virus vaccine—dried, USP XIX	Attenuated type of measles virus grown in cell cultures of chicken embryo, mixed with attenuated strain of rubella virus propagated in duck embryo cell cultures	2–8	12	Subcutaneous, one injection of 0.5 ml. Vaccine must be reconstituted from lyophilized state
Live measles, mumps, and rubella virus vaccine—dried, USP XIX	Attenuated-type measles virus and mumps virus, both grown in cell cultures of chicken embryo, mixed with attenuated strain of rubella virus propagated in duck embryo cell cultures	2–8	12	Subcutaneous, one injection of 0.5 ml. Vaccine must be reconstituted from lyophilized state
Live attenuated rubella virus vaccine—dried, USP XIX	A preparation derived from a strain of rubella virus found suitable for human immunization; virus may be grown in either duck embryo cell cultures, or rabbit kidney cell cultures	2–8	12	Subcutaneous, one injection of 0.5 ml. Vaccine must be reconstituted from lyophilized state
Live rubella and mumps virus vaccine—dried, USP XIX	An attenuated strain of rubella virus propagated in duck embryo cell cultures; mixed with a mumps strain grown in chicken embryo cell cultures	2–8	12	Subcutaneous, one injection of 0.5 ml. Vaccine must be reconstituted from lyophilized state

extensive experimentation, the 17D strain was used for human vaccination. The only serious reaction following administration of the 17D vaccine was the rare occurrence of encephalitis in infants less than one year of age; all recovered without sequelae.

The work of Enders and associates revolutionized the immunologic and epidemiologic study of poliomyelitis. With their development of the tissue culture technique, a method was devised for the first time that permitted the propagation of poliomyelitis virus in other than central nervous tissues. Poliomyelitis virus vaccine was the first produced in cell cultures; in this case, monkey kidney cells have been routinely used. Using this procedure Salk and his associates were successful in preparing a killed or inactivated vaccine that contained all three immunologic types of poliovirus. Only the attenuated poliovirus strains developed by Sabin are now produced commercially in the United States and Canada. A trivalent, live, oral poliovirus vaccine has almost entirely replaced both the inactivated type and the monovalent type of live, oral poliovirus vaccines.

Table 16–3 presents the essential data concerning a number of virus vaccines that are either currently licensed for commercial production or are in the stage of field trial research leading toward licensing for commercial production.

Rickettsial Vaccines

The preferred type of vaccine used to protect against the various rickettsial diseases has been the killed type, although a variant strain of epidemic typhus, known as "strain E," has shown great promise of providing a living rickettsial vaccine to protect against epidemic typhus fever.

Adequate quantities of rickettsiae for a typhus vaccine may be obtained from the intestines of human body lice, from rodent lungs, from tissue cultures, and from the yolk sac membranes of developing chicken embryos. Cox showed that rickettsiae of the Rocky Mountain spotted fever and typhus fever groups multiply in yolk sac membranes of developing chicken embryos. This infected tissue has been the chief source material for preparing vaccines and diagnostic reagents for a number of rickettsial diseases, such as Rocky Mountain spotted fever, epidemic typhus (louse borne), murine typhus (flea borne), and Q fever.

Table 26–4 presents the essential data concerning the two rickettsial vaccines that are manufactured on a commercial basis. A license was secured to manufacture and sell Q fever vaccine, but the product was discontinued.

Passive Immunization

Passive immunization depends on prompt administration of immune sera. From *in vitro* studies on cell cultures it became obvious that about one hour

Table 26-4

ESSENTIAL DATA CONCERNING PRODUCTS FOR ACTIVE IMMUNIZATION

Rickettsial Vaccines	Basic Preparation	Storage °C	Expiration Date, Month	Usual Dose
Rocky Mountain spotted fever vaccine, USP XIX	A sterile aqueous suspension of inactivated *Rickettsia rickettsii* prapared by growing the organisms in the yolk sac of developing chicken embryos. The vaccine is refined by chemical treatment, such as by use of ether extraction	2–8	18	Subcutaneous, 3 injections of 1.0 ml each, spaced 7 to 10 days apart
Typhus vaccine, USP XIX	A sterile aqueous suspension of the killed rickettsial organisms of epidemic typhus (*Rickettsia prowazeki*). Vaccine consists of refined material derived from an aqueous suspension of yolk sac membranes of developing chicken embryos	2–8	18	Subcutaneous, 2 injections of 0.5 each, as specified in the labeling, spaced at least 4 weeks apart

is needed for diphtheria toxin to become irreversibly bound to the cells. Therefore, during the first hour of exposure to diphtheria toxin, the cells can still be saved by washing or by addition of antitoxin. On the other hand, once a lethal dose is bound to the cells they cannot be saved by any procedure. Analogous observations were made *in vivo*. A guinea pig injected with a few lethal doses of diphtheria toxin can be quite readily saved by administration of antitoxin within 20 minutes. As time lapses, saving of the animal becomes more and more difficult and requires high doses of antitoxin. Two hours after injection, the animal can no longer be saved. In the majority of cases of diphtheria, clinical symptoms are obvious before a lethal dose of toxin is bound to tissues, whereas in most instances of tetanus a lethal dose of toxin is irreversibly bound to the tissues at the time when clinical symptoms ensue. Serum therapy is successful in diphtheria only if instituted early in the disease. Under these circumstances, antitoxin will prevent binding of the lethal dose of toxin. On the contrary, in clinically patent tetanus, serum therapy is effective only in exceptional cases. In order to be efficient, antitoxin has to be injected during the incubation period of tetanus.

Antitoxins to be used therapeutically are usually produced by active immunization of an animal, such as the horse or rabbit. Antitoxins prepared in humans are available for use in allergic individuals. The serum is processed to concentrate the antibody fraction(s) and to eliminate, reduce, or modify all other protein fractions. The basic requirements of antitoxins are (1) proper specificity, (2) high potency, (3) maximal concentration and purification, (4) adequate and proper dosage, and (5) administration by the proper route.

Table 26–5 presents the essential data concerning the various products that are commercially available for passive immunization.

Potency of an antitoxin is expressed in antitoxic units. According to Ehrlich's definition, an antitoxic unit of diphtheria antiserum is the minimal dose of the serum that is capable of neutralizing 100 MLD of diphtheria toxin. Because toxin preparations undergo spontaneous conversion into toxoid during preservation, they cannot be used as reliable standards for titration. On the other hand, antitoxin can be preserved indefinitely (at least for practical purposes) at $-70°$ C. Therefore, antitoxin has been employed as a standard for titration. Ehrlich's original antitoxin was used as the first international standard; the subsequent standard antisera were characterized in terms of this first antitoxin. The standard antitoxic serum is maintained at the State Serum Institute in Copenhagen, Denmark.

Any new diphtheria antitoxin preparation, the strength of which is to be determined, has to be compared with the standard antitoxin. This requires somewhat involved procedures. The classic procedures of titrations have used the death of a guinea pig as an "end point." The standard antiserum in an amount of one antitoxic unit is mixed with any suitable diphtheria toxin preparation at various increasing doses. Each of the mixtures is

Table 26-5

ESSENTIAL DATA CONCERNING PRODUCTS FOR PASSIVE IMMUNIZATION

	Basic Preparation	Storage °C	Expiration Date, Months	Usual Dose
Antitoxins				
Botulism antitoxin, USP XIX	A sterile solution of refined and concentrated antitoxic antibodies, chiefly globulins, obtained from the blood of healthy horses immunized against the toxins produced by the type A and type B and/or type E strains of *Clostridium botulinum*	2–8	60	Intravenous, 20,000 to 43,000 units, repeated at 2- to 4-hr intervals as necessary
Tetanus antitoxin, USP XIX	A sterile solution of the refined and concentrated proteins, chiefly globulins, containing antitoxic antibodies obtained from blood serum or plasma of healthy animals, usually horses, immunized against tetanus toxin or toxoid	2–8	60	Prophylactic: intramuscular or subcutaneous, 3000 to 10,000 units. Therapeutic, 40,000 to 100,000 units
Antivenins				
Polyvalent crotaline antivenin, USP XIX	A sterile preparation prepared by drying a frozen solution of specific venom-neutralizing globulins obtained from the serum of healthy horses immunized against venoms of four species of pit vipers, *Crotalus atrox* (western diamondback rattlesnake), *Crotalus adamanteus* (diamondback rattlesnake of southeastern United States), *Crotalus divissus terrificus* (South American rattlesnake), and *Bothrops atrox* (South American fer de lance)	2–10	70	Usual dose: intramuscular, 10 ml of reconstituted antivenin. Usual dose range—10 to 300 ml, then 10 ml every one-half to two hours, as necessary

472

Immune Serums

Antirabies serum, USP XIX	A sterile solution containing antiviral substances obtained from the blood serum or plasma of healthy animals, usually horses, that have been immunized against rabies by means of vaccine. Contains a suitable antimicrobial agent	2–8	24	Usual dose: intramuscular, 70 units per kg of body weight as a single dose. Usual dose range—40 to 120 units per kg
Pertussis immune human globulin, USP XIX	A sterile solution of globulins derived from the blood plasma of adult human donors who have been immunized with pertussis vaccine	2–8	36	Prophylactic: intramuscular, 1.25 to 2.5 ml, repeated one or two times at one-week or two-week intervals Therapeutic: intramuscular, 1.25 to 2.5 ml, repeated at one-day or two-day intervals
Tetanus immune human globulin, USP XIX	A sterile solution of globulins derived from the blood plasma of adult human donors who have been immunized with tetanus toxoid	2–8	36	Prophylactic: intramuscular, 250 units as a single dose; therapeutic: 3000 to 6000 units as a single dose
Immune human serum globulin, USP XIX	A sterile solution of globulins that contains many antibodies normally present in adult human blood	2–8	36	Prophylactic: intramuscular, 1.3 to 2.0 ml per kg; maintenance dose, 0.66 to 1.0 ml per kg, once a month

injected into a guinea pig. In this the L+ dose (*limes=* threshold; + = death) of toxin is established as the minimal dose of toxin that in the mixture with one antitoxic unit kills a guinea pig weighing 250 gm within four days. It should be realized that this dose does not necessarily contain 101 MLD since toxoid molecules present in the toxin preparation also combine with antitoxin. Thereafter, the L+ dose of toxin is mixed with various volumes of the antitoxin preparation to be titrated. Each of the mixtures is injected into a guinea pig, and the death of the animals is observed. One antitoxic unit is present in this maximal volume of the antitoxin that did not save a guinea pig from death, or, more conservatively, one antitoxic unit is present in the minimal volume of antitoxin that saved a guinea pig from death.

A similar principle for titration may be employed in a more economical way by using positive skin tests as "end points" of the titration. In this procedure appropriate antitoxin-toxin mixtures are injected intracutaneously into a guinea pig and skin reactions are observed. Finally, titration of antitoxin may be performed *in vitro* by a precipitation test. The Lf (*limes* of flocculation) of a toxin preparation is established as the dose of toxin that gives the quickest precipitation when mixed with one standard antitoxic unit. Thereafter the antitoxin under investigation is titrated against an Lf of the toxin. It is assumed that the dose of antitoxin that gives the quickest precipitation with one Lf of toxin contains one antitoxic unit. The usual strength of antisera used for therapy of diphtheria is 500 to 800 antitoxic units/ml. Exceptionally strong sera may contain up to 3000 units/ml.

The definitions for tetanus toxin and antitoxin differ from those used in diphtheria. One minimal lethal dose of tetanus toxin is the minimal dose that kills a guinea pig weighing 330 to 380 gm within four days. One antitoxic unit of tetanus antitoxin is defined as ten times the smallest volume of the serum that is capable of saving a guinea pig from 100 MLD of tetanus toxin. It should be noted that one unit of tetanus antitoxin is capable of neutralizing 1000 MLD of the toxin. Titrations of tetanus antitoxin are performed similarly to titrations of diphtheria toxin.

Antitoxic sera obtained for therapeutic purposes contain a mixture of antibodies, some of which are directed against the toxin itself, whereas others are directed against various antigenic components of the preparation used for immunization. Obviously antitoxins produced by immunization with purified toxoid preparations have fewer nonantitoxic antibodies.

Bibliography

Gell, P. G. H.; Coombs, R. R. A.; and Lachmann, P. (eds.): *Clinical Aspects of Immunology*, 3rd ed. Blackwell Scientific Publications, Ltd., Oxford, 1975.

Horsfall, F. L., Jr., and Tamm, I. (eds.): *Viral and Rickettsial Infections of Man*, 4th ed. J. B. Lippincott Co., Philadelphia, 1965.

Jenner, E.: *An Inquiry into the Causes and Effects of the Variola Vacciniae, a Disease Discovered in Some of the Western Counties of England, Particularly Gloucestershire, and Known by the Name of Cowpox.* 1798. Reprinted by Cassell & Co., Ltd., London.

Lennette, E. H.; Spaulding, E. H.; and Truant, J. P. (eds.): *Manual of Clinical Microbiology.* American Society for Microbiology, Washington, D.C., 1974.

The National Formulary, 14th ed. Mack Printing Co., Easton, Pa., published 1974, became official 1975.

Pan-American Health Organization: *First International Conference on Live Poliovirus Vaccines.* Scientific Publication No. 44. The Organization, Washington, D.C., 1959.

————: *Second International Conference on Live Poliovirus Vaccines.* Scientific Publication No. 50. The Organization, Washington, D.C., 1960.

The Pharmacopeia of the United States of America, 19th rev. Mack Publishing Co., Easton, Pa., published 1974, became official 1975.

Rose, N. R., and Friedman, H. (eds.): *Manual of Clinical Immunology.* American Society for Microbiology, Washington, D.C., 1976.

Sabin, A. B.: Properties of attenuated polioviruses and their behavior in human beings. *Spec. Pub. NY Acad. Sci.,* **5**:113–27, 1957.

Theiler, M., and Smith, H. H.: Effect of prolonged cultivation *in vitro* upon pathogenicity of yellow fever virus. *J. Exp. Med.,* **65**:767–86, 1937.

Turk, J. L.: *Immunology in Clinical Medicine.* Appleton-Century-Crofts, New York, 1971.

Wilson, G. S., and Miles, A. A. (eds.): *Topley and Wilson's Principles of Bacteriology and Immunity,* 6th ed. Williams & Wilkins Co., Baltimore, 1977.

27

Immunofluorescence and Immunoenzyme Staining

ERNST H. BEUTNER, RUSSELL J. NISENGARD, AND
BORIS ALBINI

Introduction

Immunoglobulins can be coupled to fluorescent dyes or enzymes with little or no loss in antibody activity. Many antigens can also be labeled by comparable methods. The reactions of antibodies or antigens labeled with fluorescent dyes can be rendered visible in histologic or cytologic preparations with a fluorescence microscope. Labeling with enzymes makes it possible to use histochemical methods to visualize reactions. The enzymes are permitted to catalyze reactions of substrates that yield colored reaction products. Serologic procedures based on the use of fluorescent dye markers are called fluorescent antibody techniques or immunofluorescent (IF) staining methods, and methods that employ enzyme markers are referred to as immunoenzyme (IE) staining procedures.

In order to achieve reliable results, adequately defined reagents, equipment, and methods are required. With such procedures, reasonable reproducibility can be achieved.

Principles of IF

Fluorescence and Fluorescein Isothiocyanate Labeling

From the physicochemical standpoint, fluorescent dyes or fluorochromes are a group of substances characterized by their ability to achieve elevated but unstable energy levels by absorbing light at a certain wavelength and immediately emitting light at another wavelength in the visible range of light. The absorption of light is called "excitation." Maximum excitation occurs at the absorption maximum of a fluorochrome. Excitation can, however, also be effected at other wavelengths, but to a lesser degree. Changes in the wavelength of excitation only cause insignificant shifts in the wavelength of emitted light. Emission of fluorescence occurs as excited molecules return to their lower base levels of energy 10^{-8} seconds after excitation. The efficiency with which the exciting light energy is converted to fluorescence is called the quantum efficiency. Due to a slight conversion of light energy to heat energy, a change in wavelength occurs. Since the energy of light is inversely proportional to the wavelength, the emitted light is of a longer wavelength than that of the excitation light. The relation of wavelength to energy is given by the equation:

$$E = hc/\lambda$$

where E is energy

h is Planck's constant
c is the velocity of light, and
λ is the wavelength of the light.

Several different fluorochromes are available. The most widely used fluorochrome in IF studies is fluorescein. It has a high quantum efficiency and fluoresces yellow-green, a color for which the human eye has a high sensitivity. Rhodamine, on the other hand, gives off an orange-red fluorescence and can thus afford a contrasting color, which can be helpful when two different antigens or antibodies are investigated simultaneously.

The exceptionally high capacity of fluorescein to convert to an elevated unstable energy level when it is excited by light is due to the inter-ring resonance within the molecule (Figure 27–1 *A*). The fact that this resonance is responsible for the observed fluorescence is demonstrated by the abolition of fluorescence after acetylation of the molecule (Figure 27–1 *B*). The fluorescein diacetate molecule cannot undergo inter-ring resonance and is therefore not fluorescent. Since this compound can be obtained in a pure form, it is used as a reference standard for fluorescein assays. It is readily hydrolyzed to the sodium fluorescein form by dissolving in alkali (0.1 *N* NaOH).

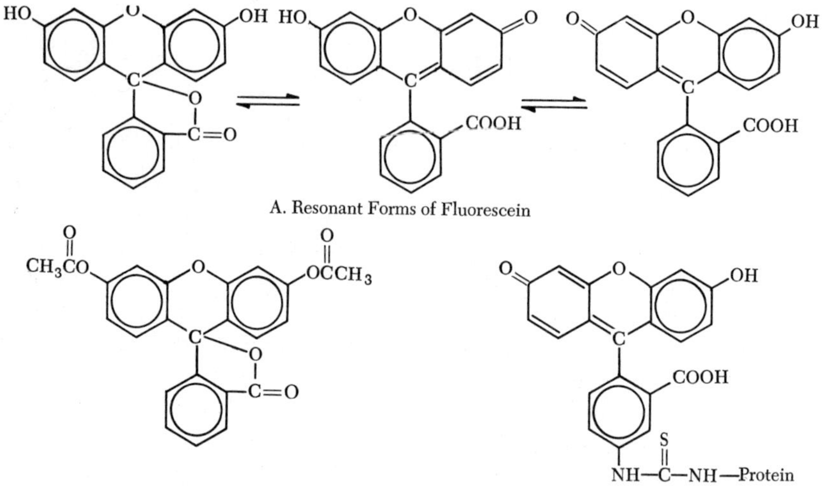

A. Resonant Forms of Fluorescein

B. Fluorescein Diacetate

C. Fluorescein Conjugate of a Protein

Figure 27-1. *A.* Three of the many resonant forms of fluorescein. The high degree of resonance of this molecule, particularly in its form as a sodium salt (at a pH of 8 or more), accounts for its unusually high level of fluorescence.

B. The diacetate form of fluorescein. This molecule cannot resonate to the carbonile form. It is a nonfluorescent colorless compound.

C. Fluorescein conjugated to a free amino group (e.g., epsilon amino group of lysine) via a thiocarbamido linkage. This linkage is formed by allowing the protein to react with FITC in an alkaline solution.

Fluorescein is usually conjugated to antibody of the IgG class or to other proteins by allowing fluorescein isothiocyanate (FITC) to react with the proteins in an alkaline buffer. The resulting reaction with the free amino groups of the protein leads to the formation of a covalent carbamido linkage:

$$\text{fluorescein-N}{=}\text{C}{=}\text{C} + \text{NH}_2\text{-protein} \longrightarrow \text{fluorescein-NH}{-}\underset{\underset{\text{S}}{\|}}{\text{C}}{-}\text{NH-protein}$$

The form of FITC shown in Figure 27–1 *C* is one of the isomer I of this compound.

Specific IF Staining

The following example shows how direct IF staining reactions with labeled antibodies may be performed. Two FITC-labeled conjugates are prepared by labeling the IgG fractions of experimentally produced rabbit antisera, one against streptococci and one against *Escherichia coli*. Two sets of smears of streptococci and of *E. coli* are made on microscope slides. One set of each is treated with serial dilution of the antistreptococcal conjugate and the other with dilutions of the same anti-*E. coli* conjugate. (For clear-cut results, it is best to absorb each conjugate with a suspension of the other strain of bacteria.) The smears are then rinsed with buffered saline, both sets of preparations receive a drop of glycerol with 10% buffered saline and a cover glass, and they are examined with a fluorescence microscope. If the set treated with the homologous conjugate gives rise to staining of the bacteria at a dilution that is at least tenfold and preferably over 100-fold greater than the lowest dilution of the heterologous conjugate that fails to cause staining, then the former may be regarded as an immunologically specific IF reaction. If this is not the case, then the immunologic basis of the observed staining is doubtful; i.e., it may be due to fluorochroming or nonspecific staining. This experiment fulfills the classic definition of an antibody, which depends on the use of an antigen both as an immunogen and as an antigenic substrate for the IF tests.

In a broader sense, the "specificity" of an IF staining reaction, i.e., its dependence on an antigen-antibody binding reaction, may be determined by the fulfillment of each of the four major characteristics (designated here as a to d) of a functional definition of an antibody. Notably, an antibody is (a) an immunoglobulin that gives (b) specific and (c) sensitive reactions in (d) serologic tests. This specificity can be tested even when the immunogen is unknown. For example, the conjugates used in the example in the foregoing paragraph can give specific IF staining if they have the following characteristics: (1) they are pure IgG; (2) their IF staining is specific for the given bacterial species; (3) their titers are at least tenfold and preferably over 100-fold higher with homologous bacteria than with the heterologous ones; and (4) the specific reactivity of the antisera from which they were prepared with the homologous strains of bacteria can be demonstrated by other IF or serologic methods. If each of these points holds true, then we can say with assurance that the conjugates give immunologically specific direct IF regardless of the origin of the antisera from which they were prepared.

The most prominent characteristic of an immunologic reaction is its specificity. In this respect, IF methods afford an additional advantage in the sense that structural localization of staining reactions constitutes a valid (but not infallible) criterion for specificity. This gains particular importance in studies of tissue immunology since IF staining makes it possible to distinguish antigenic determinants in different cells within a given tissue or in different components of given cell types. This, in part, is the reason IF staining has found its widest utilization in studies of autoimmunity (Chapter 25) and other areas of tissue immunology.

Immunofluorescence Microscopy

Sensitivity of immunofluorescence is dependent not only on the immunologic properties of the reagents, but also on the optical system employed.

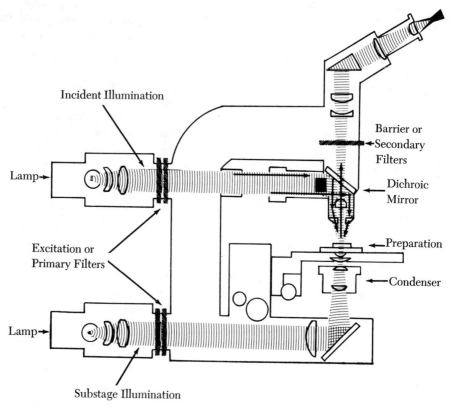

Figure 27-2. Either substage illumination through a condenser (usually of the reflecting dark-field type) or incident illumination via a dichroic mirror and through the objective lens may be employed for immunofluorescent studies.

The components of the optical system include the microscope, light source, excitation or primary filters, barrier or secondary filters, and the condenser (Figure 27–2). These components remain the same regardless of the fluorochrome utilized except for the filters. The filters, however, depend on the light source and, more important, on the excitation and emission wavelengths characteristic of each fluorochrome.

Microscope

Conventional microscopes with appropriate attachments are suitable for immunofluorescence. These microscopes contain optical glass, which transmits most of the light at more than 360 nm, the wavelength necessary for immunofluorescence. Because of this, true ultraviolet light microscopes, which transmit wavelengths of light down to 250 nm are *not* necessary.

Two basic illuminating systems are now available: the classic substage illumination through a dark-field condenser, providing transmitted light, and the newer epi-illumination which provides incident light. Microscopes are equipped with either or both systems of illumination, and both have advantages and disadvantages. An advantage of substage illumination is that it affords greater light intensity at low magnification (10 × or 25 × objectives) than incident illumination. In addition, it is usually easier to locate tissue specimens on a microscope slide. With substage illumination, however, the thickness of the specimen is of critical importance. Specimens thicker than 6 μm markedly reduce the transmitted light intensity. The intensity of light is also influenced by the magnification of the objectives. At higher magnification (40 × or greater) there is a significant reduction in the light intensity. Specimens revealing fluorescence at 10 × or 20 × are frequently negative at 100 ×. For epi-illumination, new, specially designed microscopes usually have to be purchased. These microscopes can easily be used simultaneously for both fluorescence microscopy and routine histology by addition of a bright-field condenser and tungsten light source. The thickness of specimens is not critical since it has no effect on the intensity of the incident light, and the lens creates an "optical section" of the specimen. With epi-illumination, the light intensity increases at higher magnifications [the light collection is proportional to the fourth power of the numerical aperture (NA)]. Thus, objectives with higher magnifications and a higher NA provide higher concentrations of light per optical field in incident illumination systems. However, with higher intensities of illumination, fluorescence also fades more rapidly. This is an important disadvantage when specimens must be examined with objectives 40 × or greater. Location of tissue specimens, however, can be more difficult with incident light.

Light Sources

Several light sources are available, including 50-, 100-, and 200-watt high-pressure mercury lamps, 75- 150-, and 450-watt high-pressure xenon lamps, 100-watt halogen quartz lamps, and 60-watt tungsten lamps. These differ in their relative light intensity at different wavelengths and must be selected on the basis of the fluorochrome utilized, type of illuminating system, and need for high intensity. The 200-watt high-pressure mercury lamp or the xenon high-pressure lamp provides the greatest intensity of fluorescence. The halogen quartz lamp, while providing less intensity of fluorescence, is useful with epi-illumination for many immunofluorescence applications.

Filters

For fluorescent microscopy, "excitation" or "primary" filters are placed between the light source and the microscope slide to screen out undesired wavelengths of light. The "barrier" or "secondary" filters are placed between the specimen and ocular lens to screen out undesired visible wavelengths of light. The selection of filters, therefore, depends on the excitation and emission wavelengths of each fluorochrome. FITC has its maximum excitation at 490 nm and emits at 520 nm. Tetramethyl rhodamine isothiocyanate (TRIC) is excited optimally at 540 nm and emits at 570 nm. Either colored glass filters or interference filters must be selected to provide the desired spectral characteristics for excitation and emission. Interference filters with sharp wavelength cutoffs can reduce tissue autofluorescence and yield strong specific fluorescence. For epi-illumination, a dichroic beam-splitting mirror, a type of interference filter placed at a 50° angle to the light source, is employed, which reflects excitation wavelengths and transmits emitted wavelengths into the eyepiece (Figure 27–2).

Condensers

Dark-field condensers are necessary with substage illumination. The cardioid or reflecting-type condenser provides intense illumination to a small area and is best suited for use with higher-power objectives. The wide-field condensers with toric lenses give fuller fields of illumination with $10 \times$ and $20 \times$ objectives by focusing the light as it enters the condenser.

The thickness of microscope slides is of critical importance with dark-field condensers. Generally, slides 0.75 to 1.2 mm in thickness are acceptable, but this depends on the focal length of the condenser. If the slide is too thick, it is impossible to obtain correct focusing of the condenser. If it is too thin, the column of glycerin or oil between the slide and condenser collapses and prevents critical focusing.

Characteristics of Immunofluorescence Procedures

IF methods of studying antigen-antibody reactions afford three basic advantages. First, these methods make it possible to determine the cytologic or histologic localization of antigens or antibodies in cells or tissues. Second, since whole cells or tissue sections may be examined by immunofluorescence, most, if not all, of their antigenic components are available for detection by reactions on slides. Third, a versatile group of five types of test systems can be used in IF studies (Table 27–1). These five IF test systems include (1) antibody tracing for detection of antigens on preparations; (2) antigen tracing, for detection of antibodies on microscope slide preparations; (3) immunofluorescent detection of complement; (4) blocking reactions, i.e., blocking of reactions of labeled antibodies with unlabeled antibodies; and (5) mixed immunofluorescence, i.e., double reactions of unlabeled antibodies first with given antigens on microscope slide preparation and then with the same antigen(s) in a soluble, fluorochrome-labeled form. Such mixed systems rely on the fact that antibodies are bivalent and that only one of the valencies needs to react to obtain a demonstrable fixation on a microscope preparation, thus leaving one valency free to fix to a soluble labeled-antigen molecule.

One of the limitations of immunofluorescence methods is that they are less sensitive for a given group of antigens than radioimmune assays (Chapter 29) or passive hemagglutination (Chapter 6). However, the conventional two-step indirect IF system with labeled antibodies is more sensitive than precipitation (Chapter 6) or complement fixation (Chapter 8). The estimate of antibody protein concentrations that can be detected range from 0.1 to 10 μg/ml depending on the antibody reference standards and the antigenic substrates. Another limitation is that soluble antigens tend to get lost in the washing procedures required for IF staining. Such antigens can actually become relocated due to adhesion to some other tissue components and give rise to fallacious histologic localization.

Direct and Indirect IF Staining for Antigens

The most widely used fluorescein labeling procedures are the direct, the indirect, and the complement IF staining methods. The nature of these reactions as listed in Table 27–1 and portrayed in Figure 27–3 is basically distinct. For each of these techniques, preparations must be rinsed with buffered saline between each step in processing, and the specificity of IF staining should be demonstrated by criteria of the type described above (pages 478–79).

Direct IF staining with labeled antibodies is usually an immunohistochemical test in the sense that labeled antibodies with known specificities are used to look for the corresponding antigens in smears or monolayers or sections of antigen-bearing materials.

Indirect IF staining, on the other hand, commonly serves to detect antibodies in patient and animal sera as, for example, in the fluorescent treponemal antibody (FTA) test or FTA absorption (FTA-Abs) test and in the antinuclear antibody (ANA) tests. These employ known antigens, reference sera, and antihuman IgG conjugates. The titers and patterns of IF reactions of unknown sera are read and interpreted on the basis of the staining reactions obtained with known positive and negative reference sera at selected dilutions under defined conditions. Three-step indirect IF staining for antigen can also be used to detect antigen(s) on sections, smears, or suspension (Table 27–1).

IF Staining for Antibodies and Complement IF Staining

The so-called sandwich method involves three steps as shown in Figure 27–3. It can reveal specific antibodies, e.g., in plasma cells, by first treating

Table 27-1
FIVE PRINCIPLES EMPLOYED IN DIRECT AND INDIRECT IMMUNOFLUORESCENT STAINING SYSTEMS

Type of Method	Reactants on Microscope Preparation	Reactants			Common Names of Methods	Common Uses
		A. DIRECT IF	B. INDIRECT IF SYSTEMS			
			1ST STEP	2ND STEP (AND 3RD)		
1. IF staining with antibodies	Antigens	*Ab	Ab#1	*Ab to Ig from #1 Ab producer	A. Labeled antibody FA tech. or direct IF (DIF) B. Indirect IF (IIF) C. Three-step method	Detection of unknown antigens with known antibodies Detection of unknown antibodies with known antigens Not in common use
2. IF staining with antigens	Antibodies	(*Ag)	Ag	*Ab to Ag	A. Labeled Ag IF staining B. Sandwich technique	Not commonly used because of low sensitivity Identification of antibody-producing cells in tissue
3. IF staining with complement	Antigen pre-treated with Ab	(*C)	C	*Ab to C	A. Labeled C staining B. Complement IF	Only described one time Detection of complement-fixing antibodies

		1st Step	2nd Step	3rd Step		
4. IF blocking	Antigen	Ab#1 + *Ab#2 or Ab#2 + *Ab#1	Ab#1 + Ab#2	*Ab to Ig from #1 Ab producer or *Ab to Ig from #2 Ab producer	A. IF blocking	Tests of identity or non-identity of Ab#1 and Ab#2; specificity tests
					B. Indirect IF blocking	As for IF blocking when Ab#1 and Ab#2 are of different species origin or different Ig classes
5. Mixed IF staining	Antigen	(Ab)	(*Ag) for #1 Ab (Not yet reported)		A. Mixed IF staining	Not commonly used as yet though very promising for identification of Ag
			2nd Step: Ab to Ig from #1 Ab producer	3rd Step: *Ig from 1st Ab producer	B. Mixed antiglobulin IF staining	This principle used for peroxidase labeling using Ab to peroxidase in place of 3rd step *Ig; peroxidase binding and peroxide treatment serve to visualize reaction of 1st Ab

Abbreviations: IF = immunofluorescence = FA = fluorescent antibody methods = Coons' staining
Ag = antigens; *Ag = labeled antigens (Ag to Ab in preceding step)
Ab = antibody; *Ab = labeled antibody (Ab to Ag in preceding step)
Ab to Ig from (#1 or #2) = antibodies to immunoglobulins from #1 or #2 species or individual
C   = complement component(s); *C = labeled C

485

Techniques

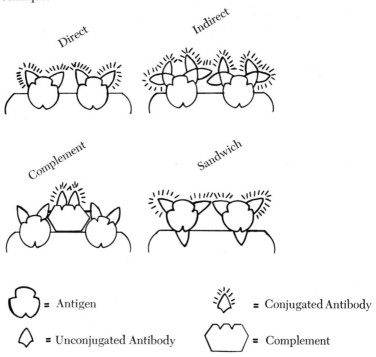

Figure 27-3. Direct immunofluorescent (IF) staining entails a simple one-step staining procedure with labeled antibodies. Multistep systems such as the indirect IF, the complement IF, and the IF "sandwich" techniques not only serve to detect diverse serologic phenomena but also are simpler to control in practice and are usually more sensitive.

frozen sections with the unlabeled specific antigen and then with labeled antibodies of the same specificity as those in the plasma cell, thus the name "sandwich technique." While direct IF staining with labeled antigen has been used successfully to detect rheumatoid factor (Chapter 25) and other antibodies in tissue, the intensity of IF staining achieved is so low that its value is doubtful.

The commonly used form of complement IF staining entails a three-step procedure (Figure 27-3). First, one uses unlabeled antibodies, just as in indirect staining. The second step consists of complement from one species (whole fresh serum), and the third, a conjugate that is specific for a complement component of that species. The method is actually a multistep procedure. It is versatile enough to detect complement-fixing antibodies regardless of specificity or species origin of the antibody. The two-step complement IF staining procedure (Table 27-1) is not practical because FITC-labeled complement is unstable. One-step IF staining with labeled anticomplement conjugates is a direct IF technique, not a complement IF procedure since it need not involve complement that is bound to antigen-antibody complexes. For example, a three-step procedure in a type 1 system consists of sequential treatment of antigen preparations with unlabeled antibodies of species A, then unlabeled antiglobulin to immunoglobulin of species A from species B, and labeled antibodies to the immunoglobulin of species B from species C.

Blocking IF and Mixed IF Staining Methods

Blocking IF was originally used as a "specificity" test for IF staining. If pretreatment of antigens with unlabeled antibodies blocked IF staining or if mixing of unlabeled and labeled antibodies did the same, this should be evidence for the "specificity" of the observed staining pattern. However, if labeled antibodies bind to different portions of the antigen molecule than the unlabeled ones, then no blocking occurs though both may be giving immunologically specific reactions. Conversely, nonspecific staining with fluorescein-labeled proteins can be "blocked" with unlabeled albumin. Thus, this IF method is not a valid criterion for specificity. The latter needs to be assessed by criteria of the type set forth earlier (pages 478–79).

Blocking IF is, however, of considerable value as a test for identity or non-identity of antigenic determinants. It assumes particular importance in IF staining in light of the fact that the identity of histologic localization does not mean identity of antigenic determinants. Either different molecules or different determinants on the same antigen molecule may, on reacting with antibodies, give rise to identical histologic or even ultrastructural pictures. Blocking IF may be carried out with direct or indirect IF tests for antigens. To obtain clearly interpretable results, it is best to mix the two types of antibodies in varying proportions so as to obtain a two-dimensional titration (one dentition for each of the antibodies). This affords unequivocal data on blocking, partial blocking, or the lack thereof. A major limitation of these methods is that steric hindrance can apparently give rise to partial blocking of two sets of antigenic determinants on one molecule that are close to each other. Thus, a monospecific anti-IgE reagent gives partial blocking of an antilight-chain conjugate.

Mixed IF staining relies on the fact that the detection of antibody IF tests for antigens requires binding of only one antibody-combining site. The remaining combining site(s) of a certain proportion of bound antibodies remains free to react with soluble FITC-labeled antigen molecules. For examples, if an indirect IF test is carried out with (1) tissue section, (2) antinuclear antibodies, and (3) unlabeled instead of labeled antihuman IgG antibodies, then antibody-combining sites on the latter remain free. The latter can be demonstrated by a third-step reaction with FITC-labeled human IgG. This gives rise to a specific ANA reaction adjusted appropriately. This principle is used in a multistep horseradish peroxidase staining method described below.

IF Techniques

IF on Sections and Smears

Most of the IF used in clinical laboratories is done by direct or indirect IF for antigens on microscope slides. Direct IF is used most commonly for frozen sections of biopsies and is performed by placing conjugates with known specificities on the sections, rinsing, mounting, and reading. Indirect IF with known antigens on slides entails placing a drop of diluted unknown serum or reference serum on the slide, rinsing, treating with an anti-Ig conjugate, rinsing, mounting, and reading.

Membrane IF Staining Technique

Most of the IF used in the clinical routine is done on tissue sections. In recent years, however, the staining of living cells in suspension has also gained importance. Cells are suspended successively in the unlabeled and/or labeled reagents and washing buffer (rather than placing reagents on sections). This group of methods known as membrane fluorescence was initiated originally by Möller. It is used to detect surface determinants of different cell classes, e.g., immunoglobulin on B lymphocytes and θ antigens on murine T cells, or to demonstrate virus-specific antigen expressed on the membrane of infected cells. In addition to its clinical use in the delineation of cell populations and a technique developed for the detection of immune complexes in sera, it is of the utmost importance in the research concerned with cell membrane composition and behavior, and function of cell membrane components. Membrane fluorescence can now be performed in a microtiter system, which makes this method usable also for routine purposes.

Technical Problems in the Control of IF

Although serologic studies with labeled antibodies are simple to perform and can offer significant advantages, failure to recognize the numerous factors that govern the observable outcome of a reaction sequence can compromise their effectiveness. But adequately controlled systems yield reproducible and interpretable results. Both nonimmunologic and immunologic variables influence the observable staining reactions. Most of the factors apply, in principle, also to enzyme labeling.

Nonimmunologic factors are the microscope, the labeling agent, and staining patterns unrelated to antigen-antibody reactions such as autofluorescence, artifactual dislocations of reactants on microscope preparations, and nonspecific staining (NSS). Differentiation between the kinds of fluorescent stains seen in a preparation is the main difficulty in interpreting results. NSS or nonimmunologic adherence of labeled proteins in a preparation is mainly due to electrostatic attraction and is more likely to occur with heavily labeled conjugates. It can frequently be differentiated from desired specific staining (DSS) by its more or less diffuse appearance, but it makes the reading of preparations difficult by depressing and sometimes even removing the background contrast. A second type of interfering staining is due to labeled antibodies to antigens in the preparation other than the antibody (antigen) sought. This is called undesired specific staining (USS) and cannot be readily differentiated from NSS. Such antibodies can, however, be removed by absorption or can be blocked by adding unlabeled antibodies with the undesired specificities to the labeled globulins. USS is usually an immunologic variable, as are the sensitivity and specificity of the conjugate as well as the type of IF system employed.

Characterization of Conjugates

At the same time that the specificity of an antiserum or its immunoglobulin fraction or a conjugate prepared from it is being established, its sensitivity also needs to be ascertained to achieve a defined IF staining system. The sensitivity of a fluorescein-conjugated globulin fraction is a function of the degree of labeling and the concentration of labeled antibody.

The degree of labeling can be determined by assaying the contents of protein (P) and fluorochrome (F), respectively. From these values the mean amount of fluorochrome per protein molecule can be calculated. This is called the F/P ratio of a conjugate and can be expressed either as a weight or as a molar measure. The molar F/P expresses the average number of fluorochrome molecules per protein molecule. In practice most work is done with conjugates with molar F/P ratios between 1.0 and 4.5 for indirect IF staining and somewhat higher for certain direct IF-staining systems, such as those used for the detection of bacteria and for membrane immunofluorescence. Ideally the F/P ratio of a conjugate should be chosen to achieve an optimum balance between the increased intensity of DSS and NSS that accompanies increased F/P ratios. A conjugate is most satisfactorily characterized if the specific antibody content (Ab/ml) is known. If this is established, then conjugates can be diluted to antibody concentrations known to be required for satisfactory IF-staining reactions.

Since the concentration of desired antibodies (Ab/ml) governs the degree of DSS with a given antigen preparation and since the concentration of fluorescein (F/ml) governs the degree of NS of a conjugate (free of undesired antibodies) on a given antigen preparation, it follows that

Ab/F is proportional to DSS/NSS

Since the relative amounts of DSS and NSS are critical in determining if and how an IF staining reaction can be interpreted, it follows that the Ab/F

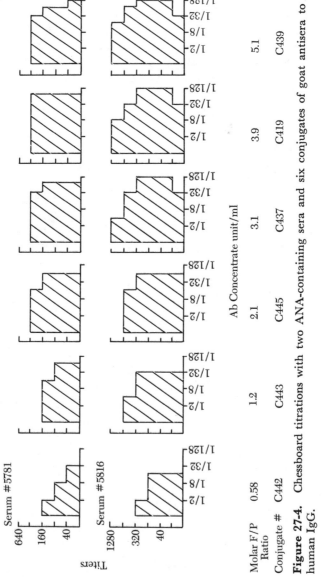

Figure 27-4. Chessboard titrations with two ANA-containing sera and six conjugates of goat antisera to human IgG.

ratio is a critical characteristic of a conjugate. The Ab/F ratio is limited by the relative antibody concentration that can be achieved. In practice even those conjugates that are prepared from purified IgG fractions of hyperimmune antisera or by absorption and elution methods rarely contain more than 30% antibody; i.e., such immunoglobulin preparations have a ratio of Ab/P of 0.3 or less. Conjugates prepared from such globulins at molar F/P ratios of 1.0 have a functionally maximal Ab/F ratio; i.e., since molar ratios can be multiplied, it follows that

$$Ab/P \div F/P = Ab/F$$

and thus

$$0.3 \div 1.0 = 0.3$$

Even such an optimal conjugate with molar Ab/F ratios of 0.3 that is free of USS can give some NSS on certain substrates such as basophils. NSS under these conditions depends on the F concentration at dilutions of conjugates that contain the desired antibody concentration.

Even defined immunofluorescence will present problems in interpreting results obtained because of concurrent NSS. The degree of NSS at given F concentrations appears to be dependent on the relative isoelectric points of the microscope preparations and the conjugates.

In practice, it is important to characterize a FITC conjugate (1) as to its *specificity*, using most conveniently immunoelectrophoresis or, more accurately, immunofluorescent staining with purified antigens; (2) as to its *sensitivity*, expressed as the F/P molar ratio and the antibody content; and finally (3) to establish the *optimal working dilution* of a conjugate for a specific antigen-antibody system, using the chessboard titration (Figure 27–4). In the chessboard titration, serial dilutions of conjugate are tested in an indirect immunofluorescence test against serial dilutions of reference sera on a known antigenic substrate. The dilution of conjugate preceding the last one still giving plateau titer values (called the plateau end point) is to be chosen for immunofluorescence tests. Conjugate concentrations may be expressed in units/ml, one unit being the end point concentration in a standard gel precipitation test (Chapter 6).

Immunoenzyme (IE) Staining

Enzymes capable of catalyzing histochemically demonstrable color reactions with selected substrates can be coupled to antibodies or other selected proteins by bonding agents such as glutaraldehyde and difluorodinitrodiphenyl sulfone as well as by other methods. Such conjugates can give rise to visible staining reactions at the site of antibody binding if tests are performed on microscope slides with frozen sections or smears of the antigens or other reactants just as for IF staining (Figure 27–3). Although a number of enzymes including glucose oxidase and alkaline phosphatase have been used in exploratory studies of this type, most of the reported work has been done with horseradish peroxidase (HRP). The substrate most frequently used to obtain permanent stained preparations with HRP-labeled antibodies is 3,3′-diaminobenzidine (DAB). The color reaction with HRP substrates is achieved after the addition of hydrogen peroxide [leucobase (DAB monomer) $\xrightarrow[\text{HRP}]{\text{H}_2\text{O}_2}$ > visible dye (DAB polymer)].

Although several methods have been used to couple HRP to immunoglobulin and to other proteins, the best appear to be two-step procedures. Thus, partial oxidation of the carbohydrate component of HRP with periodate yields aldehyde groups; these can be coupled to amino groups of immunoglobulins or other proteins to form covalent bonds (Chapter 4).

The reaction sequence with such a reagent might be as follows:

1. Two sets of smears of bacteria (a) and (b) are made on microscope slides.

2. Dilutions of a globulin fraction of an antiserum to the bacteria labeled with HRP are placed on the smears of set (a). Set (b) receives dilutions of the same conjugate after it has been absorbed with the bacteria.

3. Both sets of preparations are treated with the substrate diaminobenzidine and hydrogen peroxide to obtain the observed color reaction. If set (a) gives a titer of 10 or more and set (b) is negative, then the staining obtained with the unabsorbed conjugate may be regarded as positive.

Since the substrates used for these studies can give visible color reactions under excitation with visible light, standard light microscopy can be used as for histologic preparation. Another advantage of these methods is that the reaction products of diaminobenzidine are visible in electron microscope preparations. Thus HRP-labeled antibodies are widely used for immuno-electron microscopic studies (Chapter 28).

The disadvantage of working with HRP is that it is more costly and more time consuming than immunofluorescence methods considered above. Thus, HRP studies are used mainly for research work, although the sensitivity and the spectrum of types of reaction systems that can be used in the immunoenzyme studies are comparable to those of studies made with fluorescein labeling.

An obstacle to routine use of HRP techniques still is the lack of standardization. Only preliminary attempts have been made to define the reagents used in this test system. It seems, however, that characterization of HRP reagents may be achieved in a similar way as it has been established already for FITC conjugate.

For characterization of horseradish peroxide conjugates, the following procedures are recommended: (1) establishment of the *specificity* of conjugate as described for FITC conjugates; (2) determination of the amount of HRP in the conjugate by either biochemical or immunologic methods, and thus of the E/P ratio (*sensitivity* of the system); and (3) finding the *optimal working dilution* using the chessboard titration as described above (page 491).

The HRP staining technique is the method of choice for studies involving both light and electron microscopy. As the background staining of HRP-labeled antibodies differs from that of FITC conjugates, the use of immuno-enzyme techniques may be advantageous in some special areas of research or routine immunohistology. Finally, HRP staining methods offer the advantage of permanent staining. Therefore, preparations may be kept for a long time, which may be useful for scientific or legal reasons.

Bibliography

Andres, G. A.; Hsu, K. G.; and Seegal, B. C.: Immunologic techniques for the identification of antigens or antibodies by electron microscopy. In Weir, D. M. (ed.): *Handbook of Experimental Immunology*, 2nd ed., Vol. 2. Blackwell Scientific Publications, Oxford, 1973.

Avrameas, S.: Studies on antibody formation with enzyme markers. *Ann. NY Acad. Sci.*, 254:175–89, 1975.

Beutner, E. H.: Defined immunofluorescent staining: past progress, present status and future prospects for defined conjugates. *Ann. NY Acad. Sci.*, 177:506–26, 1971.

Beutner, E. H.; Chorzelski, T. P.; Bean, S. F.; and Jordon, R. E. (eds.): *Immuno-pathology of the Skin: Labeled Antibody Studies*. Dowden, Hutchinson and Ross, Stroudsburg, Pa., 1973.

Goldman, M.: *Fluorescent Antibody Methods*. Academic Press, Inc., New York, 1968.

Hijmans, W., and Schaeffer, M. (eds.): Fifth International Conference on Immuno-fluorescence and Related Staining Techniques. *Ann. NY Acad. Sci.*, 254:1–628, 1975.

Mellors, R. C.; Nowoslawski, A.; Korngold, L.; and Sengson, B. L.: Rheumatoid factor and the pathogenesis of rheumatoid arthritis. *J. Exp. Med.*, 113:475–84, 1961.

Nairn, R. C. (ed.): *Fluorescent Antibody Tracing*, 6th ed. Williams & Wilkins Co., Baltimore, 1976.

Nakane, P. K.: Recent progress in the peroxidase-labeled antibody method. *Ann. NY Acad. Sci.*, 254:203–11, 1975.

Schenenstein, K.; Wick, G.; and King, H.: The micro-membrane-fluorescence test: a new semiautomated technique based on the microtiler system. *J. Immunol. Meth.*, 10:143, 1976.

Shu, S., and Albini, B.: Quantitative studies of peroxidase labeled antibody. I. Indirect staining system analyzed by chessboard titrations. *J. Immunol. Meth.*, 13:341–53, 1976.

Theofilopoulos, A. N.; Wilson, C. B.; Bokisch, V. A.; and Dixon, F. J.: Binding of soluble immune complexes to human lymphoblastoid cells. II. Use of Raji cells to detect circulating immune complexes in animal and human sera. *J. Exp. Med.*, 140:1230–44, 1974.

Van Dalen, J. P. R.; Knapp, W.; and Ploem, S.: Microfluorometry of antigen-antibody interaction in immunofluorescence using antigens covalently bound to agarose beads. *J. Immunol. Meth.*, 2:383–92, 1973.

28

Immunoelectron-microscopy

BORIS ALBINI AND GIUSEPPE A. ANDRES

Introduction

Immunoelectronmicroscopy is a technique characterized by the association of various electron-dense markers with antibody or other immunoreactive macromolecules, and by the subsequent use of the electron microscope for the identification of antigen-antibody reaction at the ultrastructural level. In this chapter we will present the techniques that are currently used for conjugation of antibodies to electron-dense markers and the principal applications of these techniques in many fields of biomedical research.

In 1959, Singer conjugated globulins with ferritin without loss of immunologic activity. The introduction of the immunoferritin method extended the usefulness of Coons' technique in which fluorescein-labeled antibody is employed as an immunologic tool to identify antigens within tissues. For more than a decade, immunoferritin technique has been the mainstay of immunoelectronmicroscopy. In the last few years, the basic concepts of the original immunoferritin method have been strengthened by the addition of several new classes of labels, such as enzymes, which allow the examination of the same tissue sample by both light and electron microscopy. Further, new techniques have enriched the field of immunoelectronmicroscopy. Ferritin and enzymes have been successfully employed first as an immunizing antigen and subsequently as a marker to detect the corresponding antibody formed by the immunized animals, thereby revealing its ultrastructural location. Hybrid antibody of dual specificity has been introduced for localizing antigens through capture of free markers at the discrete site of primary immune reaction. The stereoscanning microscope has been employed for a tridimensional study of antigen-antibody reactions, and immuno-autoradiography has been improved to such an extent that it now stands as a coequal partner with the immunoferritin and immunoenzyme techniques.

Immunoferritin Technique

The immunoferritin technique is based on the principle that two protein molecules can be coupled by the use of a bifunctional reagent of low molecular weight under conditions that favor the reaction with protein molecules. Singer first employed metaxylylene diisocyanate or toluene-2,4-diisocyanate as a conjugating agent. The reaction is usually performed in two steps (Figure 28–1). In the first step ferritin is reacted with an excess of coupling agent at pH 7.5. In the second step the diisocyanate-reacted ferritin is mixed with immunoglobulin at pH 9.5. Since only part of the globulin is conjugated, specific antisera of high titer are essential. If the serum contains unwanted antibodies, it is necessary to remove them by absorption with appropriate antigens.

Ferritin is an iron-containing protein that is characterized by high electron density. It has a protein shell that envelops an inner core of ferric hydroxide micelles of 1000 to 1200 nm in diameter. The molecular weight of ferritin is 750,000. Its iron content averages 23%. The 2000 to 3000 atoms of iron in a molecule confer a high electron density to ferritin. Ferritin can be obtained from several animal sources and must be purified before conjugation in order to obtain the fraction that yields optimum results in electron microscopy. This process of purification involves repeated recrystallization in 20% cadmium sulfate and reprecipitation in ammonium sulphate at 50% saturation. Both IgG and IgM have been satisfactorily labeled (Chapter 4). Fragments I and II, obtained by papain digestion, also have been coupled to ferritin.

Many factors can affect the result of conjugation. Lack of success may be due to antisera of insufficient titer, unsatisfactory preservation of one unreactive isocyanate group in the ferritin-coupling agent preparation, or unsatisfactory quality of the coupling agent. After conjugation, portions of both antibody and ferritin remain unconjugated. It is especially important to remove the unconjugated antibody, which may react with the specific antigen, "blocking" its reaction sites and preventing the binding of the ferritin-conjugated antibody. Removal of unconjugated antibody can be achieved by ultracentrifugation. In contrast, removal of unconjugated ferritin is hardly important because it does not interfere with the specific binding of the conjugate.

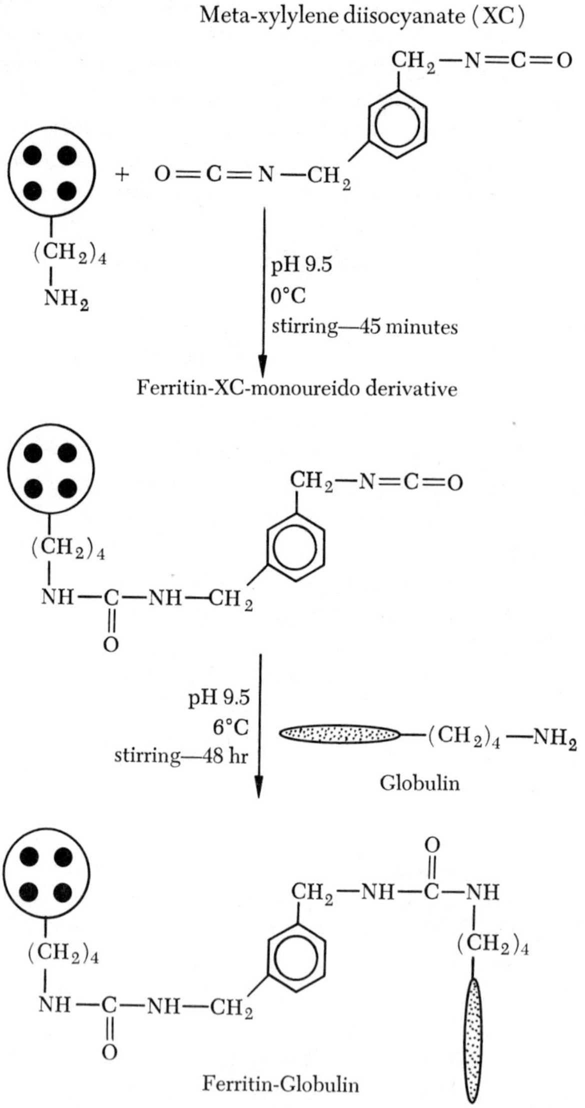

Figure 28-1. Diagram illustrating the conjugation of ferritin to globulin in a two-step reaction with XC as the coupling agent. (From Andres, G. A.; Hsu, K. G.; and Seegal, B. C.: Immunologic techniques for the identification of antigens or antibodies by electron microscopy. In Weir, D. M. [ed.]: *Handbook of Experimental Immunology*, 3rd ed., Vol. 2. Blackwell Scientific Publications, Ltd., Oxford, 1973.)

Before use in experiments with the electron microscope, the conjugates should be tested by immunoelectrophoresis in order to establish whether the "ferritin conjugate" is present and whether the conjugated antibody is still reactive with its specific antigen.

Results of immunoelectronmicroscopic study are often difficult to interpret without previous knowledge derived from the immunofluorescence technique (Chapter 27). Thus, a thorough study by the immunofluorescence technique should precede experiments in which the electron microscope is used. The potency and specificity of the antiserum used in the investigation can be readily determined with the immunofluorescence technique, and a variety of controls can be more easily performed.

Three factors must be considered in the preparation of specimens for treatment with ferritin-conjugated antibody: (1) the preservation of cellular fine structure; (2) the preservation of antigenic determinants; and (3) the penetration of large ferritin molecules between or into the cells.

The ideal solution of these problems would be to stain thin sections of embedded tissue directly, before examination in the electron microscope. The usual embedding procedure, however, greatly diminishes or eradicates the capacity of the antigen to react with antibody. Special methods have been devised to overcome these difficulties. Tissues have been embedded in water-soluble methacrylates or in bovine serum albumin cross-linked with glutaraldehyde and sectioned by ultramicrotomy. Alternatively, frozen tissues have been sectioned by cryo-ultramicrotomy, and the sections have been incubated with the ferritin-conjugated antibody. These techniques, however, are laborious and have not provided consistent results.

The methods that have been and are still most frequently used consist of the treatment of unfixed specimens with ferritin-conjugated antibody, and by postfixation and embedding. Prefixation of the specimen is frequently indispensable in order to preserve fine structure for electron microscopy. The majority of fixatives, however, quickly diminish or eradicate the capacity of the antigens to react with antibodies. The capacity of the antigens to withstand fixation depends on their chemical characteristics, the concentration of the fixative, and the duration of fixation. Before initiating experiments with the electron microscope it is advisable to test the effects of fixatives on selected specimens by using the immunofluorescence technique (Chapter 27). These preliminary experiments will suggest an acceptable compromise between preservation of fine structure and preservation of antigenicity. Among the fixatives that have been tested, only a few have proven satisfactory. One to five percent formalin or paraformaldehyde, buffered at pH 7.2, helps to maintain fine structure without inactivating antigenic determinants of immunoglobulins or basement membranes. Recently, a new fixative containing periodate, lysine, and paraformaldehyde has been used successfully to stabilize carbohydrate moieties without loss of antigenicity. After treatment with the ferritin conjugates, further fixation

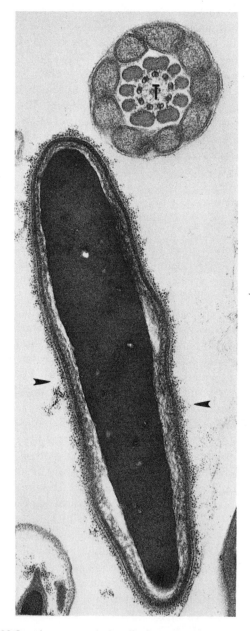

Figure 28-2. Acrosome and tail. Spermatozoa from a normal rabbit incubated with rabbit serum containing antiacrosomal antibody. The specimen was then treated with ferritin-conjugated goat antirabbit IgG. Ferritin (arrowheads) is localized on the cell membrane of a spermatozoon head but is not bound to the cell membrane of the tail (T). × 35,000.

with 1% osmium tetroxide or 2% glutaraldehyde followed by osmium tetroxide is essential in order to preserve fine structures.

The localization of surface antigens in membranes (Figure 28–2) of tissue cultured cells or suspended cells may be accomplished by simple immersion of a prefixed or unfixed specimen in the ferritin conjugate. However, due to its relatively large size, ferritin-conjugated antibody does not penetrate cells or tissues without disrupting cellular membranes or increasing tissue permeability. In order to open the plasma membrane, several methods have been employed, such as freezing and thawing, gentle homogenization of briefly fixed cells, and treatment of cells with digitonin. Localization of antigens in solid tissues can be achieved by finely mincing the prefixed tissue with a razor blade in the cold or by using a tissue chopper or a cutting machine, which consistently provides 20-μm sections of unfixed, or slightly fixed, tissues.

Three main types of controls are usually employed in order to establish the specificity of immunoferritin experiments: (1) specific immunologic "blocking" of the reaction by using an unconjugated preparation of the antibody; (2) treatment of a duplicate specimen with nonspecific ferritin conjugates; and (3) treatment of similar but normal tissue with the specific ferritin conjugate.

Recently, the immunoferritin technique has been used to localize antigens within cytomembranes. Cells or membranes are quickly chilled at 4° C, incubated with ferritin-conjugated antibody, fixed in glutaraldehyde, processed in a freeze-etching apparatus, replicated, and studied by electron microscopy.

The immunoferritin technique has been applied to a wide variety of problems, which include the identification of viral antigens; the localization of surface antigens on bacteria, red blood cells, and lymphocytes; and the production of antibodies, basement membranes, and enzymes. Furthermore, the immunoferritin technique has been used for the identification of antigen-antibody reactions in several experimental or human diseases (Chapter 25).

Hybrid-Antibody Technique

A disadvantage of the immunoferritin technique is that the ferritin–coupling agent compound can react at any site of IgG molecules and thus produce a linkage of two or more molecules without discriminating between ferritin and IgG. The resulting product of a conjugation mixture, therefore, is heterogeneous. The hybrid-antibody technique developed by Hämmerling and his colleagues partially overcomes this limitation. The method is based on Nisonoff's finding that antibody molecules of dual specificity can be obtained by combining univalent fragments of pepsin-treated antibodies of different specificities. The sequential steps of this technique are the following: Incubation of IgG immunoglobulins with pepsin produces a "cleavage" and degradation of the Fc fragment, whereas the combining activity of the antibody is preserved. Pepsin-treated antibody is a dimer $[F(ab')_2]$ of two identical units, the Fab fragments, each with one combining site linked by at least one disulfide bond (Chapter 3). Loss of the Fc fragment makes this bond highly susceptible to reduction. The bond can be selectively split, resulting in two Fab fragments. The process is reversible by mild oxidation, which reconstitutes the bivalent $F(ab')_2$ dimer. When this reconstitution takes place in a mixture of Fab pieces from antibodies of different specificities, some of the dimers so formed are "hybrids" with double specificity. This recombination occurs at random without preferential union of Fab pairs with the same serologic specificity (Figure 28–3).

A hybrid antibody with one specificity for cell-surface antigen and another for ferritin proves an ideal reagent for labeling (Figure 28–4). Also, hybrid antiferritin and anti-IgG can be made, providing a single reagent for indirect staining techniques that will locate any cell-surface antigen to which antibody is attached.

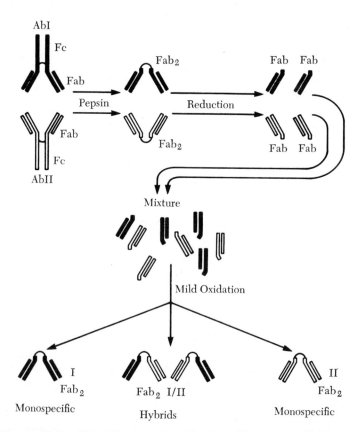

Figure 28-3. Hybridization of antibodies with two specificities (*AbI* and *AbII*).

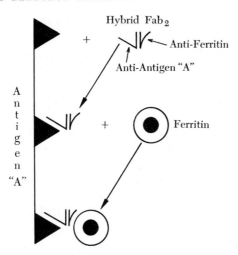

Figure 28-4. "Staining" with hybrid antibody and ferritin.

A special value of hybrid antibody technique is that visual markers other than ferritin may be used provided these are (1) of appropriate size, (2) antigenic, and (3) not proven to adsorb nonspecifically to the cell surface. Small plant viruses, such as the southern bean mosaic virus, are suitable markers in all these respects. Two hybrid-antibody preparations with specificity for ferritin in one and for a virus in the other have been used for simultaneous identification of two different antigens on the same cell.

Immunohemocyanin Technique

Hemocyanin obtained from the marine whelk *Busycon canaliculatum* is an adequate marker for electron microscopy. For preparation of hemocyanin, marine whelks are bled and the hemolymph is collected and purified. The isolated hemocyanin can be conjugated to antibody using glutaraldehyde as a coupling agent. Since hemocyanin has a molecular weight of 6×10^6, the conjugate can be used only for localization of antigens present on the cellular surface. Another application of immunohemocyanin technique is in freeze etching. These combined techniques have been used to map the distribution of Ig molecules on lymphocytes and to study the formation of "caps."

Immunoscanning Electron Microscopy Technique

The topographic tridimensional distribution of an antibody-conjugated marker localized at the cell surface can be studied by transmission electron microscopy and serial ultrathin sections of a single cells. However, this is a difficult and time-consuming procedure. In recent years, scanning electron microscopy and suitable tracers have become valuable tools for the ultra-structural analysis of cell surfaces. The main problem of immunostereo-scanning microscopy is the selection of a tracer that can be bound to antibody molecules and visualized by the scanning microscope. The relatively low resolution of the scanning microscope requires the choice of a tracer of larger size than that of ferritin or enzyme molecules. One technique that has been used is based on the property of latex particles to adsorb gamma globulin nonspecifically. If the adsorbed gamma globulins contain specific antibodies, then the latex particles may bind to specific cell-surface determinants. The antibody-coated latex is prepared by incubation of latex spheres (0.2 μm in diameter) with the antibody-containing gamma globulins at room temperature.

The indirect staining method is more efficient than the direct method. The use of latex as an ultrastructural marker has several technical limitations. First, the preparation of the immunolatex label must be performed at pH 9.2 because the gamma globulins dissociate from latex particles at pH 5.5 to 9.0 and low molarities. Second, the latex spheres tend to be hydrophobic and stick to the surface of living cells, thus requiring an aldehyde fixation of cells prior to latex labeling. Third, during preparation for scanning microscopy the shearing forces on the large latex spheres may remove them from the cell surface. This event can be minimized only by the postfixation of cells with glutaraldehyde, which stabilizes the linkage.

Fewer difficulties are found when red blood cells coated with IgG or C3 are used to identify IgG or C3 receptors on the surface of lymphocytes or other cell types. Due to their large size, erythrocytes, however, do not provide precise details concerning localization of the antigenic molecules.

Immunoautoradiography Technique

Immunoautoradiography was originally developed for the study of protein synthesis in mammalian cells. In these experiments, antibody-producing cells were incubated with the corresponding radiolabeled antigen, and the site of reaction was then identified by ultrastructural autoradiography. The first studies were performed with unfixed cells and [125]I IgG as the antigenic marker. The iodinated antibodies showed poor intracellular penetration, and only antigen that had localized in the peripheral cytoplasm was detected. Better intracellular penetration was achieved when smaller antigenic markers, prepared by papain digestion and purified by immunoadsorption, were used. At the same time, an improved preservation of fine structure was obtained by prefixation of cells.

Autoradiography with ^{125}I provides less resolution than peroxidase-labeled antibody technique. Iodination, however, is less likely to alter the immunologic specificity of the antibody molecule than conjugation with bifunctional reagents.

Use of Markers as Immunizing Agents and Subsequently as Tracers

Identification of antibody produced by lymphoid cells of actively immunized animals can be achieved by exposing the cells to the immunizing antigen, ferritin, or enzyme, and by subsequent study in the electron microscope. This method eliminates the conjugation and staining procedures. In the spleen of rabbits immunized with horseradish peroxidase, antibody first appears in the perinuclear space of hemocytoblasts where it persists through differentiation into mature plasma cells. With the full development of ergastoplasm, antibodies accumulate in the cisternae of endoplasmic reticulum and in the lamellar portion of Golgi apparatus. In mature plasma cells the antibodies are concentrated in large intracisternal granules or diffused throughout the cytoplasm.

The method of using markers as immunizing agents and subsequently as tracers is also employed for the localization of antigen-antibody complexes in allergic inflammation. In the early stage of active Arthus reaction (Chapter 19), ferritin precipitates were observed in perivascular connective tissue and to a lesser degree in venular walls but not in the lumina of the vessels. In the reverse Arthus reactions, ferritin precipitates were seen mainly in the walls of the venules, between gaps of endothelial cells and occasionally in the vascular lumina. In similar studies, ferritin has been used as antigen inducing chronic serum sickness in rabbits. Ferritin-antiferritin immune complexes were then localized by electron microscopy in glomerular structures.

Enzyme-Conjugated Antibody Method

In the last six decades, histochemical methods for the localization of enzymes in tissues have been established. These methods are based on the catalytic properties of enzymes for specific chemical reactions. In such reactions, the enzyme transforms a microscopically inconspicuous substrate into a microscopically detectable compound, which precipitates at the site of the enzyme in the tissue. To be microscopically detectable, the end product of the reaction has to be either colored, for light microscopy study, or electronopaque, for electron microscopic examination. The end product can either precipitate spontaneously or it may be precipitated by a capturing agent such as osmium tetroxide. Often, histochemical methods for the demonstration of enzymes use reactions that lead to the polymerization and cyclization of the substrate. This may increase the amount and effectiveness of conjugated double bonds in the molecule, thus modulating the color characteristics of the compound; they may change the solubility properties of the molecule and thus induce precipitation (Chapter 6).

Using bifunctional reagents that link together two protein molecules, it is possible to couple enzymes, such as acid phosphatase or horseradish peroxidase, to antibodies. Two reactions characterize these methods: first, the specific combination of the antibody-reactive site with the specific antigen; and second, the catalytic reaction of the enzyme with a substrate. The effectiveness of an immunoenzyme conjugate will depend on the specificity and avidity of the antibodies used, the reactivity of the enzyme, the availability of an adequate histochemical method to detect the enzyme, the influence of the conjugation procedures on immunologic and enzymatic reactivity of antibody and enzyme, respectively, and the conditions of the reactions of tissue staining, such as pH, temperature, and incubation time.

Immunoenzyme methods offer some advantages over immunoferritin methods. The molecular weight and the size of the conjugates can be kept lower than those of ferritin conjugates, thus facilitating tissue penetration. In many instances, visualization of immunoenzyme conjugates can be obtained by both light and electron microscopy. Increasing the time of reaction of the enzyme with the substrate improves the visibility of the end product, and thus the sensitivity of the method. On the other hand, if precipitation of the end product is too slow in comparison with its diffusion, the resolution of immunoenzyme methods may be inferior to that of immunoferritin technique.

An optimal reagent for immunocytochemistry should fulfill the following criteria summarized by Sternberger:

1. The enzyme should be easily detectable by a cytochemical method, preferably one applicable to both light and electron microscopy. In order to provide high resolution, the enzyme reaction product should not diffuse away from the production site. The cytochemical substrate should have a high turnover number with the enzyme in neutral buffers that do not induce severe tissue damage.
2. The enzyme should be available in pure form.
3. Conjugation with immunoglobulin may impair enzyme activity but should not abolish it.
4. The enzyme should be fairly stable in neutral solution.
5. The enzyme should have a relatively small molecular weight, since small enzyme-conjugated antibody penetrates tissue better than large enzyme-conjugated antibody.
6. Substrate-related enzymes should not be endogenous constituents of the tissues examined.

Horseradish peroxidase (HRP), more than other enzymes, possesses the characteristics listed above. Therefore, we will discuss more extensively the immunoperoxidase method. Other enzymes, which have rarely been used, will be mentioned briefly.

Peroxidase-Conjugated Antibody Methods

Peroxidases are hemoproteins. Histochemical methods for their localization in tissues or cells were developed by Fischel in 1910. The horseradish peroxidase is an oxidureductase with the systemic number EC 1.11.1.7 and consists of an apoenzyme and the protoporphyrin IX. It has a molecular weight of 40,000 and contains 1.27% iron. In the peroxidase-catalysed reaction, H_2O_2, methyl-00H, or ethyl-00H can be used as H acceptors, and phenols, diamines, ascorbate, leukodyes, or amino acids can function as H donors. The optimal concentration of peroxidases in substrate mixtures is 10^{-3} M. It is important to note that horseradish peroxidase is not inhibited by 70% ethanol or 10% formalin but is inhibited by NaN_3.

The use of HRP in immunoelectronmicroscopy was introduced by Nakane and Pierce. The histochemical reaction developed by Graham and Karnovsky for the visualization of the enzyme sites is based on the use of diaminobenzidine (DAB). The still hypothetic chemistry of this reaction is summarized in Figure 28–5. The polymer end product reduces and chelates osmium tetroxide, which is added as a 1% solution. This leads to the precipitation of a black, insoluble, low-valence, and electron-opaque product at the site of the enzymatic reaction.

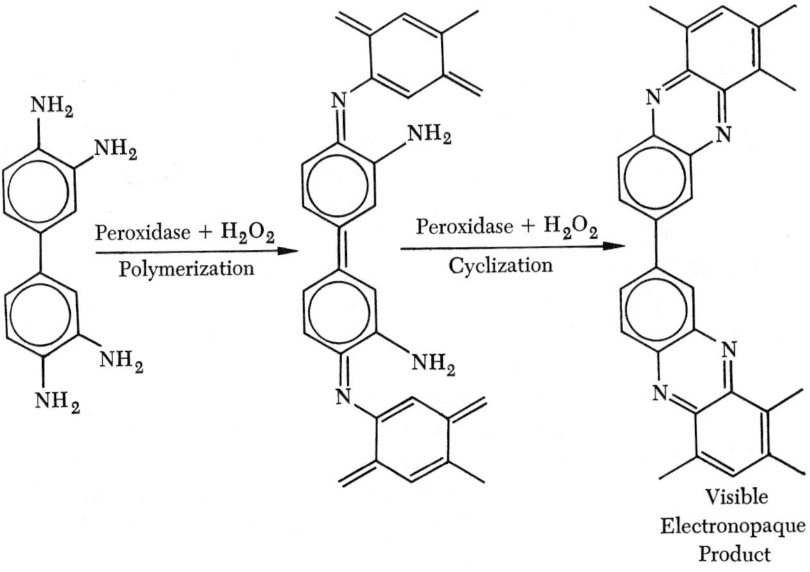

Figure 28-5. The polymerization and cyclization of diaminobenzidine (DAB).

Glutaraldehyde or 4,4'-difluoro-3,3' dinitrophenysulfone (FNPS) may be used for conjugation of peroxidase to antibody. This single-step procedure, however, has some disadvantages. FNPS reacts 66 times faster with IgG than with peroxidase; therefore, the polymerization of IgG molecules occurs much faster than the formation of IgG-peroxidase bonds. As a consequence of this event, most of the resulting product is represented by polymerized IgG, to which a few molecules of peroxidase are linked. No polymers of peroxidase are formed, and only 1 to 2% of the peroxidase originally present is conjugated to IgG.

Whereas unconjugated HRP can easily be removed from the conjugate by ammonium sulfate precipitation of the conjugated antibody, the unconjugated IgG competes for binding sites during the staining procedure and thereby decreases the capacity of the conjugate to bind to the specific antigen. The blocking of the antigenic sites by unlabeled antibody is further increased by high molecular weight of conjugates that have a higher statistical likelihood to contain peroxidase molecules. Furthermore, large molecules are at a disadvantage in terms of tissue penetration.

Conjugates obtained with the one-step method contain, at most, an average of one peroxidase molecule per three IgG molecules. After conjugation, the enzymatic activity of the conjugates is not decreased if compared with that of the enzyme prior to conjugation. In contrast, the capacity of the antibody to react with the specific antigen is usually decreased. The antibody activity during conjugation decreases by a factor of 8 to 64. These considerations explain why only highly purified antibody obtain through affinity chromatography or immunoadsorption is suitable for conjugation. Nevertheless, when employed to stain tissue sections that are studied by light microscopy, the sensitivity of the best HRP-antibody preparations is comparable to, or even higher than that of homologous FITC-conjugated antibody (Chapter 27).

A definite improvement of the immunoenzyme technique was achieved by the development of a two-step method. In the original procedure, HRP is first exposed to glutaraldehyde. In a second step, the HRP aldehyde is reacted with IgG. Although this method does not seem to increase the efficiency of peroxidase attachment to IgG, it definitely reduces the possibility of IgG polymerization.

In another similar procedure, the carbohydrate moieties of the HRP molecule are oxidized by sodium priodate to the stage of aldehydes. The aldehydes of the peroxidase molecule react in a second step with α and ε amino groups of the IgG (the α and ε groups of the peroxidase can be blocked during both steps of the conjugation with fluoronitrobenzene). This method allows an almost complete preservation of both IgG (immunologic) and peroxidase (enzymatic) activities and prevents the formation of blocking peroxidase-free IgG polymers. Almost 90 to 95% of the IgG used in the conjugation mixture is labeled with peroxidase.

HRP-conjugated antibody can be used in both direct and indirect staining methods. The indirect staining methods, which are more sensitive, are recommended. Occasionally, the direct method may be preferred because of its higher specificity.

As with the immunoferritin method, the major problems of the staining procedures for electron microscopy are (1) the fixation of the tissues, necessary for preservation of ultrastructure; (2) the preservation of tissue antigenicity; and (3) the penetration of the enzyme conjugates into tissue or cells. Excellent fixation usually precludes an effective penetration of the conjugates. Likewise, good fixation usually decreases or eradicates the capacity of the antigen to react with antibody. Finally, when optimal penetration is achieved in unfixed specimens, the preservation of fine structure is usually unsatisfactory. Thus, ideal solutions are not available, and every experiment requires an acceptable compromise between fixation of tissue, preservation of antigen, and penetration of enzyme conjugates into tissues.

In a widely used procedure, small tissue blocks (1 mm in diameter) are fixed for 2 to 4 hours at 4° C in 10% paraformaldehyde in a phosphate buffer at pH 7.2. After extensive washing in buffered saline and 4% sucrose, the tissue is frozen and sections of 20 μm are cut with a cryostat. The sections are then incubated with specific antiserum for 8 to 12 hours. After washing, a peroxidase-conjugated antibody to the immunoglobulin of the animal species providing the specific antiserum is layered on the sections and incubated for another 8 to 12 hours. The preparation is fixed in 2% glutaraldehyde for one hour. After being washed, the specimen is immersed in DAB solution without hydrogen peroxide, for one hour at 4° C. Then, hydrogen peroxide is added. After being washed in distilled water, the specimen is treated with osmium tetroxide for 60 minutes and processed according to a routine electron microscopy technique.

Nakane has recently proposed two modifications of the standard immunoenzyme technique. The first is concerned with the use of periodate-lysine paraformaldehyde as a primary fixative. The lysine cross-links the carbohydrates, thus preventing loss of polysaccharide antigens. The second modification involves freezing and thawing the fixed specimens rendering them more permeable to the conjugates.

Another method recently introduced for staining unfixed tissues is freeze substitution. With this technique, sections of 10 μm are cut in a cryostat and then stained with the conjugates. In such thin sections the penetration of the conjugates is usually satisfactory. Finally, staining of thin sections obtained from tissues prefixed with a dilute solution of paraformaldehyde and embedded in water-soluble methacrylate is also possible. The sections are placed on grids, and part of the embedding medium is removed before staining.

Staining with peroxidase conjugates can be amplified by additional incubation with antiperoxidase antibody and peroxidase. The penetration of the conjugates can be increased by using Fab fragments instead of whole IgG molecules.

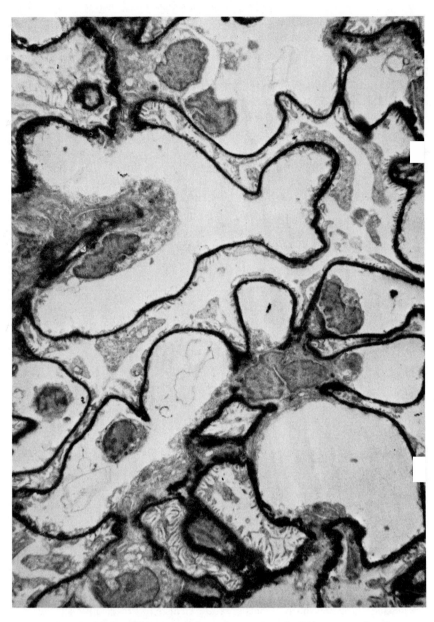

Figure 28-6. Kidney section of rat that had been rendered nephritic by the injection of rabbit antirat glomerular basement membrane serum. The tissue was first incubated with sheep antirabbit globulin serum, followed by rabbit antiperoxidase and peroxidase. The reaction product is localized in the glomerular basement membrane. × 4800.

Peroxidase-labeled antibody has been used successfully for localization of antigens in a variety of tissues and organisms. T antigens of simian virus 40 were localized in infected MA 104 cells in culture; neutral salt-soluble collagen was demonstrated in chicken leg tendons; hormones were identified in sections of rat anterior pituitary glands. In other studies, gastric parietal cell antigens and cell-surface antigens were demonstrated. Furthermore, immunoperoxidase technique was used to identify antigen-antibody reactions in experimental and human diseases (Figure 18–6) (Chapter 19).

Much remains to be done for standardization of the conjugates, fixation of the specimens, preservation of tissue antigenicity, and better penetration of the conjugates. In spite of the limitations, however, use of peroxidase-labeled antibody proved to be a valuable tool in ultrastructural immunology and immunopathology.

Other Marker Proteins in Immunoenzyme Electron Microscopy

Other peroxidases have been used as tracers in immunoenzyme methods. One of the advantages of these enzymes is a molecular weight smaller than that of HRP. This favors penetration in tissues. Cytochrome c has a molecular weight of 12,000. It is easier to purify but has an enzymatic reactivity lower than that of horseradish peroxidase. Preparation of microperoxidase, i.e., a heme-peptide fragment of cytochrome c (Mw 1,900), and use of Fab fragments make it possible to reduce the size of the conjugates to about 40,000 to 50,000 daltons.

Acid phosphatases can also be linked to antibodies, but the conjugation is more difficult. For this reason, acid-phosphate-conjugated antibodies have rarely been used in immunoelectronmicroscopy.

Unlabeled Antibody Enzyme Method

From the preceding description of the classic direct or indirect immuno-enzyme methods, it is obvious that the process of conjugation frequently decreases the reactivity of the antibody in the enzyme antibody conjugates. Therefore, immunoenzyme techniques not requiring conjugation of antibody should have certain advantages.

In the classic immunoenzyme methods, described above (pages 503–509), the link between the antibody molecule and the enzyme is established by chemical bonds. In contrast, in the unlabeled antibody enzyme method, this link is achieved by means of immune reactions. Two slightly different procedures, involving the use of HRP, have been proposed for the unlabeled antibody enzyme method (or immunoenzyme bridge technique). Both procedures are based on the use of a "bridge" antibody molecule for coupling the "primary" antibody (specific for the antigen to be detected) to the enzyme. The steps and reagents of the unlabeled antibody enzyme

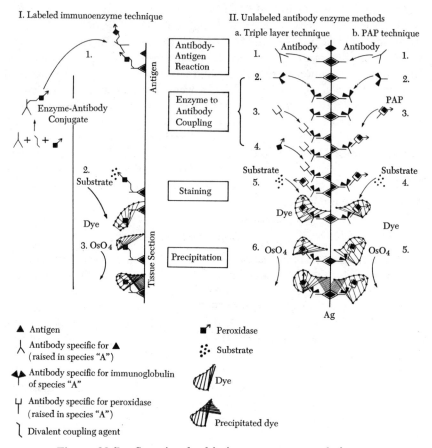

Figure 28-7. Steps involved in immunoenzyme techniques.

method are summarized and compared with the classic immunoenzyme method in Figure 28–7, which shows that both the "primary" and the antiperoxidase antibodies are raised in the same animal species. An antibody specific to immunoglobulins of this animal species is used to "bridge" the "primary" antibody to the antiperoxidase antibody. The antiperoxidase antibody is then able to capture the peroxidase molecules. It is important to note that the bridging antibody must be present in excess to allow one of the two combining sites to be free for reaction with the antiperoxidase antibody.

The first procedure of the unlabeled antibody enzyme method (triple-layer technique) is characterized by the use of antiperoxidase antibody. The antibody must be purified, as antibodies of unwanted specificity inhibit the binding of peroxidase to the site of reaction. The purification of antiperoxidase antibodies, however, is difficult, since elution by affinity-chromatography gives only a low yield. In addition, the eluted antibody is of low avidity.

For these reasons, a second method was developed in which peroxidase-antiperoxidase (PAP) complexes, instead of peroxidase antibodies, are used. The elution from affinity chromatography columns is more easily achieved if the eluted antiperoxidase antibody is kept in solution by addition of an excess of peroxidase, which favors ' the formation of antigen-antibody complexes. Such immune complexes in antigen excess are soluble. Using this procedure, virtually all the antiperoxidase antibodies can be eluted. In addition to the optimal yield, there is also the advantage that low-affinity antibodies are not preferentially selected.

The soluble PAP complex method has been used to identify several antigens including *Treponema pallidum*, ACTH in pituitary cells, cartilage collagen in chickens, and type and group-specific viral antigens.

The unlabeled PAP complex method appears 100 to 1000 times more sensitive than the immunofluorescence technique and 1000 times more sensitive than radioimmunoassay methods (Chapter 29). Nonspecific staining, although it may occur, can be controlled or prevented. Increase of polarity and hydrophobicity of the labeled end products, which inevitably occur during conjugation of enzyme to antibody, are not observed with the PAP method. The sensitivity is excellent, and thus high dilutions of reagents can be used. These characteristics make it possible to visualize by electron microscopy very small areas of antigenic reactivity, sometimes at the level of a single molecule.

Bibliography

Andres, G. A.; Hsu, K. G.; and Seegal, B. C.: Immunologic techniques for the identification of antigens or antibodies by electron microscopy. In Weir, D. M. (ed.): *Handbook of Experimental Immunology*, 3rd ed. Blackwell Scientific Publications, Ltd., Oxford, J. B. Lippincott Co., Philadelphia, 1978.

Avrameas, S.: Immunoenzyme techniques: enzymes as markers for the localization of antigens and antibodies. *Int. Rev. Cytol.*, 27:379, 1970.

De Petris, S.; Karlsbad, G.; and Pernis, B.: Localization of antibodies in plasma cells by electron microscopy. *J. Exp. Med.*, 117:849, 1963.

Essner, E.: Hemoproteins. In Hayat, M. A. (ed.): *Electron Microscopy of Enzymes: Principles and Methods*, Vol. 2. V. Nostrand Reinhold Co., New York, 1973, p. 1.

Hämmerling, U.; Aoki, T.; De Harven, E.; Boyse, E. A.; and Old, L. J.: Use of hybrid antibody with anti-g and anti-ferritin specificies in locating cell surface antigens by electron microscopy. *J. Exp. Med.*, 128:1461, 1968.

Leduc, E. H.; Avrameas, S.; and Bouteille, M.: Ultrastructural localization of antibody in differentiating plasma cell. *J. Exp. Med.*, 127:109, 1968.

Linthicum, S. D.; Sell, S.; Wagner, R. M.; and Ireft, P.: Scanning immuno-electronmicroscopy of mouse B and T lymphocytes. *Nature (Lond.)*, 252:173, 1974.

Mason, T. E.; Phifer, R. F.; Spicer, S. S.; Swallow, R. A.; and Dreskin, R. E.: An immunoglobulin enzyme bridge method for localizing tissue antigens. *J. Histochem. Cytochem.*, **17**:563, 1969.

Nakane, P. K., and Pierce, G. B.: Enzyme-labeled antibodies: preparation and application for the localization of antigens. *J. Histochem. Cytochem.*, **14**:929, 1966.

Singer, S. J.: Preparation of an electron-dense antibody conjugate. *Nature* (Lond.), **185**:1523, 1959.

Sternberger, L. A.: *Immunocytochemistry*. Prentice-Hall, Inc., Englewood Cliffs, N.J., 1974.

29

Immunoassays

Y ASUO Y AGI

Introduction

One of the recent, important contributions of immunology to other areas of life sciences is the use of immunologic principles for the analysis of minute amounts of antigenic compounds in complex mixtures such as serum and biologic fluids. These methods are called immunoassays. The specificity of antigen-antibody reactions (Chapter 5) plays an essential role in the assay in selecting the aimed molecules from many other molecules in complex mixtures. The methods utilize antigens or antibodies labeled by appropriate means. The sensitivity of the methods can be increased by the appropriate choice of labels to a level (ng – pg/ml) that cannot be attained by any other methods. The labeling is most commonly achieved by the use of radioisotopes, which can be measured readily with an extremely high sensitivity even in complex mixtures. More recently, various nonradio-isotopic labels, such as enzymes, fluorescent groups, bacteriophages, and stable free radicals, have been developed. The methods with radioisotopes are called radioimmunoassays, and those with other labels are given suitable prefixes such as enzyme immunoassays.

The radioimmunoassay was first devised in 1960 by Yalow and Berson to measure minute amounts of insulin in blood by the use of radioiodine-labeled

Table 29-1
SOME OF THE COMPOUNDS MEASURABLE BY IMMUNOASSAYS

A. *Protein and Peptide Hormones*
 Anterior pituitary
  Luteinizing hormone (LH)
  Follicle-stimulating hormone
   (FSH)
  Thyroid-stimulating hormone
   (TSH)
  Growth hormone (HGH)
  Prolactin
  Corticotropin (ACTH)

 Posterior pituitary
  Arginine vasopressin
  Oxytocin

 Parathyroid
  Parathyroid hormone

 Pancreas
  Insulin
  Glucagon

 Placenta
  Placental lactogen (HPL)
  Chorionic gonadotropin (HCG)

 Others
  Angiotensin I and II
  Gastrin
  Calcitonin
  Intrinsic factor

B. *Other Proteins and Peptides*
 Plasma
  IgE and other Igs
  Fibrinogen

  Other clotting factors

  Tumor antigens
  Carcinoembryonic antigen (CEA)
   α-fetoprotein

  Microbial antigens
   Hepatitis-associated antigens
   Other microbial antigens

C. *Haptens*
 Hormones
  Thyroxine (T_4)
  Triiodothyronine (T_3)
  Cortisol
  Deoxycorticosterone
  Aldosterone
  Testosterone
  Progesterone
  Estrogens
  Prostaglandins

 Drugs
  Morphine and codeine
  Amphetamine
  Digitoxin and digoxin
  Barbiturates
  Metadone
  Diphenylhydantoine
  Primidone
 Others
  Folic acid*
  Cyclic nucleotides*
  Vitamin B_{12}*
  Vitamin D

* Nonimmunologic.

insulin and guinea pig anti-insulin serum. The method was soon extended to other hormones of peptide nature such as glucagon and growth hormone, which otherwise could be measured only by tedious and imprecise bioassays, often with an unsatisfactory sensitivity. Subsequently, the application was further expanded not only to a number of other proteins and peptides but also to compounds of low molecular weight such as steroids and pharmaceuticals (haptens). They are not immunogenic but react with antisera prepared by immunization with their protein conjugates. Thus, within 15 years, the number of compounds that can be assayed by these methods increased greatly, and the areas of application now cover essentially all fields of biologic and medical sciences.

Table 29–1 lists some compounds of clinical interest on which the application has been reported. The same principle has been applied to some simple compounds such as c-AMP and vitamin B_{12} where specific binding proteins instead of antibodies were found.

Principles of Immunoassays

In general terms, two types of assays based on different principles are used to measure antigens in test samples. The first type utilizes labeled antigens. It was originally described by Berson and Yalow. It is called saturation assay or competitive assay and is based on the competition for a fixed amount of antibody between a labeled antigen (or hapten) and its unlabeled counterpart in the test sample. A constant amount of antibody and a constant amount of a labeled antigen as an indicator are utilized in a system. When the unlabeled counterpart is added to the system, the extent of binding of the indicator antigen to the antibody decreases as the amount of the unlabeled counterpart is increased. Thus, a reference inhibition curve is drawn by measuring the degree of antigen binding (represented by the labeled indicator antigen) at several known concentrations of unlabeled standard antigen. At the same time, the degree of antigen binding is measured on the mixtures of the indicator antigen and the test sample with the antibody. The antigen concentration in the test sample is determined by interpolation of the observed binding value into the reference curve.

The increase in sensitivity is often achieved by adding the unlabeled antigen (in the test sample) and labeled antigen sequentially to the antibody, instead of mixing the labeled and unlabeled antigen simultaneously with the antibody. The displacement of the antigen bound to the antibody with the newly added labeled antigen takes much longer time than that required for the binding of free antibody sites with the antigen. Therefore, a larger degree of inhibition can be obtained with the same amount of unlabeled antigen by such a sequential addition than by simultaneous addition.

Such competitive assays in the liquid phase have been used most extensively and have a great advantage in that minute amounts of antigens and antibodies are required. Pure antigens such as some of the peptide hormones as well as some specific antibodies of high avidity are often available only in small quantities. However, the methods require fairly long periods of incubation, usually overnight but up to one week in some cases, and some labeled peptides appear to be unstable when incubated with physiologic fluids such as plasma. In such cases, other methods utilizing solid phase antigens or antibodies may be advantageous (see below). Direct contact of labeled antigen with such interfering substances in the test samples can be avoided. Labeled antibodies generally appear to be more stable than labeled antigen when incubated for several days in high concentrations of plasma.

These competitive assays require simple methods of separating the labeled antigen that is free or is bound by the antibody as immune complexes. Antigen-antibody complexes do not form precipitates even with multivalent antigens since immunoassays are normally performed in extremely low concentrations such as 10^{-9} (ng) $\sim 10^{-12}$ g (pg) antigens/ml. A variety of separation procedures have been devised primarily dependent on the nature of antigens and the γ globulin nature of antibodies (see below). Antibodies in solid phase (immunoadsorbents containing antibody) instead of soluble antibody have also been used in a few cases by sequential addition of unlabeled antigen (test sample) and indicator antigen.

The second type of assay utilizes labeled antibodies. It has been used much less than the first type but appears to have the potential for wider application. It may be called immunometric assay. This method differs from the first type in that the antigen to be measured is assayed directly by combination with labeled specific antibodies rather than in competition with a labeled antigen for a limited amount of antibody. In this assay, samples of antigen are reacted with an excess of labeled antibody, and the amount of labeled antibody bound to antigen is determined after removing the unreacted portion of labeled antibody by adsorption on excess immunoadsorbent containing antigen. Here again, a reference curve is prepared by addition of a standard antigen in increasing amounts to a fixed amount of the labeled antibody. The concentrations of antigen in test samples are read from observed amounts of bound antibody in the reference curve. This method obviously requires labeled antibody of a high purity and the preparation of an appropriate immunoadsorbent-containing antigen. However, the same immunoadsorbent may also be utilized for preparation of antibody of a high purity prior to or after the labeling. Indeed, the antibodies can be labeled with radioiodine while they are fixed on antigen covalently bound to cellulose and then eluted with acid buffer. Such specifically purified, labeled antibody may be used successfully in subsequent immunoassays.

A variation of this principle is utilized in the immunometric assays of the "sandwich" type where multivalent antigen can be assayed. In this case, samples of antigen are incubated with an excess of immunoadsorbent containing antibody, washed, and then reincubated with an excess of the labeled antibody of the same antigenic specificity (usually from animal species other than the first antibody). Increase in the amount of labeled antibody bound to the immunoadsorbent is observed with the increase of the added antigen since the antigen serves as a bridge between the antibody in solid phase and the labeled antibody. This method has an advantage in that an increase of sensitivity may be obtained in the case of multivalent antigens since several molecules of labeled antibody can combine with a single antigen molecule previously fixed on the immunoadsorbent.

Both types of immunoassays mentioned above, competitive or immunometric, require physical separation of antigen-antibody complexes from either free antigen or free antibody. However, another approach not requiring such a separation has been devised recently for haptens labeled with some enzymes (homogeneous enzyme immunoassays). The assay depends on inhibition or activation of the enzyme activity by antibody binding. An enzymatically active morphine-lysozyme conjugate loses its activity when it combines with antimorphine antibody. When free morphine is added to the system, free hapten competes for the antibody sites with the haptenic group in the conjugate; thus the inhibition by antibody is reduced. A similar observation was made in the morphine-malate dehydrogenase system.

On the other hand, an entirely opposite phenomenon was observed with a thyroxine-malate dehydrogenase conjugate, which is enzymatically inactive. Upon combination with the antithyroxine antibody, the conjugate regained its enzymic activity. The loss and the reappearance of this dehydrogenase activity are probably due to conformational changes. Regardless of whether it is inhibition or activation, the enzymic activity in the mixtures serves for the assay of haptens without any separation steps.

Affinity and Specificity of Antibodies

The most important factor determining the sensitivity and accuracy of immunoassays is the affinity of antibodies. The sensitivity depends on the binding constant (K) between the antigen and antibody (Chapter 5). This dependence can be seen readily when one assumes model systems where a hapten and the corresponding antibody are in equilibrium in solution.

$$H + AB \rightleftharpoons H \cdot Ab \text{ (binding constant } = K)$$

$$K = \frac{[H \cdot Ab]}{[H][Ab]} = \frac{B}{F([Ab_0] - B)} \tag{1}$$

$$B/F = K[Ab_0] - KB \tag{2}$$

$$\lim_{B \to 0} F = K[Ab_0], \qquad \lim_{B/F \to 0} B = [Ab_0] \tag{3}$$

where B and F denote the concentration of bound and free hapten, respectively, and $[Ab_0]$ represents the concentration of total antibody sites.

By looking at these equations, one can see that, when a constant concentration of antibody is used, B/F is linearly proportional to B and the maximum value of B/F obtainable at an infinitely low concentration of B (and also total hapten) is equal to $K[Ab_0]$. At an infinitely high concentration of

$F(B/F \to O)$, B is obviously equal to $[Ab_0]$ (Figure 29–1). Figure 29–2 represents the change in the degree of hapten binding in relation to the total hapten concentrations added to antibodies of different affinities. One can clearly see that both the sensitivity and the accuracy of antigen detection are higher when an antibody of a higher affinity is used. With an antibody of a lower affinity, the degree of hapten binding can be increased at higher antibody concentrations, but this accompanies the loss of the sensitivity in antigen detection.

Although this simple model system is far from the actual reactions that are taking place under laboratory conditions, one can see clearly that the affinity of antibody is a major factor determining the success of sensitive immunoassays. Under normal conditions for immunoassays, the equilibrium between the antigen and antibody is not achieved completely since the concentrations of antigen and antibody are extremely low, and much longer time than practical for actual use is needed to reach the true equilibrium. Further complications are introduced by the fact that macromolecular

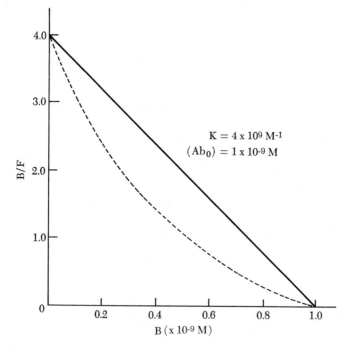

Figure 29-1. Relation between the degree of antigen binding (B/F) and the concentrations of bound antigen (B). Antibody preparations with a uniform binding constant will show a straight-line relationship (solid line, $K = 4 \times 10^9 \, M^{-1}$, $[Ab_0] = 1 \times 10^{-9} \, M$), whereas most antibody preparations that are mixed populations of antibodies with different binding constants will show concave curves (broken line).

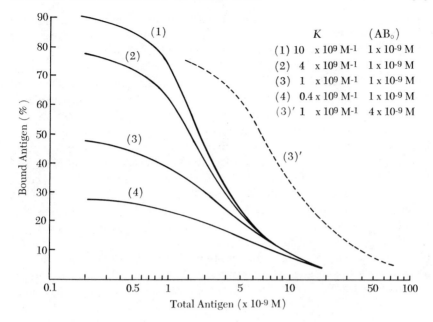

Figure 29-2. Change in the percentage of bound antigen at varying concentrations of total antigen (constant antibody concentrations). When the binding constant is lower, the slope of the curves is shallower. The maximum binding of antigen at infinitely low antigen concentration is (*1*) 90.9%, (*2*) 80%, (*3*) 50%, and (*4*) 28.6%. The curve shifts to the right, e.g., (*3*) → (*3'*), if one increases the antibody concentration in order to obtain a higher antigen binding, thus resulting in the loss of sensitivity.

antigens are multivalent and may possess different antigenic sites that react with the corresponding antibodies. The antigens or antibodies are often used in solid phase rather than in solution. Furthermore, most antibodies are extremely heterogeneous in terms of structures as well as the affinity to antigen even in the case of antibodies against a single antigenic determinant (Chapter 7). Thus, even in hapten-antihapten antibody systems, the correlation between B/F and B usually is not linear even in equilibrium and shows a concave curve as shown by the dotted line in Figure 29–1.

The heterogeneity of antibody has an important bearing in considering the immunoassays for antibodies in contrast to immunoassays for antigens. Since no two antibody preparations of presumably the same specificity are identical in the distribution of binding constants with an antigenic site, the true concentrations of antibody in a sample cannot be assayed accurately in comparison with a standard antibody preparation, particularly in a range of extremely low concentrations as in immunoassays where the equilibrium between the antigen and antibody plays a major role. (In higher concentrations of antigen and antibody, the equilibrium is shifted almost fully toward the complex formation so that antibody concentrations can be determined by appropriate means, at least for practical purposes.) On the other hand, in the immunoassays for antigens, the heterogeneity of antibody is immaterial to the validity of the assay, insofar as the antigen used to prepare the reference curve behaves in the same way as the antigen in the test samples in combination with the antibody used. In most cases, antigens are well-defined molecules, although minute differences in their structure that may be vitally important for their biologic activity may escape immunologic detection. The slightly modified molecules such as metabolites may be erroneously assayed, especially in the case of macromolecular antigens. However, such structural changes in antigenic sites usually affect the binding with the antibody and can be detected rather readily by comparing the shape of the reference curve with that obtained at various dilutions of the test samples. If the shape is different between the reference antigen and the samples, yet is the same with various test samples, one can at least estimate the relative values of the modified antigen in the test samples.

What is important in the immunoassays is the identity of the reference antigen with the antigen in the assay sample and that the labeled antigen does not need to be identical in this aspect with the unlabeled antigen used for the reference curve. In fact, various types of labels, especially the external labels such as the radioactive iodine atom, fluorescent dyes, bacteriophages, and enzymes, can affect the binding of antigen with the antibody, although the influence may differ greatly depending on the nature of labels and the antigen concerned. With the same labeled antigen, a higher sensitivity can be expected if the reference antigen has a higher affinity to the antibody than the labeled antigen.

Separation of Free Antigen and Bound Antigen

When antigen-antibody reactions are performed in solution, the separation of bound antigen (antigen-antibody complex) and free antigen poses a technical problem because extremely low concentrations of antigen and antibody are used in immunoassays (Chapter 5). No precipitate of antigen-antibody complex is formed even in a system with multivalent antigen and bivalent antibody. One of the techniques that has been used widely is the double-antibody technique. After the first incubation of antigen (labeled and unlabeled) with antibody, the bound antigen is separated from the free antigen by precipitation with an excess of an antiglobulin antibody from the second animal species ("second antibody"). Since antibodies are globulins, the antigen-antibody complexes (including bound antigen) form precipitates together with nonspecific globulins leaving the free antigen in solution.

The double-antibody technique has an advantage in that the same antiglobulin antiserum may be used in a number of assay systems in which the first antibodies come from the same animal species. However, a significant dissociation of antigen-antibody complexes may be observed during the second incubation with the antiglobulin antibody by dilution of the first incubation mixture especially in hapten-antihapten systems. Furthermore, fairly large amounts of antiglobulin antibody are required to precipitate all the globulins in biologic fluids such as plasma. For example, with a plasma sample containing 15 mg γ globulin/ml, 100 μl of the sample would usually require about 4 to 5 mg of antiglobulin antibody to achieve complete precipitation.

In addition, a variety of techniques have been used in various assay systems utilizing the difference of physicochemical properties between free antigen and bound antigen. For example, Berson and Yalow, in their original method of insulin immunoassay, utilized the fact that insulin in free form is tightly adsorbed on filter paper but insulin-antibody complex is not. Similar differences in adsorption and electric charge have been used with a variety of adsorbents such as charcoal, kaolin, silica gel, zirconium phosphate gel, and ion-exchange resins including DEAE cellulose and DEAE Sephadex. The difference in the solubility has been utilized to precipitate bound antigen (complex) by addition of salts (sodium sulfate, ammonium sulfate), acid (trichloracetic acid), and some organic solvents (ethanol, dioxan, polyethylene glycol). The difference in molecular size has been explored by gel filtration, ultrafiltration, and ultracentrifugation. The applicability of any of these techniques to a particular system depends entirely on the nature of the antigen before and after its binding to the antibody globulin.

These separation procedures may affect the apparent position of equilibrium, thus reducing the sensitivity and precision of analysis. Antigens of low affinity, such as corticosteroids, sex hormones, and certain haptenic ligands, are sensitive to disruption so that efforts must be made to minimize influencing factors such as time, dilution, and high temperature or at least to keep them constant.

Immunoadsorbents (Solid Phase Antigens and Antibodies)

A clear alternative to simplify the separation of free antigens and bound antigens (complexes) is to use solid-phase immunoadsorbents. Either the antigen or antibody can be fixed on solid material by appropriate means. With the advance of technology for such fixation, immunoassays using antigens or antibodies in solid phase have been developed rapidly and are gaining popularity. As described previously, a solid-phase antigen may be used in radiometric assays and a solid-phase antibody may be used in either radiometric assays (sandwich method) or competitive assays. An obvious requirement for this approach is that enough pure antigens or antibodies are available for preparation of immunoadsorbents.

The original technology for the fixation of antigen to solid materials started for the specific purification of antibodies. For this purpose, the effort was directed to prepare immunoadsorbents of a high antibody-binding capacity with as little adsorption of nonantibody proteins as possible in comparison with the antibody. For use in immunoassays, this high capacity may not always be needed, but the uniformity of the solid material and absence of nonspecific adsorption may be more important factors.

A variety of methods have been devised to prepare solid-phase antigens and antibodies. With proteins, insoluble antigens have been prepared by polymerization with cross-linking agents such as glutaraldehyde and carbodiimides. Such protein polymers, or antigens or antibodies fixed to naturally insoluble or artificially insolubilized protein carriers, are generally not suitable for immunoassays, since they may lose a considerable part of their immunologic activity or may be solubilized by incubation with biologic fluids (samples) during the assay.

For chemical conjugation of proteins to cellulose, cellulose was converted to derivatives with functional groups such as p-aminobenzyl cellulose (which reacts with tyrosyl residues of protein after conversion to diazonium salts) and bromoacetyl cellulose (which reacts with amino groups in protein). Other solid matrices such as beads of porous glass or plastic with functional groups are commercially available along with various cellulose derivatives. One derivative that has been popularly used is carbohydrate matrix activated with cyanogen bromide. Carbohydrates, such as filter paper, polymerized dextran (Sephadex), or agarose beads (Sepharose), are activated in alkaline pH by the addition of cyanogen bromide and can be readily conjugated to proteins in neutral pH.

The cyanogen bromide method may be used for coupling two compounds containing hydroxyl groups, e.g., two carbohydrates. For this purpose, a diamine is used as a bridging agent.

Another approach that has been used successfully for preparing immuno-adsorbents for immunoassays is physical adsorption of antigen or antibody molecules on the surface of solid matrix. For immunoassays, minute amounts of antigen or antibody are sufficient as reactants. Proteins and peptides are adsorbed tightly to solid surfaces such as glass and plastics (polystyrene, polyethylene, polyvinylchloride) and are not released under the assay conditions. A variety of physical forms such as powder, solid pieces, discs, tubes, and plastic microtiter plates have been used for such purposes.

Antiserum globulin may be fixed on the surface by standing a globulin solution of low concentration (5 to 100 $\mu g/ml$) in a polystyrene tube (10 × 75 mm) for a few hours. After removal of the globulin solution and washing by means of an aspirator (a few seconds for each step), the tube is filled with a solution of a high concentration of inert protein (e.g., 1% serum albumin) to saturate the remaining sites capable of adsorbing proteins. The tubes can be kept for a long time and may be used as solid-phase antibody after simple washing. For the assay of an antigen, the unlabeled antigen (test sample) and the labeled antigen are reacted with the tube surface either simultaneously or preferably in sequence, and the binding of the indicator labeled antigen is measured after removal of liquid phase (free antigen). The amount of globulin adsorbed on the surface is about 200 ng/cm^2, which roughly corresponds to the monomolecular film.

In the actual application of this method, a sufficient binding of the labeled antigen cannot be obtained unless the antibody titer of the antiserum is relatively high. The density of antibody on the surface probably becomes too low, and a significant portion of the adsorbed antibody molecules probably cannot bind antigen effectively because of steric interference. In such cases, the sandwich method is recommended. Instead of antiserum globulin, the tube is first coated with the antigen and then reacted with a suitable concentration of antiserum to form an antibody layer that can be used for the antigen assay in the same manner as above. This method makes it possible not only to use antisera of low titers but also to increase the sensitivity of the assay since the high-affinity antibody can be preferentially picked up from the total population to form the antibody layer under appropriate conditions. The method may also be applied to hapten systems by using the hapten-protein conjugates for coating the tubes.

Another advantage of solid-phase antigen of this type is that the antigen-coated tubes may also be used for the purification of labeled antibody for radioimmunoassays. Antibody fixed on the antigen-coated surface can be eluted readily with an acid buffer (pH 2.4). After neutralization, the eluted antibody shows a binding of 70 to 80% even when one starts from the original labeled globulin containing only a few percent of antibody. Usually, the labeled antibody eluted from one antigen-coated tube is sufficient for a large number of assays.

Labeling of Antigens and Antibodies

Labeling with Radioisotopes

Two types of labeling methods are used for radioisotopes: internal and external labeling. Internal labeling is generally used for compounds of low molecular weight (haptens) that can be chemically, or less frequently biologically, synthesized from the precursor compounds containing radioisotopes. ^{14}C and ^{3}H are most commonly used, but ^{35}S and ^{32}P may also be used for particular groups of compounds. Since the internal labeling is achieved by substitution of naturally occurring atom(s) in their structure with a radioisotope atom(s) of the same element, the internally labeled compounds behave in essentially the same manner in all physical, chemical, and biologic reactions as the unlabeled compounds. This is a great advantage for smaller compounds or small peptides over the external labels. The properties of these compounds may be considerably modified by introduction of external labels. This great advantage, however, is offset by the fact that precursor compounds are not readily available with the high specific radioactivity required for immunoassays and are generally quite expensive. If one has to perform an elaborate chemical synthesis in the laboratory, it requires special facilities and handling cautions. However, with the expanded use of radioimmunoassays for simpler compounds, a number of radiolabeled compounds are now available from commercial sources. Generally, the compounds of higher molecular weight such as proteins and large peptides cannot be synthesized chemically. They may be synthesized biologically from precursor compounds by using special enzymes, tissue/organ culture, or even living organisms, but this usually entails the need for extensive efforts for isolation and often suffers from the low yield of radioactivity that can be incorporated in the target compounds.

External labeling involves the attachment of a radioisotope atom(s) or a chemical group containing a radioisotope to the molecules. It is much more widely used than internal labeling, particularly with protein or peptide antigens and antibodies. Radioisotopes of iodide, ^{125}I and ^{131}I, are most commonly used. Iodine has several advantages as a label for radioimmunoassays. It reacts readily with proteins without altering their major properties and this linkage is stable. The radioactive iodines are readily available and iodination can be performed easily in the laboratory. Iodine has a convenient half-life (^{125}I, 60 days; ^{131}I, 8.1 days), long enough to carry out a large number of assays and short enough not to cause a problem of disposal. It can be measured readily in a crystal scintillation counter that does not require special preparation of the samples. Radioiodine is available in a carrier-free form and can be used at high levels of specific activity giving greater sensitivity.

For radioiodination, the chloramine T method devised by Hunter and Greenwood has been used most extensively. In this method, neutral protein solution is first mixed with radioactive iodine and then with chloramine T, an oxidizing agent. Iodide is converted to iodine by oxidation, and the latter reacts instantly with the tyrosine (or histidine) residues of protein molecule. After a short reaction (30 seconds to a few minutes), excess chloramine T is reduced by addition of metabisulfite, and the labeled protein is separated from unreacted iodine by a suitable method such as salt precipitation with a carrier protein or gel filtration. By this method, a few μg of protein can be labeled to levels as high as a few hundred μCi/μg.

$$I^- \xrightarrow{\text{Ch-T}} I_2 + \text{(phenol)} \longrightarrow \text{(iodophenol)} + HI$$

Another approach to radioiodination utilizes catalytic oxidation of iodide by peroxidase in the presence of trace amounts of H_2O_2. This method has been used recently to avoid possible harmful effects of oxidizing and reducing agents in the above method. The method also permits the labeling of μg quantities of proteins at a high level of specific activity. For several peptide hormones, it reportedly yields labeled preparations of better quality as judged by higher binding in routine assays.

Labeling with Enzymes

Enzymes are suitable labels for immunoassays since their catalytic properties allow them to act as amplifiers, and a number of enzymes are capable of producing more than 10^5 product molecules per minute.* Enzymatic reactions used for enzyme immunoassays are specific, and most can be

* = Per molecule of enzyme.

performed relatively easily with the equipment in the average clinical laboratory. Problems accompanying the use of radioisotopes, such as special facilities and regulations for storage, handling equipment, and waste disposal, can be avoided. On the other hand, the sensitivities of most enzyme immunoassays reported so far do not yet match the sensitivities of the corresponding radioimmunoassays. The enzymic actions may be more susceptible to interference from nonspecific factors in biologic fluids. The enzymic activity usually measured by the initial velocity of enzymic actions may be more difficult and imprecise than the measurement of radioactivity. Furthermore, the labeling procedures, particularly for proteins and peptide hormones, are more cumbersome and need more specialized expertise than those used for radioiodination. Future improvements, however, such as new enzymes as labels, more sensitive and readily applicable enzyme assays, better cross-linking procedures, and separation methods, will lead to improved assays.

The enzymes to be used as labels must be available with modest cost and in high purity. They should have a high specific activity and should be stable under conditions for storage and assays. Assay methods must be simple, rapid, sensitive, and reproducible. Enzyme, substrates, and interfering factors such as inhibitors should be absent from biologic fluids. The most common enzymes that have been used in enzyme immunoassays are horseradish peroxidase and alkaline phosphatase; glucose oxidase has also been used. Highly sensitive assay systems have been developed by the use of β-D-galactosidase and glucoamylase by spectrofluorometric methods and by the use of acetylcholinesterase with ^{3}H-acetylcholine. Lysozyme and glucose-6-phosphate dehydrogenase are used in commercially available homogeneous enzyme immunoassay kits.

For linking haptenic groups to enzymes, various functional groups that react with protein may be used, depending on the structure of haptens. It should be noted, however, that the position of the functional group on the hapten may play an important role in determining the specificity of immunologic reactions and that some functional groups may lead to inactivation of the enzymic activity by attaching to the essential residues on the enzymes.

A variety of methods have been used for linking proteins or peptides with enzymes (Chapter 28). The simplest and most widely used method is glutaraldehyde. By simply mixing the enzyme (E) and the second protein (P) in the presence of glutaraldehyde, dialdehyde, conjugates are formed through free amino groups of both proteins (E and P). The conjugates are very heterogeneous and consist of macropolymers of E-E, E-P, and P-P. The results may not be reproducible, and a considerable loss of enzymic and/or immunologic activity may be encountered. The merit of the method seems to be its simplicity compared with other methods using two-step reactions.

In a particular case of horseradish peroxidase, it reacts with only one glutaraldehyde molecule, and the second aldehyde molecule does not seem to react with the same or other peroxidase molecules. Thus, if excess glutaraldehyde is removed after reaction with the enzyme, the "activated" enzyme (E') reacts with the second protein (P) producing conjugates of E'P, $E_2'P$, and so on. This method seems to give better results than the one-step method and was successfully applied to proteins such as insulin, choriogonadotropin, and IgG. Oligosaccharide groups in horseradish peroxidase have also been used for the two-step reaction. By periodate oxidation of saccharide groups, the resulting aldehydes can form, with free amino groups of the proteins, Schiff base, which can be stabilized by reduction with sodium borohydride.

Sulfhydryl groups of β-galactosidase may be used for cross-linking with other proteins. For example, a sulfhydryl group is introduced into insulin by mercaptosuccinylation and then reacted with N,N'-o-phenylenedimaleimide. After excess reagent is removed, the "activated" insulin is coupled to β-galactosidase. Alternatively, the amino group of insulin is acetylated with m-maleimidobenzoyl N-hydroxysuccinimide ester, and the resulting maleimide insulin is conjugated to β-galactosidase through its sulfhydryl groups. Both conjugates, in conjuction with spectrofluorometric technique, yielded highly sensitive assays of insulin comparable to the radioimmunoassays.

Other cross-linking agents, such as carbodiimides, toluene 2,4-diisocyanate, cyanuric chloride, p,p'-difluoro-m,m'-dinitrophenyl sulfone, and tetrazotized o-dianisidine, have also been tried.

Summary

Utilizing the specificity of antigen-antibody reactions, a number of compounds of biologic and clinical interest may be assayed selectively in complex mixtures by remarkably simple procedures. With the appropriate choice of labels for antigens or antibodies, an extremely high level of sensitivity can be achieved. Radioisotopes have been used as labels, but the use of enzymes as labels is gaining popularity. Based on two basically different principles, competitive (or saturation) or immunometric, assays have been devised with many technical variations depending on the specific factors for each system such as effects of labeling, ease of separating antigen-antibody complexes, and availability of purified antigens or antibodies. The area is presently under active investigation for technologic progress as well as for the expansion of applications.

Bibliography

Aalberse, R. C.: Quantitative fluoroimmunoassay. *Clin. Chim. Acta*, **48**:109, 1973.
Berson, S. A., and Yalow, R. S.: Radioimmunoassay: a status report. In Good,

R. A., and Fisher, D. W. (eds.): *Immunobiology*. Sinauer Associates, Inc., Stamford, Conn., 1971, pp. 287–93.

Farr, R. S.: A quantitative immunochemical measure of the primary interaction between I-BSA and antibody. *J. Infect. Dis.*, **103**:239–62, 1958.

Garvey, J. S.: Radioisotopes and their applications. In Williams, C. A., and Chase, M. W. (eds.): *Methods in Immunology and Immunochemistry*, Vol. 2. Academic Press, Inc., New York, 1968, pp. 183–247.

Greenwood, F. C.; Hunter, W. M.; and Glover, J. S.: The preparation of ^{131}I-labelled human growth hormone of high specific radioactivity. *Biochem. J.*, **89**: 114–23, 1964.

Haimovich, J.; Hurwitz, E.; Novik, N.; and Sela, M.: Use of protein-bacteriophage conjugates for detection and quantification of proteins. *Biochim. Biophys. Acta*, **207**:125, 1970.

Leute, R.; Ullman, E. F.; and Goldstein, A.: Spin immunoassay of opiate narcotics in urine and saliva. *J.A.M.A.*, **221**:1231, 1972.

Nabarro, J. D. N. (ed.): Radioimmunoassays and saturation analysis. *Br. Med. Bull.*, **30**:1–103, 1974.

Pestka, S.; Rosenfeld, H.; and Harris, R.: Viroimmunoassays: Detection of virus-antigen/antibody complexes with an immunoadsorbent. *Immunochem.*, **11**:213–18, 1974.

Skom, J. H., and Talmage, D. W.: Nonprecipitating insulin antibodies. *J. Clin. Invest.*, **37**:783–86, 1958.

Talmage, D. W., and Radovich, J.: Labeling of antigens and antibodies. In Williams, C. A., and Chase, M. W. (eds.): *Methods in Immunology and Immunochemistry*, Vol. 1. Academic Press, Inc., New York, 1967, pp. 387–404.

Wisdom, G. B.: Enzyme-immunoassay. *Clin. Chem.*, **22**:1243, 1976.

Yalow, R. S., and Berson, S. A.: Immunoassay of endogeneous plasma insulin in man. *J. Clin. Invest.*, **39**:1157–75, 1960.

Index